The Routledge Handbook of Post-Prohibition Cannabis Research

The place of cannabis in global drug prohibition is in crisis, opening up new directions for socially engaged cannabis research. *The Routledge Handbook of Post-Prohibition Cannabis Research* invites readers to explore new landscapes of cannabis research under conditions of *legalization with, not after, prohibition*: "post-prohibition." The chapters are organized into five multidisciplinary sections: Governance, Public Health, Markets and Society, Ecology and the Environment, and Culture and Social Change. Case studies from the United States, Uruguay, Morocco, and the United Kingdom show readers alternative ways of thinking about human–cannabis relationships that move beyond questions of legality and illegality. Representing a cross-section of cannabis scholarship, the contributors provide readers with critical perspectives on legalization that are not based upon orthodoxies of prohibition. While legalization signals a global shift in the legitimacy of cannabis research, this collection identifies openings for academics, policy makers, and the public interested in ending the drug war, as well as a way to address broader social problems evident in the age of neoliberal governance within which prohibition has been entangled.

Dominic Corva is Founder and Executive Director of the Center for the Study of Cannabis and Social Policy, Co-Director of the Humboldt Institute of Interdisciplinary Marijuana Research at Humboldt State University (HSU), and Cannabis Policy Specialist for the California Center for Rural Policy at HSU. He received his PhD in geography from the University of Washington, Seattle.

Joshua S. Meisel is Professor of Sociology and Co-Director of the Humboldt Institute for Interdisciplinary Marijuana Research at Humboldt State University in Arcata, California. He is also a member of the Global Cannabis Cultivation Research Consortium. His research focuses on the sources and consequences of cannabis policy. He received his PhD in sociology from the University of Colorado, Boulder.

The Routledge Handbook of Post-Prohibition Cannabis Research

Edited by Dominic Corva and Joshua S. Meisel

Routledge
Taylor & Francis Group
NEW YORK AND LONDON

First published 2022
by Routledge
52 Vanderbilt Avenue, New York, NY 10017

and by Routledge
2 Park Square, Milton Park, Abingdon, Oxon, OX14 4RN

Routledge is an imprint of the Taylor & Francis Group, an informa business

Library of Congress Cataloging-in-Publication Data
Names: Corva, Dominic, editor. | Meisel, Joshua S., editor.
Title: The Routledge handbook of post-prohibition cannabis research : multidisciplinary perspectives / edited by Dominic Corva and Joshua S. Meisel.
Description: New York : Routledge, 2021.
Identifiers: LCCN 2020054818 | ISBN 9780367335434 (hardback) | ISBN 9781032009452 (paperback) | ISBN 9780429320491 (ebook)
Subjects: LCSH: Cannabis—Social aspects—United States. | Cannabis—Government policy—United States. | Cannabis—Law and legislation—United States.
Classification: LCC HV5822.C3 R68 2021 | DDC 362.29/50973—dc23
LC record available at https://lccn.loc.gov/2020054818

ISBN: 978-0-367-33543-4 (hbk)
ISBN: 978-1-032-00945-2 (pbk)
ISBN: 978-0-429-32049-1 (ebk)

DOI: 10.4324/9780429320491

Typeset in Bembo
by Apex CoVantage, LLC

Contents

SECTION 2
Public Health 91

SECTION 3
Markets and Society 145

Figures

Tables

Contributors

Kenza Afsahi is a lecturer in sociology at the University of Bordeaux and a researcher at the Emile Durkheim Center (CNRS) in France. Currently, she coordinates an international research program on the construction of the medical cannabis market in three countries (France-Morocco-Canada) with an interdisciplinary team. She is also co-leader of the sociology research axis of the International at the Emile Durkheim Center and a member of the editorial boards of *Cannabis and Cannabinoid Research* and the *French Journal of Visual Methods* (*Revue Française des Méthodes Visuelles*). In addition, she is associated with the Center for Sociological Research on Law and Penal Institutions (CNRS). At the University of Bordeaux, she teaches the sociology of deviance, the sociology of the cannabis market, visual sociology, issues of women's involvement in the drug market, and environmental crime.

Sunil Kumar Aggarwal, MD, PhD, FAAPMR, is a physician—medical geographer board—certified in Hospice and Palliative Medicine and Physical Medicine and Rehabilitation. He is Past Chair of the American Academy of Hospice and Palliative Medicine (AAHPM) Integrative Medicine Special Interest Group, an inaugural member of the Safe Use of Psychedelic-Assisted Therapies Forum, and was recently named as a Top 20 Emerging Leader by the AAHPM. He is an affiliate assistant professor of Rehabilitation Medicine (Clinical) and Geography and an affiliate clinical faculty with Bastyr University. He completed his MD and PhD degrees at the University of Washington (Global Health Pathway) and Residency and Fellowship at Virginia Mason, NYU, and the NIH. He is Co-founder and Co-director of the Advanced Integrative Medical Science (AIMS) Institute in Seattle, WA, a multispecialty teaching clinic and research institute offering cutting-edge care in oncology, psychiatry, neurology, rehabilitation, pain, and palliative care. He serves as Associate Hospice Medicine Director and On-Call Palliative Physician for MultiCare Health System and is an associate member of the Humboldt Institute for Interdisciplinary Marijuana Research (www.aimsinstitute.net).

Sebastián Aguiar (PhD in sociology, Universidad de la República) is a researcher and professor in the Department of Sociology, School of Social Science at the Universidad de la República, specializing in qualitative analysis. He coordinated the Monitor Cannabis Uruguay research team (School of Social Science, UdelaR). Sebastián has authored academic publications on drug policy evolution in Uruguay such as "Agenda of Rights in Uruguay. Event, Biopolitics, Immunity and Force of Law" (Spain, 2018) and "Menant la marche: l´Uruguay et ses trois lois avant-gardistes" (France 2014), as well as book chapters such as "The Green Ray" (Mexico, CIDE 2015) and "Marijuana Causes Schizophrenia" (Uruguay, CSIC 2012). He has also disseminated several works, given conferences in several countries, and participated in international conferences on drug policy.

Marcos Baudean is Senior Lecturer in Research Methodology at Universidad ORT Uruguay and Member of Monitor Cannabis Uruguay (an independent research group specialized in the monitoring and evaluation of cannabis regulation in Uruguay). He has researched extensively on Uruguayan regulation with an emphasis in health, criminal, and prison issues. His publications in the field are mostly research reports for Monitor Cannabis and the National Drug Board.

Elizabeth A. Bennett is Associate Professor of International Affairs and Director of Political Economy at Lewis & Clark College in Portland, Oregon (USA). She holds a PhD in political science from Brown University and a MALD (Master of Arts in Law and Diplomacy) in political economy and international development from The Fletcher School at Tufts University. Her research focuses on global value chains, fair trade, living wages, sustainability certifications, voluntary governance, and social sustainability, particularly in coffee, cannabis, and clothing. Her work is published in the *American Journal of Sociology, World Development, Sustainable Development, Agriculture and Human Values*, and *Globalizations*, among other journals, and she is the co-editor of *The Handbook of Research on Fair Trade* (with Laura Raynolds) and co-author of the political ethnography *The Civic Imagination: Making a Difference in American Political Life*.

Hekia Bodwitch is a postdoctoral fellow in the Natural Resource Science Department at McGill University. Hekia examines relationships between fish and agricultural production and trade regulations and producer livelihoods. She is currently working with indigenous fishers in New Zealand and small-scale cannabis growers in the Pacific Northwest on strategies to comply with environmental regulations and access markets.

Melissa Bone is a lecturer at the University of Leicester, UK, and teaches on the undergraduate criminal law and law justice and society modules in the Leicester Law School. Melissa obtained her PhD from the University of Manchester and her PhD research was funded by the Arts and Humanities Research Council (AHRC). Melissa has written a monograph for Routledge based on her PhD research entitled *Human Rights and Drug Control: A New Perspective*. As well as having research interests in the areas of drug policy and human rights law, Melissa is the co-investigator on an Economic and Social Research Council New Investigator's grant, which explores the values and opinions of people who use drugs on policy reform. Melissa's research interests additionally cover the legal landscape of cannabis social clubs throughout Europe, cannabis activism, and medical cannabis laws in the UK.

Jennifer Carah is a senior scientist with The Nature Conservancy of California. She is currently engaged in applied conservation to protect and restore stream flows and winter refuge habitat for salmonids in Northern California, as well as research on environmental flows and environmental impacts of cannabis cultivation.

Wendy Chapkis is a professor of sociology and women and gender studies at the University of Southern Maine. She also serves as the Faculty Scholar for the Jean Byers Sampson Center for Diversity. Recent articles include "The Trouble With Mary Jane's Gender: Gender Politics in the Marijuana Policy Reform Movement" (*Humboldt Journal of Social Relations*), "Cannabis, Consciousness and Healing" (*Contemporary Justice Review*), and "Productive Tensions" (*Journal of Contemporary Ethnography*). She is also the author of three books: *Dying to Get High: Marijuana as Medicine* (co-authored with Richard J. Webb, New York University Press), *Live Sex Acts: Women Performing Erotic Labor* (Routledge), and *Beauty Secrets: Women and the Politics of Appearance* (South End Press).

Mauricio Coitiño (master's degree in public policy, Universidad Católica del Uruguay) was the specialist in public policy and communication for the Monitor Cannabis Uruguay research team

(Universidad de la República). Previously, he served as a research assistant with the Latin American Marijuana Research Initiative (Universidad Católica—Florida University). He has co-authored articles on media coverage of cannabis and the Uruguayan regulation model and has presented on these matters at international conferences.

Christopher Dillis is a research affiliate of the Cannabis Research Center at the University of California-Berkeley. His dissertation research at the University of California-Davis focused on the environmental impacts of illegal logging practices in Indonesia. His current work involves modeling water use patterns of cannabis farms in Northern California and the impact of regulation on industry trends statewide.

William Dolphin is the co-author of *The Medicalization of Marijuana: Legitimacy, Stigma, and the Patient Experience* (Routledge, 2019) and a consultant to the medical cannabis patient advocacy group Americans for Safe Access. For the past 20 years, he has written primarily about medical cannabis law, policy, medical research, and the patient experience, including contributions to more than a dozen books on cannabis and drug policy. He has taught at San Francisco State University, Rhodes College, Azusa Pacific University, and the University of California, Berkeley, and currently teaches at the University of Redlands.

Trecia Ehrlich began studying the community impacts of agriculture at UC Davis, where she received a bachelor's of science in community and regional development in 2010, focusing on food sustainability and agricultural industrial change. After spending several years running rivers, Trecia came to Washington to pursue a master's degree in community-oriented public health practice at the University of Washington, where she researched the health and safety of cannabis farmworkers transitioning into a legal workspace and graduated in 2017. Since graduating, she has worked in cannabis government research, policy, and management, first as a research consultant to the Washington State Liquor and Cannabis Board and now as the hemp program manager for the Washington State Department of Agriculture. She is interested in the intersections of agricultural transformation, ecology, evolving governance, health autonomy, and biomimetics.

Marisa Lia Formosa currently works as a planner for the Natural Resources Services, a division of the nonprofit Redwood Community Action Agency, in Eureka, CA. She has a BA in politics from the University of California, Santa Cruz, and a MA in social science, environment, and community from Humboldt State University. She has over a decade of experience working on grassroots, community-based restoration, conservation, and stewardship projects. Marisa grew up in the remote, rural community of Whitethorn, located in southern Humboldt County, during the height of the green rush. Whitethorn experienced significant economic, social, and cultural impacts from illegal cannabis cultivation, and this has informed and influenced her perspective towards the cannabis industry.

Robin S. Goldstein is Principal Economic Counselor at the University of California Agricultural Issues Center, where his research focuses on the economics of regulatory policy and the prices of cannabis and other consumer products. Since 2016, he has worked with the California Bureau of Cannabis Control to evaluate the economic costs and benefits of proposed regulations. He is the author of several books, including *The Wine Trials* and *The Beer Trials*.

Erin Clover Kelly is an associate professor at Humboldt State University in the Department of Forestry, teaching policy and economics classes, as well as a field-based graduate class on rural livelihoods and well-being in the Mattole. She and her graduate students have conducted research on many topics, including forestry offset projects under the California carbon market, community conflict surrounding the creation of protected areas, and the human dimensions of scaling up forest management to address wildfire risk. She is a California Registered Professional Forester.

Chelsea E. Langer, PhD, MPH, is a project coordinator at the Center for Health and the Environment at University of California, Davis. Her work has focused on environmental and occupational epidemiology, primarily centered on agricultural workers in California.

Florencia Lemos is an undergraduate student in political science and is seeking a diploma in drug policy at the Universidad de la República. She has been a research assistant to the Monitor Cannabis Uruguay team (Universidad de la República). She is currently researching the recent evolution of drug governance in Uruguay. She has been a speaker at national and international conferences on drug policy approaches, where she has presented the Uruguayan model.

Evan Mills, PhD, is a California-based energy and climate change scientist, affiliated faculty member with UC Berkeley's Energy and Resources Group, and a member of the United Nations Intergovernmental Panel on Climate Change. He is a retired senior scientist at the US Department of Energy's Lawrence Berkeley National Laboratory, where he is now a research affiliate. He authored the definitive and widely cited peer-reviewed analysis of energy use associated with indoor cannabis cultivation in 2012. More information is available at evan-mills.com. Email: evanmills1@gmail.com.

Clara Musto (PhD in global criminology, University of Kent and University of Utrecht) currently works in the Criminology research group, School of Social Science at the Universidad de la República. Her dissertation focused on why and how Uruguay became the first country in the world to legally regulate cannabis in a comprehensive manner. She was a researcher with Monitor Cannabis Uruguay, a team specialized in the monitoring and evaluation of the new regulatory model.

Michelle Newhart, PhD, is a sociologist and author who specializes in the study of medical cannabis, health behaviors, midlife and older adulthood, and social movements. She is the co-author of *The Medicalization of Marijuana: Legitimacy, Stigma, and the Patient Experience* (Routledge, 2019) and *Understanding Research Methods, 10th Edition* (Routledge, 2017). She has presented her research at professional sociology conferences, including the Pacific Sociological Association and the Midwest Sociological Society, as well as at medical cannabis conferences and events, and has appeared on podcasts, TV, and radio shows. She is the founder of Cannabis Research in the Social Sciences (CRITSS), an informal group for researchers to share information, offer work in progress, and post research opportunities.

Whitney Ogle is an assistant professor of kinesiology at Humboldt State University and serves on the governing board of the Humboldt Institute of Interdisciplinary Marijuana Research. Her educational background spans from a clinical focus in physical therapy to a research focus on exercise physiology and the motor control of human movement. Whitney has recently focused her research efforts on understanding the relationship between cannabis and human movement by conducting interdisciplinary survey studies investigating how people use cannabis with exercise and physical therapist views and experiences with patients using cannabis products. She has organized and developed continuing education opportunities for cannabis for physical therapists. Her personal mission is to be able to take the findings from current evidence-based research on cannabis use to guide human subject research, policy, practice, and public education.

Marty Otañez is an associate professor in the Anthropology Department at the University of Colorado Denver. His research and creative work focus on labor organizing to create safer workplaces in the legal cannabis sector and policy-influential story sharing to make visible activities of tobacco farmers to counter exploitative labor practices of global tobacco companies in Malawi and other non-dominant countries. Marty teaches cannabis-related courses such as Cannabis Culture, Hemp Cultures and the Dutch Bio-Based Economy, and Worker's Rights in Cannabis Spaces. He is the producer of the community television show through Denver Open Media called "Getting High on Anthropology: A Story-Based Approach to Cannabis Research, Education and Funding" (www.FSandGreen.org).

Michael Polson, an anthropologist, is a Ciriacy-Wantrup Postdoctoral Fellow in Natural Resource Economics and Political Economy at the University of California, Berkeley. His research addresses the changing social dynamics of marijuana production in Northern California. He has published in journals and collections on political-legal anthropology, governance, environment, illegality, and neoliberalism. He is currently working on contributions to the first cannabis-themed issue of the journal *California Agriculture* and a book manuscript under advance contract with University of Minnesota Press.

Gary R. Potter is a reader in criminology at Lancaster University, UK. He has been researching illegal drug markets for over 20 years. He has a particular interest in domestic cannabis cultivation and is a founding member of the Global Cannabis Cultivation Research Consortium (www.worldwideweed.nl). His recent work has focused on those who grow cannabis for medical reasons. Key publications in this area include *Weed, Need and Greed: A Study of Domestic Cannabis Cultivation*, *World Wide Weed: Global Trends in Cannabis Cultivation and Control* (edited with Tom Decorte and Martin Bouchard) and *International Journal of Drug Policy Special Edition on Cannabis Cultivation 26* (3) (edited with Tom Decorte). He also writes and teaches about green criminology and the illegal wildlife trade.

Mary E. Power, NAS, is Professor in the Department of Integrative Biology at the University of California, Berkeley. Mary studies river food-web ecology and how ecological interactions across habitat boundaries link rivers, watersheds, and near-shore ocean ecosystems. Recently, her research focus has been on hydrologic and landscape controls on algae and cyanobacteria taxa (nutritious or toxic) that determine their seasonal production, fate, and impacts in river and estuarine food webs.

Kaitlin Reed is an assistant professor of Native American Studies at Humboldt State University. Her research interests include tribal land and water rights, traditional ecological knowledge, and environmental conflict. She is currently working on her first book project to connect the historical and ecological dots between the gold rush and the green rush, focusing on capitalistic resource extraction and violence against indigenous lands and bodies. This research examines the ecological and cultural impacts of cannabis cultivation on Yurok tribal lands, with a focus on tribal sovereignty and environmental justice.

Amanda Reiman is the founder and CEO of Personal Plants, an online educational platform to support the home cultivation and processing of therapeutic plants and fungi. She is also the Vice President of Community Development for Flow Cannabis Company, a cannabis distribution and manufacturing company that focuses on sun-grown cannabis and works with craft farmers in the Emerald Triangle. She is also the founder and CEO of Personal Plants, an online educational platform to support the home cultivation and processing of therapeutic plants and fungi. Amanda earned her PhD in social welfare from UC Berkeley in 2006 and currently lives in Ukiah, California.

Craig Reinarman is Professor of Sociology and Legal Studies Emeritus at the University of California, Santa Cruz. He was a post-doctoral fellow at the Alcohol Research Group, School of Public

Health, University of California, Berkeley. He has been a visiting professor at the University of Amsterdam and the University of Utrecht and principal investigator on research grants from the National Institute of Drug Abuse. He has served as a consultant to the World Health Organization's Substance Abuse Program and is a member of the Board of the College on Problems of Drug Dependence. Craig is the author of *American States of Mind* (Yale University Press, 1987) and co-author of *Cocaine Changes* (Temple University Press, 1991) and *Crack in America* (University of California Press, 1997). His most recent book is an anthology of critical addiction studies, *Expanding Addiction* (Routledge 2015).

Katie Kaufman Rogers is a doctoral candidate in sociology at the University of Texas at Austin, where she is also an affiliate of the Urban Ethnography Lab. Her research and teaching address the intersections of gender, race, workplace inequality, and the criminal-legal system. In her dissertation, "Breaking the Grass Ceiling: Gender, Race, and Class in the U.S. Legal Cannabis Industry," she uses in-depth interviews, field observations, and content analysis to examine women's labor experiences in a historically criminalized, masculinized cannabis industry. This work is supported by the National Science Foundation, the Rapoport Center for Human Rights and Justice, and the UT Austin College of Liberal Arts. Her research has been recognized with awards from multiple sections of the American Sociological Association and from Sociologists for Women in Society. She holds an MA in sociology from UT Austin and a BA in sociology from Colorado College.

Nathan F. Sayre is Professor in the Department of Geography at the University of California, Berkeley. He studies the history, politics, and science of natural resources and land use in the western United States. His most recent book is *The Politics of Scale: A History of Rangeland Science* (University of Chicago Press, 2017), and he is currently working on historical climatic extremes in California, particularly the mega-flood and drought of 1861–1865.

Marc B. Schenker, MD, MPH, is Distinguished Professor of Public Health Sciences and Medicine at University of California, Davis. He is the Founding Director of the Center for Occupational and Environmental Health, the Western Center for Agricultural Health and Safety, and the Migration and Health Research Center. His work has focused on numerous agricultural populations, including farmworkers and their families and farm owners and managers. His work has also focused on diverse causes of illness and injury, including agricultural dusts, pesticides, and heat.

Michelle Sexton is Assistant Adjunct Professor in the Department of Anesthesia at the University of California San Diego. She earned her doctorate in naturopathic medicine from Bastyr University in Seattle Washington, 2008. She completed a postdoctoral fellowship at the University of Washington in the Departments of Pharmacology/Psychiatry and Behavioral Sciences. Her NIH-funded predoctoral and postdoctoral research on the topic of cannabinoids and their roles in neuro-inflammation and neuro-degeneration investigated cannabis use in patients with multiple sclerosis and its impact on inflammatory markers. Michelle has presented her research internationally and published in peer-reviewed journals. Her clinical practice, research, and teaching focus is on the endocannabinoid system and potential roles for cannabis across a range of conditions and lifespan. She is a member of the International Cannabinoid Research Society, the International Association of Cannabinoid Medicine, and the Society of Cannabis Clinicians. She maintains a medical practice in San Diego, CA.

Noah Silber-Coats is a PhD candidate in the School of Geography and Development (SGD) at the University of Arizona. His dissertation research adopts a political ecology framework to examine the ongoing restructuring of the cannabis industry, with a focus on southern Oregon—a region where cultivation of the plant is linked into a variety of markets, each of which is subject to a different set of formal and informal rules. His MA, also from SGD, focused on the politics of energy and water in Mexico in the context of a boom in private industry–led hydroelectric development. His work, both sole-authored and collaborative, can be found in a variety of publications including *Water Alternatives*, *Energy Policy*, *Terrain*, and *you are here: the journal of creative geography*.

Anthony Silvaggio is an associate professor of sociology at Humboldt State University and a founding faculty member of the Humboldt Institute for Marijuana Research. His research focuses on understanding the environmental consequences of cannabis prohibition and identifying how current state legalization efforts facilitate and encourage environmental degradation. One of the first scholars in the United States to sound the alarm about the ecological impacts of industrial cannabis agriculture, he organized the *Earth Day Symposium on Marijuana and the Environment* (2013), which brought together cannabis cultivators, policy makers, land managers, tribal leaders, academics, law enforcement, and environmentalists to examine the environmental impacts of cannabis agriculture and the limits of state-level legalization efforts. His most recent work can be found in *Where There's Smoke: The Environmental Science, Public Policy, and Politics of Marijuana* (2018). His research has been featured in the *New York Times*, *The Atlantic*, *Rolling Stone*, *Al Jazeera*, and *The Nation*.

Daniel A. Sumner is the Frank H. Buck, Jr. Distinguished Professor in the Department of Agricultural and Resource Economics, University of California, Davis. Previously, Sumner was the Assistant Secretary for Economics of the US Department of Agriculture, where he supervised 1,000 professional statisticians and economists and provided economic analysis to the Secretary and other officials. His research, teaching, and outreach encompass economics of food and agricultural sustainability, often engaging multidisciplinary teams on practical questions.

David Vergara is a Switzerland-based Colombian legal assessor with an international business background. He came into contact with the cannabis space through his master's thesis at the University of East London titled "Corporate Social Responsibility in the Cannabis Industry—A Qualitative Analysis," which focused on ethical business practices within the industry. After performing his fieldwork in Colorado's cannabis sector, Vergara established connections with industry experts in the US, England, Germany, and Colombia. Currently, Vergara remains active in the cannabis industry focusing on corporate social responsibility while exploring further fields such as public health, consumer education, and drug policy reform.

Ingrid Walker is Associate Professor of American Studies at the University of Washington, Tacoma, where she studies and teaches about the politics of contemporary culture in the United States. In her 2017 book, *High: Drugs, Desire, and a Nation of Users*, Ingrid examines the dynamics that inform drug policy and medicine—dynamics between drugs, the people who use them, and social perceptions of drug use. In her TEDx talk "Drugs and Desire," she questions the social stigma of psychoactive drug use. Ingrid is focused on cultivating a more thoughtful, evidence-based drug policy research agenda. In her scholarship and advocacy, she works with researchers, policy experts, community organizers, and drug users to seek social justice for people who use drugs.

Adrianne Wilson-Poe, PhD, is a translational neuroscientist who has been studying the interaction between opioids and cannabinoids since 2004. She has been a longstanding member of the International Narcotics Research Conference and the International Cannabinoid Research Society. The National Institute on Drug Abuse has consistently funded her work throughout her career, and she is currently an assistant scientist at Legacy Research Institute in Portland, OR, with a joint appointment in the Neuroscience Department at Washington State University. Adrianne is also the CEO and co-founder of Smart Analytics, a contract research and consulting firm.

Joshua Zender is a certified public accountant (CPA) and an associate professor of accounting at Humboldt State University. He teaches corporate social responsibility, ethics, financial, managerial, cost, government, and nonprofit accounting. His research interests include cannabis tax and cost accounting matters. As an affiliated researcher of the Humboldt Institute for Interdisciplinary Marijuana Research, he has collaborated with his colleagues to produce the first Standardized Regulatory Impact Assessment (SRIA) of Regulations for Manufacturers of Adult-Use and Medical Cannabis in the State of California. This study was utilized by policy makers to design a cannabis tax system and project future governmental revenues. Through the work of his own CPA practice, he actively serves cannabis clients within the Emerald Triangle of Northern California.

Scott Zeramby is a subject matter expert who owns and operates several businesses that primarily serve the cannabis industry. In his work as a cannabis industry consultant, he collaborated in the design of a 91,000-square-foot state-of-the-art cannabis production facility in Carbondale, Illinois. He has presented to both national and international audiences on a number of cannabis-related subjects including cultivation processes, public policy, economics, and energy use.

Acknowledgements

Dominic Corva:

I am incredibly grateful to my co-editor Joshua S. Meisel, who has been an amazing friend and intellectual playmate in this project and many others that followed these last few years. His patience, kindness, humor, and formidable expertise in interdisciplinary approaches to social problems have greatly enriched my own understanding of cannabis-society relationships and nurtured this handbook as a convivial learning community. We could not have done this without the initiative and intellectually rigorous vision of our Routledge editor, Dean Birkenkamp, who has been a great support and humorous, sometimes hilarious, steward of the process.

I also want to acknowledge my core life support team: dear childhood friends Sy and Bridget Johnson, Cannabis and Social Policy Board member Aaron Varney, mother Shelia Truman, beloved cat-momma Dionea Nadir, and of course my feline companion DoctorBerry Who. This group includes my dear friend, constant support and gateway to so much, Tony Silvaggio; and his partner Kandis Kelsey. Special thanks to my CASP Board members past and present: co-founders and dear friends Michelle Sexton and Sunil Kumar Aggarwal; Naz Victoria, Don Wirtschafter, Rachel Kurtz, Joy Beckerman, Lara Kaminsky, Alison Draisin, Jason Lyddy, and Jerry Whiting.

I owe a great debt of gratitude to the people whose lives and stories led me to Southern Humboldt from where everything since has flowed. They were my introductions, guides, and early community peer reviewers: Jentri Anders, Ursi Reynolds, Kathy Epling, Paul Encimer, Douglas Fir, Mikal Jakubal, Kym Kemp, Kevin Jodrey, and William Pedro. There have been so many others along the way, and I apologize for formally acknowledging so few.

Finally, I want to acknowledge Steve Herbert and Katherine Beckett with the University of Washington Law, Societies, and Justice program, where I first created and taught a cannabis and social policy class while in graduate school. Their intellectual influence and interdisciplinary faculty community (Arzoo Osanloo, Naomi Murakawa, Angelina Godoy, and Michael McCann) made me more than a geographer and paved the way for this long, strange trip to Somewhere Else.

Joshua S. Meisel:

This project began almost a decade ago with the creation of the Humboldt Institute for Interdisciplinary Marijuana Research at Humboldt State University (www.hiimr.humboldt.edu). As a founding co-director I was introduced to the diverse research agendas of colleagues and handbook contributors Erin Clover Kelly, Whitney Ogle, Kaitlin Reed, Tony Silvaggio, and Joshua Zender. Special thanks go out to Tony Silvaggio for suggesting Dominic Corva to provide the first public talk as part of a HIIMR Speaker Series. Little did we know that that introduction would lead to this partnership 10 years later!

Leading an interdisciplinary research institute opened doors to collaborations with the following cannabis scholars who would later provide outstanding contributions to this volume: Sunil Kumar Aggarwal, Elizabeth A. Bennett, Wendy Chapkis, William Dolphin, Michelle Newhart, Marty

Otañez, Michael Polson, Amanda Reiman, and Marc B. Schenker. Other contributors found their way into this handbook through an array of shared and divergent professional networks.

Other acknowledgements include our editor at Routledge, Dean Birkenkamp, who would have known that our professional paths would cross again almost 25 years after a university tour of Cuba in 1994! I am grateful for your encouragement and thoughtful feedback as we ushered this project from concept to reality.

To my undergraduate mentor, Craig Reinarman, who opened my eyes to the racialized and class-based contours of U.S. drug policy in his infamous "Drugs and Society" course at UC Santa Cruz. Thank you Craig for seeding my lifelong interest in applying a critical constructivist lens to the study of drug issues.

To my co-editor, and HIIMR co-director, Dominic Corva, for your intellectual passion, heart, and patience in collaborating on this project and many others over the years. You bring a deep knowledge of cannabis history and geography as well as a rich tapestry of cannabis scholars and policy makers to our collaborations.

To my brother Dan for first encouraging me to focus my research interests in the emergent U.S. movements to legalize access to cannabis for medical use.

To my parents for always praising and encouraging my interests and raising me in a community, Berkeley, where I first witnessed cannabis decriminalization.

To Zachary and Noah who pushed me to reflect on parenting adolescents in the age of cannabis legalization.

And finally to my partner, Mary Virnoche, from graduate school until the present for supporting my work in more ways than you can possibly know.

1

Introduction to Post-Prohibition

Dominic Corva and Joshua S. Meisel

Keywords: cannabis, legalization, prohibition, post-prohibition, relational analyses

Post-Prohibition and Cannabis Legalization

The place of cannabis[1] in global drug prohibition, as a system of laws and policies that criminalize the production, distribution, and consumption of cannabis, opium, cocaine, and their derivatives, seems to be in crisis. At the time of this writing, Canada, Uruguay, and 15 U.S. states[2] have passed laws to license, regulate, and tax "adult-use" cannabis commodity chains from seed or clone to retail that constitute exceptions to global and national legal prohibition frameworks that emerged in the early part of the 20th century. In addition, "medicinal use" cannabis laws[3] that decriminalize and in some cases legalize certain kinds of cannabis commodity chains have been implemented around the world, and the prohibition of industrial hemp production in the United States has been lifted. The crisis of global cannabis prohibition opens up significant new directions for cannabis research in a context that is not only about legalization as a particular kind of juridical reform, but also more generalized liberalization[4] of laws and decriminalization policies governing medicinal and industrial cannabis. These shifts away from prohibition, however, remain entangled with prohibition laws and policies that pose significant limits to the kinds of freedom available to ask questions about the plant and the people who grow, distribute, and use it.

This handbook is an invitation to diverse landscapes of cannabis research opened up by the emergence of exceptions to cannabis prohibition framed relationally here as "post-prohibition": legalization with, not after, prohibition. Our purpose is to encourage critical research agendas that address the continuity of prohibition in legal cannabis frameworks as they remain entangled with what sociologists Reinarman and Levine (1997) first identified as "the continuum of global drug prohibition," later theoretically fleshed out by Levine (2003). The continuum of prohibition referred to the range of enforcement policies in any given country[5] that implement prohibition, from highly punitive to partially decriminalized: drug prohibition has geographically and historically specific varieties. Each variety poses different limits on cannabis as a subject of social and bioscientific research. The emergence of legal exceptions to prohibition creates new freedoms for developing research agendas, but the persistence of prohibition continues to limit, and

DOI: 10.4324/9780429320491-1

therefore shape, the kinds of questions that can be asked, funded, and carried out. Post-prohibition analyses identify those limits to develop and help guide research agendas through, and perhaps to, the end of prohibition.

If legalization is not currently the end of prohibition, though, what is it? Levine provided a usefully succinct operational definition: "[l]icensing production as well as sales creates cannabis legalization in one country" (151). With a little more nuance and historical perspective, we define "legalization" as a concept and practice in any given jurisdiction (not just country) that licenses and removes criminal penalties for any given self-contained supply chain from seed or clone to consumption. For our purposes, we understand legalization to have different varieties distinct from but entangled with the continuum of prohibition, from punitive criminalization to partial decriminalization. There are varieties of prohibition, and now there are varieties of legalization. Any research agenda that supports or derives from a relational analysis of the two tells us something about landscapes of post-prohibition, which, like prohibition, are geographically and historically contingent.

Partial decriminalization allows local policy and rules to govern some part of any given commodity chain without the threat of criminal enforcement. Medical decriminalization in the U.S., for example, opened up space for observational clinical research of patients who use cannabis, but not space for researchers to administer standardized doses of cannabis derivatives commonly used by those patients. Legal clinical medical cannabis research remains dependent on whatever it is the federal research farm at the University of Mississippi is growing. State-legal cannabis, however, creates an opening to recruit observational study participants that are not patients. Moreover, many kinds of social science research that do not require researchers to touch the plant are now legal, given lower human subject risks. On the other hand, institutions of higher education that get federal funding remain constrained by potential legal liability and financial risk. The varieties of prohibition continue to limit the freedom to research cannabis in legal contexts, but at those limits lie promising new fields of inquiry.

Like prohibition, approaches to legalization are political, in the sense that they have different kinds of work to do relative to locally specific prohibition frameworks and policy liberalizations within them. The age of majority with respect to legal cannabis possession and consumption, for example, is younger in some Canadian provinces than others. Some legal U.S. states have allowed for or even require the expungement or vacation of cannabis offenses of differing severity, while others do not. Some legal cannabis states incorporate medical access into their legal commodity chains rather than hybridize two systems of regulation as Colorado has done. Some legal cannabis states permit out-of-state ownership, and some do not, as Washington has done. Different jurisdictions set caps on licenses for different parts of the commodity chain. Some jurisdictions allow more vertical integration for licensees than others, and some offer more license varieties than others. Different U.S. states have different kinds of social equity programs. And medical conditions authorized for treatment with cannabis vary by jurisdiction. This is far from an exhaustive list, but it should be clear that legalization has varieties, as does prohibition.

This relational approach means that we can think about a continuum of legalization as shaped by the historical and geographical specificities of the continuum of prohibition with which they are entangled. All legalization schemes, for example, continue to prohibit and in some cases establish new criminal frameworks for non-adult cannabis consumption and distribution, but definitions of "adult" are allowed to vary by jurisdiction in Canada. All of them ban public consumption, but California permits special events where cannabis may be consumed in public. All of them zone cannabis businesses more strictly than alcohol, but zoning ordinances may vary by jurisdiction. All of them retain criminal prohibition for non-licensed production and market activities, but some have protected carve-outs for noncommercial "home grow."[6] In the U.S., all state-legal and medicinal cannabis remain subject to federal enforcement at any time, with the exception of cannabis that can be botanically classified as hemp.

How exceptions to prohibition work, including how and to what extent they liberate research questions about cannabis, constitute a new and exciting cannabis research agenda on its own. Many of the chapters in this collection operate in this register, from research on potential benefits, to research on how legal markets are constrained by ongoing prohibition laws, to considering the challenge posed by medicinal cannabis research for public health institutions that are oriented towards pharmaceutical medicine. This type of post-prohibition research agenda is primarily concerned with cannabis as a newly legitimate subject of inquiry, with political, economic, and cultural dimensions. We can call this type of approach "legal cannabis in society," because it asks questions about the integration of cannabis in society.

But Levine's theoretical model also directs researchers to consider the politics of prohibition: the uses to which they are put, especially as they relate to racialized social control, as a critical research agenda with significant implications for studying social justice landscapes. Prohibition as a system of criminal governance has had significant impacts on public health outcomes, economic development, ecological impacts, and impacts related to stigma against certain populations, especially racial and ethnic minorities but also cannabis users of any demographic. This is because criminal governance—the penal system writ large—plays a significant role in shaping the limits of liberal governance in modern societies. Liberalism, wrote Hindess (2004), may be a mode of "governing through freedom" but requires the capacity to distinguish between populations that can be governed through the "promotion of liberty" and those that "can be governed in ["illiberal"] other ways" (28). The politics of criminalized prohibition play a central role in this dynamic, as a way to identify and impact those populations (Simon 2007).

Legalization in the context of ongoing prohibition transforms, rather than necessarily eliminates, those impacts. This is the second type of research agenda indicated by post-prohibition, in which the first type is nested. The scope of this research agenda is much, much broader. It is primarily concerned with social problems, not just public health impacts of criminalization, that are widely considered across the social sciences and policy studies. Many of the chapters in this handbook add new case studies, methodological interventions, and directions for critical research agendas such as political economy, cultural studies, environmental justice, and postcolonial studies. Legal cannabis is not only embedded in problematic prohibition frameworks. It is also integrated into landscapes of economic inequality, racism, and environmental degradation that are perfectly legal and institutionalized for reasons other than prohibition. We can call this type of approach "legal cannabis and society," because it asks questions about society through the subject of cannabis.

In this introduction, and for many of the chapters collected here, research questions that are about cannabis and society are questions about the relationship between landscapes of prohibition and landscapes of neoliberalism since the 1970s. The Chicago School economists most associated with the rise of neoliberalism, particularly Milton Friedman, were not particularly fond of prohibition and saw it as antithetical to the free-market ideology their work otherwise successfully promoted (Harcourt 2011, 231–33). The tension between neoliberalism as an ideology of limited government and the massive expansion of criminal justice budgets in the U.S. since the 1980s has made unlikely bedfellows of libertarians and social justice actors behind the emergence of criminal justice reform, inclusive of cannabis liberalization, since the early 1990s.

Systemically, legalization has appeared in the landscape as one way to alleviate the tension between culturally dominant "small government" ideology and the realities of mass incarceration as "big government" penology. Legalization can therefore be seen as a somewhat belated project of neoliberal reform and/or a challenge to neoliberalism as a rationality of governance that heightens social and economic inequality. The former works to shore up neoliberal rationality so that it is more internally consistent, while the latter rejects neoliberal rationality in search of social justice.

Post-prohibition analyses, therefore, address the entanglement of prohibition and legalization through two types of relational analyses: the relationship between post-prohibition and prohibition's varieties on the continuum, from a broad historical perspective; and the relationship between post-prohibition and wider social problems for which there are already robust interdisciplinary social science research agendas.

The relational analysis that follows in four parts presents a U.S.-centric case study to provide historical context for most of the handbook chapters, rather than a comprehensive history of cannabis prohibition. The geographical focus on the U.S. allows us to define two varieties of national cannabis criminalization, economic and medical, which helps periodize the emergence of particular uses for it; how those uses changed over time in broader national political and economic contexts as well as dissent to prohibition; and how and when new uses emerged to shore up and sustain the continuity of national prohibition as part of the neoliberal order. These first three subsections set up the fourth, in which we investigate the entanglement of legalization with old and new uses for prohibition.

The U.S. case is particularly significant, given its central role in globalizing prohibition and the fact that it is here, at the source of its most punitive variety, that legal exceptions first emerged. The reader will notice that within the U.S., the historical narrative here is especially focused on California, for similar reasons. The handbook is particularly California-centric, given that the contributors were drawn from the West Coast–based editors' academic and professional network. But also, California was among the first U.S. states to prohibit cannabis, in 1913, and it is where dissent to cannabis criminalization emerged most successfully in the 1990s in local and then state medical cannabis statutes (Gieringer 2006).

Periodizing Cannabis Prohibition

We categorize two historical types of cannabis criminalization based upon the particular federal U.S. code that established it. "Prohibition 1.0" framed the cannabis commodity chain as an economic crime, as a type of public revenue evasion (1937–1969), and "Prohibition 2.0" viewed cannabis cultivation, commerce, and consumption as crimes against public health, as a controlled substance (1970–present). Within and between these two periods, criminal enforcement against different parts of the cannabis commodity chain from cultivation to consumption waned and waxed, relative to national and local socioeconomic conditions, "narcotic" drug panics, shifting demographics of use, and public support for punitive crime control at large.

Prohibition 1.0 was enacted in 1937 as a tax-and-tariff crime enforced by the Federal Bureau of Narcotics, a division of the Department of Revenue (Frydl 2013, 5–7). It was ruled unconstitutional in 1969, as a violation of the Fifth Amendment protecting citizens from self-incrimination (*Leary v United States*). For about a year and a half, cannabis was only prohibited at the state level, until it was provisionally placed in Schedule I of the 1970 Controlled Substances Act by the Nixon administration, enforced by a division of the Department of Justice, the Drug Enforcement Administration.

This placement criminalized cannabis as a Schedule I danger to public health: a drug with significant potential for abuse and no medical value. Although Nixon refused to remove cannabis from Schedule I against the recommendations of the commission he created to study the matter, ten states voted to decriminalize possession of different amounts in the 1970s (Hudak 2016, 120). The Carter administration publicly considered the national decriminalization of cannabis in the late 1970s. However, an internal scandal involving his chief drug policy advisor, Peter Bourne, removed the prospect of cannabis decriminalization from policy agendas for the next several decades (Baum 1996, 104–14). The "provisional" placement became institutionalized despite, not because, of the political environment that made it happen.

Prohibition 2.0 did not automatically lead to increased federal (and state) enforcement. That did not happen until the Reagan administration began to seriously fund drug enforcement at large, for which cannabis was initially less significant than cocaine. Federally, cannabis became a lot more punitively criminalized when the 1986 Anti-Drug Abuse Act was passed (Dufton 2017, 189–205).

At the end of the 1990s, however, cannabis prohibition became more decriminalized in the five states that passed medical cannabis decriminalization laws, starting with California in 1996, following the municipal lead of San Francisco, which passed a decriminalization statute in 1992. The first wave of medical cannabis decriminalization laws did not address or regulate production, although California Senate Bill 420 in 2003 provided loose decriminalization frameworks for medical cannabis production. A second wave of medical cannabis decriminalization laws passed in the late 2000s that increasingly regulated medical cannabis commodity chains from production to consumption.

In 2013, citing national security concerns relating to the rise of organized crime networks, Uruguay became the first country to adopt national cannabis legalization. The Uruguayan case is particularly exceptional, given that it was initiated by executive action by President José Mujica, a former left-wing guerilla, with little preexisting public support. Canada, which followed a similar medical cannabis reform trajectory as the U.S., legalized cannabis through a national legislative process in late 2018.

Cannabis Prohibition, Moral Panics, and Social Change

Prohibition 1.0 and 2.0 were clearly legislated for political, rather than scientific, reasons. In this subsection, we focus on three types of uses that seem to apply to both: political, financial, and cultural. Political uses of cannabis prohibition include the opportunity to further one's political career, whether as a bureaucrat or politician. The financial uses of cannabis prohibition refer to the opportunity to create and inflate markets involved in drug control industries (Stevens 2011), usually through the transfer of public funds to public and private sectors. And the cultural uses of prohibition relate to the symbolic representation of cannabis as a type of social threat to society that intensifies the dangerousness of other criminalized drugs and the people associated with them.

All three political uses of cannabis prohibition were pioneered for and during Prohibition 1.0, but became increasingly contested towards the end of that period and ever since, by different individuals and organizations in support of decriminalization on the one hand and legalization on the other. The sociological concept of "moral panic" (Cohen 1972) ties all three kinds of uses together.

In the 1930s, Federal Bureau of Narcotics (FBN) Director Harry Anslinger constructed a narrative about cannabis as a "terrible new drug menace . . . threatening the country, one that required immediate action by a well-funded Bureau of Narcotics," with the help of "yellow journalism" pioneer William Randolph Hearst (ibid.: 49–50). Against the testimony of the American Medical Association (AMA), Anslinger claimed that cannabis consumption caused crime, violence, insanity, and sexual deviance, including interracial miscegenation; was particularly associated with the behavior of ethnic and foreign nationals; and was especially constructed as a threat to American youth. The campaign culminated in the passage of the 1937 Marihuana Tax Stamp Act.

In short, the act was passed on the basis of a moral panic, a concept introduced by sociologist Stanley Cohen to describe a generalized feeling of public fear against groups ("folk devils") constructed as imminent threats to "societal values and interests" (Cohen 1972), about which something must be done, usually by police intervention. A crucial element of moral panics is that the hysteria they generate is disproportionate to the extent of the problem that seeds their emergence. "Politico-moral entrepreneurs" (Reinarman 1994) who inspire such drug scares, a particular type of moral panic, benefit politically and economically from what ensues, as do the budgets of police forces and the bottom lines of mass media sources that profit from sensationalist journalism (McLuhan 1964). Cultural studies pioneer Stuart Hall famously analyzed the relationship between moral panics and economic crises (Hall et al. 1978), seeing the former as particularly useful for politicians evading responsibility for the latter. In this way, a wide array of social problems can be attributed to cannabis use (Reinarman 1994).

Critical drug policy scholars often use the term "demonization" to describe the production of "folk devils" as *moral* objects of criminalized drug control. The terms "stigma" (Goffman 1963; Tyler

2020) and "stigmatization" provide similar conceptual utility, with more emphasis on how individuals manage potentially discrediting information and in turn navigate a "spoiled identity." Prohibition produces drug villains, and in so doing those associated with cannabis have generally been stigmatized and blamed for wider social problems. Both concepts are deployed in this handbook to explain how the cultural power of cannabis prohibition works.

The concept of moral panic explains the production of popular support for prohibition legislation, including movements on the continuum toward punitive enforcement against already-marginalized populations, as a function of political and economic entrepreneurialism. It is less helpful for explaining how latent configurations of power in societies that structure such entrepreneurial opportunities converge over time and in particular places or for how "panics" become institutionalized as permanent, generalized anxieties. Those configurations of power also change over time, rendering foundational uses for prohibition obscure if not irrational (Zimring and Hawkins 1992), thus creating openings for political challenges to prohibition's varieties and uses.

Certainly, the racist origins of cannabis prohibition fit the moral panic narrative, but the place of cannabis prohibition in criminalized global "narcotics" prohibition seems especially problematic. Cannabis prohibition is entangled with narcotics prohibition. Cannabis crimes are narcotics crimes, and as such they have historically been especially caught up in moral panics about heroin and cocaine, subject to the same intensifications of criminal law and enforcement that are subsequently enacted. Efforts to periodize cannabis prohibition—its varieties and its uses—must deal with this entanglement to explain changes over time.

More importantly, configurations of power in society change over time, for reasons that have little to do with cannabis and "narcotic" drug control and everything to do with shifting political and economic orthodoxies regarding the regulation, or not, of capitalism and its outcomes. We will return to this subject later, but for now we observe that since the 1980s, the ascendance of retributive criminal justice policies has shifted all sorts of activities identified with crime and urban disorder towards punitive enforcement. The uses of cannabis prohibition, as well as the politics of its dissent, have been significantly dependent on the usefulness of this turn towards retributive justice, at different times and in different places. In the next section, we examine periods of dissent to and reconsolidation of cannabis prohibition in relation to how it has been sometimes useful, and sometimes not, for the politics of "narcotic" crime control and wider dynamics of societal change.

Cannabis Prohibition 1.0: Uses and Varieties

Most scholarship on the origins of cannabis prohibition in the U.S. focus on the explicitly racist arguments popularized by the FBN director Anslinger, in the years leading up to the 1937 Marijuana Tax Stamp Act. Himmelstein (1983) first identified these as the "Mexican hypothesis" and the "Anslinger hypothesis" to explain how he successfully mobilized state and local anxieties about racialized migrant labor during the Great Depression to expand the authority and influence of his post-alcohol prohibition bureaucracy. Himmelstein, however, pointed out that such analyses fail to take into account the relationship between the political rationalities of cannabis prohibition and those of the emergent narcotics control system for which it served as a minor addition. These rationalities were also racialized, since opium-heroin was initially focused on Chinese and later, in the 1950s through the 1970s, Black populations, and cocaine was initially focused on Black populations.

The rationalities weren't just racialized—they were medicalized. Cannabis was a late addition to the category of "narcotics," created in the early 20th century as a class of drugs associated with addiction as a public health problem, and a subject of medical regulation. The origins of narcotic control emerged at the end of the 19th century in the U.S. as a reaction to the commercial exploitation of unregulated drug markets, or "patent medicines." The Pure Food and Drug Act of 1906 was the culmination of a nearly 30-year period when nearly 100 bills were introduced in

Congress to regulate food and drugs[7] by requiring accurate product labeling. The Harrison Act of 1914, by contrast, cited international obligations to implement the 1912 Hague Treaty rather than any particular domestic panic about the use of opium and cocaine (Brecher 1972). Like the 1937 Tax Stamp Act, it required registration with internal revenue collectors and imposed a special tax on "narcotics"[8] commerce. The act was immediately used by law enforcement to prosecute and jail physicians who prescribed narcotics to treat people with addiction problems (49–50). As pharmaceutical access dried up, underground commerce exploded, and major American cities like New York and San Francisco reported large increases in addiction problems, according to a 1918 Treasury Committee Report (51).

By 1936, major policy makers, including law enforcement, were applying to national narcotics prohibition the same critique that had successfully overturned alcohol prohibition (52). Anslinger's central preoccupation at the time was shoring up national narcotics control by passing the Uniform Narcotic Drug Act to transfer policing responsibility to the state budgets (Himmelstein 1983, 92): The FBN's "decision to seek a national marihuana law arose in a round-about way from its propaganda campaign on behalf of the Uniform Narcotic Drug Act and paradoxically was an unintended consequence of its attempt to avoid immediate national legislation."

From 1933, when Anslinger was appointed director of the FBN, to the early 1960s, much of America only knew about cannabis through his propaganda campaigns. Consequently, there was no popular dissent to cannabis prohibition, which was sporadically enforced against politically marginal populations, and mostly by local police forces rather than federal agents. Marginalized groups by definition are already stigmatized, and prohibition stigmas were explicitly built from existing racial animosities shared by politically powerful groups. In this sense, the propaganda campaign used by Anslinger to pass the 1937 act was useful because it led to another political technique, criminalization, for excluding stigmatized groups from society.

Criminalization did not necessarily lead to the spread of punitive enforcement against cannabis until the 1950s, when the first mandatory minimum sentencing laws against prohibited "narcotics" were passed at the federal level. The FBN became preoccupied with connecting heroin to Black populations in the 1950s, as narcotics prohibition became entangled with Cold War geopolitics. The politics of criminalized narcotics control during this period were driven by a moral panic about youth opiate use, connected geopolitically to the emergence of Cold War geopolitics because [communist] China was a significant source of opium (Bonnie and Whitebread 1999 [1974], 216). Cannabis was "along for the ride" as a legally defined "narcotic" (204–221).

In the hearings for the Boggs Act, cannabis use itself was characterized as comparatively less harmful by public health experts but first hypothesized as a "gateway" to opiate addiction (213). The "ride" that cannabis was on, however, moved cannabis criminalization more towards the punitive end of the continuum. Bonnie and Whitebread called it the "high water mark of the punitive approach to drug use" in 1974, at the time of their writing (217). The political usefulness of prohibition appears to have been strengthened by its connection with Cold War geopolitics, ethno-nationalistically constructing opiate culture and supply as a Chinese threat to which cannabis use was a gateway. The outcome, however, when this particular moral panic subsided, was that subjects of cannabis enforcement would face more highly punitive consequences than ever before.

This was not much of a problem for cannabis prohibition, since up to that point subjects of cannabis enforcement were marginalized members of society. In the early 1960s, however, cannabis use exploded across the population, drawing more and more relatively privileged members of society into its punitive web. Much has been written about the popularization of cannabis and other drug use amongst U.S. youth on college campuses in the late 1960s, as a symbol of countercultural "hippie" rebellion. That symbol was differentially connected to the proliferation of campus activism that drove White participation in the new social movements of the 1960s: the civil rights movement, the free speech movement, and the antiwar movement, especially through the institutional development of Students for a Democratic Society (SDS), in which many of the leaders of the New Left were incubated out of the legacy of the labor movement (see for example Gitlin 2003). The result was the popularization of cannabis consumption amongst White, highly educated, middle-class youth, from which emerged the first organized political challenges to prohibition.

The multi-racialization of cannabis prohibition enforcement in the 1960s may have led to a collapse in the political consensus that supported Prohibition 1.0, as more and more White, middle- and even upper-class people were prosecuted for cannabis crimes. Himmelstein referred to this as the "embourgeoisement of marihuana" (1983, 98–120). Cannabis criminalization became less and less legitimate to the public, whose increasingly direct experience with the plant contradicted the regime of knowledge Anslinger had built around it. One of them, countercultural guru and former Harvard psychiatrist Timothy Leary, was the defendant in the 1969 Supreme Court case that declared the 1937 act unconstitutional (Lattin 2010; Conners 2010).

The political usefulness of cannabis prohibition during its first period ebbed and flowed but continuously reproduced a moral panic about cannabis as a "narcotic": an explicit symbol of a racial, ethnic, demographic, medical, and geopolitical threat to society. That this happened despite the gradual accumulation of social and medical research against it (Mosher and Akins 2019, 44–54) is a testament to how useful drug prohibition at large became to "law and order" electoral politics against social movement mobilizations of the 1960s, which carried Nixon to the White House in 1968 (Goudsouzian 2019). Nixon promised the public that he would restore order to the streets, and for that he would need increased police power and funding for crime control budgets.

The recriminalization of cannabis in 1970 ran against the grain of its times. Many scholars of cannabis prohibition have reviewed the evidence connecting Nixon's hardline "law and order" politics, his overt racism,[9] and his motivation to control political enemies through legislation,[10] and the provisional placement of cannabis in the CSA's Schedule I as one of the most dangerous drugs, without accepted medical value against the recommendations of the Shafer Commission (Shafer 1972) he had created to study the matter (Mosher and Akins 2019, 1; Dufton 2017, 51–56).

Cannabis Prohibition 2.0: Uses and Varieties

The story of cannabis Prohibition 2.0 is much more complex than its predecessor, especially since it began during historical conditions that seemed to point towards imminent decriminalization. We have partitioned the story into four parts. First, we consider the political landscape of cannabis prohibition during the 1970s, when it seemed about to fall apart for good. Then, we consider two trajectories of punitive enforcement that reconsolidated the power of cannabis prohibition between 1980 and 2000: urban mass incarceration and rural militarized eradication. Finally, we consider the emergence of medical cannabis politics and liberalization policies that have once again put cannabis prohibition in crisis. Given the complex development of divergent but related policy tendencies and impacts, the narrative is historically recursive rather than linear. But all four parts investigate dimensions of relational forces that shape conditions of post-prohibition today that are relevant to the chapters collected here in the handbook.

The period when prohibition seemed on shaky grounds, between 1970 and 1980, was also a time of significant political and economic change, from postwar Keynesian orthodoxy that advocated state-managed market economies to what scholars now call neoliberalism. Ideologically, neoliberalism is associated with a return to market liberalism that was politically ascendant in the late 19th century, with a policy menu that supports deregulation, privatization of public services, fiscal conservatism, international "free trade," and the like. In practice, however, neoliberal reforms have been accompanied by a striking rise in spending on policing and incarceration (Wacquant 2009, 1–40).

The emergence of mass incarceration catalyzed by prohibition, an anti-market policy, correlates with the emergence of neoliberalism as a twin pillar of national bipartisan politics in the U.S. since the 1980s. At the time of this writing, though, both neoliberalism and the drug war, at least as the latter relates to cannabis, seem to be in crisis. We will return to that in the final subsection, after considering their co-emergence at the dawn of Prohibition 2.0.

From Shaky Grounds to New Fears

For most of the 1970s, Prohibition 2.0 held the criminalization of cannabis together *despite*, not because of, a prevailing societal consensus—including the opinion of medical experts—about cannabis as an inherently dangerous drug with no accepted medical value. Ten states passed decriminalization laws during this time period (Hudak 2016, 120), and a 1976 Supreme Court case, *Randall v U.S.*, found in favor of the defendant's claim that cannabis was medically necessary to treat his glaucoma. Since Prohibition 2.0 rests on the connection between cannabis as a dangerous drug and the assertion that it has no medical value, the Randall case disrupted that framing and paved the way for medical cannabis politics that emerged in the 1990s to challenge the legitimacy of cannabis' placement in Schedule I of the 1970 CSA ever since.

The flowering of organized dissent to cannabis prohibition between 1964 and 1980 meant that although Prohibition 2.0 provisionally reconstituted the legal basis for prohibition as a public health threat, political support for it would have to be shored up. During the 1970s, efforts to overturn it were led by people and organizations that challenged the "high potential for abuse," rather than the medical value of cannabis, as a civil libertarian issue. The National Organization for the Reform of Marijuana Laws (NORML) made significant inroads at the federal and state levels as a consumer rights organization, but rapidly declined in relevance at the end of the decade.

At the federal level, NORML lost influence with the Carter administration when its chief drug policy advisor, Peter Bourne, was allegedly caught consuming cocaine at a Washington DC NORML party (Dufton 2017, 107). His career as a cannabis policy reformer was destroyed by a media scandal that capitalized off of the generalized moral panic about dangerous drugs, this time cocaine. In the absence of federal support for cannabis decriminalization, new moral entrepreneurs gained traction in the 1970s to develop a new moral panic about cannabis and adolescent consumption.

Many scholars have identified the importance of the parent movement at the end of the 1970s and its co-optation by the Reagan Administration for the consolidation of a new moral panic about cannabis. But recent scholarship identifies how the parent movement mobilized disgust specifically with cannabis *commercialization* in the construction of the new moral panic about cannabis. Dufton (2017) explains the emergence of the paraphernalia industry at the intersection of economic crisis and the increasing acceptability of cannabis consumption across demographics and outlines how the parent movement centered on concerns about marketing paraphernalia to adolescents (123–142). For the first time, fear of commercialization—specifically as something that increases youth access—became integrated into the production of a moral panic about cannabis.

The new moral panic about cannabis commercialization was not initially connected to its usefulness for the accumulation of economic capital, as the parent movement was initially highly localized and staffed by volunteers. Nor did it necessarily support the continued criminalization of cannabis, since it mostly produced education and information explicitly designed to curb youth access. But the Reagan Administration (1980–1988) co-opted the organization and messaging of the parent movement by providing federal funding and then co-opting its cultural politics to reconsolidate cannabis prohibition into a form of globalized "law and order" politics that has become hyper-useful ever since for political parties, criminal justice budgets, public health institution budgets, and intensively reracialized social control (Dufton 2017, 143–88).

Urban Mass Incarceration as Reracialization

The Reagan Administration transitioned Prohibition 2.0 as a provisional compromise with limited public support to an integral part of a popular, globalized drug war in considerable partnership with new Democratic party politics (Corva 2008). The usefulness of moral panics about criminalized drugs as political capital ("law and order" politics) first became evidently bipartisan when the Democratic Party began shifting its platform in the 1980s to outflank the Republican Party by becoming tougher on crime and more economically liberal. This meant that Congress, led especially by New Democrats like Joe Biden, pushed the Reagan Administration further and further towards the punitive end of criminalization, especially through the 1986 and 1988 Anti-Drug Abuse Acts. The size, scale, and media sensationalism of the renewed war on drugs, including CAMP (Campaign Against Marijuana Planting) policing in California and the racialized panic around crack cocaine, caught the attention of researchers fairly quickly (Trebach 1987). But it was primarily the latter that drove the metastasization of federal funding for the drug war through the end of the Clinton Administration in 2000 (Western 2006). Unlike the 1960s and 1970s, the subjects of new politics of cannabis crime control were now primarily framed in terms of poor people of color in deindustrialized urban ghettos.

The rapid growth of punitive criminalization during the Reagan and Bush I administrations was identified in the late 1980s by comparative international criminologist Nils Christie (1991). Observing that U.S. incarceration rates per capita had become competitive with the Soviet Union, Christie connected the phenomenon to massive increases in federal funding, nationally and in block grants to states, for crime control especially related to the "war on drugs." The first edition of his book, *Crime Control as an Industry*, was subtitled with a question: "Towards Gulags, Western Style?" (1991). The second edition, published just two years later, deleted the question mark, and in the preface to the third edition published in 2000, when the prison population had reached more than 700 per 100,000, he wrote, what "was alarming in 1991, has developed into a catastrophe at the turn of the century" (8).

The twin phenomena of mass incarceration and militarized policing—both heavily racialized—resulted directly from the massive expansion of criminal penalties and related funding that poured into public budgets starting in this time period and continuing today (Balko 2014). This increase in public funding for crime and drug control ran against the grain of austerity politics associated with neoliberalism, the dominant bipartisan political ideology of the times. Criminalized drug prohibition has played a central role in the transformation from "military Keynesianism" to "carceral Keynesianism": the expansion of the carceral state through mass incarceration as a way to warehouse, rather than employ or subsidize, racialized surplus lives in the population (Gilmore 1999; Irwin 2004).

The massive shift in public spending from Keynesian social welfare programs to the prison-industrial complex (Parenti 1999), with minimal results in terms of reducing drug use or combatting illicit markets, was not lost on small government conservative and libertarian observers, including reformist law enforcement stakeholders (Masters, ed. 2004). Criminal justice reform efforts launched at the beginning of the 2000s stabilized national arrest rates and helped launch a wave of local cannabis decriminalization policies in some major American cities such as Seattle, Washington. In others, especially New York City, "broken windows," "zero tolerance," and "order maintenance" policing (Beckett and Sasson 2004, 202) intensified the rate and disparate racial composition of low-level cannabis arrests. As the growth in mass incarceration stalled out, arrests for low-level cannabis possession skyrocketed in the 2000s, albeit unevenly across the country. As arrests for all drugs peaked in 2006, arrests for cannabis continued to climb, increasing 21% between 2005 and 2010. More than 500,000 of 784,021 arrests in 2010 were made by 12 states (ACLU 2013, 39), and 29 states and the District of Columbia had higher marijuana possession arrest rates in 2010 than in 2001 (ACLU 2013, 42).

Research demonstrating the deeply racial inequities of cannabis and drug prohibition emerged in the 1990s[11] but has been most popularly synthesized by legal scholar Michelle Alexander's book

The New Jim Crow (2020 [2010]). The usefulness of the drug war, she showed, is the central role it has played in the recreation of caste dynamics to preserve dominant political and economic power hierarchies in the United States—just like legal chattel slavery and its successor, Jim Crow laws, that led to the civil rights movement in the 1950s and 1960s. Mass incarceration "caged millions of poor people and people of color and relegated millions more to permanent second-class status"[12] (ix).

Alexander examined the massive contribution of cannabis possession arrests to mass incarceration statistics as an outgrowth of "broken windows" policing starting in the 1990s (169–171). This was especially evident in large urban centers like New York City, where more than 600,000 people were arrested and jailed for possessing cannabis between 1997 and 2013, 87% of whom were Black and Brown (Levine 2013). Alexander's indictment of the war on drugs as the central driver of mass incarceration made it quite useful for cannabis legalization efforts in the 2010s. It raised the profile of legalization as a policy tool for reducing the harms of the U.S. criminal justice system, clearly framing the drug war as a social justice issue rather than an issue relating to the protection of public health (Dufton 2017, 225–48).

Two reports issued by the American Civil Liberties Union (ACLU) in 2013 and 2020 dove deep into the social justice implications of criminalized cannabis prohibition. Between 2010 and 2018, cannabis arrests declined 18%, but the overall decline included a steady increase between 2015 and 2018 (ACLU 2020, 7). They made up 43% of all drug arrests in 2018, and 89.6% of drug arrests were for simple possession. The unevenness of this pattern across the country is emphasized by a strong trend towards lower arrests in states that have decriminalized and legalized cannabis over the same period (ibid., 5). In all states, however, extreme racial disparities have not improved since 2010 (ibid., 7). The persistence of extreme racial disparities in cannabis enforcement led the ACLU to refine the way it advocated for cannabis legalization between 2013 and 2020. The 2013 report highlights racial disparities but advocates for legalization without any particular racial justice characteristics as a remedy (5), while the 2020 report advocates centering racial justice in the development of new legal frameworks and the reform of early ones (12).

The intensification of urban policing against Black and Brown people was not the only manifestation of Prohibition 2.0's shift towards the punitive end of the criminalization continuum, although it is by far the most destructive one. The Reagan administration increased federal funding for rural cannabis eradication, especially apparent in the former president's home state of California, against communities established by his (and Nixon's) political enemies from the 1960s: counterculture hippies who migrated to rural areas to go "back to the land" rather than participate in industrial modernity (Anders 1990).

Rural Militarization: Hippies, Cash Crops, and the Environment

In the late 1970s, concern about the environmental impacts of cannabis cultivation emerged, opening up a new front for both challenging and supporting criminalized cannabis prohibition. The executive director of NORML who outed Peter Bourne as a cocaine user did so in retaliation for the Carter administration's financial support for Mexico's herbicide-based aerial eradication[13] of cannabis cultivation. The "Paraquat panic" that ensued was less about impacts to the environment and more about frightening domestic cannabis users with the prospect of industrial poison (Johnson 2017, 120–22). It was so successful that U.S. cannabis consumers began to earnestly seek out domestically produced *sinsemilla*, easily distinguishable from the seeded Mexican product (Raphael 1985). Domestic wholesale prices rose dramatically for cannabis grown predominantly by hippies who had migrated to rural Northern California in the 1970s. The first "green rush" sparked a 20-year trend toward the domestication of cannabis supply in the U.S., with California overtaking Mexico shortly after the turn of the 21st century (Central Valley High Intensity Drug Trafficking Area 2010).

The period between 1980 and 2000 also featured a substantial increase and funding for militarized cannabis eradication, especially every fall harvest season (Corva 2014). This happened across the U.S. but has been documented especially well for California's annual joint federal-state-local eradication program, the Campaign Against Marijuana Planting. Outdoor eradication served as a price support, on the one hand, limiting market expansion by raising the risk of enforcement. And it served as a geographic stimulus, driving production indoors and away from each annual hotspot for CAMP activity. The most extreme example of the latter phenomenon was the way it pushed large-scale, industrial production into remote public lands.

Both of these developments had particular kinds of environmental impacts, but only the latter became integrated into the environmental politics of cannabis eradication. As the "war on terror" diverted attention and funding away from the U.S. drug war after 2001, CAMP enforcement justified its continued funding by becoming more efficient (seeking out larger operations to yield higher "plants eradicated" results) and more politically palatable by shifting the bulk of its enforcement to industrial-scale trespass grows on public lands. Between 2012 and 2014, CAMP even rebranded as CERT: Cannabis Eradication and Reclamation Teams, which significantly incorporated forest restoration into its enforcement activities (ibid.).

This particular "environmentalization" of cannabis enforcement, if not entirely its politics, was probably the most rational and widely uncontroversial—if short-lived—policy reform that emerged out of Prohibition 2.0. Environmental impacts on public lands were a real concern, supported by evidence and restorative action. The construction of the policy and the way it was (mostly) enforced was supported by many of the people engaged in unregulated cannabis livelihoods. This was especially the case for hippie populations that remained from the 1970s and medical cannabis pioneers from the 1990s, who objected strongly to industrial agriculture, regulated and unregulated, as a threat to the environment. As we will see, critiques around environmental impacts of industrial cannabis cultivation would emerge again in the politics of post-prohibition. In between, however, the emergence of medical decriminalization statutes at the end of the 1990s in response to the HIV/AIDs crisis provided considerable cultural legitimacy and some political cover for cannabis cultivation.

Medicalization and Dissent

Popular dissent to cannabis criminalization re-emerged in the United States in a very particular context: the therapeutic use of cannabis by people, usually gay men and injection drug users, dying of HIV/AIDS (Chapkis and Webb 2008). There were two indisputable ways cannabis was being used therapeutically: as a way to manage nausea as a side effect of early pharmaceutical medications, and as an experience in San Francisco Bay Area cannabis social clubs that provided relief from intersectional stigmas (sexual deviance, addiction, and cannabis demonization) prevalent outside of them. For these patients and their advocates, including medical professionals and growers, cannabis was medicinally and spiritually therapeutic.

Successful medical decriminalization initiatives opened up considerable space for other therapeutic uses to become legitimated, from cancer to epilepsy. It also opened up space for quasi-decriminalized production and distribution. As the HIV/AIDS crisis and its certainty as a death sentence receded in the 2000s, the specific proposition that medical cannabis was useful for hospice patients became generalized. Awareness of other medicinal uses for cannabis increased thanks to personal experience but also to research on how it was used historically, before the 20th century, and in other parts of the world (Mikuriya 1973; Grinspoon and Bakkalar 1997 [1993]). This trend continued to undermine consent to the proposition that cannabis has no medical value, and as more and more people gained firsthand experience with cannabis use, the proposition that it was a danger on par with opiates was also significantly weakened.

Cannabis dispensaries, an increasingly commercialized successor to the cannabis social clubs of the 1990s, proliferated in every state that passed medical cannabis initiatives. This phenomenon was probably intensified by the financial crisis of the late 2000s, but no formal research on this connection has been done to this point. There is, however, a great deal of research[14] on the connection between informal drug market participation and exclusion from the formal economy. These formally unregulated retail storefronts provided an increasingly public face for cannabis commerce, none of which was taxed. Stymied by medical cannabis statutes that broadly decriminalized medical use, federal prosecutors turned to the Obama administration for guidance.

In 2009, Deputy Attorney General David Ogden issued a memorandum to clarify what should and should not be prosecuted in medical cannabis states. Cases that demonstrate "clear and unambiguous compliance with applicable state law" would not be prosecuted, but specific characteristics of any given case, including sales to minors, unlawful possession of firearms, and significant commercial activity, defined cases that could be subject to federal criminal enforcement. The "Ogden memo" (Ogden 2009) resolved a contradiction between punitive cannabis prohibition and medical cannabis decriminalization by getting more prescriptive about which cannabis crimes could be regarded by the Department of Justice as subject to federal enforcement.

Medical cannabis entrepreneurs, focused on compliance with state laws as a guideline for evading criminal prosecution, saw the Ogden memo as implied consent to go forward from the federal government, especially for proposed legislation to regulate and tax medical cannabis supply chains (Washington 2011 Senate Bill 5073[15]) and in California, an adult-use initiative (2010 Proposition 19[16]). The former was passed by the state legislature but gutted by then-governor Christine Gregoire, and the latter failed in the electoral process. The sense that legal cannabis commerce was around the corner, combined with a lack of economic opportunity during "the Great Recession," provided the necessary conditions for a new and much more public "green rush."

The public proliferation of cannabis commercialization after the Ogden memo led Ogden's successor, James Cole, to issue another memorandum in 2011 (Cole 2011), clarifying that cases involving large amounts of cash and financial transactions were fair game for federal prosecutors. A crackdown on medical cannabis dispensaries in California ensued, scattering many operators to other states. The moral panic legitimating Prohibition 2.0 once again related to the profitability of unregulated medical cannabis commerce. The nonprofit ethos of 1990s' medical cannabis statutes significantly remained but became increasingly buried by sensational headlines, stories, television shows, and books celebrating the green rush (see for example Regan 2011; Campbell 2012).

Fears about the commercialization of medical cannabis fed directly into arguments for legalization, especially as an effort to capture untaxed revenues and stimulate economic development. Decriminalized medical markets were characterized as competitors to regulated and taxed adult-use markets, but that tension was managed differently by state. Washington effectively gutted its medical cannabis laws in 2016, the earliest opportunity for its legislature to change laws passed by initiative (Washington 2015 Senate Bill 5052). By contrast, Colorado maintains a dual system to this day, albeit with more medical cannabis taxation and regulation.

Uses and Varieties of Legalization

Like prohibition, legalization has varieties ranging on a continuum, with different types of rules and regulations that carve out differential legal exceptions to prohibition. Everywhere we look, we see legal cannabis contingencies that can only be explained by acknowledging and examining their relative entanglement with the continuity of prohibition. These entanglements happen when geographically and historically specific varieties of prohibition encounter varieties of legal exceptions to prohibition. Post-prohibition landscapes are complex, but they can be modelled at the intersection of these two tendencies.

Cannabis legalization is entangled with cannabis prohibition at different scales than the aforementioned federal-state example. The U.N. treaties governing drug control, for example, limit the kinds of legal cannabis commodity trade that can occur across national borders. And within U.S. states that have legalized cannabis, "local control" allows counties and cities to opt out of regulated commerce, which not only limits where cannabis can be legally produced and sold but stimulates unregulated cannabis market activity and consumption. Canada also allows provinces and territories to set added restrictions around possession limits, minimum age, public use, and personal cultivation.[17]

The varieties of legalization, from a technocratic standpoint, are shaped to accommodate rather than overturn federal prohibition. The governors of the first two states to pass legalization initiatives, Washington and Colorado, immediately asked the Obama administration for guidance. In response, James Cole issued his second memo, outlining eight specific conditions that would prevent federal intervention and enforcement of the Controlled Substances Act (Cole 2013). These were preventing distribution to minors; preventing criminal organizations from directly profiting "from the sale of marijuana"[18]; preventing diversion to other states; preventing legal cannabis businesses to be used to launder illegal cannabis revenue; preventing violence and the use of firearms in the cultivation and distribution of cannabis; preventing the exacerbation of adverse public health outcomes; preventing environmental damage especially on public lands; and preventing cannabis possession or use on federal property.

Each state was free to figure out how their system would be designed to prevent each of these federal concerns, none of which seem to be necessarily connected to Prohibition 2.0's medical scheduling logic. Rather than a moral panic, the federal guidelines constituted a more rational approach to drug policy with broad flexibility for local interpretation and implementation. The memo did, however, construct a discourse of fear around cannabis that singled it out as a dangerous commodity that would require "strong and effective regulatory and enforcement mechanisms that will address the threat that those state laws could pose to public safety, public health, and other law enforcement interests."

The memo's focus on prevention excluded any interest that states might have in maximizing therapeutic access, for example; preventing monopolies or monopolistic licensing schemes; or minimizing law enforcement participation in the design or implementation of regulations. In fact, Cole emphasized a distinction between his first memo's warning that large-scale, commercial medical cannabis enterprises were fair game for federal enforcement and this memo, for which "the size or commercial nature of a marijuana operation" should necessarily be considered problematic. The memo also implicitly conscripted public safety, public health, and law enforcement interests in the design and implementation of laws that they had played no part in passing; all were passed by voter initiative until 2020 when the Illinois legislature became the first state body to legalize adult use. Still, the memo provided a broad informal policy framework for states to experiment with different approaches.

While legitimate experiments, in the popular imagination, take place in laboratories, it was not long before the metaphor of states as "laboratories of democracy" popularized by Supreme Court Justice Louis Brandeis in 1932 became associated with cannabis legalization. In 2016, the Democratic Party articulated this discourse in its national platform:

> We believe that the states should be laboratories of democracy on the issue of marijuana, and those states that want to decriminalize marijuana should be able to do so. We support policies that will allow more research to be done on marijuana, as well as reforming our laws to allow legal marijuana businesses to exist without uncertainty. And we recognize that our current marijuana laws have had an unacceptable disparate impact, with arrest rates for marijuana possession among African-Americans far outstripping arrest rates among whites despite similar usage rates.
>
> *(Democratic Platform Committee 2016, 14)*

The "laboratories of democracy" metaphor deployed in the platform was less prophylactic than the 2013 Cole memo. The Democratic National Party platform outlined three social benefits, not just prevention of harms, that state regulation could offer: more research (not just research into harms); sustainable industry (not just the replacement of unregulated markets); and racial justice. These three justifications for cannabis legalization were prevented from incorporation into federal policy when Republican Donald Trump won the 2016 election.

This development was compounded when Trump's Attorney General, Jeff Sessions, issued a 2018 memo that cancelled those of Cole and Ogden, effectively leaving federal cannabis enforcement up to the discretion of federal prosecutors. The previous memos, Sessions wrote, undermined "the rule of law and the ability of our local, state, tribal, and federal law enforcement" to "reduce violent crime, stem the tide of the drug crisis, and dismantle criminal gangs." The logic of moral panic that underwrote the "provisional" placement of cannabis in Schedule I by the Nixon Administration in 1970 was back, but the varieties of legalization continued to develop. The "bipartisan consensus" around cannabis criminalization that characterized most of Prohibition 2.0, however, is not as evident as it once was.

The varieties of legalization have also become increasingly contested, from below, by the rise of the Black Lives Matter Movement (2014–present) that pushed racial and social justice issues to the forefront globally. Some states that legalized after 2012 incorporated some element of "social equity" policy into their frameworks, although none so far have much to show for it (ACLU 2020). Social equity policies include provisions and/or mandates for misdemeanor cannabis convictions to be vacated or expunged; special licensing windows for individuals to apply from communities impacted by cannabis criminalization; assistance to equity applicants to help navigate complex regulation schemes and/or develop business education; and direct funding from cannabis tax revenue and/or general funds to communities impacted by cannabis criminalization (Nani, ed. 2020). The provision of special licenses for equity applicants has been made more urgent by the fact that legal cannabis ownership to this point is predominantly White, male, and already wealthy. This is exacerbated by the politics of enforcement against unregulated markets that are predominantly Black, Brown, and poor, sometimes lobbied for by legal industry participants and trade associations that see them as competition (Youth Forward and Getting It Right From the Start 2020).

The chapters collected in this handbook reflect the many ways to research how the varieties and uses of legalization reproduce patterns of social exclusion and inclusion incubated by Prohibition since the beginning of the 20th century, as well as systemic patterns of inclusion and exclusion that have been perfectly legal, especially since the 1970s. The latter means that our U.S. contributors are often critical of the institutions that have been in charge of evaluating potential legalization harms outlined in the second Cole memo. The varieties of legalization that are entangled with prohibition are ill-equipped to optimize many beneficial aspects of the human–cannabis relationship that have become apparent to generations of activists.

But policy makers that implement cannabis legalization, so far, seem largely uninterested in and/or incapable of minimizing the harms of punitive criminalization to which they must defer. The vast majority of lifelong harms related to mass incarceration come from cannabis felonies, not misdemeanors that have been decriminalized and sometimes vacated from records, and there is no movement yet to clear cannabis felonies or release people with felonies from prison. The focus by legalization advocates on legalizing adult consumption, rather than or in lieu of decriminalizing cultivation or distribution, may be partly responsible for this. Anxiety about unregulated commercialization may be another contributing factor, since many arguments for legalization construct unregulated market participants as violent criminals and international drug cartels (Trujillo 2011). Such discourses are never based on rigorous research[19] into the demographic composition of unregulated cannabis market participants, and as such fit the definition of moral panics explored earlier.

Illegal cannabis and other drug markets are a sector of the informal economy that has helped people and communities be resilient in the face of declining or nonexistent economic opportunities (see Weisheit 1993 and Bourgeois 2003 for rural and urban contexts, respectively). This is especially salient given the emergence of two major global economic crises in the last ten years. The systematic exclusion of these actors from legal cannabis ownership and jobs is a problem for legalization, especially when more enforcement is called for as a way to protect licensed operators from competition. Strict regulations, high taxes, restrictive zoning, and license caps associated with legal cannabis regulation keep ownership *and* prices out of reach for many. And policy mandates focused on preventing hypothesized public safety harms from legal cannabis feed back into, rather than clearly break from, the moral panic underpinning punitive cannabis and drug prohibition.

Conclusion

Post-prohibition research agendas are at least attentive to, if not center, the entanglement of legalization with prohibition. In this conclusion, we review how that works broadly in each of our five sections. This handbook invites researchers to a landscape of entanglement with five interdisciplinary social issues entangled in policies and practices of legalization: Governance; Public Health; Markets and Society; Ecology and the Environment; and Culture and Social Change. Our conclusion ends with a review of these themes by section as they relate to the concept of post-prohibition laid out in this introduction.

The Organization of the Handbook

Governance

We use the term "governance" (rather than "government") to include the ways that cannabis prohibition shapes life and livelihood outcomes, not only through punitive enforcement but as a way of reproducing the persistence of illiberal outcomes in liberal societies today (Hindess 2004). For decades, cannabis legalization has been promoted as a horizon of individual freedom not yet reached in societies that have otherwise made considerable progress liberating other ways of being different than those previously considered immoral and deviant. Seen this way, the right for adults to legally consume cannabis is akin to the achievement of same-sex marriage protections in the 21st century. But as we have seen, cannabis prohibition has rarely been about restricting the ability of privileged members of society to consume cannabis. Rather, it has been useful for a wide variety of ways to maintain social order by excluding stigmatized demographics from social and economic mobility, and it has been useful for people and institutions that profit from the expansion of drug control spending. The legalization of adult-use consumption does not inherently address broader problems of modern governance—cultural exclusion, socioeconomic inequality, and bloated security budgets—for which cannabis prohibition has served a complementary role.

The chapters in this section contribute to analyses of legalization at its jurisdictional and social justice limits. Reinarman addresses the deep roots and continuity of exclusionary politics that have historically made use of cannabis prohibition, and he grapples with new concerns about legal cannabis commercial exploitation as a challenge to legalization going forward. Polson locates contemporary resistance to cannabis liberalization at the local scale in the neoliberal politics of exurban gentrification. Chapkis identifies the increasing influence of corporate interests on state cannabis policy in Maine, where legacy medical cultivators are structurally excluded from ownership. Reed mobilizes a postcolonial critique of cannabis legalization as a project of settler colonialism. Baudean evaluates the outcomes related to social policy goals set forth by the Uruguayan government at the beginning of its legalization process, which did not initially have majority public support. And Bone and

Potter examine dynamics of inclusion and exclusion in legalized medical cannabis markets in the United Kingdom.

Public Health

Public health professionals and institutions have come a long way, from being significant objects of "narcotics" prohibition governance to significant stakeholders in government-funded research that has been almost exclusively focused on justifying the Schedule I classification of cannabis as a drug with high potential for abuse and no medical value. The importance of Schedule I as a rationale for punitive criminalization may be overstated, since cocaine and methamphetamines for example have been significant objects of punitive criminalization despite being Schedule II. Arguments about whether cannabis has medical value have developed away from a general, if irrational, denial into a maze of debates about botanical versus pharmaceutical medicine; modes of ingestion; what role recreation and spirituality play in individual health outcomes; and even the calculus of health harms created by punitive criminalization versus harms associated with use.

The chapters in this section contribute to analyses of legalization that highlight how public health and prohibition remain entangled and also emphasize new ways of thinking about and researching cannabis as a public health benefit despite limits to public health research posed by its entanglement with prohibition. Aggarwal takes on the subject of public health as an institution of Western pharmaceutical interests, arguing that they marginalize non-Western approaches to the spiritual dimensions of human health and happiness. Wilson-Poe addresses the potential of cannabis use as a harm reduction tool by providing a comprehensive review of opiate substitution literatures. Ogle opens up the subject of cannabis use as wellness practice for exercise and sports, a subject that was abandoned in the 1970s. Ehrlich reflects on the importance of developing public health research agendas that are informed by the everyday experiences of research subjects. And Schenker and Langer examine the emergence of health and safety regulations for cannabis workers in legal cannabis landscapes.

Markets and Society

The proliferation of cannabis markets because of, rather than despite, punitive enforcement against them has posed a special problem for erstwhile "market societies" associated with the rise of neoliberalism since the 1970s. Prohibition is anti-market governance, but prohibition markets are perhaps the most free-market economic sectors available in capitalist societies. This makes "strict control" licensing schemes especially difficult to implement, if one of the goals of legalization is to protect the public through extremely bureaucratic regulation. At the same time, broad support for strict control seems to be based on the assumption that free markets (in some things) lead to forms of commercial exploitation that prioritize profits over public safety. Neoliberal societies may have a problem, after all, with unregulated capitalism. This underlying anxiety about "industry" does not distinguish between large-scale, financialized industry stakeholders and legacy small-scale cannabis livelihood stakeholders that have become prevalent since the emergence of medical cannabis commodity chains in the 1990s.

The chapters in this section examine the entanglement of cannabis markets, legal and otherwise, within existing landscapes of capitalism. Goldstein and Sumner detail how landscapes of strict state regulation in California limit the development of legal markets while stimulating unlicensed markets. Zender's research highlights how federal prohibition shapes the business forms chosen by legal cannabis firms and significantly limits their profitability. On a more critical note, Otañez directs researchers to center legal cannabis worker health and safety in landscapes of industrial cannabis production. Similarly, Otañez and Vergara highlight the need for critical research on corporate social responsibility branding in legal cannabis markets. Bennett examines the potential, or lack of it, of "ethical consumerism" to promote environmentally friendly cannabis supply chains in Portland, Oregon. And Silber-Coats introduces researchers to the complex landscape of medicinal "hemp" markets as escape valves for traditional cannabis producers in Oregon.

Ecology and the Environment

Questions about the relationship between cannabis control and environmental protection are both a lot simpler, politically at least, and a lot more complex in post-prohibition analyses. Domestic cannabis cultivation in the U.S. comes from a countercultural demographic with radical environmental politics, many of whom developed a critique of environmental impacts associated with large-scale industrial agriculture decades before such critiques became mobilized by law enforcement agencies. Contemporary discourses about the environmental impacts of cannabis cultivation, however, rarely scrutinize new impacts made possible by licensing energy-intensive, large-scale cultivation. For example, the spread of commercial cannabis genetics developed since the 1970s in the global North to globally historical cannabis cultivation landscapes in the global South operates much the same as the spread of genetically modified seeds, distorting and displacing peasant livelihoods.

The chapters in this section examine how cannabis production landscapes connect with themes of conservation and environmental change. Dillis et al. situate emergent landscapes of licensed cannabis production in California's industrial agriculture landscape. Silvaggio examines the complex landscape of environmental impacts in California, identifying ways in which eradication has structurally produced the problems that it claims to address under conditions of legalization. Mills and Zeramby delve deeply into the energy politics of indoor cultivation, arguing that cannabis policy and environmental policy are politically decoupled from each other. Kelly and Formosa complicate our understanding of the relationship between cannabis livelihood production and commercial exploitation by locating values and practices of environmental stewardship in legacy production areas that could be useful again under conditions of legalization, if given opportunities to transition. Finally, Afsahi connects the commercialization of cannabis seed commodity chains to transformations in rural Moroccan cultivation landscapes.

Culture and Social Change

Cannabis as a subject of culture and social change bookends the handbook's starting focus on governance through law by focusing on the cultural politics of prohibition, which mainly work to stigmatize cannabis use and users, often in connection with the stigmatization of marginalized populations in society. The opposite of stigmatization is often referred to as "normalization," but normal cultural values are not free of discrimination or even aspired to by cultural communities associated with cannabis production, distribution, and consumption under conditions of prohibition. Cannabis meant dissent to normal values when its use first became widespread in the 1960s. The fact that entrepreneurialism developed from the counterculture should not obscure how objectionable the values of crass commercialism, militarism, bureaucracy, resource exploitation, and even Western medicine were to the hippies and their cultural descendants. Prohibition culture, the idea that cannabis and people who grow, distribute, and use it are inherently immoral, both preceded formal prohibition and endures through the stigma embedded in value systems that limit the power of legalization to make the changes it promises. Cultural studies about cannabis prohibition constitute a sort of "final frontier" for post-prohibition studies. Irrational fear of cannabis and its users will remain long after the last laws based on such fears are repealed.

The chapters in this section examine the entanglement of cultural values promoted by and through cannabis liberalization (medical and legal reforms) with broader cultural values that developed and continue to thrive under conditions of prohibition. Newhart and Dolphin address the management of intersectional stigmatization by contemporary medical cannabis patients, for whom the normalization of adult recreational use poses structural challenges to the legitimacy of patient identity. Walker critiques the politics of adult-use "normalization" by interrogating the limits of recreation as a problematically normalized subjectivity in consumerist societies. Rogers examines the mobilization of privileged identities in advertising to "normalize" legal cannabis use as particularly White, upper class, and female. Aguiar et al. interrogate the positive role of media framing to significantly increase public support for cannabis legalization in Uruguay. Sexton identifies the proliferation of unsupported claims about the therapeutic use of cannabis, particularly CBD products, as entrepreneurial marketing fills the gap created by restrictions on clinical research. Finally, on a more positive note, Reiman advocates for a more intentional integration of legal cannabis values with those associated with social movements of the 1960s: civil rights, environmentalism, and gender justice.

The chapters collected in all five sections model research agendas that are less about an "after" for prohibition than a collection of directions for researching cannabis legalization as it is related to ongoing problems in society, including the continuity of prohibition laws, policies, and attitudes. Legalization is the beginning of opportunities to understand the place of cannabis in society, rather than a historical moment in which it is liberated from the power dynamics that were useful for its criminalization. There is much to celebrate about the progress that legalization represents, but perhaps its greatest value for interdisciplinary research are the agendas upon which they are finally able to embark.

Notes

1 We use "cannabis" to refer to *Cannabis sativa L.* as a single genus with distinct biotypes bred for fiber/food/fuel purposes ("industrial hemp") as well as medicinal/drug (cannabinoid) properties (Clarke and Merlin 2013, xvi).

2 Alaska, Arizona, California, Colorado, Illinois, Maine, Massachusetts, Michigan, Montana, Nevada, New Jersey, Oregon, South Dakota, Vermont, and Washington.

3 At the time of this writing, 46 U.S. states have passed some variation of medicinal cannabis decriminalization (Americans for Safe Access 2020).

4 We use "liberalization" as a category that includes cannabis decriminalization and legalization reforms.

5 Levine's geographical unit of varietal differentiation was "country," given the relationship between UN treaties and nation-state territoriality. Given the development of cannabis legalization in the U.S., where cities and counties retain local control to opt out of legal frameworks, we consider "varieties" to refer to any given jurisdiction that implements prohibition: cities, counties, states/provinces, nation-states, and potentially regional trade zones as well as bilateral agreements.

6 Within California, though, home-grow provisions are limited by local zoning ordinances that vary by canopy limits and parcel sizes, among other things.

7 www.fda.gov/about-fda/fdas-evolving-regulatory-powers/part-i-1906-food-and-drugs-act-and-its-enforcement

8 The act created "narcotics" as a class of dangerous drugs, rather than a scientifically rational class of drugs with "narcotic" effects, by classifying cocaine, a drug with decidedly nonnarcotic properties, as a narcotic.

9 "Every one of the bastards that are out for legalizing marijuana is Jewish. What the Christ is the matter with them?" (Nixon in Dufton 2017, 50); and "[President Nixon] emphasized that you have to face the fact that the whole problem is really the blacks. The key is to devise a system that recognizes this while appearing not to" (Nixon aide H.R. Haldeman in Baum 1996, 13).

10 "The Nixon campaign in 1968, and the Nixon White House after that, had two enemies: the antiwar left and black people. You understand what I'm saying? We knew we couldn't make it illegal to be either against the war or black, but by getting the public to associate the hippies with marijuana and blacks with heroin, and then criminalizing both heavily, we could disrupt those communities. We could arrest their leaders, raid their homes, break up their meetings, and vilify them night after night on the evening news. Did we know we were lying about the drugs? Of course we did" (Nixon White House Counsel and Chief Domestic advisor John Ehrlichman in Baum 2020).

11 See for example Lausanne 1991; Reinarman and Levine 1997; Wacquant 2009.

12 Alexander's thesis goes way, way beyond the presentation of crime control statistics, such as per capita incarceration, to explore the societally constitutive nature of our punitive criminal justice system, including its racially disparate cannabis enforcement. The book is less a critique of prohibition than a sweeping critique of "colorblind" neoliberalization in America since the 1960s. The caste system to which she refers includes poor people of any color swept up in the criminal justice system, and the moral entrepreneurs she indicts for creating and maintaining it include Black elites and institutions.
13 It should be noted that the U.S. also used herbicidal eradication in Vietnam against cannabis cultivation extensively between 1969 and 1974 (Johnson 2017, 120).
14 See for example Portes et al. 1989; Bourgeois 2003; Weisheit 1993; Campbell 2009.
15 WA State E2SSB 5073.2011. URL: http://lawfilesext.leg.wa.gov/biennium/2011-12/Pdf/Bills/Session%20Laws/Senate/5073-S2.SL.pdf#page=1, accessed November 12, 2020.
16 Not to be confused with the 1972 California Proposition 19, which was the first statewide cannabis legalization initiative (Brady 2013).
17 Cannabis Act. 2018. Accessed November 20, 2020. URL: https://laws-lois.justice.gc.ca/eng/acts/C-24.5/page-1.html.
18 This appears to direct states to curb unregulated cannabis markets, whether or not they are connected to legal cannabis markets.
19 That sort of research is fairly risky under conditions of prohibition, but not impossible, as some of our chapters demonstrate.

References

ACLU. 2013. *The War on Marijuana in Black and White*. American Civil Liberties Union. www.aclu.org/report/report-war-marijuana-black-and-white.

———. 2020. *A Tale of Two Countries Racially Targeted Arrests in the Era of Marijuana Reform*. American Civil Liberties Union. www.aclu.org/report/tale-two-countries-racially-targeted-arrests-era-marijuana-reform.

Alexander, Michelle. 2020 [2010]. *The New Jim Crow: Mass Incarceration in the Age of Colorblindness*. New York and London: The New Press.

Americans for Safe Access. 2020. *2020 State of the States*. https://american-safe-access.s3.amazonaws.com/sos2020/StateoftheStates20_Spreads.pdf.

Anders, Jentri. 1990. *Beyond Counterculture: The Community of Mateel*. Pullman, WA: Washington State University Press.

Balko, Radley. 2014. *Rise of the Warrior Cop: The Militarization of America's Police Forces*. Public Affairs: ebook.

Baum, Dan. 1996. *Smoke and Mirrors: The War on Drugs and The Politics of Failure*. Boston, New York, Toronto and London: Little, Brown and Company.

———. 2016. "Legalize it All." *Harpers*. Accessed July 24, 2020. https://harpers.org/archive/2016/04/legalize-it-all/.

Beckett, Katherine, and Theodore Sasson. 2004 [2000]. *The Politics of Injustice: Crime and Punishment in America*. Thousand Oaks, CA: Sage Publications.

Bonnie, Richard J., and Charles H. Whitebread. 1999. *The Marijuana Conviction: A History of Marijuana Prohibition in the United States*. New York: The Lindesmith Center.

Bourgeois, Philippe. 2003 [1995]. *In Search of Respect: Selling Crack in El Barrio*. New York: Cambridge University Press.

Brady, Emily. 2013. *Humboldt: Life on America's Marijuana Frontier*. New York: Grand Central Publishing.

Brecher, Edward, and the Editors of Consumer Reports. 1972. *Licit and Illicit Drugs: The Consumers Union Report*. Boston, ON: Little, Brown and Company.

Campbell, Greg. 2012. *Pot, Inc.: Inside Medical Marijuana, America's Most Outlaw Industry*. New York: Sterling.

Campbell, Howard. 2009. Drug War Zone: Frontline Dispatches from the Streets of El Paso and Juarez. Austin: University of Texas Press.

Central Valley High Intensity Drug Trafficking Area [HIDTA]. 2010. *Marijuana Production in California*. Washington, DC: U.S. Department of Justice National Drug Intelligence Center.

Chapkis, Wendy, and Richard J. Webb. 2008. *Dying to Get High: Marijuana as Medicine*. New York and London: New York University Press.

Christie, Nils. 2000 [1991, 1993]. *Crime Control as Industry*. London and New York: Routledge.

Clarke, Robert C. and Mark Merlin. 2013. *Cannabis Evolution and Ethnobotany*. Berkeley and Los Angeles, California: University of California Press.

Cohen, Stanley. 1972. *Folk Devils and Moral Panics: The Creation of the Mods and Rockers*. London: MacGibbon and Kee.

Cole, James. 2011. *Memorandum for United States Attorneys*. U.S. Department of Justice. Accessed November 12, 2020. www.justice.gov/sites/default/files/oip/legacy/2014/07/23/dag-guidance-2011-for-medical-marijuana-use.pdf.

———. 2013. *Memorandum for All United States Attorneys*. U.S. Department of Justice. Accessed November 12, 2020. www.justice.gov/iso/opa/resources/3052013829132756857467.pdf.

Conners, Peter. 2010. White Hand Society: The Psychedelic Partnership of Timothy Leary and Allen Ginsberg. San Francisco: City Lights Books.

Corva, Dominic. 2008. "Neoliberal Globalization and the War on Drugs: Transnationalizing Illiberal Governance in the Americas." *Political Geography* 27 (2): 176–93.

———. 2014. "Requiem for a CAMP: The Life and Death of a Domestic U.S. Drug War Institution." *International Journal of Drug Policy* 25 (1): 71–80.

Democratic Platform Committee. 2016. *Democratic Party Platform*, 4. Online Document. Accessed August 25, 2020. https://democrats.org/wp-content/uploads/2018/10/2016_DNC_Platform.pdf.

Dufton, Emily. 2017. Grass Roots: The Rise and Fall and Rise of Marijuana in America. New York: Basic Books.

Frydl, Kathleen. 2013. *The Drug Wars in America, 1940–1973*. New York: Cambridge University Press.

Gieringer, Dale. 2006. "The Origins of Cannabis Prohibition in California." *Contemporary Drug Problems* 25 (2).

Gilmore, Ruth Wilson. 1999. "Globalisation and U.S. Prison Growth: From Military Keynesianism to Post-Keynesian Militarism." *Race and Class* 40 (2/3): 171–88.

Gitlin, Todd. 2003. *The Whole World Is Watching: Mass Media in the Making and Unmaking of the New Left*. Berkeley, CA: University of California Press.

Goffman, Erving. *Stigma: Notes on the Management of Spoiled Identity*. New York: Simon & Schuster.

Goudsouzian, Aram. 2019. *The Men and the Moment: The Election of 1968 and the Rise of Partisan Politics in America*. Chapel Hill: University of North Carolina Press.

Grinspoon, Lester, and James Bakkalar. 1997 [2003]. *Marihuana: The Forbidden Medicine*. New Haven and London: Yale University Press.

Hall, Stuart, Chas Critcher, Tony Jefferson, and Brian Roberts. 1978. *Policing the Crisis: Mugging, the State and Law and Order*. London and Basingstoke: MacMillan Press.

Harcourt, Bernard. 2011. *The Illusion of Free Markets: Punishment and the Myth of the Natural Order*. Cambridge, MA and London: Harvard University Press.

Himmelstein, Jerome. 1983. The Strange Career of Marijuana: Politics and Ideology of Drug Control in America. Westport, CT: Greenwood Press.

Hindess, Barry. 2004. "Liberalism—What's in a Name?" Chapter in *Global Governmentality: Governing International Spaces*, edited by W. Larner and W. Walters. London and New York: Routledge.

Hudak, John. 2016. *Marijuana: A Short History*. Washington, DC: Brookings Institution Press.

Irwin, John. 2004. *The Warehouse Prison: Disposal of the New Dangerous Class*. Los Angeles: Roxbury.

Johnson, Nick. 2017. *Grass Roots: A History of Cannabis in the American West*. Corvallis: Oregon State University Press.

Lattin, Don. 2010. *The Harvard Psychedelic Club*. New York: Harper Collins Books.

Lausanne, Clarence. 1991. *Pipe Dream Blues: Racism and the War on Drugs*. Boston: South End Press.

Levine, Harry. 2003. "Global Drug Prohibition: Its Uses and Crises." *International Journal of Drug Policy* 14: 145–53.

———. 2013. "The Scandal of Racist Marijuana Arrests—and What to Do About It." *The Nation*, October 30. Online article Accessed July 22, 2020. www.thenation.com/article/archive/scandal-racist-marijuana-arrests-and-what-do-about-it/

Masters, Sheriff Bill, ed. 2004. *The New Prohibition: Voices of Dissent Challenge the Drug War*. Lonedell, MO: Accurate Press.

McLuhan, Marshall. 1964. *Understanding Media*. New York: McGraw Hill Education.

Mikuriya, Tod H., ed. 1973. *Marijuana: Medical Papers: 1839–1972*. Oakland, CA: Medi-Comp Press.

Mosher, Clayton, and Stuart Akins. 2019. *In the Weeds: Demonization, Legalization, and the Evolution of U.S. Marijuana Policy*. Philadelphia: Temple University Press.

Nani, Christopher. 2020. *Understanding Social Equity*. Denver, CO: SSRN. https://papers.ssrn.com/sol3/papers.cfm?abstract_id=3622268.

Ogden, David. 2009. *Memorandum for Selected United States Attorneys*. U.S. Department of Justice. Accessed November 12, 2020. www.justice.gov/archives/opa/blog/memorandum-selected-united-state-attorneys-investigations-and-prosecutions-states.

Parenti, Christian. 1999. *Lockdown America: Police and Prisons in the Age of Crisis*. London: Verso.

Portes, Alejandro, Manuel Castells, and Lauren Benton, eds. 1989. *The Informal Economy: Studies in Advanced and Less Developed Countries*. Baltimore and London: The Johns Hopkins University Press.

Raphael, Ray. 1985. *Cash Crop: An American Dream*. Mendocino, CA: Ridge Times Press.

Regan, Trish. 2011. *Joint Ventures: Inside America's Almost Legal Marijuana Industry*. Hoboken, NJ: John Wiley and Sons.

Reinarman, Craig. 1994. "The Social Construction of Drug Scares." In *Constructions of Deviance: Social Power, Context, and Interaction*, edited by Patricia A. Adler and Peter Adler, 155–165. Boston, MA: Wadsworth Publishing.

Reinarman, Craig, and Harry Levine, eds. 1997. *Crack in America: Demon Drugs and Social Justice*. Berkeley, CA: University of California Press.

Shafer, Raymond, chair. National Commission on Marihuana and Drug Abuse. 1972. *Marihuana: A Signal of Misunderstanding*. The First Report of the National Commission on Marihuana and Drug Abuse. Washington, DC: U.S. Government Printing Office.

Simon, Jonathan. 2007. *Governing Through Crime: How the War on Crime Transformed American Democracy and Created a Culture of Fear*. New York: Oxford University Press.

Stevens, Alex. 2011. *Drugs, Crime and Public Health*. Oxfordshire, Canada and New York: Routledge.

Trebach, Arnold. 1987. *The Great Drug War*. New York: Palgrave Macmillan.

Trujillo, Colin William. 2011. "Marijuana, Mexico and the Media." MA Thesis, Humboldt State University. http://dspace.calstate.edu/handle/2148/722.

Tyler, Imogen. 2020. *Stigma: The Machinery of Inequality*. London: Zed Books.

Wacquant, Loïc. 2009. *Punishing the Poor: The Neoliberal Government of Social Insecurity*. Durham and London: Duke University Press.

Weisheit, Ralph. 1993. "Studying Drugs in Rural Areas: Notes from the Field." *Journal of Research in Crime and Delinquency* 30 (2): 213–32.

Western, Bruce. 2006. *Punishment and Inequality in America*. New York: Russell Sage Foundation.

Youth Forward and Getting It Right From the Start. 2020. *California Cannabis Tax Revenues: A Windfall for Law Enforcement or an Opportunity for Healing Communities?* Public Health Advocates. https://phadvocates.org/wp-content/uploads/2020/06/YouthForward_CannabisTaxReport2020_REV060820.pdf.

Zimring, Franklin, and Gordon Hawkins. 1995 [1992]. *The Search for Rational Drug Control*. Cambridge: Cambridge University Press.

Section 1
Governance

The purpose of this opening section is to stimulate research agendas about cannabis legalization as a governance reform that breaks from, rather than defers to, assumptions, practices, and injustices associated with prohibition governance. This starts with identifying and coming to terms with the harms of prohibition as a social problem for which legalization is meant to be a political answer. For many legalization initiative supporters, for example, that social problem has mostly been experienced as a lack of reliable access to cannabis for medicinal, therapeutic, and adult-use consumption. For critical drug policy scholars and communities impacted by criminalization, on the other hand, prohibition is a system of authoritarian social control that extends way beyond cannabis, into human rights issues exacerbated by the role that militarized policing and drug war profiteering play in maintaining the social order. The former is a particular relational problem with cannabis prohibition in free societies, while the latter is a broader relational problem with governance in societies that may not be as free as advertised.

The varieties of legalization that have emerged so far are differentially democratic in the sense of who is included and who is excluded in the making of local legal frameworks and policy implementation. "Who is excluded" from legalization is important for historical reasons, because they reflect the same demographics of those who have been explicitly excluded from freedom through prohibition: people of color, "countercultural" people, indigenous people, dispossessed people making livelihoods in the informal sector, and young people, among others. The chapters presented in this section offer a range of theoretical frameworks, methodologies, and research agendas for exploring the promise of legalization as a liberation movement, but also its limits under conditions of ongoing prohibition. We are interested here in research that investigates the discourse and practice of legalization as a means for liberalizing governance, rather than an end in and of itself that defeats authoritarian, racially disproportionate prohibition.

Sociologist Craig Reinarman opens our section on Governance by locating recent developments in cannabis policy liberalization in the long history of U.S. drug prohibition as a technique of social control in different ways and at different times against marginalized and vulnerable communities for the sake of raising political capital. In "Notes on a Post-Prohibition Research Agenda," Reinarman argues that reformist calculations of the costs and benefits of cannabis legalization rarely consider the benefits of ending drug prohibition's systematic suppression of human rights. This, he says, renders the project of cannabis legalization vulnerable to prohibitionist discourse that keeps the public debate focused on drugs, rather than people. The legalization of cannabis as a revenue-producing commodity, rather than a symbol of authoritarian social control, also suppresses broader systemic critiques of legal drug market commercialization. Reinarman's contribution tells us something about the necessity for research agendas that remain attentive to the continuity of prohibition, but also suggest new directions for post-prohibition inquiry that delve into the integration of legal cannabis markets with capitalism.

In "Legalization and Prohibition: Breaks, Continuities, and the Shifting Terms of Racial-Capitalist Governance," anthropologist Michael Polson shows the potential for developing political economy critiques of post-prohibition landscapes using ethnographic methods. His work in rural Northern California landscapes situate processes of legal implementation in conditions of ongoing federal prohibition, on the one hand, and the cultural continuity of prohibition in local power dynamics, on the other. On the ground, the emergence and contestation of legal market implementation are shaped by historically continuous discourses and practices of economic development, governed through land use ordinances and, increasingly, environmental politics. Polson's chapter invites researchers to consider post-prohibition dynamics as embedded in local power dynamics that are constitutive of, rather than independent from, the development of capitalist modernity.

Sociologist Wendy Chapkis also invites researchers to investigate the political economy of cannabis legalization from below by considering tensions between grassroots cannabis activists and the state politics of legal market implementation in Maine. In "Growing Pains: Marijuana Legalization in Maine," Chapkis provides a case study to highlight the continuity of "legalization" as a phenomenon that grew out of medical cannabis legalization in the late 1990s. Chapkis's mixed-methods approach utilizes media content analysis and interview data to materialize and center the increasingly marginalized politics and livelihoods of medical cannabis people. In doing so, she complicates the relationship between political mobilization and market commercialization in the face of adult-use cannabis regulation that seems to favor capital accumulation over livelihood preservation. Is there room for restorative and reparative justice, she wonders, in the governance of legal cannabis markets?

In "Cannabis, Settler Colonialism, and Tribal Sovereignty in California," Native American Studies scholar Kaitlin Reed takes readers interested in the tension between justice and cannabis markets on a deeply postcolonial journey. This indigenous people's critique of cannabis legalization is not so much interested in the continuity of prohibition in landscapes of legalization as how the continuity of coloniality is reflected in the recent spread of cannabis markets regardless of governance type. Neither prohibition governance nor legal cannabis statute considered the interests of tribal sovereignty in design and implementation. As a result, both types of governance and the markets they produce reflect and reproduce the continuity of settler colonialism. Reed's decolonial critique opens up a potentially rich research agenda about cannabis governance beyond the national juridical landscape.

Policy scholar Marcos Baudean's chapter, "Five Years of Cannabis Regulation: What Can We Learn From the Uruguayan Experience?" provides researchers with a unique case study of Uruguay's experience with legalization in 2013. First, it provides a case study of legalization's global varieties, of particular interest since it emerged in Uruguay at the tail end of Latin America's decade of "left turns."[1] Second, legalization was catalyzed by presidential initiative, despite initial lack of popular support (see Aguiar et al. Chapter 27, this volume). Baudean identifies the government's hypothesized effects of legalization on security and public health and evaluates their actual outcomes five years later, using existing quantitative data. His case study not only is an excellent primer on Uruguayan legalization, but also models a question for researchers investigating other varieties of legalization to ask: what should the public expect from legalization as a jurisdictional social policy, and are those expectations met? Research agendas attentive to this question can reveal much about degrees of accountability built into varieties of legalization.

In "Medical Cannabis in the UK: The (False) Dawn of a New Era?," legal scholar Melissa Bone and criminologist Gary R. Potter conclude our Governance section by considering the international dimensions of post-prohibition as a phenomenon characterized by legalization with, not after, prohibition. In the UK, medical cannabis legalization remains the dominant domain of cannabis criminal justice reform, rather than the governance of adult use. As a result, the authors point towards research agendas about uneven access to public health. They highlight an emergent tension between controlled substance scheduling reform and human rights: Like recreational cannabis dynamics, political liberalization provides uneven benefits between economically marginalized patients and pharmaceutical gatekeepers.

Together, these chapters offer paths forward for critical research about cannabis legalization that rejects prohibition discourses and practices but connects with broader concerns about inclusion and exclusion in the legal landscape. As such, they also connect with well-established literatures across the social sciences that are critically engaged with the politics and practice of democratic governance in modernity. They enlarge our sense of what cannabis legalization does, where it is, and how it becomes entangled with other structures of power in society.

Note

1 The "left turns" refers to the wave of left-wing governments that were elected to power in the 2000s that all shared a critique of neoliberalism, on the one hand, and U.S. imperialism—often related to the war on drugs—in Latin America, on the other (see Dangle 2010; Cameron and Hershberg, eds. 2010).

References

Cameron, Maxwell A., and Eric Hershberg. 2010. *Latin America's Left Turns: Politics, Policies, & Trajectories of Change*. Boulder, CO: Lyn Rienner.

Dangl, Benjamin. 2010. *Dancing with Dynamite: Social Movements and States in Latin America*. Oakland, CA: AK Press.

2

Notes on a Post-Prohibition Research Agenda

Craig Reinarman

Keywords: cannabis, marijuana, prohibition, legalization, regulation, commercialization

Introduction

On June 6, 1932, John D. Rockefeller Jr. released a public letter to Nicholas Murray Butler, president of Columbia University, announcing Rockefeller's surprising support for a resolution Butler was proposing for the Republican Party platform: *repeal of alcohol prohibition*. It caused a political sensation.

This did not come easily for Rockefeller. "I was born a tea-totaler; all my life I have been a tea-totaler on principle," he wrote, noting that neither he nor his parents or grandparents had "ever tasted a drop of intoxicating liquor." His mother and grandmother had been temperance crusaders who prayed "on their knees in the saloons" to save men from the "horrors of drunkenness." The letter shocked anti-liquor crusaders because for years prior to prohibition, Rockefeller and his father had been prominent backers of the Anti-Saloon League, the powerful lobby most responsible for the passage of national alcohol prohibition (McGirr 2016, 237–38). They ardently hoped the new law would eliminate alcohol and the many problems attributed to it. Millions of Americans shared that hope. The crusade against drink was the utopian fantasy of many native-born, white middle-class Protestants, but it was the largest social movement in the US at the beginning of the 20th century (Gusfield 1963; Levine 1985; Okrent 2010; McGirr 2016).

After a dozen years of national alcohol prohibition, however, Rockefeller came to the "profound conviction" that whatever benefits prohibition brought were "more than outweighed by the evils" that were "likely to lead to conditions unspeakably worse than those which prevailed before." He found

> that drinking generally has increased; that the speakeasy has replaced the saloon . . . that a vast army of lawbreakers has been recruited and financed on a colossal scale; that many of our best citizens, piqued at what they regarded as an infringement of their private rights, have openly and unabashed[ly] disregarded the Eighteenth Amendment; that as an inevitable result respect

DOI: 10.4324/9780429320491-2

> for all law has been greatly lessened; that crime has increased to an unprecedented degree—I have slowly and reluctantly come to believe.[1]

In the crisis context of the Great Depression, alcohol prohibition made less and less sense to more and more people. Urban Democrats supported repeal. Some key Republicans were joining them, including newspaper baron William Randolph Hearst. Rockefeller saw that Republicans were losing support by backing prohibition and wrote that he hoped to take alcohol policies "out of the field of partisan politics."

Rockefeller understood that after decades of demonizing alcohol it would be "difficult for our people as a whole to agree in advance" on a new alcohol control system. So he asked his top adviser, Raymond Fosdick, to set up a public policy institute to study the alternatives and draft a model alcohol control law that might guide local governments. They recommended a flexible "local option" model that allowed states to set specific alcohol regulations. The 18th Amendment was repealed in 1933, and within two years nearly all states had their own alcohol control systems that closely followed the model law (Levine and Reinarman 1991). To some extent, the states had become, in Justice Brandeis's famous phrase, "laboratories of democracy" with regard to alcohol policy.

Here in 2020, Americans again find themselves at an historic inflection point, this time about cannabis policy. Through the political haze we can see the rough contours of a post-prohibition paradigm coming into view. First, there has been a *generational shift in experience*, from a tiny sliver of the population having used cannabis in 1960 to half the adult population having done so by 2010 (NIDA 2019). Second, this has led to a *discursive shift* in the culture from a discourse shaped by temperance and prohibition, drug wars, and "just say no" campaigns, to one in which the ingestion of consciousness-altering substances, cannabis in particular, is commonly understood not as deviance, disease, addiction, or mental illness but simply something many ordinary people *do* (e.g., Parker, Aldridge, and Measham 1998; Eisenbach-Stangl, Moskalewicz, and Thom 2009). Cannabis use is a cultural practice, one among many technologies of the modern self deployed for pleasure, against pain, or both (see Walker 2017). This shift in attitudes can be measured many ways but is most obvious in opinion polls and voting behavior showing majoritarian support for cannabis legalization.

Third, there has been a *political/policy shift* in which state and local policies have been enacted as if national cannabis prohibition was a thing of the past. Despite federal law, at the time of this writing voters and legislators in 34 states have legalized medical marijuana and in 16 of these states have legalized adult use. As officials now enact various reforms to regulate cannabis, the "laboratories" of the states are in effect conducting novel post-prohibition policy experiments. Several additional states have taken steps toward decriminalization, and more legalization initiatives are gaining support. Cannabis is a burgeoning industry, providing tens of thousands of jobs and many millions in tax revenue. In politics and policy, cannabis has undergone a moral passage into legitimacy. Together, these shifts mark the early stages of *de facto* repeal of cannabis prohibition.

Although the trend line seems clear, the forces favoring cannabis prohibition run very deep in American culture; they are unlikely to slink away in defeat, political tails between their legs. To sustain the trend toward the legal regulation of cannabis, advocates will need research that addresses the questions that defenders of prohibition will continue to raise.

Rockefeller's observations about the unintended consequences of alcohol prohibition 90 years ago hold for drug prohibition today. The lessons that led to repeal of the 18th Amendment, however, have only recently and partially been applied to cannabis and other criminalized drugs. Drug prohibition was largely invented by anti-alcohol crusaders and alcohol prohibition agents who were zealous in their attempts to suppress other drugs after repeal of alcohol prohibition. The new Federal Bureau of Narcotics stoked race and class prejudices, creating fears of "alien" drugs and "dangerous classes" of users in a process I call *reciprocal demonization* (Duster 1970; Musto 1973; Bonnie and

Whitebread 1974; Epstein 1977). From their inception, drug laws were deployed as mechanisms for the social control of the "other."

The cumulative effects of drug prohibition continue to cloud public understanding, creating fear and moral condemnation that are then mobilized into political support for continued prohibition. It is still taken as "common sense" that drugs cause crime, disease, and overdose deaths. It is less well understood that such claims are partly self-fulfilling. "Drug-related crime" is caused as much by the dehumanizing funnel of narrowing options shaped by prohibition as by addiction *per se* (Rosenbaum 1981). The spread of HIV/AIDS and hepatitis-C among people who inject drugs stems from syringe sharing, which has more to do with the criminalized context of drug use than with drugs themselves. Most opiate overdose deaths are more a function of the lack of potency labeling and quality controls in illicit markets than of the alleged depravity of "junkies."

In short, the dangers citizens have been led to fear most about illicit drugs are as much the predictable effects of drug *policy* as the effects of drugs. Prohibition helped create the conditions under which drug use is more likely to be problematic, and thus helped create the consequences that then appear to confirm the need for prohibition.

The Drug Policy Reform Movement

As the costs and consequences of drug prohibition climbed in the 1980s, activists forged a drug policy reform movement from a growing array of public health officials, physicians, attorneys, elected officials, researchers, and religious leaders who challenged prohibition. They made drug policy contested terrain. Elements of this first emerged internationally. Dutch reformers created licensed cannabis retail shops. British drugs workers set up syringe exchanges. Swiss and German officials created safe consumption spaces and opiate maintenance programs. Then Portugal, Belgium, Denmark, Australia, Spain, Argentina, Uruguay, and Canada all moved away from the hardline prohibitionist policies advocated by US and UN drug control agencies and toward decriminalization and harm reduction.

In the US, the National Organization for the Reform of Marijuana Laws began pushing for cannabis legalization in the 1970s. In the 1980s drug policy reformers joined with AIDS activists to establish syringe exchanges, which were adopted as crucial public health measures to reduce the spread of HIV/AIDS (e.g., Kerr et al. 2010) and hepatitis-C in 150 or more US cities, despite federal laws prohibiting them. In the 1990s the Drug Policy Alliance and medical marijuana advocates began to win state-level laws. Since 2000, the drug war's disproportionate damage to communities of color has made drug policy reform a top priority for civil rights and racial justice organizations, from the NAACP and the Congressional Black Caucus to Black Lives Matter (Burns 2019). These strands of drug policy reform activism may be understood as green shoots of citizen resistance to the state apparatus of prohibition. The wide range of reforms, innovations, and policy experiments now underway make this an epochal moment in the history of drug policy, with cannabis leading the way.

The drug policy reform movement faced substantial opposition, not least from a drug control industrial complex that lobbied hard for prohibitionist policies and funding (e.g., Frydl 2013). For years, reformist discourse about drugs was suppressed and key policy questions were excluded from scientific forums. Scientists were warned that they should avoid using even the term "harm reduction" if they wanted their research papers accepted and their grants funded. There is a growing medical literature on the therapeutic potentials of cannabis (Institute of Medicine 1999), but the scientific studies necessary to demonstrate its precise efficacy for specific types of patients have been systematically blocked by the Drug Enforcement Administration (which then cites the lack of scientific evidence of efficacy as the reason for their blockage).

The National Institute on Drug Abuse is the principal source of funding for research on drug issues. But as its name implies, NIDA focuses primarily on the physiological, neurological, and psychological aspects of *individual abuse*, addiction, and treatment. Equally important research on the *social context* of drug use and drug-related problems—including the impact of prohibitionist policies—is rarely funded. More important for the post-cannabis prohibition epoch now dawning, studies of what users have found *beneficial* about cannabis, their rules and rituals for self-regulating use, protective practices, and strategies for natural recovery, have received very little support. Until recently, studies of the therapeutic potentials of cannabis for cancer patients or of MDMA or LSD for veterans with post-traumatic stress disorder have not been funded (see Pollan 2018; Giffort 2020). These are among the scientific casualties of the drug war.

This distortion of public discourse about drugs in the service of state orthodoxy about prohibition has been toxic to both science and democratic policymaking. In such a fear-ridden, heavily moralized policy arena, a more open knowledge production process will be essential for evaluating reform policies. The antidote is to crank open the analytic aperture, conduct solid research on previously *verboten* questions, and have honest discussions of the evidence. Since at least Galileo, politically inconvenient scientific knowledge has often been buried. One core task facing post-prohibition researchers is to excavate such knowledge.

In 2011, the Global Commission on Drug Policy issued its report on the War on Drugs. It recommended what is now coming to pass with cannabis: "robust experimentation with harm reduction, decriminalization and legal regulatory policies." The first "principle" articulated in the report is, "Drug policies must be based on solid empirical and scientific evidence. The primary measure of success should be the reduction of harm to the health, security, and welfare of individuals and society." Drug prohibition's true costs and benefits have never been systematically compared to those of legal regulation according to this criterion. But this is now possible for cannabis. Given the carefully cultivated fears about drugs and the resistance to drug policy reform, research on cannabis legalization and other alternatives to prohibition must be especially rigorous. The more reforms are adopted, the more important it is for research to identify their limitations and unintended consequences. In this way research can help create an evidence-based feedback mechanism so that cannabis regulations and other reforms can be evaluated, adjusted, and made more effective.

Playing Defense

Reforms of all sorts are never safely set in stone; sooner or later they always require defending. In recent years, democratic civil society movements in Eastern Europe and in developing nations moved forward only to get pushed backward. In the US at this writing, key elements of the New Deal from the 1930s—labor rights, bank regulation, Social Security—are under attack from a renascent Right. The civil rights movement has had to win its victories for racial justice again and again; even now the Voting Rights Act of 1965 is being eviscerated. Legal reforms alone often remain vulnerable if the political values behind them are not woven into culture and institutionalized.

In drug policy, the Netherlands successfully pioneered a licensed cannabis sales system but has been pressured by neighboring nations to constrict it. England partially decriminalized cannabis but then reversed course. In the US, research has clearly established the cost-effectiveness of treatment in lieu of incarceration for drug offenders (Rydell and Sohler Everingham 1994; Caulkins et al. 1997; McVay, Schiraldi, and Ziedenberg 2004; Ettner et al. 2006), yet police unions, prison guards, and prosecutors still oppose this and push for harsher punishments. Even with unequivocal evidence of their safety and efficacy (e.g., Kerr et al. 2010; California Department of Public Health 2018), syringe exchange programs continue to face local opposition. Despite polls showing majority support for medical marijuana laws and legalization (e.g., Hartig and Geiger 2018), dispensaries and retail outlets still face zoning, regulatory, and other challenges. In short, cannabis policy reforms will surely require defending, and research will be the front line of that defense.

A post-prohibition research agenda should begin with a *human rights perspective* on drug use, namely the presumption that sovereign individuals—not the state—have the right to decide what they put into their own bodies.[2] This perspective is also fundamental to rigorous scientific research on drug policies, for drug users have essential expertise about their drug use and how it affects their lives. No matter how troubled or troubling some of them may seem (particularly in a prohibitionist context), people who use drugs must be seen presumptively as full citizen subjects rather than pathologized objects of social control—part of "us," not "them." To understand the risks and rewards of drug use, researchers must be able to understand how citizens who use drugs react to the evolving constellation of conditions they confront.

Is Availability Destiny?

The drug control industry and other opponents of cannabis legalization have for many years confidently predicted that greater availability would inevitably lead to greater cannabis consumption and, therefore, more problems (for a useful overview, see Room et al. 2010). An early clue about this claim came in the 1970s, when 11 US states passed limited forms of marijuana decriminalization. Several evaluations showed that neither use prevalence nor drug-related problems increased more in those states than in similar states that did not decriminalize (Johnston, Bachman, and O'Malley 1981; Maloff 1981; Single 1981). Since the 1980s, the Netherlands has had up to 400 "coffee shops" licensed to sell cannabis (Beileman and Goeree 2000). Dutch rates of cannabis use prevalence, however, have remained on par with or below those of most neighboring countries that prohibit cannabis and at just over half the prevalence rate in the US (Reinarman, Cohen, and Kaal 2004; Room et al. 2010).

In 1996, California voters passed Proposition 215, a medical marijuana initiative that spawned a sprawling system of dispensaries and dramatically expanded availability. Opponents worried that this would lead to an upsurge of use by youth (e.g., Levy 2013). Yet marijuana use by California high school students *declined* slightly for nearly a decade and remained below pre-1996 levels longer (Skager and Austin 2004). After Colorado, Washington, Oregon, and Alaska legalized adult recreational use, the percentage of their high school students who reported past-month cannabis use remained stable or declined (Washington State Department of Health 2016; Colorado Department of Public Health 2017; Oregon Health Authority 2019; Brooks-Russell et al. 2019; Anderson et al. 2019). A recent analysis of European data (Stevens 2019) showed no statistically significant association between cannabis policy liberalization and use by young people. Availability is not destiny.

But the fact that the sky has not fallen does not mean that questions about the effects of increasing availability are settled. Unlike illicit markets, licensing and regulation provide strong economic incentives for cannabis dispensaries and retail outlets to enforce age restrictions scrupulously. Of course, many young people still consume cannabis. But if keeping it out of the hands of youth is a worthy policy objective, then post-prohibition research should explore how some youth get around age restrictions, the frequency and quantity of their use, and whether they experience problems. And what if cannabis consumption *does* increase over time under regulated sales? This in itself would not constitute a self-evident evil, but it would be important for researchers to determine whether increased prevalence led to an increase in *problematic* use and, equally important, whether increased use of cannabis had any positive collateral impacts such as a decrease in opioid or alcohol consumption.

Of Markets and Regulations

As with post-repeal alcohol control, states that have legalized cannabis have replaced prohibition with regulated markets. This can take various forms. After alcohol prohibition was repealed, taxes were structured to favor milder beverages, and "dram shop" laws limited the size of drinks and the hours saloons could be open. Other regulations were designed to prevent the liquor industry from agglomerating excessive market power through vertical integration (controlling production and sale).

Opponents of cannabis legalization raise the specter of "Big Cannabis" *a la* "Big Tobacco" and "Big Pharma," arguing that unfettered market forces tend to result in industry concentration and undue wealth and political influence that could disadvantage public health. Traditional underground growers who produced cannabis under prohibition also worry about "Big Cannabis" squeezing them out and obtaining corporate patents on strains of cannabis.

Beyond limiting sales to adults, on which there is broad consensus, what exactly should be regulated and how should such regulations be enforced? When Dutch *de facto* legalization led to greater commercialization, more coffee shops, and advertising that glamorized cannabis, use became more prevalent among youth. The Dutch government tightened their rules; now coffee shops cannot display so much as a marijuana leaf in their windows. Youth prevalence edged back down (MacCoun and Reuter 2001). In the US, state-level legalization has led to billboards promoting cannabis stores along major freeways. Millions have been spent on clever cannabis marketing. Anyone visiting a licensed cannabis outlet will notice the extraordinary variety of products and paraphernalia on offer. Should there be limits on cannabis commercialization? If so, what kinds? Who decides?

Unless regulations are thoughtful and enforced, the drive for more profits will likely yield more promotion and larger grow operations to maximize economies of scale. In any industry, big players tend to push out or acquire smaller players, leading to a concentration of capital. Large growers will advocate for the right to do whatever will maximize crop yields and profits. In some areas with good growing climates, there has been a land rush and tree clearance. There are already private equity firms that invest solely in cannabis-related businesses, and multinational conglomerates are being formed. What are the implications of all this for the workers who tend, clip, and ship the plants? For consumers? Neighbors? In post-prohibition spaces where the artisanal is becoming corporate, people who worry about "Big Cannabis" aren't just being paranoid.

News headlines hint at some of the potential risks of commercialization. Big Pharma firms Purdue and Johnson & Johnson have agreed to pay billions in settlements for having misleadingly promoted Oxycontin and its chemical cousins, which helped create the opioid epidemic (Hoffman 2019). The prominent corporate consulting firm McKinsey advised Johnson & Johnson to "turbocharge" sales by getting "more patients on higher doses of opioids" and to study techniques "for keeping patients on opioids longer" (Bogdanich 2019). A leading manufacturer of nicotine vaping devices, Juul Labs, apparently targeted schools and youth camps to promote use of e-cigarettes, which they marketed in candy flavors and in the handy form of rechargeable USB drives (Kaplan 2019). The Centers for Disease Control report a 13-fold rise in the use of e-cigarettes among high school students since 2011 (Cullen et al. 2018).

The industry, the state, and cannabis consumers now face a question that has long confronted alcohol policy: *Should we allow a consciousness-altering drug to be marketed just like any ordinary commodity?* Both before and after repeal of alcohol prohibition, the answer has been various forms of "No." The trick is to find the optimal balance of licensing requirements, fees, taxes, labor safeguards, environmental protections, and retail regulations—without so burdening the legal industry that small businesses are priced out and the black market resurges. However, some noncommercial production and distribution (home grows and other "gray market" transactions) may serve as a brake on both monopolization and excessive enforcement. The post-prohibition research agenda will have to include questions about the political economy of cannabis and the modes of governmentality being invented to regulate it.

Finally, will the deepening immersion of cannabis in the whirlpool of advanced capitalism affect the ceremonial or sacred aspects of cannabis long treasured by users? Marx wrote that in the ceaseless churn of capitalism "all that is solid melts into air, all that is holy is profaned." Weber noted that capitalist modernity brings a relentless efficiency, an "iron cage" of rationality (from which, ironically, cannabis has often served as a valued escape). Norman Zinberg (1984) argued that the *culture* surrounding drugs is intrinsic to their powers—that the psychological set of user expectations and the structure of the social settings in which it is used are fundamental parts of their effects and the meanings we inscribe upon those effects. If so, then post-prohibition researchers might also ask, how will the altered states of consciousness themselves be altered by the increasing commodification of cannabis?

Notes

1 Quotes from the Rockefeller letter were taken from Levine (1985, 10–11), based on the Rockefeller Family Archives, 1920s–1930s.

2 Whether and to what degree this principle should hold for other market participants, e.g., "dealers," would depend on the cannabis product type, the scale of operation, whether it was medically authorized, other applicable regulatory rules, etc. Answers will require much public debate and a far more complicated analysis than space allows here.

References

Anderson, D. Mark., Benjamin Hansen, Daniel I. Rees, and Joseph J. Sabia. 2019. "Medical Marijuana Laws and Teen Marijuana Use: New Estimates from the Youth Risk Behavior Survey." *JAMA Pediatrics* 173 (9): 879–81. https://jamanetwork.com/journals/jamapediatrics/article-abstract/2737637.

Beileman, Bert, and P. Goeree. 2000. *Coffee Shops Geteld: Aantallen Verkooppunten van Cannabis in Nederland [Coffee Shops Counted: Numbers of Points of Sale of Cannabis in the Netherlands]*. Groningen, NL: Stichting Intraval.

Bogdanich, Walt. 2019. "McKinsey Advised Johnson & Johnson on Increasing Opioid Sales." *The New York Times*, July 25, sec. Business. www.nytimes.com/2019/07/25/business/mckinsey-johnson-and-johnson-opioids.html.

Bonnie, Richard J., and Charles H. Whitebread. 1974. *The Marihuana Conviction: A History of Marihuana Prohibition in the United States*. Charlottesville, VA: University Press of Virginia.

Brooks-Russell, Ashley, Ming Ma, Arnold H. Levinson, Leo Kattari, Tom Kirchner, Erin M. Anderson Goodell, and Renee M. Johnson. 2019. "Adolescent Marijuana Use, Marijuana-Related Perceptions, and Use of Other Substances Before and After Initiation of Retail Marijuana Sales in Colorado (2013–2015)." *Prevention Science: The Official Journal of the Society for Prevention Research* 20 (2): 185–93. https://doi.org/10.1007/s11121-018-0933-2.

Burns, Janet. 2019. "As Congress Hears Cannabis Testimony, Advocates Form Powerful Coalition for Racial Justice." *Forbes*. www.forbes.com/sites/janetwburns/2019/07/10/as-congress-hears-cannabis-testimony-advocates-form-powerful-coalition/.

California Department of Public Health. 2018. *Issue Brief: Syringe Access Policies for California Syringe Exchange Programs*. Sacramento, CA: Office of AIDS, California Department of Public Health.

Caulkins, Jonathan P., C. Peter Rydell, William L. Schwabe, and James Chiesa. 1997. *Mandatory Minimum Drug Sentences: Throwing Away the Key or the Taxpayers' Money?* Santa Monica, CA: The RAND Corporation.

Colorado Department of Public Health & Environment. 2018. *Data Brief: Colorado Youth Marijuana Use 2017*. Healthy Kids Colorado Survey. https://drive.google.com/file/d/1M3XdmqznZDl2y6D7Hz6iDGwTFTHSGrtP/view.

Cullen, Karen A., Bridget K. Ambrose, Andrea S. Gentzke, Benjamin J. Apelberg, Ahmed Jamal, and Brian A. King. 2018. "Notes from the Field: Use of Electronic Cigarettes and Any Tobacco Product Among Middle and High School Students—United States, 2011–2018." *MMWR. Morbidity and Mortality Weekly Report* 67 (45): 1276–77. https://doi.org/10.15585/mmwr.mm6745a5.

Duster, Troy. 1970. *The Legislation of Morality: Law, Drugs, and Moral Judgment*. New York: Free Press.

Eisenbach-Stangl, Irmgard, Jacek Moskalewicz, and Betsy Thom. 2009. *Two Worlds of Drug Consumption in Late Modern Societies*. Surrey, UK: Ashgate Publishing, Ltd.

Epstein, Edward Jay. 1977. *Agency of Fear: Opiates and Political Power in America*. New York: Putnam.

Ettner, Susan L., David Huang, Elizabeth Evans, Danielle Rose Ash, Mary Hardy, Mickel Jourabchi, and Yih-Ing Hser. 2006. "Benefit—Cost in the California Treatment Outcome Project: Does Substance Abuse Treatment 'Pay for Itself'?" *Health Services Research* 41 (1): 192–213. https://doi.org/10.1111/j.1475-6773.2005.00466.x.

Frydl, Kathleen J. 2013. *The Drug Wars in America, 1940–1973*. New York: Cambridge University Press.

Giffort, Danielle. 2020. *Acid Revival: The Psychedelic Renaissance and the Quest for Medical Legitimacy*. Minneapolis: University of Minnesota Press.

Global Commission on Drug Policy. 2011. *The War on Drugs: Report of the Global Commission on Drug Policy*. www.globalcommissionondrugs.org/wp-content/uploads/2017/10/GCDP_WaronDrugs_EN.pdf.

Gusfield, Joseph R. 1963. *Symbolic Crusade: Status Politics and the American Temperance Movement*. Urbana, IL: University of Illinois Press.

Hartig, Hannah, and Abigail Geiger. 2018. "About Six in Ten Americans Support Marijuana Legalization." *Pew Research Center*, October 8. www.pewresearch.org/fact-tank/2018/10/08/americans-support-marijuana-legalization.

Hoffman, Jan. 2019. "Johnson & Johnson Ordered to Pay $572 Million in Landmark Opioid Trial." *The New York Times*, August 26, sec. Health. www.nytimes.com/2019/08/26/health/oklahoma-opioids-johnson-and-johnson.html.

Institute of Medicine. 1999. *Marijuana as Medicine: Assessing the Science Base*. Washington, DC: National Academy Press.

Johnston, Lloyd D., Jerald G. Bachman, and Patrick M. O'Malley. 1981. *Marijuana Decriminalization: The Impact on Youth, 1975–1980*. Monitoring the Future Occasional Paper 13. Ann Arbor, MI: University of Michigan, Institute for Social Research.

Kaplan, Sheila. 2019. "Juul Targeted Schools and Youth Camps, House Panel on Vaping Claims." *The New York Times*, July 25, sec. Health. www.nytimes.com/2019/07/25/health/juul-teens-vaping.html.

Kerr, Thomas, Will Small, Chris Buchner, Ruth Zhang, Kathy Li, Julio Montaner, and Evan Wood. 2010. "Syringe Sharing and HIV Incidence Among Injection Drug Users and Increased Access to Sterile Syringes." *American Journal of Public Health* 100 (8): 1449–53. https://doi.org/10.2105/AJPH.2009.178467.

Levine, Harry G. 1985. "The Birth of American Alcohol Control: Prohibition, the Power Elite, and the Problem of Lawlessness." *Contemporary Drug Problems* 12: 63–115.

Levine, Harry G., and Craig Reinarman. 1991. "From Prohibition to Regulation: Lessons from Alcohol Policy for Drug Policy." *Milbank Quarterly* 69: 461–94.

Levy, Sharon. 2013. "Effects of Marijuana Policy on Children and Adolescents." *JAMA Pediatrics* 167: 600–2.

MacCoun, Robert J., and Peter Reuter. 2001. "Evaluating Alternative Cannabis Regimes." *British Journal of Psychiatry* 178: 173–78.

Maloff, Deborah. 1981. "A Review of the Effects of Decriminalization of Marijuana." *Contemporary Drug Problems* 10: 307–22.

McGirr, Lisa. 2016. *The War on Alcohol: Prohibition and the Rise of the American State*. New York, NY: W. W. Norton & Company.

McVay, Doug, Vincent Schiraldi, and Jason Ziedenberg. 2004. *Treatment or Incarceration? National and State Findings on the Efficacy and Cost Savings of Drug Treatment vs. Imprisonment*. Washington, DC: Justice Policy Institute. www.justicepolicy.org/uploads/justicepolicy/documents/04-01_rep_mdtreatmentorincarceration_ac-dp.pdf.

Musto, David. 1973. *The American Disease: Origins of Narcotics Control*. New York: Oxford University Press.

National Institute on Drug Abuse. 2019. *National Survey on Drug Use and Health*. Washington, DC: National Institutes of Health. www.drugabuse.gov/national-survey-drug-use-health.

Okrent, Daniel. 2010. *Last Call: The Rise and Fall of Prohibition*. New York: Simon & Schuster.

Oregon Health Authority. 2019. *Youth Marijuana Use, Attitudes, and Related Behaviors in Oregon*. February. Oregon Health Authority. www.oregon.gov/oha/PH/PREVENTIONWELLNESS/MARIJUANA/Documents/fact-sheet-marijuana-youth.pdf.

Parker, Howard, John Aldridge, and Fiona Measham. 1998. *Illegal Leisure: The Normalization of Adolescent Recreational Drug Use*. London: Routledge.

Pollan, Michael. 2018. *How to Change Your Mind: What the New Science of Psychedelics Teaches Us About Consciousness, Dying, Addiction, Depression, and Transcendence*. New York: Penguin Press.

Reinarman, Craig, Peter D. A. Cohen, and Hendrien L. Kaal. 2004. "The Limited Relevance of Drug Policy: Cannabis in Amsterdam and San Francisco." *American Journal of Public Health* 94: 836–42.

Rockefeller Archives, and John D. Rockefeller, Jr. *Miscellaneous Correspondence on Prohibition and Related Issues, 1920s–1930s*. New York, NY: Rockefeller Center.

Room, Robin, Benedikt Fischer, Wayne Hall, Simon Lenton, and Peter Reuter. 2010. *Cannabis Policy: Moving Beyond Stalemate*. Oxford, UK: Oxford University Press.

Rosenbaum, Marsha. 1981. *Women on Heroin*. New Brunswick, NJ: Rutgers University Press.

Rydell, C. Peter, and Susan S. Sohler Everingham. 1994. *Controlling Cocaine*. Santa Monica, CA: Drug Policy Research Center, RAND Corporation. Prepared for the Office of National Drug Control Policy and the United States Army.

Single, Eric W. 1981. "The Impact of Marijuana Decriminalization." *Research Advances in Alcohol and Drug Problems* 6: 405–24.

Skager, Rodney, and Gregory Austin. 2004. *10th Biennial California Student Survey: Drug, Alcohol and Tobacco Use, 2003–04*. Sacramento, CA: Office of the Attorney General.

Stevens, Alex. 2019. "Is Policy 'Liberalization' Associated with Higher Odds of Adolescent Cannabis Use?" *International Journal of Drug Policy* 66: 94–99.

Walker, Ingrid. 2017. *High: Drugs, Desire, and a Nation of Users*. Seattle and London: University of Washington Press.

Washington State Department of Health. 2017. "2016 Washington State Healthy Youth Survey Data Brief: Marijuana." www.doh.wa.gov/Portals/1/Documents/8350/160-NonDOH-DB-MJ.pdf.

Zinberg, Norman E. 1984. *Drug, Set, and Setting: The Basis for Controlled Intoxicant Use*. New Haven, CT: Yale University Press.

3

Legalization and Prohibition

Breaks, Continuities, and the Shifting Terms of Racial-Capitalist Governance

Michael Polson

Keywords: Ethnography, Law, Social Practice, Political Economy, Neo-prohibition

Introduction

I quietly entered the board of supervisors meeting just as the sheriff heaped praise upon his retiring deputy, a man who had spent the majority of his career, 25 years, eradicating marijuana in this rural Northern California county. Having seized "well over 1 million illegal marijuana plants and billions of dollars' worth of illicit drugs," according to the sheriff, the deputy was honored as a "bulldog" and a patriot. Whether on local news or a cable TV series, he trumpeted marijuana's dangers for years. Once the deputy tearfully thanked the board for their recognition, the sheriff presented his latest report on marijuana eradication and enforcement efforts, highlighting seizure statistics, interagency collaborations, and the positive effects of the Drug Awareness and Resistance Education (DARE) program on the county's youth. That day was the 17th time county supervisors voted to renew a "state of emergency" declaration on cannabis cultivation. At least one supervisor was getting antsy, asking the sheriff what, if anything, this enforcement approach to cannabis had yielded. Municipalities in the supervisor's district were opting to regulate recreational and medical cannabis and the county's virtual prohibition was becoming untenable. The sheriff, suddenly on defense, retreated into a rhetoric of concern for "the children," the future of the county, whose interest must be defended by continuing moral and legal enforcement against cannabis, a plant the sheriff once called "public enemy #1."

This scenario unfolded in 2019, three years after California legalized recreational cannabis and 23 years after voters approved medical marijuana. It highlights the fraught coexistence of prohibition and legalization, which appear as differing, even opposed, ways of governing cannabis. Yet, together they comprise the everyday terms of cannabis governance. In the US, international treaties and federal laws prohibit; state laws might prohibit, decriminalize, medicalize, or commercialize; counties, tribal governments, and cities might opt in or out of state or federal rules; and any number of agencies—water boards, planning commissions, natural resource bureaus, drug enforcement agencies—may intervene across these jurisdictions, civilly or criminally, wielding federal, state, or local

 DOI: 10.4324/9780429320491-3

codes, depending on its mandates. The closer one looks, divisions between prohibition and legalization are fuzzier than they seem. In this chapter, I will argue that cannabis research needs to attend to the differences *and* the continuities between prohibition and legalization. Doing so illuminates the degree to which the transition to legalization *substantively* alters or maintains the power relations that secured prohibition itself.

What dynamics are unique to—and shared by—prohibition and legalization? Under prohibition, rich social worlds developed, even if they were severely constrained by socio-legal forces. Similarly, legalization holds many liberalizing potentialities, even as it calls forward new, often hidden and mundane, forms of power over people and nature. Though clearly different, each policy regime can functionally, discursively, and materially sustain power relations in ways that evacuate the regime shift of meaning. These continuities illustrate the potentials and limits of legalization within liberal-capitalist societies. In order to expropriate value from laboring humans and nature, capitalist societies depend upon the structured devaluation of people and places (Gilmore 2007; Harvey 1996; Massey 1984), whether through moralizing labels, criminal sanctions, designations of waste, or racialized sorting. These mechanisms of devaluation are often shrouded by "universal" liberal precepts like justice, private property, sobriety, productivity, and moral comportment (Hill 1996; Hirschman 1997; Losurdo 2014; Thompson 1975)—the violation of these precepts justifies devaluation (e.g. as criminals, derelicts, waste, racialized inferiors) and conceals the necessity of these inequalities for capitalist production. If this dynamic of liberal capitalism exists across prohibition and legalization, how might prohibition's crude power mechanisms show up in legalized settings, perhaps in new garb?

I approach this matter in two ways. I investigate how each regime works by looking at its *effects*—administrative techniques, everyday practices, subjectivity formation, the enabling or limiting of capacities, territorial configuration, and so on. Then, I explain the role that each policy regime plays in its historical-social context, a role that may mark a departure from or symmetrical rearticulation of one another.

Throughout, I draw on ethnographic research I have conducted since 2010 in Northern California, a period and place that saw a drastic transformation in the social circulation of cannabis, as it was inducted into formal legal, political, and economic relations. Ethnography has value in assessing the messy overlay of prohibition and legalization. In attending to the everyday rhythms and practices that coagulate meanings and cement social relations, ethnography assembles from the ground up realities that other analytic modes can miss. For instance, to know prohibition through enforcement statistics, public statements of officials, and writings of advocates and detractors—not to mention ideas of criminal deviance that structure many of those accounts—would not only miss how those accounts travel and are reproduced to varying effects but also obscure the whole range of alternate, unofficial understandings that people create in otherwise illegible, inaccessible, or illegalized realms. Ethnography helps to see *between* analytic concepts into the place where meanings, structures, and relations come together in social life (Geertz 1974; Asad 1986; Munn 1990). Prohibition and legality are not given. They are produced, are reproduced, achieve effects, and make visible and invisible elements of reality to differently situated people. By understanding the multiple perspectives that constitute social reality (Haraway 1988), ethnography depicts what prohibition and legalization are in any given time and place. It is through ethnographic methods that the insights of this article became clear, where the intricacies of legalization and prohibition and their messy convergence revealed themselves in the daily rhythms of social life.

Prohibition

Prohibitions, according to many (Douglas 1966; Freud 1913; Lévi-Strauss 1949), are moments in which social strictures override individual behavior, forming a foundation for social interaction. Yet, prohibitions do more than restrict—they generate collective forms of life (Foucault 1990). Cannabis prohibition does not simply proscribe behavior, it generates administrative apparatuses, innovates conceptual vocabularies, shapes social relations (e.g. in the family, between ethnic groups, among "strangers"), and much more. If one views prohibition as simply repressive, one misses what it has produced. Though some regard the War on Drugs as a failed attempt to control, it constantly *succeeds* in producing social dynamics. Even if prohibition officially ends, the patterns it established linger, with varying afterlives (Garriott 2011). In short, prohibition *is* what it generates.

In liberal capitalist societies, ideologically premised as they are on the free barter, truck, and trade of goods, prohibition is a unique mode of governance. It creates and regulates market action not through regulatory code but through juridical action. The placement of prohibited realms beyond regulatory reach enables them to develop their own social systems, with their own symbolic codes, languages, ethics, circuits of knowledge, and such. Prohibition also requires a governance apparatus for its material-discursive administration. In California's Emerald Triangle,[1] eradication teams made cannabis visible and material (Polson 2018). Enforcement statistics and prohibition-mandated researchers made it knowable in official ways. A primary governing mechanism of supply-side cannabis prohibition was price (cf. Roitman 2005). Designed to discourage consumption, prohibition inflated prices by inducing risks (Polson 2013), thus attracting people into production, effectively calling into formation the very thing it sought to prohibit. Price, as a central organizing force of social life, organized everyday practices and subjectivities in market terms—they were "marketized." Even as people continued acting out of communal, political, or (counter)cultural motivations, increased prices (and risks) pushed people to conceive of themselves in market terms—buyers, sellers, utility-maximizers (cf. Corva 2008). Prohibition's marketizing force even colored political expression. Cultivators and activists opposed prohibition primarily in free-market, often libertarian, political registers of hemp, property, and civil rights. In the Emerald Triangle, prohibition's government-at-a-distance (Rose and Miller 1992) emerged within particular political-economic dynamics. Amidst the decline of the 150-year-old timber industry, cannabis provided livelihoods to rural residents, serving as a sponge for the unemployed and a means of government-shaped redistribution at a time of decreasing access to welfare. Instead of entitlements or worker protections, this "shadow Keynesian" system of governance operated via risk, reward, and the omnipresent possibility of incarceration and loss of freedom and rights (Polson 2018).

In California's Sierra Foothills, prohibition operated in different yet generative ways. Amidst several decades of exurban residential expansion, prohibition served to conjure spatial imaginaries of a nostalgically rural and implicitly white refuge from urban, racialized, and criminal danger. In Calaveras County, the sheriff propagated this imaginary through high-profile anti-cannabis policing and eradication practices and consolidated it into institutional-political power. The sheriff's actions projected an exclusionary imaginary of rural defense—of moral values and property values—that appealed to exurban in-migrants and wedded them to both cannabis prohibition and continued residential development. In doing so, the sheriff spearheaded opposition to other county factions, which were advancing an alternative political-spatial imaginary centered on conservation, tourism, and transparent deliberative government. This worked until the 2008 mortgage crisis brought this developer-driven, police-defended imaginary into crisis. At that time, medical marijuana activists found political traction in challenging the sheriff's power, effectively halting prohibitionist techniques and reworking the fabric of exurban life to incorporate cannabis (Polson 2020).

These two examples show the importance of understanding the specific techniques and apparatuses that comprise prohibition as well as the political-economic projects to which they are bound. It is possible to imagine other directions in the study of prohibition. One might attend to the ways individuals and communities live under prohibition (August 2012; McCubbrey 2007; Weisheit 1990) or how prohibition creates certain modes of land tenure and value capture (Carrier and Klantschnig 2006; Halvaksz 2007; Polson 2013). One might also attend to the organization of productive relations, specifically to the role of race, ethnicity, and tribal status (Polson 2016; Polson and

Petersen-Rockney 2019), the allocation of risk and reward (Polson 2013), and the forms of care, trust, and power that suffuse labor relations and commodity chains under prohibition (Hafley and Tewksbury 1995; Laudati 2016; Potter 2006).

In sum, prohibition can be considered a kind of marketizing government-at-a-distance. It incites self-governance, incentivizes and sanctions actions, and administrates social life through calculative techniques and enforcement institutions. The question in assessing prohibition is not simply what it proscribes but also what it produces. Any analysis of legalization—why it might fail, succeed, or take on particular dynamics—must first grasp what prohibition generated. Legalization is not simply a corrective to what prohibition failed to do; it is, conspicuously or not, an encounter with all that prohibition succeeded in achieving.

Legalization

Legalization may be defined as a moment of policy regime shift, coming in several forms (e.g. decriminalization, medicalization, commercialization). It may also be defined as a process through which an object (e.g. an act, a commodity, a group of people) acquires legal meaning. This occurs not just in authoritative policy actions but in everyday contexts and institutional settings, where legal meanings are encountered and (re)produced (Comaroff and Comaroff 2008; von Benda-Beckmann, von Benda-Beckmann, and Griffiths 2012). Who generates and mobilizes these meanings, with what effects, and bound to what kinds of political-economic projects?

In Humboldt County on California's North Coast, legalization became an object of anticipation. People formulated and projected developmental visions of what legalization could entail and, wielding these imagined futures, sought to guide legalization in certain directions (Polson 2017). Marijuana's shift from criminal to legal circuitry coincided with the final collapse of the timber industry in the late 2000s. Freed from the timber-developmental regime that dominated county life since its colonization in the mid-1800s, two visions emerged from two political blocs. One was premised on an idea of sustainability and localist "smart growth," which embraced cannabis as a new, job-producing anchor industry. The other, based among actors variously invested in prohibition for political and economic purposes (property owners, developers, law enforcement, timber operators, even some cannabis growers), begrudgingly made marginal space for legal cannabis within a broader vision of a *rentier* economy dominated by property development and speculative appreciation. This anticipatory political visioning still ramifies in debates over jobs, sustainability, and property values, even as both visions mobilized local energies to become the first to enact a full framework to regulate cannabis after statewide legalization. Here, "legalization" was more than a policy moment—it was a social and political process and struggle through which cannabis acquired legal meanings, which continue to shape everyday life and relations.

In Amador County in the Sierra Foothills, cannabis was translated to legal forums through the register of "land use." With a shift in jurisdiction from law enforcement to the planning commission, a set of political claims were made newly audible. Activists, articulating demands and medical needs in this new institutional forum, could be recognized as citizen-residents rather than criminals. Issues of poverty, addiction, injury, and medical necessity were presented publicly, lending legitimacy and legibility to claimants and necessitating new responses and rationales from administrative institutions and surprised politicians. Yet, other sets of claims were also activated by marijuana's jurisdictional shift, namely those of the county's well-represented property owners, who demanded cannabis be considered a nuisance and abide by civilly aesthetic norms of propriety (Polson 2015; cf. Blomley 2005). Cultivators, most of them low-income whites, were met with new techniques of control—blight-spotting, complaints, inspections, abatements, etc. Following statewide legalization, these civil techniques have been leveraged in other counties to enact de facto and official bans on cannabis commerce generally (Polson and Petersen-Rockney 2019), lending new shape to legalized cannabis.

Legalization generates unique social forms. It rearranges the logics, agencies, and techniques that govern cannabis and makes possible new kinds of political capacities and legibilities, community and territorial dynamics, and modes of self-understanding. Yet, legalization necessarily builds from the patterns routinized under prohibition. After all, if "legalization" can be considered a process through which an object acquires legal meanings and relations, "prohibition" is just another way marijuana is made into a legal object, albeit in criminalizing terms.

Prohibition and Legalization

As jurisdictional mandates, prohibition and legality coexist across space, and, as modes of regulating economic action, they both serve similar social-regulatory functions. Moreover, each shapes the other. In the US, legalization haltingly emerges in various places, yet prohibition recursively constricts the terms in which it can be realized, as it did when localities halted regulatory efforts under threat of federal intervention (Polson 2017) or when agricultural agencies cite federal funding worries to deny cannabis cultivators assistance (Polson and Petersen-Rockney 2019). Conversely, prohibitionist strategies are reworked as legalization advances, as happened when the federal government retrenched its jurisdictional authority over public parks when support for widespread cannabis prohibition flagged in California (Polson 2019).

The environmental politics around cannabis provide a clear example of the coincidence of prohibition and legalization—and the possibilities for a post-prohibition environmental politics of cannabis. In Northern California, law enforcement has historically framed cannabis as an environmental threat requiring prohibitionist responses, namely eradication. Pollution, danger, violence, and cartels were commonly invoked in discourses of environmental defense, often in ways that racialized cannabis production in order to rally environmental publics to the cause of prohibition—despite an admitted lack of proven links to actual cartels in the region (Mozingo 2012). As cannabis was brought under medical and, later, commercial regulation, these material discourses persisted as environmental status demarcated the line between good/responsible and bad/irresponsible cultivators—a distinction made not only by policy makers but by cultivators themselves, who had to perform their suitability for legal recognition. This eco-ethical sorting, which I trace in Mendocino County (Polson 2019), reproduced existing inequalities along racial, class, and cultural lines, even as it allowed some well-resourced actors to consolidate claims on the emerging economy. Humboldt County, however, made attempts to draw upon the expertise of cannabis market actors in formulating land use regulations. This facilitated a broader debate about the terms of sustainability and also generated forces that eventually shaped statewide environmental protections around cannabis (Polson 2019). Though these robust environmental regulations are exceptions to agricultural regulation generally, the question remains whether they will erect high barriers to market entry, exclude broad swaths of historical cannabis market actors, and facilitate industrial consolidation with its own sets of environmental issues (see Bodwitch et al. In press for recent findings). Regardless, prohibition-tinged environmental logics are now being invoked to justify federal, state, and local efforts to ban or eradicate cannabis, recriminalize some farmers, and discipline the plant into private land markets.

This is evidently the case in Siskiyou County on the Oregon border, where the sheriff is leveraging environmental agencies and civil enforcement capacities to substantively recriminalize cannabis. The effort got its start when the county moved to regulate cannabis for the first time in 2015 (nearly 20 years after medical cannabis passed at the state level). The move to regulate emerged amidst public controversy over the presence of Hmong-American farmers, who began moving in relatively large numbers to grow cannabis in this sparsely populated county. The resulting civil codes seemed to be applied most readily to Hmong Americans, who not only lived on highly visible subdivided lots that were easily susceptible to complaints of blight and nuisance (by neighbors and government officials), but whose cultural and linguistic difference made them more salient to complainants. The sheriff, whose pleas to protect children were mentioned in the introduction, urged and won passage of a county moratorium on cannabis commerce, prohibitive requirements on self-provisioning, and a unique emergency declaration over an influx of cannabis cultivators. He assumed enforcement powers from the county's underfunded civil enforcement agencies and has rallied various land use agencies to his side, ranging from fire prevention, fish and wildlife, and county planning offices to toxic substances control and water regulators, which collectively wield civil and criminal sanctioning powers. The effect of this neo-prohibitionist resurgence in a post-legalization setting has been to shut down and criminally stigmatize Hmong-American, countercultural, ill, and poor white and Native growers in unincorporated lands. Meanwhile, several municipalities in the county are licensing cannabis operations to those able to navigate regulatory requirements and leverage resources to (re)locate there (Polson and Petersen-Rockney 2019), leading to a filtered stratification among cannabis market actors.

Though some predicted legalization efforts would produce economic benefits that would convince even the most morally conservative and revanchist jurisdictions to reverse course, this market logic has not conquered all—and, even if it did, "free" markets do not in themselves deliver social or environmental justice. Whether in terms of property aesthetics, environmental protection, or fear of cartels or invasive outsiders, there are many new articulations of post-legalization prohibitionisms, and they intricately connect to broader political-economic and racial projects to protect land values, privilege various sectors and groups, and control subdominant populations. While perhaps this is merely a "transitional" process of cultural-social adjustment, it is very possible that cannabis, like any psychotropic substance, will continue to generate political contestation over social order and its potential negation in liminal realms (cf. Turner 1967).

New research can illuminate the manifold and often implicit connections between prohibition and legalization. For instance, how do legalizing policies draw on prohibitionist meanings? Whether as a vice, a public health threat, a prescribed medicine, a recreational substance, an agricultural crop, or a substance that enriches wellness, like herbal supplements, marijuana's framing matters tremendously for how it is governed, perceived, produced, and consumed. Also, new research can bring attention to populations once governed by prohibition that cannot find a place in legalized markets. What new illegal or informal markets take shape, either with cannabis or in lieu of it? What new systems of social control emerge to govern those who built the cannabis economy but are now excluded in its operation? One might look to studies of other collapsed and rearticulated systems of governance, like post-welfare poverty management (Goode and Maskovsky 2001) and the management of deindustrialized populations (Cowie, Heathcott, and Bluestone 2003). Given the global scope of cannabis prohibition and commodity flows, these matters are as relevant in California as they are in Mexico, Paraguay, Morocco, South Africa, Afghanistan, and other traditional producer nations, especially as countries from Spain to South Korea, Australia to Thailand, Uruguay to Canada and the US, the main purveyor of global prohibition, "legalize" cannabis in various ways.

Conclusion

In this chapter, I argued that prohibition and legalization produce distinct modalities of governance yet they also overlap, coexist, and give form to one another in practice. Legalization does not emerge as a clean slate—it comes into existence through the social relations crafted and routinized under prohibition. I showed how prohibition and legalization can be understood: first, through their effects; second, through their articulation in political-economic projects; and third, through ethnographic methods.

If society has determined that cannabis is in fact a legal substance—and that the precepts underlying its prohibition are misplaced—then the persistent (and insidious) logics underlying prohibition must be identified and uprooted. Legalization may bring unique freedoms and social dynamics, yet it also produces and justifies inequalities and practices of environmental exploitation that may or may not derive from prohibition. What happens to political action in this transition? As some of my interlocutors have argued, does it become unnecessary as the irresistible, ineluctable logic of the market takes over? To the contrary, politics abound, whether sublimated in new civil terms, expressed in languages of competition and market survival, or rearticulated in claims to medical access, racial and social equity, environmental stewardship, drug reform, heritage or appellation status, economic development, or agricultural transformation. Legalization will not, in itself, break with racial-capitalist systems of domination, yet it can become a social reality in more or less destructive or restorative ways. If legalization can be unhitched from prohibitionist logics and assumptions about the ways legal markets necessarily work, it offers a chance to do things differently.

Note

1 A geo-cultural and agricultural area that spans Humboldt, Trinity, and Mendocino Counties. See Leeper (1990) and Meisel (2017).

References

Asad, T. 1986. "The Concept of Cultural Translation in British Social Anthropology." In *Writing Culture: The Poetics and Politics of Ethnography*, edited by J. Clifford and G. Marcus, 141–64. Berkeley, CA: University of California Press.

August, K. D. 2012. "Playing the Game: Marijuana Growing in a Rural Community." Master's thesis, Humboldt State University, Arcata, CA.

Blomley, N. 2005. "The Borrowed View: Privacy, Propriety, and the Entanglements of Property." *Law & Social Inquiry* 30 (4): 617–61.

Bodwitch, H., M. Polson, E. Biber, G.M. Hickey, and V. Butsic. In Press. "Why Comply? Farmer Motivations and Barriers in Cannabis Agriculture." *Journal of Rural Studies*.

Carrier, N., and G. Klantschnig. 2006. "Illicit Livelihoods: Drug Crops and Development in Africa." *Review of African Political Economy* 43 (148): 174–89.

Comaroff, J., and J. L. Comaroff, eds. 2008. *Law and Disorder in the Postcolony*. Chicago: University of Chicago Press.

Corva, D. 2008. "Neoliberal Globalization and the War on Drugs: Transnationalizing Illiberal Governance in the Americas." *Political Geography* 27 (2): 176–93.

Cowie, J, J. Heathcott, and B. Bluestone, eds. 2003. *Beyond the Ruins: The Meanings of Deindustrialization*. Ithaca, NY: Cornell University Press.

Douglas, M. 1966. *Purity and Danger: An Analysis of Concepts of Pollution and Taboo*. New York: Routledge and Keagan Paul.

Foucault, M. 1990 [1978]. *The History of Sexuality*. New York: Vintage.

Freud, S. 1918 [1913]. *Totem and Taboo*. Translated by A. A. Brill. New York: Moffat, Yard and Co.

Garriott, W. 2011. *Policing Methamphetamine: Narcopolitics in Rural America*. New York: New York University Press.

Geertz, C. 1974. "'From the Native's Point of View': On the Nature of Anthropological Understanding." *Bulletin of the American Academy of Arts and Sciences*: 26–45.

Gilmore, R. W. 2007. *Golden Gulag: Prisons, Surplus, Crisis and Opposition in Globalizing California*. Berkeley, CA: University of California Press.

Goode, J. G., and J. Maskovsky, eds. 2001. *New Poverty Studies: The Ethnography of Power, Politics, and Impoverished People in the United States*. New York: New York University Press.

Hafley, S. R., and R. Tewksbury. 1995. "The Rural Kentucky Marijuana Industry: Organization and Community Involvement." *Deviant Behavior* 16 (3): 201–21.

Halvaksz, J. A. 2007. "Cannabis and Fantasies of Development: Revaluing Relations through Land in Rural Papua New Guinea." *The Australian Journal of Anthropology* 18 (1): 56–71.

Haraway, D. 1988. "Situated Knowledges: The Science Question in Feminism and the Privilege of Partial Perspective." *Feminist Studies* 14 (3): 575–99.

Harvey, D. 1996. *Justice, Nature and the Geography of Difference*. Oxford: Blackwell.

Hill, C. 1996. *Liberty Against the Law: Some Seventeenth-Century Controversies*. New York: Viking Adult.

Hirschman, A. O. 1997. *The Passions and the Interests: Political Arguments for Capitalism Before its Triumph*. Westport, CT: Greenwood Publishing Group.

Laudati, A. A. 2016. "Securing (in) Security: Relinking Violence and the Trade in Cannabis Sativa in Eastern Democratic Republic of Congo." *Review of African Political Economy* 43 (148): 190–205.

Leeper, J. 1990. "Humboldt County: Its Role in the Emerald Triangle." *California Geographer* XXX: 93–109.

Lévi-Strauss, C. 1969 [1949]. *The Elementary Structures of Kinship*. Boston: Beacon Press.

Losurdo, D. 2014. *Liberalism: A Counter-History*. New York: Verso Books.

Massey, D. 1984. *Spatial Divisions of Labor: Social Structures and the Geography of Production*. London: Methuen.

McCubbrey, J. P. 2007. "Impacts of Illicit-Drug Policy on Community Cohesion: A Case Study of the Campaign Against Marijuana Planting in Southern Humboldt County, California." PhD dissertation, Western Institute for Social Research, Berkeley, CA.

Meisel, J. 2017. "Hidden in Plain Sight: Cannabis Cultivation in the Emerald Triangle." *California Geographer* 56: 3–26.

Mozingo, J. 2012. "Roots of Pot Cultivation in National Forests Are Hard to Find." *LA Times,* December 26. www.latimes.com/archives/la-xpm-2012-dec-26-la-me-mexican-marijuana-20121226-story.html.

Munn, N. 1990. "Constructing Regional Worlds in Experience: Kula Exchange, Witchcraft and Gawan Local Events." *Man* 25 (1): 1–17.

Polson, M. 2013. "Land and Law in Marijuana Country: Clean Capital, Dirty Money, and the Drug War's Rentier Nexus." *PoLAR: Political and Legal Anthropology Review* 36 (2): 215–30.

———. 2015. "From Outlaw to Citizen: Police Power, Property, and the Territorial Politics of Medical Marijuana in California's Exurbs." *Territory, Politics, Governance* 3 (4): 387–406.

———. 2016. "Through the Gateway: Marijuana Production, Governance, and the Drug War Détente." Doctoral dissertation, City University of New York, New York.

———. 2017. "Planning for Marijuana: Development, Governance, and Regional Political Economy." In *The Illicit and Illegal in Regional and Urban Governance and Development*, edited by F. Chiodelli, T. Hall, and R. Hudson, 167–89. New York: Routledge.

———. 2018. "Marketing Marijuana: Prohibition, Medicalization, and the Commodity." In *Economy, Crime and Wrong in a Neoliberal Era*, edited by J. Carrier, 140–71. New York: Berghahn Books.

———. 2019. "Making Marijuana an Environmental Issue: Prohibition, Pollution, and Policy." *Environment and Planning E: Nature and Space* 2 (2): 229–51.

———. 2020. "Buttressed and Breached: The Exurban Fortress, Cannabis Activism, and the Drug War's Shifting Political Geography." *Environment and Planning D: Society and Space* 38 (4): 626–45.

Polson, M., and M. Petersen-Rockney. 2019. "Cannabis Farmers or Criminals? Enforcement-First Approaches Fuel Disparity and Hinder Regulation." *California Agriculture* 73 (3): 185–93.

Potter, G. 2006. "Weed, Need and Greed: Domestic Marijuana Production and the UK cannabis Market." Doctoral dissertation, University of Sheffield, Sheffield, England.

Roitman, J. 2005. *Fiscal disobedience: An Anthropology of Economic Regulation in Central Africa*. Princeton: Princeton University Press.

Rose, N., and P. Miller. 1992. "Political Power Beyond the State: Problematics of Government." *British Journal of Sociology* 23 (2): 173–205.

Thompson, E. P. 1975. *Whigs and Hunters*. New York: Pantheon.

Turner, V. 1967. *The Forest of Symbols: Aspects of Ndembu Ritual*. New York: Cornell University Press.

Von Benda-Beckmann, F., K. von Benda-Beckmann, and A. Griffiths, eds. 2012. *The Power of Law in a Transnational World: Anthropological Enquiries*. New York: Berghahn Books.

Weisheit, R. A. 1990. "Domestic Marijuana Growers: Mainstreaming Deviance." *Deviant Behavior* 11 (2): 107–29.

4

Growing Pains

Marijuana Legalization in Maine

Wendy Chapkis

Keywords: Cannabis legalization, Maine marijuana policy, small cannabis cultivators, cannabis regulation, legalization implementation

Introduction

In 2015 at a Maine Marijuana Summit, just months before this U.S. state would vote on legalization, a progressive state representative, Diane Russell (D-Portland) urged activists not to become distracted or divided over the question of who would make money after prohibition ended. In the face of the need to end the War on Drugs, she said, "conversation about who makes profits off this industry is irrelevant" (Russell 2015b).

I have come to disagree. I entered the conversation about marijuana legalization in the 1990s, writing an ethnography of one of the very earliest medical marijuana patient collectives in the US, the *Wo/men's Alliance for Medical Marijuana* (*WAMM*) in Santa Cruz, California.[1] For the members of *WAMM*, cannabis was a medicine, not a money tree. In fact, the co-founder of the organization, Valerie Leveroni Corral, was affectionately known to the membership as the "anti-profit." Valerie, Michael Corral, and a group of seriously ill and terminally ill patients, collectively cultivated, harvested, and processed a small crop of cannabis and redistributed it *without charge* to the 200 or so patient members.

This glorious, and fraught, experiment in the provision of medicine outside a cash economy survived for more than 25 years[2] despite the challenges of relying largely on volunteer labor and in the face of the very significant threats from the federal government. In 2002, in an early morning raid by the federal Drug Enforcement Administration, the collective's garden was destroyed, the co-founders were taken into custody by armed agents, and the seriously ill membership was traumatized. Valerie and Michael engaged in years of legal battles in the federal courts before winning important concessions. Early medical marijuana activists, then, were not only doing the work of patient care and cannabis provision but were also on the front lines doing battle against prohibition.

Writing about *WAMM* made clear to me that, while their marijuana was free, it certainly was not without cost to the people who cultivated and distributed it. Now, in the early decades of

 DOI: 10.4324/9780429320491-4

cannabis legalization, the debt owed to those early activists is being repaid instead to venture capitalists who are cashing in on a safer investment climate. And, as prominent drug policy reform advocates observe, it is reshaping the movement. Just months before the 2016 election (in which medical marijuana would extend its reach by becoming legal in over half of all states in the US, and in which voters would legalize adult recreational use in four more states—California, Nevada, Massachusetts and Maine) the founder of the national *Drug Policy Alliance*, Ethan Nadelmann, warned that it might be the "last year in which drug policy reform organizations, driven primarily by concerns of civil liberties and civil rights and other good public policy motivations, will be able to significantly shape the legislation. [. . .] as the years progress, various industry forces will loom larger" (Lopez 2015). The same year, the national policy director for the Marijuana Policy Project Dan Riffle resigned because, he said, "the industry is taking over the legalization movement" (Warner 2015).

How Did We Get There From Here? Marijuana Legalization in Maine

For more than 40 years, Maine has been at the forefront of efforts in the US to end the war on cannabis. In 1976, it was the third state to decriminalize marijuana. In 1999, Maine became the first state east of the Mississippi to legalize the medical use of marijuana. And, a decade later, in 2009, the state created a loosely regulated system for licensing small grower/caregivers.

The 2009 law also created a very limited dispensary system, authorizing only eight for the entire state of Maine—half of which were awarded to one company, *Wellness Connection*—creating various interconnected dissatisfactions. The dispensaries were subject to much more stringent regulation than small growers, including inspections, product testing, and security requirements, a fact that dispensary lawyers and lobbyists frequently complained about. Caregivers, on the other hand, who were allowed to cultivate no more than 30 plants (five each for up to six patients), scoffed at the notion that they were unfairly advantaged by the rules, pointing to the monopoly dispensaries enjoyed on large-scale cultivation and distribution.

The law that limited the number of plants, and patients, for each caregiver, also prohibited small growers from selling any portion of their crop to the licensed dispensaries. Dispensaries were required to be vertically integrated, growing and processing everything they distributed. State Representative Diane Russell acknowledged that "the state artificially created a system that created friction [between dispensaries and small growers] when they could have actually created a system that was synergistic or symbiotic" (Russell 2015a).

Despite the bother and expense of producing a more regulated crop, the dispensaries did well. Their sales showed impressive growth year after year. In 2014, dispensary sales rose by 40% and, in 2015, by another 46% (Miller 2017).

Meanwhile, caregivers, attempting to operate within the legal constraints of 30 plants and 6 patients, struggled. As Russell noted, "It's hard to be a caregiver and follow the rules because you don't make any money. I mean, if you're a good farmer you can develop a huge crop off of one plant. What do you do when you can only sell so much to your 6 patients?" (Russell 2015a).

Things changed for caregiver cultivators in 2016, when they agreed to increased regulation in exchange for the right to legally sell their harvest to any number of authorized patients. In addition, they were allowed (with municipal approval) to open small retail shops (in effect, small dispensaries). The effect was dramatic: the number of licensed caregivers increased by almost 43% in 2017 to more than 3,000; about half of Maine's estimated 51,000 patients began securing their cannabis through small caregiver cultivators (Overton 2017).

The eight larger dispensaries still saw growth in their sales, but at a much slower rate of increase. The president of the Maine Dispensary Operators Association, Timothy Smale, complained "They [patients] get all this information. They get all these products. They buy from us for a while, and we never see them again after a few more months because they find a better price" (Overton 2017).

Tensions between the large- and small-scale cultivator/distributors were reproduced in efforts to legalize recreational adult-use of marijuana. At least two legislative proposals failed in the legislature in part because the sponsors of the measures (Diane Russell and Mark Dion, both Democratic Representatives from Portland) were unable to secure the support of both the caregivers and the dispensaries. "Both sides," Russell argued, "want exclusivity in the new market. But the real crux is that I'm trying to bring accountability and oversight to the industry. That's what the caregivers hate about my bill" (Russell 2015a). Paul McCarrier, the lobbyist for the caregiver community, on the other hand, argued that the proposals, especially Rep. Dion's, were "a dispensary monopoly model bill. It's not like you're trying to say 'look, let's put some fair regulations on this [small grower caregiver] sector of the industry to make sure it's abiding by the laws and the rules'" (McCarrier 2015a).

In an effort to take control of the conversation over what would constitute "fair regulations," and specifically to protect the interests of small growers, Paul McCarrier, working with a group of caregivers, drafted a citizen's initiative to legalize marijuana. *Legalize Maine*'s tagline was "save small farmers, keep profits local." The national *Marijuana Policy Project* had already spearheaded two successful local legalization initiatives (in the cities of Portland and South Portland) and was eager to add Maine to the list of states that had legalized adult-use. But because of concerns that the local group, *Legalize Maine*, was too intransigent and too unprofessional to win a campaign, the *MPP* began collecting signatures for their own competing initiative to "*Regulate Marijuana Like Alcohol*."

In many ways, the *Legalize* and the *Regulate* initiatives were more different in tone than in substance. Both initiatives, for example, provided for home cultivation and on-site consumption in licensed retail settings. *Legalize Maine*'s proposal, however, included a total cultivation cap of 800,000 square feet, setting aside 40% of those licenses for small growers. The *Regulate* campaign believed that a cultivation cap would be too limiting and instead attempted, in their initiative, to protect locals from out-of-state investment through a temporary residency requirement.[3]

As the deadline to submit signatures approached, it appeared both initiatives might qualify for the ballot, likely dooming both to defeat by splitting the vote. At the last moment, the national Marijuana Policy Project agreed to drop their initiative and throw their weight and resources behind the local campaign. MPP's decision may have been influenced by the fact that national momentum seemed threatened after Ohioans rejected a corporate-cannabis funded initiative. As the International Business Times reported, "the specter of the failed initiative will likely haunt the cannabis scene for a long time. Looking back, people may see what happened in Ohio as a turning point in the cannabis crusade, the moment when the national dialogue around legalization shifted in ways that might not bode well for marijuana advocacy" (Warner 2015). In short, national marijuana legalization organizations could ill afford another loss in Maine.

While the merger of the two campaigns increased the likelihood of the measure passing, it set off alarms among members of the caregiver community who were suspicious of the intentions of the national organization. Paul McCarrier of the *Legalize* campaign admitted:

> "We did too good of a job demonizing them [the *Regulate* campaign]. And people don't really understand the initiative process so they're under the impression that, because *MPP* will be running the campaign, that they can just arbitrarily change the language after it's passed. But it doesn't work like that. The legislature does not change the wording of citizen's initiatives if the language is cut and dry"
>
> *(McCarrier 2015b)*

But, in fact, the legislature did exactly that. After the initiative passed (by a less than one percent margin)[4], the Maine legislature significantly rewrote the law before allowing it to be implemented.

In fact, the 2016 legislature, changed—or outright repealed—every one of the citizen's initiatives that had passed that year.[5] The changes to marijuana legalization included removing some of the more innovative elements of the law including on-site consumption at "social clubs." In addition, the legislature changed the provisions in the law specifically intended to protect small growers from out-of-state corporate competition. The cultivation cap was eliminated, making unlimited cultivation licenses available, thus removing the requirement that 40% would be set aside for small growers. The legislature instead turned to language in the abandoned *Regulate* initiative, adding a temporary state residency requirement for owners and investors with controlling interest in Maine marijuana businesses. The state Office of Marijuana Policy explained that the residency rule would "help prevent large, out-of-state companies" from "controlling the Maine recreational market" and "help Maine residents" keep the industry "rooted in Maine" (Overton 2019b).

Then, just days before the legislature was set for a final vote on the new rules, the largest dispensary group in the state, *Wellness Connection* threatened to sue over the residency requirement for controlling investment in a marijuana business (Valigra 2019). Of particular concern to them were provisions making it difficult for out-of-state companies to hide behind the "corporate veil" of complex ownership structures to disguise out-of-state control (Mistler 2019). The threatened lawsuit would indefinitely delay implementation of the already 3 year old law.[6]

The stakes were clear to small growers who urged the Maine legislature to stand firm and "keep out-of-state interests from gobbling up the state's marijuana market, and keep whatever profits are to be made from it in the hands of Mainers" (Overton 2019a). The owner of one small dispensary, Glenn Peterson, supported the residency requirement because, he said, "We want to give Maine residents a chance before the big boys come in" (Overton 2019a).

Nonetheless, within days of the threatened suit, the legislature agreed to revise the residency rules. *Wellness Connection*'s attorney Dan Walker, told the press, "We can work with the changes that were made. We do not feel we need to bring a lawsuit" (Mistler 2019). The legislature passed the regulations and implementation commenced. The state began to approve licenses and cities and towns began the process of opting in and granting local licenses.

But, one year later, just before the first recreational retail sales were set to begin, *Wellness Connection* reversed course and sued to remove all remaining residency restrictions.[7] The timing of the lawsuit was striking, coming just three days after a state of civil emergency was declared in Maine following the first confirmed cases of COVID-19. The Governor's safer-at-home quarantine triggered mass unemployment and widespread concern about the long-term consequences on the important tourist economy in "Vacationland" (as Maine license plates read). The lawsuit filed by *Wellness Connection* threatened the one bright spot on the economic horizon: projected increases in tax revenues from legal marijuana sales. In 2019, retail sales of medical marijuana reached over $111 million dollars making it the third largest industry in the state (Valigra 2020). Based on the experiences of other states with legalized medical and recreational adult-use, sales in Maine were projected to increase to $180 million dollars in the first year (Overton 2020b). The *Wellness Connection* lawsuit which halted implementation represented a very real threat to that much needed tax revenue in the state. Within six weeks of the suit being filed, the state Attorney General's office acceded, refusing to defend the residency restrictions in court (Shepherd 2019).

The Future of Small Cultivation in the State of Maine

Currently, over 75% of medical marijuana sales in Maine are in the hands of small grower caregivers; the other 25% is controlled by the large dispensaries, most notably *Wellness Connection* with half of all those licenses. For now, the medical marijuana sector remains separate from the recreational one, regulated under a separate set of rules. This could give small medical marijuana growers and retailers a limited advantage, at least initially. As David Boyer of the *Regulate* campaign points out, some communities that have already allowed limited cultivation and distribution of *medical* marijuana by caregivers and small dispensaries may balk at authorizing recreational retail stores: "some towns will ban retail [because] they don't want people specifically coming into your town to buy drugs. That's how they think about it" (Boyer 2015). This could help drive business to caregivers and existing small dispensaries. One small marijuana business owner argues, "in the early days of legalization, buying marijuana in Maine will likely mean long drives for many. [. . .] that will likely result in more people seeking a medical use card" (Whittle 2019).

But the distinctions between the medical and recreational sectors are being whittled away. The same month as the *Wellness* lawsuit against residency requirements was filed, the Maine legislature imposed new testing requirements on medical marijuana products to make them more consistent with the recreational market (Overton 2020a).[8] Expensive testing requirements are likely to force small growers and producers out of business, or into investor-controlled economies of scale.

Paul McCarrier (Lobbyist, small grower, and cannabis business owner):

> I think at least 60% of caregivers think that the law that passed is not good. People tell me, they'll say, 'you ruined my life because now the price is going down and I can't make it.' A lot of people are going to lose out because what the legislature did; they made it where there's going to be an unlimited amount of cultivation. But we're selling a unique commodity that can't legally cross state lines. And what you'll see when you have unlimited licenses and a limited market, is a race to the bottom with prices. The farmers lose. And because we don't have access to traditional financing methods [like small business bank loans], if you're a small farmer, you're at the mercy of capital. That's why, in our law [the voter-approved initiative], we tried to have limited licenses and to ensure that they first went to people who were already in the medical marijuana industry. That would have given those farmers leverage in negotiations with capital when it came to interest rates and equity. But now, if you have the capital, you can go out and get your own license. Why do you need me? You'll just go out and get the license and say 'hey Paul, I'll pay you $10 an hour to be my weed farmer' as opposed to 'hey Paul, I'll lend you the million dollars you need to successfully develop your company in the foreseeable future but I want 50% equity.' And you could have said, 'I want 51%; you can have 49%, and then I'll take your million.' So, you could say we are coming to the end of the first Golden Age of cannabis in Maine. I mean, money is going to get involved with this no matter what you do. You can't stop the flow of money; it's like stopping the flow of water. It will always get where it wants to go.

With the coming wave of corporate cannabis, much is riding on the consumer. As Mark Barnett of the Maine Craft Cannabis Association observes: "It's going to be up to Maine consumers to do a little education to learn where their marijuana is coming from. Do they want to support the out-of-state bully that sued the state when it didn't get what it wanted, or do they want to support small Maine businesses" (Overton 2020b).

Diane Russell, for her part, is placing her hope on "niche markets": "You'll see niche markets in both the medical and adult use sides. I think that's where the caregivers are going to come into play. Because there are a lot of folks out there that all they want to do is grow their bud. They are really obsessed with growing their bud. It's a calling. And there will always be people looking for them. But the question is, can they compete? That's the scary thing" (Russell 2015a).

Competition from corporate cannabis is an especially unfair match under the current conditions of federal prohibition. As McCarrier notes, small growers can't sell their crop across state lines and cannabis businesses are not eligible for business loans from banks. They also cannot open lines of credit and are unable to write-off business expenses (Fertig 2019). To finance a cannabis business under these conditions means either taking out a personal loan using a family home as collateral, or, for the big players, relying on large private loans from venture capitalists.

Already in some states with legalized marijuana, like Oregon, massive overproduction by large corporate cultivators has led to a glut of marijuana and a collapse in the price (Associated Press 2018; Foden-Vencil 2019; Schaneman 2018). The large cannabis businesses are able to take the losses in the interest of market capture while small cannabis farmers, ineligible for crop insurance and bankruptcy protection, will lose their farms and homes (Fertig 2019).

What to Do—Directions for Future Research

More research needs to be done on the effects of corporate cannabis on small growers, especially in rural areas where cannabis cultivation under conditions of prohibition blunted the effects of deindustrialization by providing an alternative source of income. Alongside a regional class focus, future research must also stay focused on questions of race. The War on Drugs has specifically targeted people of color[9] while the benefits of legalization are being unequally distributed by race. It is a shocking indictment that, for example, only one percent of legal storefront marijuana businesses in the US are currently owned by Black Americans (Chicago-Lewis 2016).

The "early adopter" states for marijuana legalization, like Colorado and Washington state, did not include provisions to address those inequalities. However, more recent forms of legalization legislation in California, Illinois, Massachusetts, Michigan, and Oregon—but notably not (as of this writing) Maine—do include specific social equity provisions. The most important of these is expungement of cannabis convictions. Other provisions have focused on producing more equitable distribution of the economic opportunities of cannabis legalization, such as no-interest start-up business loans or licensing frameworks that give priority to individuals and communities most heavily impacted by the criminalization of cannabis.

These social equity provisions are an important focus of future research; knowledge about best practices will inform better marijuana legalization legislation going forward. But even well-crafted cannabis laws can offer only limited benefit in repairing the massive harms done by the War on Drugs—and the massive diversion of government resources to fight it.

Since 1971, the War on Drugs has cost US taxpayers an estimated $1 trillion dollars; marijuana prohibition, alone, costs $7.7 billion a year (Pearl 2018). In a post-prohibition era, researchers could turn their attention to a "peace dividend," examining how best, and most equitably, to allocate resources to repair the widespread damage done in the name of a "drug-free America."

But, despite progress in ending cannabis prohibition, the War on Drugs is far from over. Even the war on cannabis has not ended. Marijuana remains illegal in many states as well as under federal law; as recently as 2018, about 4 in every 10 drug arrests were for marijuana offenses (Gramlich 2020). Even in states that have legalized marijuana, like Maine, implementation often seems designed to ensure that some growers and producers will be forced outside the law. It is worth emphasizing that this is not what voters intended by legalization. As Mark Barnett of the Maine Craft Cannabis Association observes, marijuana legalization as implemented in 2020, "leaves Maine voters with almost nothing we voted for in 2016. Mainers did not want corporate marijuana, but that is exactly what we'll be getting now. It's going to be a race to the bottom" (Overton 2020b).

If access to legal, affordable, and accessible weed was the only goal of legalization, marijuana will surely have completed its journey from movement to market. "Users" will simply become "consumers," and "growers" and "dealers" will be replaced by large corporate entities like Wellness

Connection/Acreage Holdings. Meanwhile, groups that have faced disproportionate risk, and experienced disproportionate punishment, during the War on Drugs will continue to pay the price.

"Tom" (former small grower and formerly incarcerated drug law offender):[10]

"I'm from Bellflower, Maine. Used to be called Bellflower Mills; they changed the name after there were no more mills. From the age of 10, I saw that the only way you were ever going to make something of yourself was if you grew weed. The weed that was grown in my town was from necessity. Mainly we didn't even get to smoke it, the good weed. The good stuff got sent away immediately and sold for top dollar. It's like the town knew that our weed that we grew was too good for us to smoke because we needed it financially. Everybody enjoyed that money. People would get work done on their cars and the automotive people would be happy. People that worked on houses, a guy would have a good grow and fix his roof. It was a really romantic time to be a grower because it was make or break. It was like you can have all those things, like I said: fix your house, buy a truck. Or you could end up in jail. So, I'm kind of on the fence about legalization; I hope maybe some folks in my community can make legalization work for them. But there's still no work up there; growing marijuana is like the last thing we are clinging to, to be able to maintain our way of life. I worry that some people will think 'well alright; we won. It's legalized.'"

Acknowledgements

Thank you to Elizabeth Lowell for research assistance, and to Gabriel Demaine, Erica Rand, Dominic Corva, and Joshua S. Meisel for thoughtful comment on the manuscript.

Notes

1 For more information about WAMM, see Chapkis and Webb (2008).

2 The Corrals were forced to sell their land; this challenged the model under which they were operating. Currently WAMM is securing licenses and permits from the City of Santa Cruz and the State of California to reopen as a plant therapy center that will include medical marijuana provision.

3 As David Boyer noted, under the cultivation cap, less than 150 licenses would be available for small growers, which would create intense competition among the more than 3,000 licensed medical marijuana caregivers who might want to enter the recreational market (Boyer, 2015).

4 The narrow margin was due in part to the fact that areas of the state where cannabis is cultivated (Down East, interior, and northern Maine) all voted against legalization. This suggests that small growers remained suspicious. The high levels of support for legalization in urban areas, like Portland, helped tip the balance in favor of legalization, but only barely (New York Times 2017).

5 In the same election, voters had also approved a new state tax of 3% on those earning more than $200,000 to benefit education; a ranked choice voting system for state and federal elections; and a raise in the state minimum wage. The legislature repealed the new 3% tax and significantly weakened both the ranked choice voting law and the minimum wage increase. Legislators then turned their attention to rewriting the marijuana legalization law (Mistler 2017).

6 In 2019, controlling interest in Wellness Connection was held by one of the world's largest cannabis corporations, Acreage Holdings, based in New York. According to their website, *Acreage Holdings* is "a leading, vertically integrated multi-state operator" controlling 1.2 million square feet of cultivation and manufacturing in 20 states. Their board includes John Boehner (R-Ohio), former Canadian Conservative Prime Minister Brian Mulroney, and former Massachusetts Republican Governor William Weld. https://www.acreageholdings.com/.

7 The revised regulations required that, through 2024, a majority ownership be held by persons who resided in the state for at least half of the year and had paid taxes in Maine for the past 4 years. Officers, directors, managers, and general partners in Maine marijuana businesses also were required to be Maine residents.

8 Previously, small caregiver medical marijuana businesses were only required to test their products to support advertising claims such as "pesticide-free" or percentage of THC. The new regulations will now require the same potency-testing used in the adult-use recreational market.

9 As is frequently noted, Blacks and Whites use cannabis and other drugs at similar rates, but Blacks have been almost 4 times as likely to be arrested for marijuana offenses (ACLU 2013). See also Duchemin (2017) on the disproportionate arrest of People of Color in states after the enactment of some decriminalization.

10 Tom's name and his town have been changed to protect his anonymity (Tom 2015).

References

American Civil Liberties Union. 2013. "The war on marijuana in Black and White." June. https://www.aclu.org/report/report-war-marijuana-black-and-white?redirect=criminal-law-reform/war-marijuana-black-and-white.

Associated Press. 2018. "Marijuana prices crashing in Oregon after state stoked weed glut." *CBS News*, May 31. https://www.cbsnews.com/news/marijuana-prices-crashing-in-oregon-after-state-stoked-weed-glut/.

Boyer, David. 2015. Interview. June 4. Portland, Maine.

Chapkis, Wendy and Richard J. Webb. 2008. *Dying to Get High*. New York: New York University Press.

Chicago-Lewis, Amanda. 2016. "How Black People are Being Shut Out of America's Weed Boom." *BuzzFeed*, March 16. https://www.buzzfeed.com/amandachicagolewis/americas-white-only-weed-boom?utm_term=.ynJQDOVr1#.nhyr3oJbV.

Duchemin, Ashley. 2017. "The Fragility of Legalization: Who's Cashing in on Marijuana?" *Bitch Media*, October 26. https://www.bitchmedia.org/article/marijuana-legalization/what-we-gain-expense-people-color.

Fertig, Natalie. 2019. "How Legal Weed Is Killing America's Most Famous Marijuana Farmers." *Politico Magazine*, June 4. https://www.politico.com/magazine/story/2019/06/04/humboldt-county-marijuana-farmers-regulations-227041.

Foden-Vencil, Kristian. 2019. "Oregon Is Producing Twice as Much Cannabis as People Are Using." *Oregon Public Radio*, January 31. https://www.opb.org/news/article/oregon-cannabis-surplus-2019/.

Gramlich, John. 2020. "Four-in-Ten U.S. Drug Arrests in 2018 Were for Marijuana Offenses, Mostly Possession." *Pew Research*. https://www.pewresearch.org/fact-tank/2020/01/22/four-in-ten-u-s-drug-arrests-in-2018-were-for-marijuana-offenses-mostly-possession/.

Lopez, German. 2015. "Big Marijuana Is Coming and Even Legalization Supporters Are Worried," *Vox*, December 2. https://www.vox.com/policy-and-politics/2015/12/2/9831980/marijuana-legalization-industry-business.

McCarrier, Paul. 2015a. Interview June 22. Augusta Maine.

———. 2015b. Interview. January 23. Augusta, Maine.

Miller, Kevin. 2017. "Medical Marijuana Providers Seek First Chance at Retail Sales." *Portland Press Herald*, April 25. https://www.pressherald.com/2017/04/25/medical-marijuana-providers-seek-first-chance-at-retail-sales/.

Mistler, Steve. 2017. "All Voter-Approved Initiatives from 2016 Ballot in Flux in Legislature." *Maine Public Radio*, January 19. https://www.mainepublic.org/post/all-voter-approved-initiatives-2016-ballot-flux-legislature.

———. 2019. "Maine's Largest Dispensary Group Threatens to Sue State over Proposed Marijuana Rules." *Maine Public and Bangor Daily News*, June 10. https://bangordailynews.com/2019/06/10/news/state/maines-largest-dispensary-group-threatens-to-sue-state-over-proposed-marijuana-rules/.

New York Times. 2017. "Maine Question 1—Legalize Marijuana—Results: Approved." *New York Times*, August 1. https://www.nytimes.com/elections/2016/results/maine-ballot-measure-1-legalize-marijuana.

Overton, Penelope. 2017. "Sales Growth at Maine's Medical Marijuana Dispensaries Slows Drastically." *Portland Press Herald*, May 12. https://www.pressherald.com/2017/05/12/sales-growth-at-maines-medical-marijuana-dispensaries-slows-drastically/.

———. 2019a. "Maine's Biggest Marijuana Company Threatens to Sue State If It is Shut Out of Recreational Market." *Portland Press Herald*, June 10. https://www.pressherald.com/2019/06/10/wellness-connection-shut-us-out-maine-and-well-sue/.

———. 2019b. "Adjusted Pot Rules Would Relax Residency Requirements for Marijuana Companies." *Portland Press Herald*, June 13. https://www.pressherald.com/2019/06/13/adjusted-pot-rule-proposal-would-relax-residency-requirements-for-marijuana-companies/.

———. 2020a. "Industry Wins Some, Loses Some in Changes to Medical Marijuana Reform Bill." *Portland Press Herald*, March 12. https://www.pressherald.com/2020/03/12/industry-wins-some-loses-some-in-medical-marijuana-reform-bill-changes/.

———. 2020b. "Maine Drops Residency Requirement for Recreational Pot Businesses." *Portland Press Herald*, May 11. https://www.pressherald.com/2020/05/11/maine-drops-residency-requirement-for-recreational-pot-businesses/.

Pearl, Betsy. 2018. "Ending the War on Drugs: By the Numbers." *American Progress*, June 27. https://www.americanprogress.org/issues/criminal-justice/reports/2018/06/27/452819/ending-war-drugs-numbers/.

Russell, Diane. 2015a. Interview. June 24. Portland, Maine.

———. 2015b. Remarks at the Maine Marijuana Summit, December 5. Maple Hill Conference Center, Hallowell, Maine.

Schaneman, Bart. 2018. "Washington State Cannabis Oversupply Spurs Calls for Change." *Marijuana Business Daily*, January 10. https://mjbizdaily.com/washington-state-cannabis-supply-hits-new-low-spurs-calls-change/.

Shepherd, Michael. 2019. "What's Holding Up Maine's Latest Attempt to Make Legal Marijuana Possible." *Bangor Daily News*, June 12. https://bangordailynews.com/2019/06/12/politics/daily-brief/whats-holding-up-maines-latest-attempt-to-make-legal-marijuana-sales-possible/.

Tom. 2015. Interview. July 24. Portland, Maine.

Valigra, Lori. 2019. "How the First Year of Maine's Recreational Marijuana Market Will Likely Roll Out." *Bangor Daily News*, June 17. https://bangordailynews.com/2019/06/17/business/how-the-first-year-of-maines-adult-use-marijuana-market-will-likely-roll-out/.

———. 2020. "Maine Marijuana Company Sues State Over Residency Requirement." *Bangor Daily News*, March 24. https://bangordailynews.com/2020/03/23/news/lewiston-auburn/maine-marijuana-company-sues-state-over-residency-requirement/.

Warner, Joel. 2015. "Marijuana Legalization 2015: Major Pot Activist Quits Marijuana Policy Project, Says Industry Is Taking Over Movement." *International Business Times*, December 1. https://www.ibtimes.com/marijuana-legalization-2015-major-pot-activist-quits-marijuana-policy-project-says-2203385.

Whittle, Patrick. 2019. "Legal Pot Is Coming, But Will There be Enough Places to Puff?" *Portland Press Herald*, June 17. https://www.pressherald.com/2019/06/16/legal-pot-is-coming-but-will-there-be-enough-places-to-puff/.

Bio Note:

Wendy Chapkis is a Professor of Sociology and Women & Gender Studies at the University of Southern Maine. Her recent publications include "From Harm Reinforcement to Harm Reduction" (*Deviant Behavior*); "The Trouble with Mary Jane's Gender: gender politics in the marijuana policy reform movement" (*Humboldt Journal of Social Relations*), "Cannabis, Consciousness and Healing" (*Contemporary Justice Review*), and "Productive Tensions" (*Journal of Contemporary Ethnography*). She is also the author of three books: *Dying to Get High: Marijuana as Medicine* (co-authored with Richard J. Webb, New York University Press); *Live Sex Acts: Women Performing Erotic Labor* (Routledge); and *Beauty Secrets: Women and the Politics of Appearance* (South End Press).

5

Cannabis, Settler Colonialism, and Tribal Sovereignty in California

Kaitlin Reed

Keywords: Settler colonialism, tribal sovereignty, Native Americans, tribal nations, California

Introduction

The plant genus *Cannabis*—encompassing both the textile fiber known as hemp (*Cannabis sativa*) and the medicinal flower (*Cannabis indica*)—was instrumental in the colonization of North America. Columbus's so-called discovery of the New World would have been impossible without sails and ropes made of hemp (Museum). Early settlers to North America grew "hemp fiber in exchange for safe transit to the New World," and the wealth of America's "founding fathers"[1] was built by hemp production (Lee 2012, 16; Deitch 2003). In California, Spanish missionaries forced California Indians to cultivate hemp for the Catholic Church (Mosk 1939). *Cannabis* has long been both aid and witness to the colonization of what would become the United States.

This chapter focuses on commercial cannabis production and its impact on Native nations in California. Drawing on discourse analysis and concepts from the interdisciplinary field of Native American Studies, I demonstrate how the commercial cannabis industry in California, thus far, enacts a continuation of settler colonialism via exploitation of Native lands and the exclusion of sovereign Native nations from the state cannabis market. This is not to say that cannabis is a unique commodity in that regard, but rather to suggest that questions of tribal sovereignty and settler colonialism have largely been ignored within cannabis policy and discourse.

While Native nations are developing commercial cannabis industries in numerous states (see Smith 2015; Ramirez 2018; Bartlett 2019), a specific examination of commercial cannabis in California is warranted. In addition to a long legacy of cannabis production, California has a large Native American population. There are currently 109 federally recognized Native American tribes in California and 78 tribes petitioning for recognition. The geographic and demographic diversity of California allows for an examination of a wide range of concerns for tribal nations.

This chapter examines the diverse experiences of tribal nations in California, including the Yurok Tribe in northwestern California, the Pit River Tribe in northeastern California, and an organization comprising several tribal nations, the California Native American Cannabis Association (C-NACA). The Yurok Tribe has struggled to protect their natural resources and cultural resources from cannabis

DOI: 10.4324/9780429320491-5

cultivation. For the Yurok Tribe, cannabis cultivation is a continuation of a settler colonial pattern of resource extraction and presents worrisome concerns to both tribal lands and cultural resources. In contrast, both the Pit River Tribe and C-NACA insist upon their sovereign right to provide regulated and legal cannabis products to California consumers. The development of commercial cannabis policy and regulation in California is forcing both the state government and tribal nations to confront important questions about tribal sovereignty and tribal jurisdiction, and the continuation of settler colonial patterns of natural resource extraction. To grapple with these questions, we must turn to two critical concepts in Native American Studies: settler colonialism and tribal sovereignty.

Engaging Native American Studies

Native American Studies (NAS) is an academic discipline born of political activism and drawn from Indigenous intellectual traditions developed over millennia (Kidwell and Velie 2005). While Native peoples have long been present in American universities—stored in boxes of anthropology departments' basements or lining the shelves of a linguist's office—for most of the 19th and 20th centuries, Native people were treated as objects to be studied, not intellectuals capable of conducting research. In the 1960s and 1970s, Native scholars rejected stereotypical and racist depictions of Native peoples perpetuated by historians, anthropologists, and the like. "For Native knowledge to acquire power for its carriers . . . [NAS] had to be systematically organized into a discipline. Its beneficiaries would be Indian Nations" (Cook-Lynn 1997, 10). Inherently interdisciplinary, NAS empowers Native bodies of knowledge and strives to protect Native nationhood. To understand the impact of the cannabis industry on Native nations in California, I rely on two concepts from NAS: settler colonialism and tribal sovereignty.

Settler colonialism is a form of colonialism wherein settlers create a new home for themselves. This differs from extractive colonialism wherein colonial powers seek to extract natural resources and human bodies for wealth accumulation and labor. In the process of settler colonialism, settlers destroy and/or remove Indigenous populations to replace them with reproduced settler colonial structures and populations (Arvin, Tuck, and Morrill 2013). Ideological conceptions of *terra nullius*[2] marked the landscape of North America as open for business, and notions of Manifest Destiny engendered moral justifications to colonize and pillage territories. Settler colonialism is an inherently violent process because "people do not hand over their land, resources, children, and futures without a fight, and that fight is met with violence" (Dunbar-Ortiz 2014, 8). This process in unending, and in this way settler colonialism should be understood not as an event that occurred in the past and is now complete, but rather as a structure that must be continually perpetuated and reproduced (Wolfe 2006). As such, there is a continual insistence on "settler sovereignty over all things in their new domain" (Tuck and Yang 2012, 5). Through legal battles and treaty agreements—none of which have been fully upheld by the United States (Deloria Jr. 1969)—Native leaders fought for the recognition of their rights within the settler state framework. This is referred to as tribal sovereignty.

Tribal sovereignty is a key concept of Native American Studies. While NAS scholars remain critical of its ideological origins (see Alfred 2005; Barker 2005; Deloria Jr. 1979), sovereignty is the legal framework through which tribes assert and defend their rights.[3] Tribal sovereignty describes a historically specific relationship between tribal nations[4] and the United States federal government established in a series of Supreme Court decisions known as the Marshall Trilogy (1823–1832). The Marshall Trilogy relegated tribes as "domestic-dependent nations" that exist within the boundaries of the United States. In other words, Marshall recognized tribes as sovereigns—but not to the same degree as the United States or foreign nations. For Marshall, the relationship between tribal nations and the federal government was akin to a ward to his guardian (Barker 2005; Deloria Jr. and Lytle 1984). This relationship has been further defined as a "trust relationship" wherein the United States is obligated to act in the best interest of tribes. Simultaneously, however, the United States possesses plenary powers "which includes the ultimate power to terminate the federal/tribal relationship. There is an inherent tension in these positions" (Williams and Hoover 1999, 31). Kevin Bruyneel refers to this tension as colonial ambivalence, wherein the United States federal government plays both guardian and conqueror. Despite the trust relationship, the United States has historically acted in ways that lessen Native Indigenous political and economic power (Echo-Hawk 2010; Bruyneel 2007). As such, the "history of conflict between the United States and the Indian tribes has revolved around the question of preserving the right to self-government and the attributes of Indian sovereignty as suggested in Marshall's decision" (Deloria Jr. and Lytle 1984, 17).

Tribal sovereignty—much like how settler colonialism is continually reproduced—is continually asserted, contested, and reconfigured.

> The imposition of colonial rule denotes the effort of the United States to narrowly bound indigenous political status in space and time, seeking to limit the ability of indigenous people to define their own identity and develop economically and politically on their own terms. In resistance to this colonial rule, indigenous political actors work across American spatial and temporal boundaries, demanding rights and resources from the liberal democratic settler-state while also challenging the imposition of colonial rule on their lives.
>
> *(Bruyneel 2007, xvii)*

In so doing, Bruyneel argues, tribal nations occupy a third space[5] of sovereignty that is neither part of nor apart from the settler state. Within this liminal space, Native nations garner rights through their special relationship with the federal government while simultaneously seeking self-determination outside of the American purview. In other words, tribal governments may critique the legitimacy of the settler state's existence while simultaneously advocating for the recognition of their rights within that same framework. But struggles and contestations over what tribal sovereignty entails does not occur within a theoretical vacuum; rather, interpretations and limits of tribal sovereignty are debated over specific issues—for example, tribal fishing rights in the 1970s and tribal casinos in the 1990s (Deloria Jr. and Lytle 1984; Wilkinson 2005). Today that issue may be cannabis. The cannabis industry is relevant to Native nations and NAS scholars because the acknowledgement of tribal sovereignty within the cannabis market, or lack thereof, could ultimately influence how the settler state interprets our rights and ability to self-govern on other issues in the future. Therefore, my analysis of the cannabis industry in California cannot be separated from an understanding that Native nations throughout California still have legitimate claim to (and the knowledge to sustainably steward) these lands.

Cannabis, Settler Colonialism, and the Yurok Tribe

In northwestern California, the Yurok Tribe has lived along the Klamath River since time immemorial. Within Yurok epistemology, the River is a living being and Salmon are relatives. Since the Euroamerican invasion of Yurok homelands beginning with the genocidal gold rush of the 1800s (Norton 1979), numerous settler activities have since threatened both the River and the Salmon—from hydraulic mining and mercury pollution from the gold rush, to clear-cutting forests, to commercial fisheries, to the construction of hydroelectric dams. Today, patterns of resource extraction continue as the Yurok deal with the environmental and cultural impacts of cannabis cultivation[6] on tribal lands[7] (Reed 2019). The environmental impacts of cannabis cultivation on Yurok tribal lands—namely the pollution and theft of tribal lands and waters—constitute a continuation of settler colonial violence that further degrades the health of Yurok lands and bodies.

Since 2014, the Yurok Tribe Environmental Program (YTEP) have detected numerous environmental harms directly caused from cannabis cultivation on Yurok tribal lands and ancestral territory, including human waste pollution, solid hazardous waste, non-point source pollution, and water diversion (Thiesen and Plocher 2014; Thiesen and Plocher 2016). Human waste pollution has been detected at numerous abandoned cultivation sites. Many sites lack sanitation facilities, while some construct outhouses over the creek so that water flushes waste away. During growing months, YTEP has detected increased levels of coliform and *E. coli* at various monitoring stations along the Klamath River and its tributaries (Reed 2019). Solid and hazardous waste includes household garbage, abandoned vehicles and trailers, petroleum products, batteries, plastics, spent irrigation lines, air conditioners, and refrigerators. If left on the landscape, these materials will degrade over time, creating additional contamination for future generations. Non-point source pollution includes fertilizers, spent soils, and pesticides. Numerous toxic chemicals have been recovered at cultivation sites by YTEP, including rodenticides and over-the-counter fertilizers (Reed 2019). Near the Trinity River—the principal tributary of the Klamath River—the Department of Environmental Health in Trinity County issued a quarantine of a private parcel used for cannabis cultivation. Following a search warrant executed by the California Department of Fish and Wildlife on October 2, 2018, several pesticides used for cultivation were recovered that are currently banned in the United States, including carbofuran,[8] methamidophos,[9] and avermectin B1[10] (Kemp 2018). Pollution from cannabis cultivation—in myriad forms—is adversely affecting Yurok water and soil quality, as well as impacting environmental and human health in ways yet unknown (Reed 2019).

The various sources of pollution from cannabis cultivation harm Yurok tribal lands, waters, and bodies. As a land-based people, interactions with a contaminated and toxic landscape could cause an array of unknown human health impacts. Tlingit scholar Anne Spice argues that toxicity must be understood within a context of settler colonialism:

> Toxicity and the invasive infrastructures it spills from separate us from the land by damaging our relations to it. If our lands are toxic, the more we engage in our cultural practices, the more we risk harming our bodies. Toxicity . . . eliminates us as Indigenous peoples by making Indigenous practices dangerous. Don't eat the fish, don't drink the water, don't gather the berries. It does the work of settler colonialism by destroying to replace.
>
> *(Spice 2018)*

As Salmon People, Yurok are obligated to protect Salmon relatives and depend upon Salmon for subsistence and cultural practices. By contaminating and diverting water for cannabis agriculture in an already overtaxed Klamath River Basin, cannabis cultivation presents a worrisome threat to the health and vitality of salmon populations for Yurok and future generations.

Water diversions for cannabis cultivation have dewatered entire streams on the Yurok Indian Reservation and impacted tribal drinking water; evidence of water diversion (e.g. irrigation and water storage infrastructure) is evident at numerous abandoned cultivation sites (Reed 2019). In a 2015 study based in northwestern California, Bauer et al. found that "water demand for marijuana cultivation exceeds streamflow during the low-flow period . . . diminished streamflow is likely to have lethal or sub-lethal effects on state- and federal-listed salmon and steelhead trout and to cause further decline of sensitive amphibian species" (Bauer et al. 2015, 1). In Redwood Creek South, located in Yurok ancestral territory, the data indicated the estimated water demand for cannabis cultivation in 2015 was 165% of the annual seven-day flow (Bauer et al. 2015, 13).

Like the Water Protectors at Standing Rock (Estes and Dhillon 2019), Yurok people understand that water is life, and it is no coincidence that the most pressing environmental concern of cannabis cultivation is water. Water diversions from the Klamath River and its tributaries are worrisome to the Yurok Tribe for two key reasons. First, cannabis-related water diversions—on top of already allocated water diversions for agricultural interests—add stress on an overtaxed river basin and takes additional water away from salmon and other aquatic species. In 2002, the Klamath River became home to the largest fish kill in American history (LaDuke 2005). That trauma continues to impact Yurok people, and cannabis cultivation presents yet another threat to salmon. Second, water quantity and water quality are fundamentally linked. When stream flows have been reduced, the impacts on water quality from chemical pollution and human waste are magnified.

Yurok elders have long said that Yurok people are "merely a reflection of the river, and will never be healthy again until it is" (Yurok Tribe 2016, 70). In other words, what damages our River or Salmon simultaneously damages our bodies and culture. Potawatomi scholar Kyle Powys Whyte argues, "settler colonialism can be interpreted as a form of environmental injustice" because it "wrongfully interferes with and erases the socioecological contexts required for Indigenous populations to experience the world as a place infused with responsibilities to humans, nonhumans and ecosystems" (Whyte 2016, 159). Yurok people have a reciprocal relationship with salmon: we steward the river and fish for salmon and salmon sustain our generations. Activities that harm our salmon—from damming the river to irrigating for alfalfa and cannabis—prevent salmon from returning home or create a toxic river in which salmon cannot survive; therefore, Yurok people cannot fulfill their physical, social, and spiritual commitments to salmon.

Yurok people have been avid protectors of the River and the Salmon. Through a collaborative cannabis eradication campaign called Operation Yurok, the Yurok Tribe—in collaboration with county, state, and federal law enforcement—have drastically reduced the amount of cannabis cultivation occurring within the Yurok Indian Reservation. The new issue facing the Yurok Tribe is legal permitted cultivation within ancestral territory. Because ancestral territory is within Humboldt County's jurisdiction, the county is legally able to site cultivation activities within ancestral territory. This is problematic for the Yurok Tribe because numerous gathering sites and sacred sites are outside the reservation boundary. Moreover, the Yurok Tribe must put financial and human resources toward cannabis permitting (e.g. review permit applications or conducting site visits). However, the Yurok Tribe does not receive any of the permit fees or other financial resources that Humboldt County does to conduct this work. Therefore, the Yurok Tribe is paying the brunt of the environmental consequences without seeing any of the economic benefits of the legal cannabis industry.

Cannabis, Tribal Sovereignty, and the Pit River Tribe

On July 8, 2015, dozens of law enforcement agents from the Bureau of Indian Affairs and the Federal Drug Enforcement Agency invaded a tribal cannabis operation located on Pit River tribal land in Modoc County, California (NoiseCat 2015). According to the former Pit River[11] Tribal Council Chairman Mickey Gemmill Jr., some tribal members were subjected to excessive police force, severely injured, and arrested during the search (Pit River Tribe 2015). Agents destroyed plants, seized processed cannabis, and confiscated confidential patient information and other documents (Eid 2015; Armitage 2015). Three months prior to this invasion—on April 6, 2015—the Pit River tribal government adopted a tribal medical marijuana program under tribal law that was also consistent with California's medicinal cannabis laws (Pit River Tribe 2015). Gemmill Jr. spoke out after the raid to criticize the federal government and the Bureau of Indian Affairs specifically. Speaking on behalf of the Pit River Tribe, Gemmill Jr. declared, "We have been transparent in our conversations with the federal government and made no secret of our intent to exercise our sovereignty in the manner we believe appropriate" (Pit River Tribe 2015, 2). The Pit River Tribe provided the U.S. Attorney's Office with their Medical Marijuana Program Ordinance, and during consultations with the federal government, the tribe "asked the U.S. Attorney's office to identify any concerns and to advise the tribal government before taking any enforcement action against the tribal project" (Pit River Tribe 2015, 2). The U.S. Attorney's Office declined to do so.

The Pit River Tribe issued a press release on July 9, 2015, titled "Federal Government Fails to Respect Tribal Self Governance."

> We are very disappointed with the decision of the Bureau of Indian Affairs, as the lead federal agency, to descend on sovereign land with an army of nearly fifty law enforcement officers . . . that the BIA would take such a disrespectful approach to an Indian tribe on its own land is a serious assault to the Tribe's right to self-governance. We believe that it is important to remind the BIA of its responsibility to protect Indian tribes, not to undermine legitimate tribal efforts to create jobs and improve the health and welfare of tribal members.
>
> *(Pit River Tribe 2015, 2)*

The Bureau of Indian Affairs (BIA) is the federal agency responsible for upholding the United States' trust relationship with Native nations. Their mission is to "enhance the quality of life, to promote economic opportunity, and to carry out the responsibility to protect and improve the trust assets of American Indians, Indian tribes and Alaska Natives" (Bureau of Indian Affairs 2019). Gemmill Jr.'s critique of the BIA highlights the imposition of colonial rule over California Indians and the ways in which the settler state continually narrows the abilities of Native nations to develop politically and economically on their own accord, despite federal obligations to protect the economic well-being of tribes.

This is emblematic of Bruyneel's notion of "colonial ambivalence." The settler state reserves the privilege of choosing when to be a guardian and when to be a conqueror. The very agency responsible for protecting tribes is responsible for the invasion into sovereign territory, theft of product, and violence against and imprisonment of tribal members. The Pit River Tribe, then, in resistance, is operating within a third space of sovereignty—simultaneously demanding rights from the settler state (sovereign right to develop a Medical Marijuana Program Ordinance; BIA's responsibility to protect Indian tribes) *and* challenging the very imposition of colonial rule (establishing a cannabis operation in violation of federal law).

While Pit River has served as a cautionary tale of sorts for other California Indian tribes, the necessity for economic development on many rural Native reservations has led tribal governments to pursue participation in the state cannabis market. Proposition 64—the legislation that legalized recreational cannabis in California—does not include, incorporate, or even address Native American tribes. Former executive director of the California Growers Association, Hezekiah Allen, suggested that "tribal cannabis is probably the last big unsettled question[12] in California cannabis policy" (quoted in Lewis 2016). State policy makers argued that addressing tribes in Proposition 64 would be too complicated and time consuming and, instead, they would retroactively address tribes later on.

In response to the exclusion of tribes from the California state market, the California Native American Cannabis Association formed in 2017. As of 2019 C-NACA represents 25 tribes in California. Their mission is to "protect tribal sovereignty and promote tribal self-reliance by assisting California tribes in designing and implementing comprehensively regulated, legal cannabis and hemp enterprises that benefit tribal communities" (C-NACA 2017). On behalf of the member tribes, C-NACA has gone to state regulatory agencies and voiced tribal concerns and frustrations on being excluded from the state cannabis market. But currently, there is no mechanism for tribes to participate in the state cannabis market without waiving sovereign immunity and submitting to unfettered regulatory jurisdiction on tribal land and licensing authority to the state (California Code of Regulations, Title 16, Division 42, Section 5009).

Representing tribal governments, C-NACA aimed to negotiate with California to reach a fair and equitable agreement for tribal participation in the state cannabis market. Using agreements in Oregon, Washington, and Nevada as models, C-NACA helped develop Assembly Bill 924 to provide tribal access to the state's legal cannabis market. Similarly to tribal gaming, AB 924 would allow a tribal government to enter into a regulatory agreement or compact with the governor to develop a tribal cannabis regulatory commission. Under AB 924, tribes would still agree to comply with state regulations—but tribes would remain the regulatory authority. However, the state pushed for complete regulatory jurisdiction on tribal lands and to keep any taxes levied by the tribe[13] (Levitan 2019). Moreover, proposed amendments to the bill by the California legislature would have forced tribes to waive sovereign immunity, receive approval from local government, and defer jurisdiction to state regulators (Herrington 2019). These terms were unacceptable to C-NACA and its membership tribes. The bill was killed in a Senate committee meeting in November 2018. California Indian tribes continue to be excluded from the state cannabis market. The necessity for C-NACA and AB 924 prove that Native tribes remain subjected to colonial rule—but simultaneously demonstrate how tribal governments resist this imposition and work within what Bruyneel refers to as a third space of sovereignty.

Both the exclusion of tribes from the California state market and the prohibition enforcement efforts experienced by the Pit River Tribe are fundamentally different than other exclusions and prohibition enforcement efforts in non-Native communities. First, in California (and throughout the United States), we are on Indian land[14]—regardless of whether a space is officially demarcated as a reservation—because, quite simply, *all* land is Native land (Goeman 2013). Therefore, all cannabis production in the United States is occurring on Native land—and Native peoples in California are not benefitting from it. Second, as just as importantly, we maintain a unique relationship with the United States that differs from the experience of other populations within the United States. Tribal governments are sovereign nations with a right to self-determination, and the upholding of this relationship serves as the basis for the United States government's legitimacy. If states refuse to engage in government-to-government relationships with tribes, and if tribal sovereignty is not acknowledged and taken seriously within the California commercial cannabis industry, it could set a dangerous precedent for the exercise of tribal sovereignty in other capacities and ultimately put tribal rights in jeopardy. Tribal nations have much at stake because our sovereign right to determine our own laws is critical to our livelihoods and collective continuance as culturally and politically distinct peoples. Therefore, it is critical to make space for tribal sovereignty discourse within cannabis policy.

Reflections and Future Directions

These seemingly opposite narratives of some tribes fighting to protect their lands from cannabis agriculture while some tribes struggle to break into the cannabis market both demonstrate that Native people are not benefiting from the cannabis industry. This is not to say, however, that other populations are not also disenfranchised by the settler state or the California cannabis market, but it does demonstrate that the settler state continues to wield power over Native peoples in unique and harmful ways. Future work that engages both Native peoples and cannabis research is sorely needed. Specific questions include: Will the environmental regulations of cannabis production at both the state and the county level adequately protect tribal lands and cultural resources? What additional protections will be necessary to ensure protection of these resources? How should the local jurisdictions and the state engage with tribes regarding cannabis permitting with ancestral homelands? Will tribal participation in the cannabis industry prove useful for tribal economic and community development?

Cannabis represents a new avenue through which tribal sovereignty will be negotiated and may influence the relationship between Native nations and the settler state moving forward. Moreover, economic development predicated on natural resource extraction, like commercial cannabis, poses concerning sustainability questions for the future—especially considering upcoming climate-driven changes to land and water. It is important for all participants of the cannabis industry—and everybody else that occupies Native lands—to engage with their role (and often, complicity) in settler colonialism and recognize the tribal sovereignty of California's Indigenous peoples. The most ambitious question the cannabis industry can reflect upon going forward is how the cannabis industry can aid in the ultimate project of decolonization.

Notes

1 Thomas Jefferson, however, allegedly abandoned cannabis cultivation because "he felt it was too hard on his slaves" (Deitch 2003, 19).

2 Latin for "nobody's land," *terra nullius* was used as a justification for conquest and continued state occupation within international law.

3 This is not to say that the settler state "granted" tribal sovereignty to Native nations. Native nations exercised autonomous self-governance over their territories long before the European invasion of North America, and Native sovereignty predates the formation of the American nation-state.

4 Tribal nation refers to Native American sovereigns that have a formal nation-to-nation relationship with the United States federal government. Tribal nations are variously called tribes, nations, band, pueblos, communities, and Native villages. There are currently 573 (federally recognized) tribal nations located across 35 states (NCAI 2019). I use tribal nations and tribes interchangeably throughout.

5 Bruyneel derives this concept from Homi Bhabha's concept of "third space of enunciation"—an intervention in literary and cultural productions (see Bhabha 1994). Edward Soja has also used this concept within urban cultural geography (see Soja 1996).

6 It is worth noting here that cannabis cultivation in northwestern California is diverse and cannot be homogenized. While some grow cannabis for personal use and attempt to coexist "with the natural world . . . [and] emulate Native ways" (Robinson Bosk 2000, x), many grow cannabis for profit on a large scale. The environmental impacts of cannabis cultivation examined in this chapter are largely the result of for-profit cultivation, and said impacts have intensified within the past decade.

7 The Yurok Tribe has a zero-tolerance policy on cannabis cultivation on the Yurok Indian Reservation—so all cultivation on the reservation is illegal. Yurok tribal lands, however, refers to both the Yurok Indian Reservation and Yurok ancestral territory. Yurok ancestral territory, however, falls within Humboldt County's jurisdiction, and there is a combination of legal cultivation, illegal trespass cultivation, and noncompliant cultivation.

8 Carbofuran is a Class 1 pesticide (meaning it is extremely hazardous) that is primarily used to control insects on crops. Carbofuran is very toxic to birds and has been illegally used to intentionally kill wildlife. For humans, carbofuran has one of the highest acute toxicities of any insecticide; carbofuran poisoning can lead to death. Banned in both Canada and the European Union, carbofuran was supposed to be banned by the Environmental Protection Agency in 2006, but the US manufacturer of carbofuran is fighting the EPA's decision (Pesticide Action Network 2010).

9 Also a Class 1 pesticide, methamidophos is used on crops. Methamidophos is rapidly absorbed through the stomach, lungs, and skin of humans and is very toxic to both birds and aquatic organisms (Extension Toxicology Network 1995).

10 While avermectin B1 (and other avermectin pesticides) is relatively non-harmful to mammals, it is highly toxic to fish and aquatic invertebrates. It is also highly toxic to bees (Extension Toxicology Network 1994).

11 The Pit River Tribe is federally recognized and composed of 11 autonomous bands. The targeted operation was producing medicinal cannabis.

12 Tribal attorney Mark Levitan argues that if the state does not address the tribal situation in California, the state cannot fulfill the purposes of Proposition 64. The purpose and intent of Proposition 64—as outlined in the legislation—is to establish a comprehensive system to legalize and regulate the production of cannabis across the State of California. If tribal governments continue to be ignored, there will be large gaps all over the state and inconsistent regulations (Levitan 2019).

13 An equal power dynamic is certainly at play here. California is the sixth-largest economy in the world, and Native American reservations endure the most extreme poverty rates in the country.

14 Justifications for colonization are based on legal fictions (i.e. Doctrine of Discovery). In California specifically, the 18 treaties negotiated with various California Indian tribes were never ratified by the United States Senate. So, arguably, the United States does not have a rightful claim to California.

References

Alfred, Taiaiake. 2005. "Sovereignty." In *Sovereignty Matters: Locations of Contestation and Possibility in Indigenous Struggles for Self-Determination*, edited by Joanne Barker, 33–50. Lincoln: University of Nebraska Press.

Armitage, Lynn. 2015. "Pot Raid Has Pit River Tribe Fuming; Rips BIA." *Indian Country Today*, July 17. http://indiancountrytodaymedianetwork.com/2015/07/17/pot-raid-has-pit-river-tribe-fuming-rips-bia-161119.

Arvin, Maile, Eve Tuck, and Angie Morrill. 2013. "Decolonizing Feminism: Challenging Connections Between Settler Colonialism and Heteropatriarchy." *Feminist Formations* 25 (1): 8–34.

Barker, Joanne. 2005. *Sovereignty Matters: Locations of Contestation and Possibility in Indigenous Struggles for Self-Determination*. Lincoln: University of Nebraska Press.

Bartlett, Brad A. 2019. "Tribes and Cannabis: Reaching New Highs in the Burgeoning Cannabis Marketplace." *Federal Lawyer* 66 (2): 49–52.

Bauer, Scott, Jennifer Olson, Adam Cockrill, Michael van Hattem, Linda Miller, Margaret Tauzer, and Gordon Leppig. 2015. "Impacts of Surface Water Diversions for Marijuana Cultivation on Aquatic Habitat in Four Northwestern California Watersheds." *PloS One* 10 (3).

Bhabha, Homi. 1994. *The Location of Culture*. New York: Routledge Press.

Bruyneel, Kevin. 2007. *The Third Space of Sovereignty: The Postcolonial Politics of U.S.-Indigenous Relations*. Edited by Robert Warrior and Jace Weaver, *Indigenous Americans*. Minneapolis: University of Minnesota Press.

Bureau of Indian Affairs (BIA). "Bureau of Indian Affairs (BIA): Mission Statement." Accessed August 25, 2019. www.bia.gov/bia.

California Code of Regulations, Title 16, Division 42, Bureau of Cannabis Control, Section 5009. Sacramento, CA.

California Native American Cannabis Association (C-NACA). 2017. "Our Commitment." https://cnaca.us/cnaca-activity.

Cook-Lynn, Elizabeth. 1997. "Who Stole Native American Studies?" *Wicazo Sa Review* 12 (1): 9–28.

Deitch, Robert. 2003. *Hemp—American History Revisited*. New York: Algora Publishing.

Deloria Jr., Vine. 1969. *Custer Died for Your Sins: An Indian Manifesto*. New York: University of Oklahoma Press.

———. 1979. "Self-Determination and the Concept of Sovereignty." In *Economic Development in American Indian Reservations*, edited by Roxanne Dunbar-Ortiz, 22–28. Albuquerque: University of New Mexico Native American Studies.

Deloria Jr., Vine, and Clifford M. Lytle. 1984. *The Nations Within: The Past and Future of American Indian Sovereignty*. New York: Pantheon Books.

Dunbar-Ortiz, Roxanne. 2014. *An Indigenous Peoples' History of the United States*. Boston, MA: Beacon Press.

Echo-Hawk, Walter R. 2010. *In the Courts of the Conqueror: The 10 Worst Indian Law Cases Ever Decided*. Golden, CO: Fulcrum Publishing.

Eid, Troy A. 2015. "Federal Narcotics Laws Can Still Trump Tribal Sovereignty." *Law 360*, July 20.

Estes, Nick, and Jaskiran Dhillon. 2019. *Standing with Standing Rock: Voices from the #NoDAPL Movement*. Minneapolis: University of Minnesota Press.

Extension Toxicology Network. 1994. "Abamectin." Cornell University http://pmep.cce.cornell.edu/profiles/extoxnet/24d-captan/abamectin-ext.html.

———. 1995. "Methamidophos." Cornell University http://pmep.cce.cornell.edu/profiles/extoxnet/haloxyfop-methylparathion/methamidophos-ext.html.

Goeman, Mishuana. 2013. *Mark My Words: Native Women Mapping Our Nations*. Minneapolis: University of Minnesota Press.

Herrington, A. J. 2019. "CA's Tribal Nations Are Shut Out of the Legal Cannabis Industry." *High Times*. https://hightimes.com/news/what-about-social-equity-cas-tribal-nations-kept-out-of-legal-cannabis-market/.

Kemp, Kym. 2018. "Potentially Dangerous Pesticides Spilled into Mill Creek Which Flows into the Trinity River." *Redheaded Blackbelt*, October 3. https://kymkemp.com/2018/10/03/potentially-dangerous-pesticides-spilled-into-mill-creek-which-flows-into-the-trinity-river/.

Kidwell, Clara Sue, and Alan Velie. 2005. *Native American Studies*. Edited by Robert Con Davis-Undiano, *Introducing Ethnic Studies*. Lincoln: University of Nebraska Press.

LaDuke, Winona. 2005. "Klamath Land and Life." In *Recovering the Sacred: The Power of Naming and Claiming*, 47–66. Cambridge, MA: South End Press.

Lee, Martin A. 2012. *Smoke Signals: A Social History of Marijuana—Medical, Recreational, and Scientific*. New York: Scribner.

Levitan, Mark. 2019. "Tribal Participation in the California Cannabis Market." Bureau of Cannabis Control Cannabis Advisory Committee Meeting, Los Angeles, June 28.

Lewis, Amanda Chicago. 2016. "How Black People are Being Shut Out of America's Weed Boom: Whitewashing the Green Rush." *Buzzfeed News*, March 16. www.buzzfeednews.com/article/amandachicagolewis/americas-white-only-weed-boom.

Mosk, Sanford A. 1939. "Subsidized Hemp Production in Spanish California." *Agricultural History* 13 (4): 171–75.

Museum, Hash Marihuana & Hemp. "Columbus and Cannabis." Hash Marihuana & Hemp Museum. https://hashmuseum.com/en/collection/columbus-and-cannabis.

National Congress of the American Indian. 2019. *Tribal Nations & the United States: An Introduction*. Washington, DC: National Congress of the American Indian.

NoiseCat, Julian Brave. 2015. "Native Tribes Want Pot Business, But Financial Gain May Cost Their Sovereignty." *The Guardian*, October 9. www.theguardian.com/commentisfree/2015/oct/09/native-tribes-want-pot-marijuana-business-financial-gain-may-cost-sovereignty.

Norton, Jack. 1979. *When Our Worlds Cried: Genocide in Northwestern California*. San Francisco: The Indian Historical Press.

Pesticide Action Network. 2010. "Undue Influence." www.panna.org/resources/undue-influence.

Pit River Tribe. 2015. *Federal Government Fails to Respect Tribal Self Governance: Pit River Tribe Disappointed in Enforcement Action Against the Tribe's Lawful Medical Marijuana Project*. Burney, CA.

Ramirez, Matthew. 2018. "New Mexico Tribal Cannabis: Policy, Politics, & Guidelines for Government-to-Government Cooperation in State-Tribal Cannabis Compacting." *Natural Resources Journal* 58 (1): 75–124.

Reed, Kaitlin. 2019. "The Environmental and Cultural Impacts of Cannabis Cultivation on Yurok Tribal Lands." PhD dissertation, Native American Studies, University of California, Davis, CA.

Robinson Bosk, Beth, ed. 2000. *The New Settler Interviews: Vol. I: Boogie at the Brink*. White River Junction, VT: Chelsea Green Publishing Company.

Smith, Melinda. 2015. "Native Americans and the Legalization of Marijuana: Can the Tribes Turn Another Addiction into Affluence?" *Indian Law Review* 507 (2): 507–52.

Soja, Edward. 1996. *Thirdspace: Journeys to Los Angeles and Other Real-and-Imagined Places*. Malden, MA: Blackwell Publishers.

Spice, Anne. 2018. "Processing Settler Toxicities: Part II." *Footnotes*, June 23. https://footnotesblog.com/2018/06/23/processing-settler-toxicities-part-ii/.

Thiesen, Stan, and Orrin Plocher. 2014. *DRAFT: Sampling and Analysis Plan for Illegal Marijuana Cultivation Sites on the Yurok Reservation*. Arcata, CA: Freshwater Environmental Services.

———. 2016. *Water Demand Estimate for Marijuana Cultivation within the Yurok Indian Reservation*. Arcata, CA: Freshwater Environmental Services.

Tuck, Eve, and K. Wayne Yang. 2012. "Decolonization is Not a Metaphor." *Decolonization: Indigeneity, Education & Society* 1 (1): 1–40.

Whyte, Kyle Powys. 2016. "Indigenous Experience, Environmental Justice and Settler Colonialism." In *Nature and Experience: Phenomenology and the Environment*, edited by Bryan E. Bannon. London: Rowman & Littlefield International.

Wilkinson, Charles. 2005. *Blood Struggle: The Rise of Modern Indian Nations*. New York: W. W. Norton & Company.

Williams, Susan, and Kathryn M. Hoover. 1999. "Assaults on Tribal Sovereignty: Signs of a New Era in Federal Indian Policy." *Indigenous Woman* 2 (6): 31–33.

Wolfe, Patrick. 2006. "Settler Colonialism and the Elimination of the Native." *Journal of Genocide Research* 8 (4): 387–409.

Yurok Tribe. 2016. "Yurok Tribe Scoping Comments on the Klamath Hydroelectric Project EIR." January 29, State Water Resources Control Board, Sacramento, CA.

6

Five Years of Cannabis Regulation

What Can We Learn From the Uruguayan Experience?

Marcos Baudean

Keywords: Cannabis regulation, Uruguay, evaluation, results

Introduction

The Uruguayan experience regulating[1] cannabis has attracted international attention because

- It involves all possible uses of the product, including recreational and medicinal consumption as well as industrial applications and scientific research.
- It is nationwide in scope.
- It provides state control of the registry of users and dispensary-based distribution allowing price control, potency control, and production quality standards.
- It is focused on promoting health, safety, and justice by centering notions of harm reduction and human rights.

Before the regulation of cannabis for adult use by Canada in 2018, Uruguay was the only country that had legalized cannabis at the national level. Law 19172 passed in December 2013, and implementation began in 2014. The law regulates adult (recreational), medical, and industrial uses. Regarding adult use, the law establishes three legal avenues to access cannabis: domestic cultivation, cannabis clubs, and pharmacies. Users can only obtain cannabis from one of these three sources. Domestic cultivation and cannabis club registries opened in 2014. However, registration and sale through pharmacies started as late as July 2017.

Despite the great expectations internationally from the results, there has been limited evaluation of the Uruguayan initiative. At the time of this writing (February 20, 2020), a title search on "Uruguay" and "cannabis" in SCOPUS yielded 13 articles. The topics dealt with in these papers focus specifically on the Uruguayan model and its challenges (Pardo 2014; Room 2014; Garat 2016; Cerdá and Kilmer 2017; Walsh and Ramsey 2018), comparative results on specific issues (Decorte et al. 2017; Hughes 2018), public opinion (Cruz, Boidi, and Queirolo 2018a, 2018b), cannabis clubs

DOI: 10.4324/9780429320491-6

(Queirolo, Boidi, and Cruz 2016; Decorte et al. 2017), and other specific issues (Boidi, Queirolo, and Cruz 2016; Evans 2016).

There is little research, however, on the general results of the regulation of cannabis for adult uses.[2] This chapter seeks to fill the void by providing a general perspective on the progress towards regulation as well as assessing the projected outcomes in two objectives of regulation: public health and security.

The Analytical Framework for the Evaluation of Cannabis Regulation in Uruguay

In 2014, the National Drug Board (JND),[3] the Uruguayan Drugs Observatory (OUD), staff of various ministries, staff of the Institute for the Regulation and Control of Cannabis (IRCCA), officials of the Judicial Power,[4] national and international experts, and Monitor Cannabis Uruguay (MCU) developed a system of indicators for the evaluation of cannabis regulation. The "Uruguayan Cannabis Regulation Indicator System" (UCRIS) originated in a series of documents prepared by the JND in collaboration with ministries (JND 2014a, 2014b, 2014c, 2014d). Those documents were discussed in two international seminars held in 2014 (Fesur 2014).

Monitor Cannabis Uruguay proposed an analytical framework for the evaluation of cannabis regulation results based on JND documents and international seminars. In this section, I present a summary of that framework and related hypotheses concerning cannabis regulation impacts on health and security. In the discussion, I will associate each result with the corresponding hypothesis as it was formulated in 2014.

The UCRIS is a very complete collection of indicators that can be analyzed from different perspectives. As I established in the previous section, Uruguayan regulation is a policy based on notions of harm reduction and human rights. These notions have consequences for the health and security objectives pursued by cannabis regulation. As Pablo Galain has put it, Uruguay defended its regulation at the United Nations General Assembly Special Session (UNGASS) 2016 as a policy directed to facilitate safe consumption of cannabis in terms of the quality of the product and the means of obtaining it (Galain 2018, 40). It implies that an expected result of regulation is

> to replace, or at least compete with, the illegal or black market in supplying the regulated drug as well as reducing the harm linked to consumption by offering a better quality product than that of the illegal market. Thus, the fundamental goals of a harm reduction policy should be a regulated market that offers improvement in quality, reduction in price and increase in security.
>
> *(Galain 2018, 49)*

This focus means that regulation is intended to reduce harms caused by consuming bad-quality products, harms related to exposure to violence when buying the product, and inequalities in access to better-quality products. Therefore, the evaluation of the policy needs to consider more aspects than the traditional indicators of prevalence, adverse effects, and mortality (public health) or systemic homicides and evolution of prosecutions (security).

In the first place, the assessment of results in public health needs to consider how regulation facilitates access to better-quality products than what is offered by the illegal market. Second, there has to be no inequalities in access to the best cannabis products. It is important to assess how users from different socioeconomic backgrounds access the product. Third, security aspects should consider not only public safety issues; regulation should eliminate the risk of violence—from traffickers and the police—that users face when buying the product.

Hypothesis in Public Health and Security

Hypotheses in Public Health

The UCRIS established that a legal market for recreational cannabis should produce changes in five dimensions of public health: health risk, risk of problematic drug use, health benefit (only those 18 years or older),[5] adverse effects, and mortality. The hypotheses developed in 2014 for each of the public health dimensions are presented next.

HEALTH RISK

1. There will be an initial increase in marijuana use due to the greater availability and legitimacy of the substance.
2. The separation of markets (legal, illegal) and the lower exposure to the supply of other drugs will produce a decrease in the experimentation and subsequent use of other substances.
3. The existence of prevention programs with a focus on cannabis will cause an increase in the risk perception of the substance.

RISK OF PROBLEMATIC DRUG USE

4. The process of "normalization" of cannabis should make easier the self-recognition of problematic use, therefore the demand for treatment will increase.
5. The process of "normalization" of cannabis will result in an increase in the demand for cannabis treatment in absolute terms and in the proportion of problematic consumers who demand care.
6. Regulation will not cause an increase in the risk behaviors of the adult (ICD-10[6]) or teen (CAST[7]) population using cannabis with the methods used to measure them.

HEALTH BENEFIT

To understand health benefit hypotheses, it is important to frame Uruguayan cannabis regulation as a harm reduction policy (Galain 2018). One of the reasons for policy makers to foster cannabis regulation was to improve users' health by facilitating access to a better product. Cannabis flower/buds are considered much better than the traditional illegal product: pressed cannabis.[8] In the first place, cannabis sold in pharmacies is of mandatory organic cultivation. Second, the comparison of samples of homegrown cannabis and pressed cannabis showed that the former does not contain the various toxic substances found in samples of pressed marijuana (contaminants, fungi, additives).[9] For those reasons, the displacement of the illegal product by the legal one is considered a health benefit. This reasoning justifies the following hypotheses (7–9):

7. The number of people who declare obtaining cannabis from the illegal market will decrease as they obtain the product through legal mechanisms.
8. The illegal market will decrease gradually as the registration of legal mechanisms increases.
9. The migration of users from the illegal market to the legal market will depend on two main factors. One is the legitimacy that users conferred to the system. The second is the benefits perceived by users of the illegal market for being in the legal market.

ADVERSE EFFECTS

10. In a regulated context, cannabis-related reports to the Toxicology Information and Advice Center will increase, as exposure to the substance increases.

MORTALITY

11. In a regulated context, the number of drug-related deaths will not vary.

Security Hypotheses

Law 19.172 is one of the initiatives implemented by the Uruguayan government in response to the security problems that the country was going through at the beginning of the decade. In 2012, the government proposed the "Strategy for Life and Social Harmony" (Gabinete de Seguridad 2012), including a series of actions aimed at comprehensively dealing with security problems such as interpersonal violence, the escalating homicide rate, and the alleged deterioration of social relations.

However, prior literature affirms that cannabis markets are not necessarily violent. As Room and colleagues established, most cannabis purchases are between friends, "with purely market transactions as a secondary source of acquisition" (Room et al. 2010, 61). Research on cannabis-buying practices in Uruguay confirms the international acquisition pattern rooted in social networks (Fesur 2015). In 2014, according to a national survey, only 23% of the users bought cannabis directly from traffickers in the last year, 44% of these buyers reported sometimes being fearful when purchasing cannabis, and 17% reported experiencing violence while purchasing cannabis (Fesur 2015).

Law 19.172 was intended to reduce drug-related violence in two aspects: violence derived from the link between users and traffickers and from conflicts between actors involved in organized crime. In Article 4, the legislature established that the law

> aims to protect the inhabitants of the country from the risks derived from the links with the illegal drug trade and trafficking, through the intervention of the State, attacking the devastating health, social and economic consequences of the problematic use of psychoactive substances, and reducing the incidence of drug trafficking and organized crime.
>
> *(JND 2014d, 56)*

The proposed reduction in drug trafficking (and related violence) should derive from displacing the illegal cannabis market, an important portion of the total drug market (Musto 2018; Fesur 2014; Repetto 2014).

In 2014, experts and government officials considered that a regulated market for recreational cannabis might reduce violence associated with drug trafficking in the long term. The hypothesized mechanism was the following:

12. If legal markets displace illegal sources, the latter will decrease in number of consumers and sales volume.
13. If the illegal cannabis market is reduced, the presence and activity of drug trafficking in Uruguay will be weakened because cannabis is an important part of that business.
14. In the *short term*, therefore, it is possible that changes in the market due to regulation will produce an increase in "systemic homicides."[10] In the *long term*, the presence and activity of drug trafficking should decrease and the number of systemic homicides linked to gang disputes should be reduced.

An increase in systemic homicides may occur as drug traffickers compete to replace profits lost to the legal sector from the cannabis trade. This loss leads them to dispute territories with increasing intensity in order to recover profits, otherwise known as a "strangulation mechanism" (Fesur 2014). Therefore, to justify the intensification of the conflict due to the regulation of cannabis, it is necessary for regulation to displace, almost completely, illegal actors from the cannabis market.

Methods

In 2016, Monitor Cannabis Uruguay[11] implemented a strategy for monitoring and evaluating the impact of cannabis regulation in Uruguay. The data collected covers the period 2013–2018.

MCU proposed a specific methodological approach that considered the implementation of evaluative research on the results and impacts of the policy, as well as on the instruments used to implement it. In this chapter, I present data to evaluate the impact of the legal market on health and security-related objectives. The performance of selected quantitative indicators are analyzed using descriptive statistics. The implementation of the recreational cannabis market is examined, drawing on semi-structured interviews between 2015 and 2018 with users, traffickers, police officers, politicians, and researchers.

Existing data from a variety of sources is also used. Health data is collected from National Drug Surveys[12] implemented by the National Drug Board (2001–2018), MCU Survey on the Use of Cannabis (2017),[13] Toxicology Information and Advice Center (CIAT), Uruguayan Drug Observatory, and Institute for the Regulation and Control of Cannabis. Security and Justice data comes from the National Drug Board, Ministry of Interior, Judicial Power, and interviews conducted with users, traffickers, and police officers. Finally, this study relies on national newspaper coverage between 2014 and 2018.

The Adult-Use Cannabis Market in Uruguay

When legal access was first implemented, the government expected that the creation of a legal market would largely displace the illegal cannabis market. Distribution through pharmacies was the most important tool designed to supply the market. The evaluation strategies proposed in 2014 assumed that measures of public health, security, and justice would be positively impacted by the gradual establishment of the legal market (Fesur 2014). Therefore, the first point to consider when assessing the results of the regulation in Uruguay is to determine to what extent the legal market has developed. This is important because the size of the legal market is related to the health benefits of regulation. As I established in the previous section, consuming a better-quality cannabis product is an important part of a harm reduction policy. In this section, the aim is to establish the following:

- The legal market is an important source of supply in Uruguay, but not through pharmacies, as expected in 2014. Instead, domestic cultivation, legal and illegal, has become one of the most important sources of cannabis supply.
- The total demand for cannabis in Uruguay is satisfied through a combination of a legal market, an illicit market, and an emerging "gray market" (legally registered users who give away or sell their surplus).
- Illicit actors continue to satisfy the demand for cannabis. However, the illegal market now consists of two types of actors.

    - The first type, the traditional cannabis trafficker, imports and sells pressed cannabis from Paraguay. Since 2017 they have added flower buds according to police seizure data (Baudean 2019).[14]
    - The second type includes unregistered local producers who sell their product directly to consumers. These local producers are not necessarily criminals. In fact, police do not consider them as a target. Most of them can be considered entrepreneurs who take advantage of the opportunity to prosper (Baudean 2019; Queirolo 2020).

According to Law 19.172, legal cannabis users can register as either home growers, pharmacy buyers, or members of a cannabis club. Users can register to obtain cannabis from only one source. Every registered user can have access to up to 40 grams of cannabis per month. MCU National Drug Survey data shows that 257,432 Uruguayans (15% of the population between 15 and 65 years old) report having used cannabis at least once in the past year. The 47,067 registered users who buy or grow cannabis include 36,487 pharmacy buyers, 7,163 home growers, and 3,417 cannabis club members (IRCCA, n.d.). Sharing cannabis is legal in Uruguay. Registered users are known to share cannabis with other users. The IRCCA estimates that 30% of last year's users accessed legal cannabis in an undetermined quantity (JND-Presidencia 2019).

Using different sources, MCU estimated the volume and value of the national adult-use cannabis market for 2017 (see Table 6.2). The data came from the MCU National Survey on the Use of Cannabis (2017) and IRCCA (relative to the number of people registered as legal cannabis users).[15] MCU estimated value using the price of legal cannabis and established the potential of the legal market assuming that every channel produces the total amount permitted for every user (40 grams per month). The estimated national cannabis market is 39.8 tons, which represents US $45.5 million a year. The potential of the legal market is 22.6 tons per year, which represent US $25.9 million.

According to this data, the legal market could capture 57% of the total national market, once it is producing at its legal maximum. However, it is not easy to determine the total amount of legal cannabis produced because the exact production of legal home growers remains unknown. The only available data is the quantity of cannabis sold through pharmacies between 2017 and early 2019, which amounted to 2 tons and 254 kilos of cannabis (IRCCA 2019). In order to get an idea of the gap between the potential demand and the legal market supply, I examined available pharmacy data. From July 2017 to January 2019 there were 29,028 pharmacy users who made at least one purchase. That represents a maximum demand of 20 tons and 900 kilos (assuming each user consumed the legal limit of 40 grams per month). In the period between July 2017 and January 2019, legal production yielded 2 tons. According to these figures, the potential demand is ten times the actual legal production. The implication is that pharmacy shoppers have on average two sources of cannabis.[16]

Surveys and interviews with users confirm that cannabis from local producers (whether it was given away or sold) are important sources of provision (Baudean 2018c; Queirolo, Boidi, and Cruz 2018). According to the JND survey, in 2018 36% of last year's users accessed cannabis mostly through sharing or buying to unregistered growers or cannabis social clubs members (Junta Nacional de Drogas and Observatorio Uruguayo de Drogas 2019). In 2014, 58% of users in the prior year reported using pressed cannabis. In 2017, 22% of the prior year's users declared pressed cannabis as the most frequent product used and 12% in 2018.[17]

Local producers are not related to trafficking networks. Some producers give away their surplus, and others have established small businesses supplying a relatively small network of users (Baudean 2019; Queirolo 2020). There were more than 45,000 home growers in 2017 (Aguiar, Lemos, and Musto 2019), three times the amount reported by the Sixth National Drug Survey (2014) three years earlier. The control of small producers is still weak, since they are not a target of the police and the IRCCA has a limited capacity for inspections. It is noteworthy that illegally grown local flower buds have a place in the market, even though it is much more expensive than legally cultivated flowers[18] and pressed cannabis. There are at least three reasons why illegal local flower is in higher demand than legal sources: users prefer flowers, tourists demand them (and can pay much more than the local users), and growers offer a greater variety of genetics and potency not available from legal producers.

From the perspective of harm reduction and human rights (Galain 2018), access through legal, "gray market" or unregistered local producers is a positive result for two reasons. First, the product in those three channels is a better product than the traditional cannabis from Paraguay. Second, the transactions are free from violence.

Public Health Objectives Results

Five years after the national regulation of cannabis began, several indicators show that regulation has its strengths and weaknesses. On the one hand, most users access healthy products (flower buds) cultivated locally, and direct contact with traffickers has decreased. An important result is that, although cannabis use prevalence rates increased among adults and teenagers, there have been no changes in the problematic use of cannabis and drug-related deaths. On the other hand, there are inequalities in access to cannabis insofar as consumers of traditional and less expensive, pressed cannabis are more likely to be of low socioeconomic status.

Health Risk

As expected, there has been an increase in the use of cannabis among adults and adolescents. As can be seen in Table 6.1, cannabis remains the third most consumed psychoactive substance, as it was before regulation, behind alcohol and tobacco. Adult prevalence rates for cannabis use increased significantly from 9% in 2014 to 15% in 2017 (last year users).[19] There is no variation between 2017 and 2018 surveys. In the long run, alcohol, cocaine, and ecstasy use has increased significantly. Among adults, there has been a moderate decrease in the perception of great risk due to the consumption of cannabis several times a week, from 62% in 2014 to 51% in 2017 (chi square: $p < .001$). The user base is widening to include a greater percentage of women and older users. The proportion of women using cannabis has almost doubled from approximately 6% in 2014 to 12% in 2017 (chi square: $p < .001$). Likewise, the proportion of those over 36 years old using cannabis has increased from 3% in 2014 to 7% in 2017 (chi square: $p < .001$). Cannabis remains the third most consumed psychoactive substance, as it was before regulation.

A disappointing result is that the consumption of alcohol or other drugs has not decreased among the adult population. However, if we compare the people who started their consumption in the period between measurements, there is a decrease in prevalence of alcohol, tobacco, and cocaine,[20] although the differences are not statistically significant (Baudean 2018c).

Among teenagers, in the first decade of the century, cannabis use increased from 8% to 13% (last year prevalence) (Junta Nacional de Drogas and Observatorio Uruguayo de Drogas 2011). Table 6.2 shows that after regulation cannabis use continued to increase, and it stabilized between 2016 and 2018, around 20% (last year use). Alcohol is the most important drug consumed; since 2003 around 70% of students declared using it in the last year (with the exception of the 2014 survey). There was a moderate increase in benzodiazepines and tobacco use after regulation, and stability in the rates of other drug use. There was a 3% increase in the perception of great risk due to the consumption of cannabis several times a week between 2014 and 2016 (chi square: $p < .001$). Prevalence rates for teenage females increased, almost equaling the prevalence rate for teenage males.

Cannabis use rates among Uruguayan teenagers increased after regulation, as Table 6.2 shows. These results are not consistent with cannabis prevalence rates among youth in the United States.

Table 6.1 Last year prevalence of the main substances monitored (adult's survey)

	2001	*2006*	*2011*	*2014*	*2017*	*2018*
Alcohol	71.4%	66.5% ****	74.0% ****	71.1% ***	69.4%	77.1% ****
Tobacco	36.8%	36.9%	33.9% ****	33.0%	36.5% ***	32.7% ***
Cannabis	1.4%	5.5% ****	8.3% ****	9.3%	15.4% ****	14.6%
Cocaine	0.2%	1.6% ****	1.9%	1.6%	2.9% ****	2.0%
Cocaine base paste	–	0.3%	0.4%	0.2%	0.4%	–
MDMA / Ecstasy	–	0.1%	0.2%	0.4%	0.9% ****	0.9%

Source: III, IV, V, VI, and VII National Household Survey on Drug Use, JND (2001–2018). Monitor Cannabis Uruguay Survey on the Use of Cannabis (2017)

Comparisons: * $p < .05$; ** $p < .01$; *** $p < .005$; **** $p < .001$ (chi-square tests)

Table 6.2 Last year prevalence of the main substances monitored (student's survey)

	2011	*2014*	*2016*	*2018*
Alcohol	69.9%	60.2% ****	69.3% ****	72.1% ***
Tobacco	20.2%	15.5% ****	18.5% ****	18.0%
Cannabis	12.0%	17.0% ****	19.8% ****	19.7%
Cocaine	1.4%	2.1% ***	2.5%	2.2%
Cocaine base paste	0.4%	0.5%	0.5%	0.6%
Benzodiazepines (with and without prescription)	7.7%	7.1%	10.9% ****	11.9%
Stimulants (Ritalin, Cedrin, etc.) (with and without prescription)	1.8%	1.4%	1.5%	1.6%

Source: IV, VI, VII, and VIII National Survey on Drug Use in Middle School Students, JND

Comparisons: *p < .05; **p < .01; ***p < .005; ****p < .001 (chi-square tests)

According to the Colorado Department of Public Safety baseline report on the impacts of marijuana legalization, use of cannabis among youths under 18 has remained stable since legalization (CDPS 2018, 101–22). Washington State presents similar results (Dilley et al. 2018; NWHIDTA 2017). However, it is important to note that cannabis use rates were high before regulation began in Uruguay. In fact, Uruguay ranks second after Chile in cannabis use among adolescents according to UNASUR.[21]

A plausible explanation for the increase in cannabis use among adolescents in Uruguay may be the accessibility of cannabis. According to the National Drug Board's last report, students have access to cannabis almost in the same proportion through purchase (37%) or through other users who give them the product as a gift (36%) (Junta Nacional de Drogas and Observatorio Uruguayo de Drogas 2020).[22] A recent research note in *JAMA Pediatrics* speculates that the stability or decline in youth consumption in the states that passed cannabis laws (medicinal or recreational) is due to the difficulties in accessing cannabis after legalization "as drug dealers are replaced by licensed dispensaries that require proof of age" (Anderson et al. 2019, 881). In Uruguay, the illegal sale of cannabis has not been displaced completely by the legal market. Instead, new illegal actors have emerged, and this situation facilitates access to the product. Teenagers can buy cannabis from dealers or from growers. What is most important is that growers represent less risk of violence or deception than do traffickers in general.

Risk of Problematic Use

Cannabis remains the least frequent reason for requesting treatment among people who use drugs: 8% of total requests in 2018.[23] Nevertheless, the absolute number of users in Uruguay who demand treatment almost doubled between 2013 and 2018, from 51 to 95 cases. Likewise, the proportion of those seeking drug treatments specifically for cannabis use increased from 6% in 2013 to 8% in 2018.[24] One important issue regarding problematic use is the evolution of potency in the market (Room et al. 2010). In the United States, prices have declined and potency increased (Kilmer and Kleiman 2018). There is no systematic registration of potency in Uruguay. However, it is highly probable that average potency increased in the last five years, because today the main product is flower buds, not pressed cannabis (which has a low percentage of THC). National Drug Survey 2014 (JND) and MCU Survey 2017 asked prior-year cannabis users if they know the potency of the cannabis they usually smoke. If the respondent knew the potency, then they were asked about the average potency of the cannabis they smoke. Data show an increase in the proportion of users who know cannabis potency, from 23% in 2014 to 36% in 2017 (chi square: $p < .001$). There was also a moderate increase in the average potency of cannabis reported by users. The majority of users consume medium-potency products and only a minority consume high-potency products.[25] Data show stability in risk of problematic use in adults (using ICD-10), from 17% (2014) to 16% (2018) of last year's users. Among students, risk is also stable. According to CAST, about 12% of last year's users were at risk of problematic use in 2014, 2016, and 2018 (Junta Nacional de Drogas and Observatorio Uruguayo de Drogas 2020).

Health Benefit (Among Those 18 and Older)

The proportion of the population that has registered as cannabis users increased over the five years since legalization, but it is still far from the total number of users. Registered or not, users obtain cannabis from various sources. On average, they have access to cannabis from two types of sources: the legal and the non-legal and gray market. Only 27% of users access cannabis exclusively through either legal or non-legal means. The most important result is that users who directly or indirectly buy (as the most frequent product) pressed cannabis from traffickers descended from 58% (2014) to 12% (2018) (Junta Nacional de Drogas and Observatorio Uruguayo de Drogas 2016, 2019).

One weakness of regulation is that not everybody has the same access to better products (flowers/bud). As seen in Table 6.3, consumption of flower buds and pressed cannabis differs significantly by socioeconomic status. Users who only consume pressed cannabis are more likely of lower socioeconomic status (SES).

Adverse Effects

As expected, there was a moderate increase in the rate of adverse effects due to the use of cannabis. There are two general data sources to evaluate adverse effects. The Toxicology Information and Advice Center registers intoxication cases in hospital emergencies. The other source of information about adverse effects comes from hospital discharge records.[26]

According to the CIAT, requests involving drugs increased from 3.5% to 5.8% between 2010 and 2015. In cases of intoxication, there is a polydrug use pattern (Negrín 2017). In fact there were 413 cases and 594 substances involved in those cases in 2010. In 2015 there were 574 cases and 877 substances involved. In this period, the number of substances increased more than the number of cases (48% more substances compared to 39% more cases), suggesting an increase in the polydrug use pattern. In this context, the presence of cannabis increased from 63 cases in 2010 to 121 cases in 2015. Cannabis remained the fifth most common substance mentioned during consultations (after alcohol, cocaine, cocaine paste, and benzodiazepines).[27] Cannabis consultations are mostly associated with alcohol, cocaine, and cocaine paste.

Table 6.3 Summary of total products consumed by socioeconomic status (last year users)

Products Used	*Total (n = 338)*	*Socioeconomic Status*		
		Low (n = 72)	*Middle (n = 176)*	*High (n = 90)*
Flowers and pressed cannabis	21%	23%	22%	18%
Flowers only	63%	47%	65%	71%
Pressed cannabis only	14%	29%	12%	6%
DK/NA	2%	0%	1%	5%
Total	100%	100%	100%	100%

Source: Monitor Cannabis Uruguay Survey on the Use of Cannabis (2017)

Chi square $p < .001$

According to hospital discharge records, between 2011 and 2017, there was great stability in drug-related cases (about 1% of total discharges). There was an increase in "Mental and behavioral disorders due to the use of cannabinoids" between 2013 and 2017, from 20 to 75 cases. However, this figure represents less than 2% of total drug-related cases in 2017.[28]

Drug-Related Mortality

The available data confirm the hypothesis that the number of drug-related deaths would not change after regulation. According to OUD statistics, less than 1% of total deaths were related to narcotics between 2012 and 2017.[29]

Security Objectives Results

Results are organized around the discussion of the four hypotheses related to impacts on security.

Hypothesis: The Illegal Marijuana Market Will Decrease in Number of Consumers and Volume

The landscape is much more complex than expected. The use of the traditional product (pressed cannabis) has declined, but new illegal products have appeared. The number of pressed cannabis users declined from 58% in 2014 to 22% in 2017 and 12% in 2018. Traditional traffickers compete with legal cannabis and with non-legal local growers who sell their product. The lack of accurate estimates of the volume of each product consumed (flowers and pressed cannabis) makes it difficult to evaluate change in the scale of the illegal market. The only available measurement for the presence of pressed cannabis comes from seizures data. This indicator remained stable at 2.7 tons on average each year over the period 2013–2017. Traditional trafficking has survived, but regulation has reduced its market control; 23% of prior-year users bought directly from traffickers in 2014 compared to only 13% in 2017. This is a positive result because less contact with traffickers is less exposure to the risk of violence and to the offer of other drugs when buying.

Hypothesis: The Presence and Activity of Drug Trafficking Should Decrease After Regulation Because Cannabis Is an Important Part of the Whole Drug Business

Regulation and new competitors have reduced traffickers' participation in the market, but they still consider it a profitable activity. Some evidence suggests that there have been changes in the traditional illegal business. The police report that cannabis from Paraguay enters through the Brazilian border using automobiles lined with bricks of pressed cannabis. These shipments contain from 100 to 300 kilos while, prior to 2013, it was common for police to detect 500-kilo shipments entering Uruguay in small aircraft. This data suggest that there are no dominant importers in the business of pressed cannabis from Paraguay. It seems that small actors with the potential to distribute cannabis are undertaking the entry of the substance into the territory. Before the regulation of cannabis, these small actors used to buy the product from importers with the financial resources to sustain a large import operation.

Hypothesis: In the Short Term, an Increase in Systemic Homicides Might Occur (Homicides Between Members of Organized Gangs of Drug Traffickers). In the Long Term, Systemic Homicides Linked to Narcotics Should Be Reduced.

As expected, the number of homicides grew during the period 2013–2018, but I propose that cannabis regulation did not contribute to this violence.

First, it is difficult to establish that cannabis regulation preceded the increase in criminal conflict because it began before the regulation. Homicides related to criminal conflicts peaked in 2012 (Garat 2015; Müller Sienra and Draper 2017). That is an indication that causes of conflict were prevalent in the illicit drug markets, even before regulation.

Second, it is also difficult to establish a correlation between cannabis regulation and the outbreak of criminal conflict. The regulatory law was approved in December 2013 and the regulatory decrees were established in 2014 (for recreational and industrial cannabis) and 2015 (for medicinal cannabis). The implementation of regulations for home growers and clubs began in 2014. However, the first cannabis clubs were not approved until 2015 (IRCCA 2018). Cannabis sales through pharmacies started in July 2017. Total pharmacy sales (since 2017) reached 2.2 tons in January 2019. Therefore, regulation progressed very slowly in Uruguay, but the amount of criminal conflict rose steadily from 2012 to 2018 (see Table 6.4). The homicide rate in the country grew from 7.7 per 100,000 inhabitants in 2012 to 11.8 in 2018. Most importantly, homicides due to criminal conflict is the only category that increased during the study period; conflicts between criminals represented 29% of all homicides in 2012 and 47% in 2018 (see Table 6.4).

Third, there is insufficient legal supply to satisfy market demand. As a result, traffickers still have a market niche, though their product is less preferred by users. Interviews with traffickers confirm that cannabis remains an important product for them, but it is not the main source of profit (which are cocaine and cocaine paste base). Therefore, there is little support for the notion of regulation initiating a strangulation effect among traffickers.

Fourth, alternative hypotheses may give a better explanation for the criminal conflict associated with the illicit drug markets. Parallel to regulation, the Ministry of Interior has followed a policy of systematic persecution of micro-traffic. Micro-traffic is an important security problem due to the criminal acts surrounding the outlets. These outlets often sell more than one drug, and it is common to find cocaine, cocaine paste base, and illegal cannabis. Prior research shows that this kind of enforcement policy tends to produce violence in drug markets (Werb et al. 2011). This policy encourages criminal conflict among those who want to grow at the expense of competitors and interacts with preexisting conflicts over territorial control. Territorial control is one of the most important triggers of conflict in the drug market (El País 2017; Dos Santos 2018; Baudean 2018b). Furthermore, this policy forces distributors to articulate business with retailers to secure their market share. Retailers who try to deal with more than one distributor are punished. Other sources of violence in the drug market include

- Theft among distributors or owners of retail outlets. This is so common that retail outlets have security cameras to prevent attacks.

Table 6.4 Homicides, by motive or circumstance (total country, 2013–2018)

	2012	*2013*	*2014*	*2015*	*2017*	*2018*
Conflicts between criminals	29%	31%	35%	37%	45%	47%
Mugging/theft	14%	23%	17%	19%	13%	11%
Domestic violence	17%	17%	18%	18%	13%	12%
Spontaneous disputes	18%	12%	17%	11%	16%	12%
Conflicts because of debts/properties	–	2%	–	–	–	–
Other motives	8%	5%	5%	6%	5%	3%
Unknown motive	14%	11%	8%	10%	8%	15%
Total	**100%**	**100%**	**100%**	**100%**	**100%**	**100%**

Source: Ministry of Interior

- Disputes between members at different levels of the same organization (for example, when a member at the base wants to start growing his or her own business).
- Debts related to drug business or drug use. These debts may have originated in prison.
- Kidnapping of narcotraffickers for ransom.
- Violence caused by interpersonal disputes. Gang members are armed; therefore, personal disputes with others for reasons unrelated to the drug market can be resolved with violence.

In sum, violence is necessary to ensure product sales and market share and to send "costly signals"[30] (Gambetta 2009) in a market where credit is one of the most important tools used to grow influence (from importers to distributors, from distributors to retailers, and from retailers to consumers).

No direct effects of the reform on criminal violence have been observed. As discussed earlier, violence within drug markets has complex and multiple sources. On the one hand, the increase in micro-trafficking repression pushes market players to integrate vertically to protect their businesses (distribution and retail). On the other hand, the proliferation of small groups makes the control of drug sale territories unstable. It is unlikely that the advent of the regulation of only one illicit drug could alleviate existing tensions. All this suggests that criminal conflict in the drug market cannot be addressed effectively with the regulation of cannabis.

Conclusions

As I said at the beginning of the chapter, notions of harm reduction and human rights inspired Uruguayan regulation of cannabis. The policy is respectful of the individual consumption decision and aims to improve the quality of the product consumed, reducing access risks. Concomitantly, it has objectives related to security and the enforcement of drug laws. What has regulation achieved? What is there left to do? What can we learn from the experience so far? Those questions I will try to discuss here.

A general assessment of cannabis regulation for adult use in Uruguay can be divided into two main components. On the one hand, the so-called Uruguayan experiment shows that state regulation is a good institutional arrangement to legalize previously illicit drugs at a national level. Even when regulation has not been fully implemented, as in Uruguay, public health results show that positive changes outweigh negative ones. Since the start of cannabis regulation five years ago, users have gained access to better products and user contact with traffickers has been reduced by displacing illicit trade networks. Furthermore, no health crisis has emerged. Therefore, cannabis regulation seems to improve the legal situation of users, keeping them away from the criminal justice system and from traffickers, as well as causing no harm in terms of adverse public health effects. On the other hand, the Uruguayan experiment shows that the regulation of a single substance is not enough to contain the violence of drug markets. Violence is embedded in the functioning of drug markets. The regulation of cannabis is still far from having succeeded in suppressing the conditions that give rise to violence in these contexts. In the following discussion, I develop this general assessment.

Legal market. The establishment of a legal market is a key mechanism for the achievement of expected results under regulation. This point appears as one of the weaknesses of the Uruguayan experience. There are currently only 16 pharmacies distributing in the country, and none of them can use the banking system. The limited number of pharmacies makes access to cannabis unequal. Most of the pharmacies are concentrated in the capital of the country (6 of 16), and even within Montevideo the number of pharmacies is limited in low-income areas. There are several reasons for this result. The bidding process to choose companies that produce legal cannabis is long and complex. Quality standards for cannabis distributed in pharmacies constrain supply. The international financial system also restricts the development of the distribution of the product. It is clear that satisfying the demand for recreational cannabis through a legal market is more challenging than anticipated in 2013.

Harm reduction and human rights. Indicators of harm reduction and human rights suggest positive results associated with Uruguayan regulation. Users can access products of better quality than they could before regulation, and the exposure to traffickers and violence has declined. Considering that the legal market is still under construction, how did this happen? The Uruguayan experience shows that, in the absence of dispensary supply, local growers assume the role of supplying the market. These local growers have no links to traditional drug trafficking, and consequently, the exposure of cannabis users to drug trafficking networks has declined. This situation was not anticipated in 2013 when the law was drafted and the main concern of policy makers was how to use state distribution to displace drug trafficking. There has been a marked decrease in the number of customers engaging with illicit markets controlled by drug traffickers because users buy or obtain their cannabis from local growers. Given these results, several questions arise. Is it necessary for the state to be the main supplier in a regulatory scheme? Or is it better to allow sourcing through local growers by increasing control over their production and marketing activities? If the goal is to displace traditional drug trafficking networks and ensure that the user has access to cannabis without being exposed to criminal networks, either option can ensure the result.

Public health. Prior to the regulation of cannabis, dire predictions of a health crisis were made in Uruguay (Garat 2015; Müller Sienra and Draper 2017). These predictions were unfounded. Though cannabis use prevalence rates have increased among adults, they are not even close to the level for alcohol and tobacco. Among adolescents, cannabis use has increased, and currently has the same prevalence rate as tobacco. Based on the experiences in Colorado and Washington, increased adolescent use in Uruguay might be explained by underdeveloped distribution through pharmacies. When the state becomes the main supplier, traffickers and local producers will not be able to compete in price. In such a scenario, it will be more difficult for adolescents to obtain cannabis. The risk of problematic use is stable in both populations. The most commonly abused drug is still alcohol. The hypothesized decrease in legal and illegal drug consumption as a result of cannabis regulation is yet to be confirmed in the case of Uruguay. However, many questions remain. How does cannabis regulation influence the consumption of other legal and illegal drugs? In order to be able to evaluate the link between cannabis and other drugs, more longitudinal research needs to be conducted.

Security. The Uruguayan case shows that systemic violence associated with drug markets has not decreased with the legalization of cannabis. Expectations of drastic changes in rates of systemic violence in the drug markets should therefore be reconsidered. Five conclusions can be drawn from the Uruguayan experience on this matter.

First, it is important to harmonize the whole security policy carried out by the state. The regulation of a substance does not necessarily imply a change in traditional drug policies focused on the repression of micro-trafficking. Such policies generally encourage criminal conflict. In Uruguay, the increase in repression of micro-trafficking since 2015 has interacted with preexisting conflicts between gangs. Additionally, the successful capture of drug trafficking leaders from opposing gangs has transformed prisons into places of conflict due to distribution rivalries.

Second, trafficking is a form of employment. While regulation in Uruguay removes an existing source of income, it does not offer a legal alternative. Trafficking networks try to adapt quickly to the new situation and look for substitutes for cannabis commerce. Therefore, the big challenge in reducing trafficking is how to offer legal and economically viable alternative employment to those involved.

Third, it seems that the pattern of conflict in the drug markets is not dependent on the substances. Instead, it depends on the kinds of relationships that illicit markets produce. Unregulated drug markets are characterized by patterns of relationships that often lead to conflict. The impossibility of resolving conflicts between competitors through legal means is an important one. Another factor is that there are multiple sources of conflict: growth through territorial expansion, debts due to credit sales, and theft among distributors, among others. In Uruguay, conflict is concentrated in the most vulnerable areas of Montevideo and big inland cities. While the homicide rate in 2017 was 12 per 100,000 inhabitants in Montevideo, the homicide rate in the most violence-prone areas ranged from 17 to 20 per 100,000 inhabitants (Baudean 2018c). In those areas, inhabitants consider the drug business very attractive and a way of survival or social mobility. Regulation of one substance does not eliminate conflicts that arise from other illegal substance trafficking. That is why the legalization of a single drug may not be sufficient to stop violence.

Fourth, it is necessary to propose policies to reduce criminal recidivism for people linked to the illicit drug business. In Uruguay, drug law violators are mainly prosecuted for drug trafficking or supply. Prisons are a key environment in which the construction of criminal networks and staff recruitment can occur (Pereyra 2016; Losa 2018). Even when the police capture a gang leader, the gang's business can still be managed from prison. Many times wives or younger relatives direct the operations in their territory. Sometimes these operators are more prone to violence. It is necessary to think about how to work with people in prison and what rehabilitation strategies will be used to generate changes in drug trafficking networks. The discussion of this topic has been absent from the debate. During the period analyzed, laws that increase penalties for drug offenses (making exceptions for cannabis) have been enacted (Baudean 2018a). These policies increase the time offenders remain in prison, making it even more difficult for them to reintegrate into legal activities. Finally, Uruguay has a growing incarcerated population[31] and, although cannabis is one of the main drugs used by inmates, they have no legal access to it (OPS 2016).

In closing, Uruguay has drafted one of the most advanced laws on cannabis regulation, but it has had a difficult implementation experience. As a consequence, it faces significant challenges in the short term. On the one hand, the weakness of Uruguayan regulation is the underdevelopment of licensed retail. Currently, a significant portion of the supply remains illegal (mainly unregistered local producers). Traffickers have been displaced as main suppliers because their product is of poor quality. However, traffickers are trying to find a way to stay in the cannabis business. There are indicators of this attempt, such as the increasing number of flower buds in police seizures. On the other hand, the slow growth of participation by pharmacies in the legal business is a crucial problem for the future of regulation. More importantly, and as of this writing, the right-wing coalition is in office and very critical of sales through pharmacies. Finally, most local growers are not registered. For that reason, when they sell their product, they commit a crime. Until March 2020, the police did not consider these producers a target. However, the promise of the new government is greater repression of trafficking at all levels. If the police decide to target local producers and it produces scarcity in illicit cannabis supply, while there is no improvement in the legal supply, who will step in to satisfy demand?

Until now, the key role played by local cannabis growers has remedied implementation flaws. Decision makers are aware of the situation and in possession of adequate information and analysis to enable the improvement of cannabis regulations. However, the future is uncertain because the political context has changed in Uruguay. Implementation time has been extended to three governments since the law was passed in 2013. Two governments on the left and one on the right (as of 2020). During this time, regulation has faced more resistance from the Ministry of Health (a key agency) than from citizens or politicians. In addition, the current minister of health comes from the far-right party "Cabildo Abierto." This political party is the only one, along with the evangelist deputies, that advocates for the repeal of the cannabis law on moral grounds. Thus, it is unlikely that there will be an improvement in the present circumstances.

Notes

1 I use the term regulation as it is defined by Transform Drug Policy Foundation as "a set of legal rules and enforcement infrastructure designed to control or govern certain types of products and conduct . . .

Activities that take place beyond the parameters of a given regulatory framework remain prohibited and subject to legal sanctions" (Rolles 2009, 19).

2 See for a rare example Obradovic 2019, comparing Colorado, Washington, and Uruguay.

3 In this document, I retain the Spanish acronym to help readers locate the original sources.

4 In Uruguay, the Supreme Court, the judiciary, and the administration of the courts are together in the Judicial Power.

5 The UCRIS considers that there are no benefits derived from cannabis consumption in the population under 18.

6 International Statistical Classification of Diseases and Related Health Problems, 10th edition.

7 Cannabis Abuse Screening Test.

8 Pressed cannabis is the traditional illicit product in Uruguay; it is also consumed in Brazil, Argentina, and Chile. Pressed cannabis is produced in Paraguay. It enters Uruguay mainly through the border with Brazil. The product combines flowers with other parts of the plant. For that reason, its potency is variable, but in general it is considered a low-potency product. Cannabis and other products are pressed together to form bricks. The composition of non-vegetal products varies, and it is scarcely known. The mechanism of pressing the product facilitates international traffic.

9 A preliminary analysis of the Interdisciplinary Group of Cannabis Studies (Medical School and Chemistry faculty at the Universidad de la República, the major university in the country) identified 52 toxic agents in pressed cannabis (Delgado 2015).

10 Systemic homicides are homicides between members of organized gangs of drug traffickers (Goldstein 1985).

11 Monitor Cannabis Uruguay is an independent research team working at the School of Social Science of Universidad de la República (Montevideo, Uruguay).

12 There are two main surveys: one for students and the other for the adult population. The target population of the Student Survey is adolescents from 13 to 17 years old who attend secondary school in cities with 10,000 or more inhabitants. A representative sample of the target population and the five regions of the country is obtained based on a two-stage stratified sampling. In the first stage the schools and in the second stage the classes were the sampling units. Finally, the totality of the students of the selected classes completed the survey questionnaire. I use the VI and VII edition of the survey (2014 and 2016) to discuss the results of regulation. The target population of the Adult Survey is persons between 15 and 65 years of age living in urban areas with 10,000 or more inhabitants. A random sample is drawn stratified by conglomerates in several stages of selection. I compare VI edition of the survey (2014) with MCU Survey on the Use of Cannabis (2017) to discuss the results of cannabis regulation. Recently the JND has communicated results from the Student and from the Adult Survey, 2018 edition. I will use the available data of the new edition of both surveys.

13 Monitor Cannabis administered a survey in November and December of 2017 to a representative sample of 2,181 residents between the age of 15 and 65 in towns with 10,000 or more inhabitants in Uruguay. A team of researchers from Monitor Cannabis, the University of the Republic, the Catholic University of Uruguay, University ORT Uruguay, and the University of California Davis prepared the questionnaire.

14 Traffickers perceive flower buds as having less risk of seizure by the police; there is no need for international contacts to obtain the product, and it is preferred by users.

15 The estimation came mainly from the MCU National Survey. The survey asks for the total quantity the person consumed in the last month. Interviews were conducted with respondents to calibrate the questionnaire wording. Images were used to represent 1 gram of cannabis. Interview responses were consistent with user reports obtained through other questionnaires (frequency, for example). Responses were also consistent with an RDS Survey implemented by Catholic University of Uruguay with weekly users (Queirolo, Boidi, and Cruz 2018). As Robin Room and colleagues argue, self-report population surveys to replicate total consumption systematically underestimate the market. Self-report population surveys provide an estimate of about two thirds of total consumption (Room et al. 2010, 61).

16 Data comes from MCU Survey 2017. The average ways of access to cannabis for pharmacy buyers is 1.8 with a standard deviation of 1.3.

17 According to the most recent edition of JND Adult Survey (2018).

18 In January 2019, 1 gram of legal flowers cost US $1.15, while 1 gram of illegal flowers cost US $5.01 and a gram of pressed cannabis US 0.57. Sources: Interview with users (2017–2018), Monitor Cannabis Uruguay Survey on the Use of Cannabis (2017), IRCCA, the Police.

19 A recent report by the JND estimated prior year use in 15% of adult population (Junta Nacional de Drogas and Observatorio Uruguayo de Drogas 2019).

20 This relates to those who started using cannabis between 2011 and 2014 compared to those who started using cannabis between 2014 and 2017.

21 It is a ranking developed by UNASUR, based on data provided by each South American state. UNASUR (Unión de Naciones Suramericanas) is the Union of South American Nations. The organization was created in 2008 to propel regional integration on issues including democracy, education, energy, environment, infrastructure, and security and to eliminate social inequality and exclusion.

22 The proportions remain stable if compared with the previous report (Junta Nacional de Drogas and Observatorio Uruguayo de Drogas 2018).

23 The source is the Uruguayan Drug Observatory system of information "Tratamiento registra." It covers 66% of the total number of clinics specialized in drug treatment. There is no other source of data in Uruguay. The data presented are updated as of December 2018.

24 Data reflects total consultations according to "Tratamiento registra." It is not based on a sample.

25 In 2017, 36% of users reported using products with a range of 6%–9% THC, while 7% reported using products with 20% or more THC.

26 This data refers to the complete universe of hospital discharges; it is not based on a sample.

27 In 2015, the presence of the most important substances reported were the following: alcohol 38%, cocaine 35%, cocaine paste 27%, benzodiazepines 22%, and cannabis 21%.

28 Data comes from the Uruguayan Drug Observatory.

29 The OUD produces data based on the vital statistics of the Ministry of Health. The reference universe is the total number of deaths recorded in the country between 2012 and 2017.

30 This refers to actions designed to inform and give credibility to the information being conveyed. That is why they are "costly" (Gambetta 2009).

31 According to World Prison Brief, Uruguay ranks 34th in a list of 222 countries according to its population in prison (295 prisoners per 100,000 inhabitants) (World Prison Brief n.d.).

References

Aguiar, Sebastián, Florencia Lemos, and Clara Musto. 2019. "In the Backyard: Cannabis Self-Cultivation in Uruguay 2014–2018." Presentation at the 13th. International Society for the Study of Drug Policy Conference, Paris School of Economics, Paris, May 2019.

Anderson, D. Mark, Benjamin Hansen, Daniel I. Rees, and Joseph J. Sabia. 2019. "Association of Marijuana Laws with Teen Marijuana Use: New Estimates from the Youth Risk Behavior Surveys." *JAMA Pediatrics* 173 (9) (July): 879–81.

Baudean, Marcos. 2018a. "Línea de base para la evaluación y monitoreo de la regulación del cannabis recreativo en Uruguay. Objetivo Aplicación de la Justicia." *Monitor Cannabis*. http://monitorcannabis.uy/informe-sobre-el-objetivo-aplicacion-de-la-justicia-de-la-regulacion-del-cannabis-recreativo-en-uruguay-linea-de-base/.

———. 2018b. "Línea de base para la evaluación y monitoreo de la regulación del cannabis recreativo en Uruguay. Objetivo Seguridad y Convivencia." *Monitor Cannabis*. http://monitorcannabis.uy/informe-sobre-el-objetivo-seguridad-de-la-regulacion-del-cannabis-recreativo-en-uruguay-linea-de-base/.

———. 2018c. "Una primera lectura sobre los resultados de la regulación del cannabis en Uruguay a cinco años de promulgada la ley 19.172." Presentation at Congreso Cinco años de la regulación del cannabis, Facultad de Ciencias Sociales, Montevideo, December 2018c.

———. 2019. "Five Years of Cannabis Regulation in Uruguay: What Are the Changes in Health, Security and Justice? What Can We Learn from the Uruguayan Experience of Regulation?" Presentation at the 13th. International Society for the study of Drug Policy Conference, Paris School of Economics, Paris, May 2019.

Boidi, María Fernanda, Rosario Queirolo, and José Miguel Cruz. 2016. "Cannabis Consumption Patterns among Frequent Consumers in Uruguay." *International Journal of Drug Policy* 34 (June): 34–40.

CDPS. 2018. *Impacts of Marijuana Legalization in Colorado*. Denver, CO: U.S. Colorado Department of Public Safety, Division of Criminal Justice, Research Report.

Cerdá, Magdalena, and Beau Kilmer. 2017. "Uruguay's Middle-Ground Approach to Cannabis Legalization." *International Journal of Drug Policy* 42 (April): 118–20.

Cruz, José Miguel, María Fernanda Boidi, and Rosario Queirolo. 2018a. "Saying no to Weed: Public Opinion Towards Cannabis Legalization in Uruguay." *Drugs: Education, Prevention and Policy* 25 (1) (November): 67–76.

———. 2018b. "The Status of Support for Cannabis Regulation in Uruguay 4 Years after Reform: Evidence from Public Opinion Surveys." *Drug and Alcohol Review* 37 (April): S429–S434.

Decorte, Tom et al. 2017. "Regulating Cannabis Social Clubs: A Comparative Analysis of Legal and Self-Regulatory Practices in Spain, Belgium and Uruguay." *International Journal of Drug Policy* 43 (February): 44–56.

Delgado, Nicolás. 2015. "La Universidad crea laboratorio para investigar la marihuana." *El Observador*, September 21.

Dilley, Julia A. et al. 2018. "Prevalence of Cannabis Use in Youths after Legalization in Washington State." *JAMA Pediatrics* 173 (2) (December): 192–93.

Dos Santos, Camilo. 2018. "Quién es quién entre los narcos uruguayos." *El Observador*, November 25.

El País. 2017. "Los muertos que llora el 40 Semanas." *El País*, April 9.

Evans, Von Jennifer. 2016. "Uruguay's Cannabis Policy: Pharmacists as Legal Dealers." *Pharmazeutische Zeitung* 161 (21) (May).

Fesur. 2014. *Estrategia para la evaluación de resultados y monitoreo de implementación de la ley 19.172*. Edited by Baudean Marcos, Gustavo Robaina, Clara Musto, and Martín Collazo. Montevideo: Uruguay. Fesur, Research Report.

———. 2015. *El módulo sobre Cannabis en la 6ta. Encuesta Nacional sobre Consumo de Drogas en Hogares*. Edited by Baudean Marcos, Gustavo Robaina, and Martín Collazo. Montevideo: Uruguay. Fesur, Research Report.

Gabinete de Seguridad. 2012. "Estrategia por la vida y la convivencia." *Presidencia*. https://medios.presidencia.gub.uy/jm_portal/2012/noticias/NO_E582/Estrategia.pdf.

Galain, Pablo. 2018. "The Uruguayan Model of Regulating Cannabis-Legal and Geopolitical Questions." *Zeitschrift fur die gesamte strafrechtswissenschaft* 130 (3) (October): 1–50.

Gambetta, Diego. 2009. *Codes of the Underworld. How Criminals Communicate*. Princeton, NJ: Princeton University Press.

Garat, Guillermo. 2015. *El camino. La regulación del cannabis en Uruguay según sus actores políticos y sociales*. Montevideo: Fesur.

———. 2016. "Uruguay: A Way to Regulate the Cannabis Market." In *Drug Policies and the Politics of Drugs in the Americas*, edited by Beatriz Caiuby Labate, Clancy Cavnar, and Thiago Rodrigues, 209–26. Manhattan, NY: Springer.

Goldstein, Paul J. 1985. "The drugs/Violence Nexus: A Tripartite Conceptual Framework." *Journal of Drug Issues* 39 (October): 143–74.

Hughes, C. E. 2018. "The Trajectories of Cannabis and Tobacco Policies in the United States, Uruguay, Canada and Portugal: Is More Cross-Substance Learning Possible Outside of the United States?" *Addiction* 113 (4) (August): 603–5.

IRCCA. 2018. *Mercado Regulado del Cannabis*. Informe al 05/04/18. Montevideo: Uruguay. IRCCA, Research Report.

———. 2019. *Mercado Regulado del Cannabis*. Informe al 30/01/19. Montevideo: Uruguay. IRCCA, Research Report.

———. N.d. "IRCCA." Accessed June 30, 2019. www.ircca.gub.uy/.

JND—Presidencia. 2019. "Comercio ilegal de cannabis se redujo más de cinco veces entre 2014 y 2018." *JND*. www.gub.uy/junta-nacional-drogas/comunicacion/noticias/comercio-ilegal-cannabis-se-redujo-cinco-veces-entre-2014-2018.

JND. 2014a. *Dimensión aplicación de la justicia con equidad. Aportes al diseño de evaluación y monitoreo de la ley 19.172*. Edited by Latorre Laura and Marcelo Brito. Montevideo: Uruguay. Junta Nacional de Drogas, Research Report.

———. 2014b. *Dimensión seguridad ciudadana y convivencia. Aportes al diseño de evaluación y monitoreo de la ley 19.172*. Edited by Latorre Laura and Ricardo Fraiman. Montevideo: Uruguay. Junta Nacional de Drogas, Research Report.

———. 2014c. *Dimensión Salud. Aportes al diseño de evaluación y monitoreo de la ley 19.172*. Edited by Suárez Héctor, Jessica Ramírez, and Leticia Keuroglian. Montevideo: Uruguay. Junta Nacional de Drogas, Research Report.

———. 2014d. *Ley 19.172*. Montevideo: Junta Nacional de Drogas.

Junta Nacional de Drogas and Observatorio Uruguayo de Drogas. 2011. *Sobre ruidos y nueces Consumo de drogas legales e ilegales en la adolescencia*. Montevideo: JND—OUD.

———. 2016. *VI Encuesta Nacional en Hogares sobre Consumo de Drogas*. Montevideo: JND—OUD.

———. 2018. *VII Encuesta Nacional sobre consumo de drogas en estudiantes de enseñanza media*. Montevideo: JND—OUD.

———. 2019. *VII Encuesta Nacional sobre Consumo de Drogas en población general*. Montevideo: JND—OUD.

———. 2020. *VIII Encuesta Nacional sobre consumo de drogas en estudiantes de enseñanza media*. Montevideo: JND—OUD.

Kilmer, Beau, and Mark A. R. Kleiman. 2018. "Navigating Cannabis Legalization 2.0." *The Hill*, December 4. https://thehill.com/blogs/congress-blog/healthcare/419627-navigating-cannabis-legalization-20.

Losa, Guillermo. 2018. "Mujeres en el narcotráfico: herederas en una guerra iniciada por hombres." *El Observador*, September 25.

Müller Sienra, Christian, and Guillermo Draper. 2017. *Marihuana oficial. Crónica de un experimento uruguayo*. Montevideo: Sudamericana.

Musto, Clara. 2018. "Regulating Cannabis Markets. The Construction of an Innovative Drug Policy in Uruguay." PhD dissertation, University of Kent/Universiteit Utrecht. https://kar.kent.ac.uk/id/eprint/68477.

Negrín, Alba. 2017. "Variedades de cannabis, patrones de uso y escenarios de riesgo." *JND*. www.gub.uy/junta-nacional-drogas/comunicacion/noticias/actividad-academica-evidencia-sobre-beneficios-y-riesgos-de-la-utilizacion-de.

NWHIDTA. 2017. *Washington State Marijuana Impact Report*. Vol. 2. Seattle, WA: U.S. Northwest High Intensity Drug Trafficking Area, Research Report.

Obradovic, Ivana. 2019. "From Prohibition to Regulation: A Comparative Analysis of the Emergence and Related Outcomes of New Legal Cannabis Policy Models (Colorado, Washington State and Uruguay)." *International Journal of Drug Policy*. Doi.org/10.1016/j.drugpo.2019.11.002.

OPS. 2016. *Salud y enfermedad en condiciones de privación de libertad: diagnóstico epidemiológico*. Edited by Levcovitz Eduardo, Fernández Galeano Miguel, Rodríguez Buño Ricardo, and Benia Wilson. Montevideo: Uruguay. OPP, Research Report.

Pardo, Bryce. 2014. "Cannabis Policy Reforms in the Americas: A Comparative Analysis of Colorado, Washington and Uruguay." *International Journal of Drug Policy* 25 (4) (July): 727–35.

Pereyra, Gabriel. 2016. "Bandas criminales. El crímen organizado ya está aquí." *El Observador*, May 23.

Queirolo, Rosario. 2020. "Uruguay: The First Country to Legalize Cannabis." In *Legalizing Cannabis. Experiences, Lessons and Scenarios*, edited by Tom Decorte, Simon Lenton, and Chris Wilkins. New York: Routledge.

Queirolo, Rosario, María Fernanda Boidi, and José Miguel Cruz. 2016. "Cannabis Clubs in Uruguay: The Challenges of Regulation." *International Journal of Drug Policy* 34 (August): 41–48.

———. 2018. "El impacto de la regulación de la marihuana en los consumidores frecuentes en Uruguay." Presentation at Congreso Cinco años de la regulación del cannabis, Facultad de Ciencias Sociales, Montevideo, December 2018.

Repetto, Lorena. 2014. "Regulación del cannabis ¿un asunto de seguridad? Entrada y mantenimiento en agenda de un problema de política pública." *Revista Uruguaya de Ciencia Política* 23 (1) (December): 119–41.

Rolles, Stephen. 2009. *After the War on Drugs: Blueprint for Regulation*. Bristol: Transform Drug Policy Foundation.

Room, Robin. 2014. "Legalizing a Market for Cannabis for Pleasure: Colorado, Washington, Uruguay and Beyond." *Addiction* 109 (3) (March): 345–51. Doi:10.1111/add.12355.

Room, Robin et al. 2010. *Cannabis Policy: Moving Beyond Stalemate*. New York: Oxford University Press.

Walsh, John, and Geoff Ramsey. 2018. "Cannabis Regulation in Uruguay: An Innovative Law Facing Major Challenges." *Journal of Drug Policy Analysis* 11 (1) (June).

Werb, Dan et al. 2011. "Effect of Drug Law Enforcement on Drug Market Violence: A Systemic Review." *International Journal of Drug Policy* 22 (2) (March): 87–94.

World Prison Brief. N.d. "Highest to Lowest." Accessed October 5, 2019. https://prisonstudies.org/highest-to-lowest/prison-population-total.

7

Medical Cannabis in the UK

The (False) Dawn of a New Era?

Melissa Bone and Gary R. Potter

Keywords: Cannabis, drug policy, medicine, criminal law, medical cannabis, human rights

Introduction

Officially, since November 2018, medical cannabis in the UK has been legal if authorised by a specialist physician. In reality, while access to CBD products[1] is widespread (and does not need authorisation by a doctor), legal access to preparations containing THC[2] remains highly constrained. However, demand for medical cannabis products is high, and many thousands of people do use cannabis medicinally but remain dependent on illegal sources. While the 2018 change in the law initially offered hope to those using medical cannabis illegally, the practical impact of the changes thus far has been infinitesimal. Those for whom medical cannabis may be beneficial continue to face a stark choice: either suffer the symptoms that could be treated were cannabis legally available or resort to committing criminal offences in pursuit of relief from their conditions.

In this chapter we discuss access to medical cannabis in the UK. We start with an overview of the demand for medical cannabis in the UK and how this demand has, under prohibition, been met by relying on criminal activity. We then outline the legal situation regarding medical cannabis in the UK following the changes of November 2018. Finally, we speculate on future developments, asking whether the 2018 changes really are the beginning of a new era of legal access to medical cannabis or merely a political sop to media and public pressure with little genuine impact for those who could benefit from medical cannabis.

The Demand for Medical Cannabis in the UK

Although now known primarily as an illegal recreational drug, there is a long history of medical cannabis use in the UK. As a tincture in alcohol, cannabis was a readily available and widely used medicine until 1971 when it was removed from the pharmacopeia (Nutt 2014). Under the Misuse of Drugs Act 1971 (MDA), cannabis possession, supply, cultivation, production and importation became criminal offences with no differentiation under the law between medical and nonmedical use.

DOI: 10.4324/9780429320491-7

Despite the risk of prosecution and potential imprisonment, it has been estimated that over 30,000 people use cannabis for medical purposes on a daily basis in the UK (Nutt 2014) and that this number could rise to over 1,000,000 if medical cannabis were legally available (APPG 2016). Medical users range from those who turn to cannabis only after diagnosis and failure to find effective legal treatment for their conditions to those who were already using cannabis recreationally but have come to recognise medical benefits on top of their original (nonmedical) reasons for using (Klein and Potter 2018). Cannabis is reported by UK users to alleviate a wide variety of mental and physical health conditions ranging from common, minor ailments to rare and serious illnesses (UPA 2016; Hakkarainen et al. 2015; see Table 7.1).

With very few exceptions, the tens of thousands of medical cannabis users in the UK are regularly committing criminal offences. Under s5(2) of the MDA the possession of cannabis is a criminal offence which carries a maximum penalty of five years' imprisonment, an unlimited fine or both. Procuring cannabis involves a greater degree of criminal involvement. Medical users, like recreational users, have a range of options. They can buy their cannabis from stereotypical drug dealers operating in the open market (cf. Hough and Natarajan 2000, 4), thus facilitating drug supply offences and possibly supporting the serious and organised crime that can overlap with commercial criminal markets.[3] Obtaining cannabis from these sorts of dealers poses many risks. In this scenario, buyers face a greater risk of coming to the attention of the criminal justice system and of being ripped off or otherwise victimised by the dealers they turn to. They also face uncertainties over the

Table 7.1 Top medical conditions for which cannabis users self-report medicinal use in two UK surveys

UPA (2016)		*Hakkarainen et al. (2015)*	
Condition	*Respondents (%*)*	*Condition*	*Respondents (%*)*
Depression	30.0	Depression/other mood disorders	52.5
Anxiety	26.3	Anxiety or panic disorders	36.1
Pain	24.1	Chronic pain (e.g., fibromyalgia)	31.1
Arthritis	12.7	Inflammation of the joints (arthritis)	29.7
Insomnia	10.9	Migraines and headaches	26.5
Fibromyalgia	9.1	Bowel problems	16.4
PTSD	6.6	PTSD	9.1
Spinal damage	6.6	Asthma	8.2
IBS	6.3	Hypertension	7.8
Trauma/injury	5.9	ADHD	6.8
Multiple sclerosis	5.6	Dependence and withdrawal from other drugs	6.4
ADHD	4.8	Autism and Asperger's syndrome	5.5
Migraines	4.5	Cancer	4.1
Neuropathy	4.2	Anorexia	2.7
Cancer	4.0	Eye disease (glaucoma)	2.3
Sciatica	3.0	Nausea (e.g., after chemotherapy)	2.3
Crohn's	3.0	Multiple sclerosis	2.3
Asthma	2.6	Hepatitis	1.8
Bipolar disorder	2.2	HIV/AIDS	0.9
		Schizophrenia	0.5
		Tourette's	0.5
		Other	40.2

Sources: UPA (2016); Hakkarainen et al. (2015)

* Percentages total more than 100 as many respondents report multiple conditions.

quality, potency and purity—and, thus, the medical efficacy—of what they are buying (Potter and Klein 2020). For those already vulnerable—and often desperate—due to their medical conditions, being structurally forced into contact with criminal dealers is far from ideal (Klein and Potter 2018).

For those with the right connections, cannabis can be secured by suppliers who are not involved in other types of crime and who do not seek to exploit their customers—that is, 'friendly businesses' or 'social supply' networks (see, e.g., Potter 2009; Werse and Bernard 2016). This minimises exposure to risks associated with the open market and links to more serious criminals, but these approaches to supply are usually focused on recreational users and may not provide the best product for those seeking medical benefit.

Another option for medical users is to grow their own cannabis or to get other people to grow cannabis for them (Potter 2010; Potter et al. 2015). This allows them some control over the product—experienced growers tailor the cannabis they produce, by selecting different strains and controlling the growing environment, to have the combination of cannabinoids that work best to treat their symptoms (Klein and Potter 2018; Hakkarainen et al. 2015). It also removes the need to rely on 'real' dealers (i.e., those who are driven by profit and are involved in other criminal activity; cf. Parker 2000; Potter 2009) and the risks associated with participating in the open drug market. However, growing cannabis—at least, of the quality needed to maximise the medical benefits—needs skill, specialist equipment, time and space—resources that may not be available to all medical users, especially those who have crippling conditions or limited incomes because of their ill health (Potter and Klein 2020). Depending on more able friends or family to grow on their behalf carries the extra moral burden of having others break the law on their behalf, and the economic costs still have to be borne by either the grower or the user (Klein and Potter 2018).

A final option is to import medical cannabis from countries where it is legally available, an approach that has been reported in the press and to parliamentary committees seeking evidence to support possible changes to the law (see, e.g., Health and Social Care Committee 2019b). This involves the time and money needed for international travel and the legal challenges of bringing such products back into the UK.

Caught between the criminal law and their own illnesses, it is perhaps not surprising that medical users have become increasingly proactive in their efforts to enable access to cannabis. Two trends are particularly noteworthy here. First, many medical users form their own mutual supply networks enabling access to known-quality cannabis for those in need without them having to contact the sorts of drug dealers who are linked to other types of crime[4] (Potter 2010; Klein and Potter 2018; Pardal et al. 2020). However, involvement in growing, supplying or importing cannabis all carry more serious penalties under the MDA than simple possession—whether done by mutual supply networks or organised crime groups. It is an irony that altruistically motivated efforts to support medical users in avoiding the criminal market involve greater levels of criminality—and the risk of more serious criminal penalties—than simple possession (Potter and Klein 2020). It is noteworthy that UK law does not recognise medical use as an acceptable justification for possession, cultivation or supply: in a 2005 judgment, the Court of Appeal of England and Wales held that the common law defence of necessity was not available to defendants cultivating or possessing cannabis for personal use, or to defendants who intended to supply cannabis to others, for the purposes of alleviating pain (see, e.g., R v. Quayle and Others 2005[5]; see also Bone 2020 for a detailed overview of cannabis case law in the UK).

A second, parallel (and often overlapping) trend has seen patient groups emerge as increasingly vociferous campaign organisations lobbying for legal access to medical cannabis (see, e.g., www.upalliance.org; www.endourpain.org; www.carlysamnesty.org). Notably, in recent years, these campaigns have received the backing of a number of high-profile figures, including current and former politicians, celebrities, and respected medical and criminal justice professionals. Already bolstered by the increasing body of scientific evidence for the efficacy of medical cannabis to treat a range of conditions (see, e.g., Barnes and Barnes 2016) and the legalisation of medical cannabis in a growing number of jurisdictions around the world, the campaign for medical cannabis in the UK received a further boost in 2018 when two cases of young boys (Billy Caldwell and Alfie Dingley) with severe forms of epilepsy received extensive sympathetic media coverage. Both boys had responded well to cannabis treatment but were unable to continue using their medicines legally in the UK. The groundswell of public support following these cases is credited as the tipping point that led to the 2018 change in the law (Bone 2020). These changes were initially hailed by campaigners, with Jon Liebling, the Political Director of the United Patients Alliance, describing November 1, 2018, as "a long overdue and historical day for medical cannabis in the UK" (Liebling 2019). However, initial enthusiasm quickly waned as it became apparent that the change in the law was likely to apply only to a tiny number of medical cannabis users, leaving most having to continue committing criminal offences if they were to treat their conditions with cannabis.

The Emergence of—and Limits to—Legal Medical Cannabis

International law calls for countries to prohibit the use of cannabis and to criminalise its production and supply, except for medical or scientific purposes (Dorn and Jamieson 2000). Cannabis, cannabis resin, extracts and tinctures of cannabis are grouped together in Schedule I of the United Nations Single Convention on Narcotic Drugs (1961), with the cannabis plant and cannabis resin also included in Schedule IV. Substances in both schedules are considered under the Single Convention to be particularly liable to abuse and to have little or no therapeutic value.

Historically, UK drug policy has been closely aligned to the UN conventions with, if anything, stricter domestic laws than necessary to fulfil obligations under the international legislation (Dorn and Jamieson 2000). In the UK, possession, supply, cultivation, production, importation and exportation of cannabis are criminal offences under the MDA. Until recently, cannabis was placed in Schedule 1 of the Misuse of Drugs Regulations (2001) (MDR), a restrictive schedule which, like the international legislation, considers the drug to have little or no therapeutic value. However, the accumulating scientific evidence, legalisation of medical cannabis in other jurisdictions, and cases such as Alfie Dingley and Billy Caldwell led to the UK government reviewing the scheduling of cannabis under the MDR and the medical potential of cannabis formally being acknowledged in UK law.

Following a review conducted by Professor Dame Sally Davies, the chief medical officer (CMO) for England, and agreed upon by the Advisory Council on the Misuse of Drugs (ACMD), it was decided that cannabis-based products for medicinal use (CBPMUs) should reside in the less restrictive Schedule 2 of the MDR (Davies 2018). Consequently, on the November 1, 2018, the Misuse of Drugs (Amendments) (Cannabis and Licence Fees) (England, Wales and Scotland) Regulations (2018) (the 2018 Regulations) amended previous regulations, moving CBPMUs to Schedule 2. Effectively, this means that there is now a legal route for cannabis-based products for medicinal use to be prescribed by specialist clinicians. A "cannabis based product for medicinal use" has been defined by the UK government as a medicinal product or a substance used in the preparation of a medicinal product, which contains cannabis, cannabis resin, cannabinol or a cannabinol derivative, produced for medicinal use in humans (see s3 of the 2018 Regulations).

This legal change does not explicitly state which medical conditions could benefit from cannabis medicines. In theory, any patient with a medical condition where there is clear published evidence of benefit, and where all other licensed treatment options have been exhausted, is potentially eligible for medicinal cannabis (see the 2018 Regulations; Department of Health and Social Care 2018). These criteria are clearly ambiguous. In practice, the early professional guidance is focused on cannabis use for a very small number of medical conditions, including chemotherapy-induced nausea and vomiting, pain (both neuropathic and in a palliative care context), spasticity in multiple sclerosis, and paediatric epilepsy conditions (British Paediatric Neurology Association (BPNA) 2018; Royal College of Physicians (RCP) 2018). Initially, it is likely that these conditions will be seen as more suitable for unlicensed CBPMUs. Indeed, the National Institute for Clinical Excellence (NICE) guidance (2019a) affirms the narrow focus on prescribing recommendations for the aforementioned medical conditions, effectively excluding other medical conditions until further evidence becomes available.

Though the law has a broader applicability in theory than the very small number of medical conditions focused on in the guidance, in practice specialist clinicians are erroneously interpreting the existing guidance on prescribing as proscriptive, thus excluding whole categories of patients for whom cannabis could have a therapeutic effect (see The Medicinal Cannabis Clinicians Society and the APPG on Medical Cannabis under Prescription 2019). Excluding general practitioners (GPs) from prescribing also reduces the availability and accessibility of medicinal cannabis in practice, since cannabis is seen as a symptom treatment as opposed to a cure for many conditions. General practitioners would therefore be better placed than specialist clinicians to adopt a more holistic approach to medical cannabis prescribing (ibid.).

The legal definition of a CBPMU also leads to a further discrepancy between the availability and accessibility of medical cannabis in theory and in practice. Since a CBPMU is defined as 'a medicinal product', a clear distinction is drawn between CBPMUs residing in Schedule 2 of the MDR and 'street' cannabis which continues to reside in Schedule 1, with criminal sanctions under the MDA still attached. With cannabis products not clearly recognised as CBPMUs still criminalised and the cost of prescribing a distinct (licensed or unlicensed) CBPMU, the availability and accessibility of medicinal cannabis in practice has remained severely limited.

In the UK, all CBPMUs, apart from nabiximols (marketed as Sativex®), Epidyolex® and Nabilone, are currently unlicensed. In theory, a specialist clinician is able to prescribe an unlicensed CBPMU, Nabilone, Epidyolex® or Sativex® (a product which has a market authorisation and resides in Schedule 4 of the MDR). However, in practice, National Institute for Health and Clinical Excellence guidelines (NICE 2014) do not recommend that Sativex® is prescribed on the National Health Service (NHS) due to its high cost. The prescription of Nabilone is also infrequent: it is a synthetic cannabinoid and only recommended when other treatments have failed and under the close supervision of a specialist doctor (NHS 2018). NICE's draft guidance on medical cannabis further recommended that Epidyolex® should not be prescribed on the NHS for children with two severe forms of epilepsy due to the lack of evidence of its clinical efficacy, the fact that its long-term effect remains unclear, and concerns about its cost (NICE 2019b, 2019c). At the time of writing, however, NICE has since recommended that Epidyolex® be prescribed on the NHS, despite the previous concerns (GW Pharmaceuticals 2019). Additionally, NHS Trusts and Clinical Commissioning Groups have reportedly told clinicians in some instances that CBPMUs are too expensive to prescribe, since each prescription is on a 'named patient' basis and has to be individually imported, until bulk supply can be made available in the UK (MCCS and APPG 2019).

It has been acknowledged that the lack of access to medicinal cannabis in the UK has likely left many medical users having to buy 'street cannabis' (Health and Social Care Committee 2019a, Q194), or to otherwise grow their own (see Klein and Potter 2018), as was the situation before the rescheduling of CBPMUs. Under the current legal framework, this situation is likely to continue for some time in the UK because an overarching reason for the general reluctance to prescribe is a perceived lack of guidance and information for health professionals (see Bone 2020). As of March 2019, only six private prescriptions for a CBPMU have been issued in the UK and not a single NHS prescription has been dispensed (MCCS and APPG 2019). While this figure is likely to rise, with reports of " 'hundreds' seeking private clinics for medical cannabis" (Bettiza 2019), the numbers likely to be able to access medical cannabis on prescription remain insignificant in the context of the many thousands using medical cannabis illegally. (It is worth noting that the cost of going private means this route to access is further constrained.)

The problem here is attaining the standard of evidence required to recognise the medical benefits of cannabis for different conditions. The existing guidance considers the evidence base for the efficacy and safety for most cannabis medicines to be extremely limited, and there is a clear preference for reliance on randomised control trial (RCT) data (BPNA 2018; RCP 2018). While RCTs are recognised as constituting the 'gold standard' for evidence, a recent parliamentary report on medicinal cannabis acknowledges that RCTs can take up to four years to complete. This could be perceived as "unfair on patients and their families if they are asked to wait years for research to be conducted and for clinicians to prescribe" (Health and Social Care Committee 2019b, para. 60). An activist from the campaign group End Our Pain, Peter Carroll reports:

> Dame Sally Davies herself said that we have to wait maybe three or four years before that kind of high-quality, gold-standard data is with us. How do you explain that to the parent sitting behind me now who is—and you may disapprove of this—sourcing a full plant extract cannabis, bringing it into the country and treating her child with it, and the child has improved dramatically?
>
> *(ibid.)*

Though the parliamentary committee recognise the dangers in using anecdotal evidence, they report that impassioned arguments are being made by parents and clinicians who supported them for observational trials to be conducted alongside RCTs. Arguably, practical reasoning dictates that externally observed medical statistics (i.e., RCT data) and internal observation studies ought to inform each other to gain a more complete picture—helping to build a body of research in this area and improve a clinician's education (see Sen 2004; Bone 2020). Indeed, when considering the provision of medical cannabis around the world, a rather peculiar evidential picture is presented. It has often been the case that bottom-up anecdotal evidence and activist campaigns (as opposed to top-down quantitative RCTs) initially alerted the medical community to the plant's potential therapeutic use, given the restrictive scheduling constraints placed upon research (see Bone, Klein, and Potter 2018, introducing a special issue in *Drugs and Alcohol Today* that includes human stories from cannabis activists and patients).

Futures

To summarise the current situation, medical cannabis is legally available in the UK but only for a tiny proportion of those who may find medical cannabis beneficial. Access to legal supplies is restricted to a small number of conditions and further constrained by administrative, economic and evidential constraints. This leaves the previous situation of most medical users having to resort to criminal activity virtually unchanged. It is no surprise that the initial enthusiasm of campaign groups for the November 2018 rescheduling has been replaced by cynicism and frustration.

Moreover, the potential success of future legal challenges in the UK remain unlikely. While R v. Quayle and Others (2005) effectively closed down the viability of the medical necessity defence in relation to the medical use of cannabis, it also foreclosed the option of a human rights challenge to drug prohibition on the basis of medical use. Article 8(1) of the European Convention on Human Rights (ECHR) is incorporated into UK law via the Human Rights Act (1998) and provides, "Everyone has the right to respect for his private and family life". The right to private life is closely related to the right to health, and it could therefore ground a negative health obligation on behalf of the state not to interfere with a person's health choices (Bone 2020). Although Article 8 of the ECHR was narrowly applied in *Quayle* as the Court of Appeal were only required to consider the application of Article 8 in relation to extending the common law defence of medical necessity, the latter case *R* v. *Altham* (2006) closed down a broader Article 8 and an Article 3 challenge—prohibiting torture or subjecting a person to inhuman or degrading treatment. The Court of Appeal ruled that the state had done nothing to subject Altham to inhuman or degrading treatment by prohibiting cannabis for medicinal use, and following *Quayle*, that a broader Article 8 challenge, assessing the compatibility of cannabis laws with Article 8 human rights, was not open to him.

It is therefore unlikely that patients will be able to use human rights provisions contained within the ECHR to argue that the state has a negative health obligation not to interfere with a person's health choices in the immediate future.[6] Though it is worth noting that Article 8 of the ECHR is much broader in scope, since the sphere of 'private life' extends to broader autonomy-based human rights as well (Bone 2020). While there are landmark cases in Mexico and South Africa which have successfully argued that prohibitive cannabis laws infringe complainants' human rights to health, self-ownership, the free development of personality and privacy (see Amparo in Review 237/2014, 548/2018; *Prince and Others* 2018), this line of reasoning is unlikely to be successful in the UK. UK judges predominately defer to the legislature when cannabis laws and human rights laws conflict and are more constrained procedurally and legally than are judges in comparable jurisdictions. Under the Human Rights Act (HRA) (1998), the UK courts are required to interpret drug control legislation in a compliant way (s3 HRA), or else make a declaration of incompatibility (s4 HRA), in contrast to cannabis case law in other jurisdictions where judges can declare laws prohibiting cannabis to be unconstitutional and take steps to actively create drug policies shaped from a human rights perspective (see the Canadian cases of *R* v. *Parker* 2000; *Hitzig* v. *Canada* 2003).

Finally, while it is generally recognised that there is no right to treatment in the UK (Bone 2020; see also Wicks 2007), there is a right to procedural proprietary, as the European and domestic case law indicates that individuals are entitled to expect some minimal procedural requirements when their health care access is decided by the government and/or the medical profession. Since medical cannabis is neither available nor accessible in practice, it could potentially be open to individuals to argue that their human rights are infringed, as there is a failure in practice to provide an *accessible* and *effective* procedure to establish whether a patient can access medical cannabis at this time (see *A B and C* v. *Ireland* 2010[7]—an ECHR case which applied this reasoning in relation to the provision of abortion under Irish law; see also Bone 2020). Again, it is unlikely that this argument will garner much success in future cases as doctors are reluctant to prescribe at present due to the aforementioned perceived lack of RCT data and other evidence demonstrating the efficacy of medical cannabis and due to resource allocation issues within the NHS. Indeed, public pressure and growing media interest has proved to be more successful thus far in relation to changing the legal situation.

The question is whether the changes that have already taken place represent the thin edge of a wedge that will, over time, see greater access to legal medical cannabis, or are they a political sop in response to media and public pressure following the high profile stories of Alfie Dingley and Billy Caldwell with minimal tangible impact on the wider medical-cannabis using public. We believe that there are some good grounds for optimism for those campaigning for greater access to medical cannabis. The very fact of rescheduling cannabis under the MDR is legally significant, even if this significance has not yet been realised practically. Previously, the underlying principle was that cannabis was not recognised as having therapeutic value at all; to establish the category of CBPMUs as a Schedule 2 drug provides legal recognition that cannabis does indeed have medical potential. RCTs may be slow to follow, but this change removes some barriers to RCTs being conducted at all. Meanwhile, RCT evidence is accumulating in other countries that have greater access to medical cannabis—and this evidence will feed into expanding the range of conditions for which the benefits of CBPMUs may be recognised even if RCTs remain limited in the UK. Further, although RCTs are the gold standard evidence, removal of the blanket assumptions that cannabis has no medical potential and should be subject to criminal prohibition should also open the way to the accumulation and recognition of other types of evidence, including anecdotal evidence and individual GP case reports.

What is more, change at the international level may further encourage the loosening of UK regulation of medical cannabis. In January 2019 the World Health Organization's (WHO) Expert Committee on Drug Dependence (ECDD) recommended changing the scheduling of cannabis in recognition of the increasing body of evidence demonstrating the plant's medicinal value (WHO 2019). The ECDD also clarified that CBD is not subject to international control under the convention and addressed longstanding inconsistencies in scheduling. The ECDD noted that cannabis use is not associated with 'a significant risk of death', unlike other substances included in Schedules I and IV such as fentanyl analogues, heroin and other opioids (ibid.: 41). In December 2020, the UN Commission on Narcotic Drugs (CND) followed the WHO's recommendation and voted to remove cannabis from Schedule IV—finally acknowledging its medicinal potential (CND, 2020). This could have far reaching implications for national regulatory landscapes.

Notes

1 CBD (cannabidiol) is a cannabinoid that does not have psychoactive properties and falls outside of the global drug regulation framework as confirmed by the World Health Organization's (2019, 53–54) *Expert Committee on Drug Dependence*.

2 THC (tetrahydrocannabinol) is the main psychoactive ingredient of cannabis.

3 The role of serious and organised crime in cannabis markets is often exaggerated by media and law enforcement representations. Most people involved in growing or supplying cannabis in the UK avoid violence and involvement in other forms of crime. Nevertheless, serious and organised crime does exist in relation to drug markets—and dealers of this type are more likely to operate in open markets. See Potter and Klein (2020) for a detailed discussion.

4 That is, crimes other than possession, cultivation, production or supply of cannabis.

5 In UK and commonwealth criminal cases, R (*rex* or *regina*—i.e., the king or queen) is used to denote the Crown (i.e., the state) as prosecutor or plaintiff. In criminal cases it is usually the CPS (Crown Prosecution Service) who bring the action against the defendant on behalf of the state.

6 While the human right to health can manifest as the *positive* legal duties a state has to provide us with basic health care, the human right to health can also afford individuals the *negative* right to live and construct their own lives as they see fit, free from external constraint by the state (for more detail see Bone 2020).

7 A B and C are letters assigned to represent the three women in the case heard before the European Court of Human Rights in order to protect their identity.

References

APPG [All Party Parliamentary Group for Drug Policy Reform]. 2016. *Access to Medicinal Cannabis: Meeting Patient Needs*. London: APPG. https://drive.google.com/file/d/1mx0Q33DCm4OsGnw3L3GDYpMHvwOq7nVw/view?usp=sharing.

Barnes, M. P., and J. C. Barnes. 2016. *Cannabis: The Evidence for Medical Use*. London: APPG. https://drive.google.com/file/d/0B0c_8hkDJu0DUDZMUzhoY1RqMG8/view.

Bettiza, S. 2019. "'Hundreds' Seek Private Clinics for Medical Cannabis." *BBC News*, August 16. www.bbc.co.uk/news/health-49333826.

Bone, M. 2020. *Human Rights and Drug Control: A New Perspective*. Oxon, UK: Routledge.

Bone, M., A. Klein, and G. Potter. 2018. "Introduction: Cultivation, Medication, Activism and Cannabis Policy." *Drugs and Alcohol Today* 18 (2): 73–9.

British Paediatric Neurology Association. 2018. *Guidance on the Use of Cannabis-Based Products for Medicinal Use in Children and Young People with Epilepsy*, October 31. www.bpna.org.uk/userfiles/BPNA_CBPM_Guidance_Oct2018.pdf.

Commission on Narcotic Drugs. 2020. "Press Statement – 2 December 2020 CND votes on recommendations for cannabis and cannabis-related substances (2 December 2020)." https://www.unodc.org/documents/commissions/CND/CND_Sessions/CND_63Reconvened/Press_statement_CND_2_December.pdf.

Davies, S. C. 2018. *Cannabis Scheduling Review Part 1, the Therapeutic and Medicinal Benefits of Cannabis Based Products—a Review of Recent Evidence*. London: Department of Health and Social Care.

Department of Health and Social Care. 2018. "Letter Guidance on Cannabis Based Products for Medicinal Use (October 31, 2018)." www.england.nhs.uk/wp-content/uploads/2018/10/letter-guidance-on-cannabis-based-products-for-medicinal-use.pdf.

Dorn, N., and A. Jamieson. 2000. *Room for Manoeuvre: Overview of Comparative Legal Research into National Drug Laws of France, Germany, Italy, Spain, the Netherlands and Sweden and Their Relation to Three International Drugs Conventions*. London: DrugScope.

GW Pharmaceuticals. 2019. "GW Pharmaceuticals Receives Positive NICE Recommendation for EPIDY-OLEX® (cannabidiol) Oral Solution for the Treatment of Seizures in Patients with Two Rare, Severe Forms of Childhood-Onset Epilepsy (November 10, 2019)." http://ir.gwpharm.com/news-releases/news-release-details/gw-pharmaceuticals-receives-positive-nice-recommendation.

Hakkarainen, P., V. Asmussen Frank, M. J. Barratt, H. V. Dahl, T. Decorte, K. Karjalainen, S. Lenton, G. Potter, and B. Werse. 2015. "Growing Medicine: Small-Scale Cannabis Cultivation for Medical Purposes in Six Different Countries." *International Journal of Drug Policy* 26: 250–56.

Health and Social Care Committee. 2019a. "Oral Evidence: Drugs Policy: Medicinal Cannabis, (March 26, 2019)." HC 1821. House of Commons. http://data.parliament.uk/writtenevidence/committeeevidence.svc/evidencedocument/health-and-social-care-committee/drugs-policy-medicinal-cannabis/oral/98822.html.

———. 2019b. "Drugs Policy: Medicinal Cannabis Sixteenth Report of Session 2017–19 (June 18, 2019)." HC 1821. House of Commons. https://publications.parliament.uk/pa/cm201719/cmselect/cmhealth/1821/182102.htm.

Hough, M., and M. Natarajan. 2000. "Introduction: Illegal Drug Markets, Research and Policy." In *Illegal Drug Markets: From Research to Prevention Policy Crime Prevention Studies Volume 11*, edited by M. Natarajan and M. Hough, 1–17. Monsey, NY: Criminal Justice Press.

Klein, A., and G. R. Potter. 2018. "The Three Betrayals of the Medical Cannabis Growing Activist: From Multiple Victimhood to Reconstruction, Redemption and Activism." *International Journal of Drug Policy* 53: 65–72.

Liebling, J. 2019. "Medicinal Cannabis Guidelines." https://darlingcognitions.wordpress.com/2018/11/01/press-release-medicinal-cannabis-guidelines/#more-672.

The Medical Cannabis Clinicians Society and the All Party Parliamentary Group on Medical Cannabis under Prescription. 2019. "Written evidence from The Medical Cannabis Clinicians Society and the All Party Parliamentary Group on Medical Cannabis under Prescription (March 26, 2019)." DMC0088. http://data.parliament.uk/writtenevidence/committeeevidence.svc/evidencedocument/health-and-social-care-committee/drugs-policy-medicinal-cannabis/written/97723.html.

National Health Service. 2018. "Medical Cannabis (and Cannabis Oils)." www.nhs.uk/conditions/medical-cannabis/.

National Institute for Clinical Excellence. 2014. "Multiple Sclerosis in Adults: Management Clinical Guideline (October 8, 2014)." Clinical guideline [CG186]. www.nice.org.uk/guidance/cg186.

———. 2019a. "Cannabis-Based Medicinal Products (November 11, 2019)." NICE guideline [NG144]. www.nice.org.uk/guidance/ng144.

———. 2019b. "Cannabidiol with Clobazam for Treating Seizures Associated with Lennox-Gastaut Syndrome. Appraisal Consultation Document." www.nice.org.uk/guidance/gid-ta10410/documents/129.

———. 2019c. "Cannabidiol for Adjuvant Treatment of Seizures Associated with Dravet Syndrome. Appraisal Consultation Document." www.nice.org.uk/guidance/gid-ta10274/documents/129.

Nutt, D. 2014. "Medicinal Cannabis: Time for a Comeback?" *The Pharmaceutical Journal* (November 19). www.pharmaceutical-journal.com/opinion/comment/medicinal-cannabis-time-for-a-comeback/20067185.article.

Pardal, M., T. Decorte, M. Bone, Ò. Parés, and J. Johansson. 2020. "Mapping Cannabis Social Clubs in Europe." *European Journal of Criminology*. doi: 10.1177/1477370820941392.

Parker, H. 2000. "How Young Britons Obtain Their Drugs: Drugs Transactions at the Point of Consumption." In *Illegal Drug Markets: From Research to Prevention Policy Crime Prevention Studies Volume 11*, edited by M. Natarajan, and M. Hough, 59–81. Monsey, New York: Criminal Justice Press.

Potter, G. 2009. "Exploring Retail-Level Drug Distribution: Social Supply, 'Real' Dealers and the User/Dealer Interface." In *Old and New Policies, Theories, Research Methods and Drug Users Across Europe*, edited by Zsolt Demetrovics, Jane Fountain, and Ludwig Kraus. Lengerich, Germany: Pabst.

———. 2010. *Weed, Need and Greed: A Study of Domestic Cannabis Cultivation*. London: Free Association Books.

Potter, G., M. J. Barratt, A. Malm, M. Bouchard, T. Blok, A.-S. Christensen, T. Decorte, V. Asmussen Frank, P. Hakkarainen, A. Klein, S. Lenton, J. Perälä, B. Werse, and M. Wouters. 2015. "Global Patterns of Domestic Cannabis Cultivation: Sample Characteristics and Patterns of Growing Across Eleven Countries." *International Journal of Drug Policy* 26 (3): 226–37. doi:10.1016/j.drugpo.2014.12.007.

Potter, G., and A. Klein. 2020. "Coming Out of the Closet: Risk Management Strategies of Illegal Cannabis Growers." In *Risk and Substance Use: Framing Dangerous People and Dangerous Places*, edited by S. MacGregor and B. Thom. London: Routledge.

Royal College of Physicians. 2018. "Recommendations on Cannabis-Based Products for Medicinal Use." October 31. www.rcplondon.ac.uk/projects/outputs/recommendations-cannabis-based-products-medicinal-use.

Sen, A. 2004. "Health Achievement and Equity: External and Internal Perspectives." In *Public Health, Ethics and Equity*, edited by S. Anand, F. Peter, and A. Sen. Oxford: Oxford University Press.

UPA [United Patients Alliance]. 2016. *All-Party Parliamentary Group for Drug Policy Reform: Medical Cannabis Patient Survey*. London: UPA/APPG. www.upalliance.org/s/UPA-Patient-Survey-2016.pdf.

Werse, B., and C. Bernard, eds. 2016. *Friendly Business: International Views on Social Supply, Self-Supply and Small-Scale Drug Dealing*. Wiesbaden, Germany: Springer.

Wicks, E. 2007. *Human Rights and Healthcare*. Portland, OR: Hart Publishing.

World Health Organization. 2019. *Expert Committee on Drug Dependence: Forty-First Report*. WHO Technical Report Series, No. 1018. https://apps.who.int/iris/bitstream/handle/10665/325073/9789241210270-eng.pdf?ua=1.

Case Law

A, B and C v. Ireland [GC], no. 25579/05 (2010).

Amparo in Review, 237 (2014).

Amparo in Review, 548 (2018).

Hitzig v. Canada, CanLII 30796 (ON C.A.) (2003).

Minister of Justice and Constitutional Development and Others v. Prince (Clarke and Others Intervening); National Director of Public Prosecutions and Others v. Rubin; National Director of Public Prosecutions and Others v. Acton., (CCT108/17) ZACC 30 (2018).

R v. Altham, EWCA Crim 7 (2006).

R v. Parker, 188 DLR (4th) 385 (2000).

R v. Quayle; R v. Wales; R v. Taylor and another; R v. Kenny; Attorney General's Reference. (No 2 of 2004) EWCA Crim 1415 (2005).

Legislation

The European Convention on Human Rights (1950).

The Human Rights Act (1998).

The Misuse of Drugs Act (1971).

The Misuse of Drugs (Amendments) (Cannabis and Licence Fees) (England, Wales and Scotland) Regulations (2018).

The Misuse of Drugs Regulations (2001).

Single Convention on Narcotic Drugs (1961).

Section 2
Public Health

The shift towards creating regulated cannabis and related systems of control not only poses challenges for governance, as discussed in the previous section, but also creates space for research on cannabis as both a therapeutic and spiritual plant. The relationship between legal cannabis and public health is particularly fraught, given that Prohibition 2.0 was initiated in the late 1960s by declaring cannabis an exceptional public health threat. The legacy of this conflict between criminalization and medicalization is still evident as prohibition-era assertions of the physiological dangers of the plant and moral degradation of users has yet to be fully addressed in cultural and political discourse. This tension has fairly radical implications for how societies govern medicine and medical research in a post-prohibition era. Institutions of public health have become tasked—usually reluctantly—with identifying how to regulate, fund, and administer the consumption of cannabis as a net public health benefit. The recent (re)designation of cannabis as a potential therapeutic in most U.S. states and many countries (see Silber-Coats Chapter 18, this volume) disrupts the prior dominant public health messaging that defined cannabis as a dangerous drug of abuse.

Interdisciplinary approaches to public health examine the social systems that prevent disease and promote health. In specialized harm reduction literatures, prohibition itself is understood as harmful to public health (Emerson and Haden 2018). Legalization and regulated cannabis create research opportunities that widen the focus of public health research scholarship to address prohibition as a public health problem, on the one hand. On the other hand, legalization opens up opportunities to research how cannabis use may promote spiritual health, harm reduction, and wellness. The emergence of medical cannabis provides a direct critique of public health orthodoxies by pushing research and policy to entertain the possibility that cannabis can also improve well-being rather than exclusively be viewed as a source of public harm. Legal cannabis also creates conditions conducive for alternative modes of inquiry and sample populations.

Public health research agendas related to cannabis begin with a call for public health professionals to accept spiritual and inner exploration as essential elements of health and wellness. In "Deep Respect After Profound Neglect: Spiritual Health and Safety for Use of Cannabis and Other Entheogens in an Integrative Public Health System," physician and medical geographer Sunil Kumar Aggarwal provides an auto-ethnographic examination of the entheogenic uses of cannabis in which spiritual health is reimagined as a cornerstone of physical and mental wellness. This chapter also questions the cultural and legislative marginalization of cannabis internationally and provides solid historical footing on which cannabis specifically, and altered states of consciousness more broadly, can be understood as a part of the pursuit of wellness. Aggarwal asks how the public health profession would change if prevention of the existential threats of climate change and global nuclear war became priorities for public health scholars, policy makers, and practitioners. Importantly, this chapter calls for future research to examine the ways in which spiritual wellness might be related to physiological and psychological wellness.

Contesting public health orthodoxies regarding cannabis as a drug of abuse opens therapeutic possibilities. In "Opioids and Substance Abuse: Cannabis as a Harm Reduction Tool," neuroscientist Adrianne Wilson-Poe provides an overview of how cannabis can be used as a harm reduction strategy to address opioid dependency and overdose deaths. This chapter identifies funding and supply barriers to public health research examining cannabis as a harm reduction tool. Wilson-Poe describes the state of knowledge—and research gaps—relating to cannabis as either an adjunct or alternative to opioids for those struggling with opioid dependency, withdrawal, and the ongoing need for the treatment of chronic pain. While there is mounting evidence demonstrating the efficacy of cannabis as part of an exit strategy from opioid dependency, Wilson-Poe underscores the need for research examining the use of cannabis for treating acute pain, opioid withdrawal in comparison to FDA medications, and the relative efficacy of variable cultivars and modes of ingestion.

The therapeutic potential of cannabis is further explored by kinesiologist Whitney Ogle in "Cannabis in Exercise and Sport." In reviewing the research evidence—and gaps—in scientific knowledge regarding the use of cannabis in exercise and competitive sports, Ogle provides an important addition to how discourses of cannabis therapeutics are challenging the prohibition frame of cannabis as a drug of abuse and to where vestiges of prohibition persist, such as in professional sports. Similar to Wilson-Poe's call for rigorous research into the effects of dosage, potency, and mode of ingestion on chronic pain and opioid withdrawal, Ogle proposes that human performance is an understudied area for cannabis scholars in the public health space. She highlights the need for researchers in this subject area to return to questions that were first asked in the 1960s and 1970s but were abandoned as Prohibition 2.0 limited cannabis research opportunities. Ogle offers a clear agenda for research examining how cannabis may enhance performance and recovery.

The subsequent chapter by public health scholar Trecia Ehrlich shifts our focus to examine how the cannabis research methods selected maintain dominant models of "legitimate" cannabis scholarship. In "Utilizing Community-Based Participatory Research in Cannabis Knowledge Formation," Ehrlich traces how prohibition ideology historically shaped the creation and dissemination of public health knowledge related to cannabis. This knowledge, as others have highlighted, views cannabis as a drug of *abuse* with no therapeutic benefits. In the absence of empirical data supporting medicinal uses of cannabis, a window of opportunity has been opened for the cannabis industry to provide a counternarrative. Public health professionals are left to reconcile these often conflicting narratives. In order to transcend the historic fear of government intervention and social stigma associated with cannabis cultivation and use, Ehrlich proposes that community-based participatory research (CBPR) be deployed to better inform public health messaging to promote safe cannabis use. In this chapter, Ehrlich draws on her experience using CBPR to gather information from cannabis workers about their exposure to UV radiation and reflects upon the utility of this methodology as an alternative to top-down models of institutional public health research.

Cannabis workers are also the focus of public health scholars Marc B. Schenker and Chelsea E. Langer's exploration of the "Health and Safety of Cannabis Workers." In their chapter, Schenker and Langer describe the variable occupational risks faced by those workers involved in regulated cannabis cultivation and processing. As cannabis work becomes recognized as a major agricultural activity, they suggest that research consider the occupational and personal safety (e.g., workplace harassment/violence) hazards faced by workers. Given the limitations of health and safety data relating to even licensed growers, Schenker and Langer call for research agendas that move beyond describing potential risks to also quantify, using rigorous methods, the actual hazards, susceptibility factors, and health outcomes faced by cannabis workers. Such knowledge will be necessary to develop effective workplace safety protocols, policies, and prevention technologies. Their chapter dovetails with contributions in the Markets and Society section on cannabis corporate social responsibility (see Otañez and Vergara Chapter 16) and ethical consumerism (see Bennett Chapter 17) in the United States, in which the promise of regulated cannabis markets for protecting worker health and safety faces resistance from ongoing federal prohibition and the cannabis capitalist class (see Otañez Chapter 15).

The chapters in this section ask researchers to consider prohibition itself as a public health problem while regulated cannabis cultivation, commerce, and consumption create new research possibilities in which medical cannabis represents a specific critique of public health. Taken together, the focus of these chapters is on minimizing the myriad of potential harms to the physiological and mental health of workers and consumers associated with the cultivation, processing, and consumption of cannabis.

Reference

Emerson, Brian, and Mark Haden. 2018. "Public Health and the Harm Reduction Approach to Illegal Psychoactive Substances." In *Reference Module in Biomedical Sciences*, B9780128012383662000. Elsevier. https://doi.org/10.1016/B978-0-12-801238-3.66208-6.

8

Deep Respect After Profound Neglect

Spiritual Health and Safety for Use of Cannabis and Other Entheogens in an Integrative Public Health System

Sunil Kumar Aggarwal

Keywords: cannabis, entheogens, spiritual health, psychedelics, public health

Cannabis, Entheogens, and Spirituality in Public Health

Cannabis is a botanical revered in numerous religious traditions as an entheogen, or substance that can induce awe or inspiration. It is lauded for its ability to promote inner peace, heighten the experience of the present moment, and aid in meditation to attune a partaker to a Higher Self consciousness. A critical point is that even those who may not be utilizing cannabis as part of any kind of recognized religion may still be using it in a manner consistent with spiritual intents or as an expression of the spiritually related concept of freely exercising sovereignty over one's consciousness. Cannabis use referred to as 'recreational'—literally, to 're-create' or 'renew'—may be better understood under the wider category of spiritual well-being related use, given that the pursuit of pleasure, happiness, and connection are all aspects of the fulfillment of human spirituality. Similarly, medical use of cannabis for health, well-being, and fulfillment of hope in the face of existential threats to survival and life quality that disease and disability present integrally involves a spiritual health dimension, in addition to physical and mental ones.

In 1983, the World Health Organization (WHO) first recognized the implicit spiritual dimension in health, and in 1998, the WHO executive board added "spiritual" to the definition of health itself, resolving, "Health is a dynamic state of complete physical, mental, spiritual and social well-being and not merely the absence of disease or infirmity" (Chirico 2016, 13). Spiritual health or spiritual well-being, a corollary concept, has been defined as "a state of being where an individual is able to deal with day-to-day life in a manner which leads to the realization of one's full potential; meaning and purpose of life; and happiness from within" (Dhar et al. 2011). Spiritual health is increasingly being addressed in palliative care for patients with serious and life-threatening illness, and there is an

DOI: 10.4324/9780429320491-8

ongoing need for this across the full spectrum of health services. To help guide clinicians, in 2009 the US National Consensus Project developed this definition of spirituality which goes beyond religious concerns to include philosophical and existential ones:

> Spirituality is the aspect of humanity that refers to the way individuals seek and express meaning and purpose and the way they experience their connectedness to the moment, to self, to others, to nature, and to the significant or sacred.
>
> *(Puchalski et al. 2009, 887)*

In the US public health sector, spiritual issues have mostly focused on respecting select groups' religious practices with regards to participation in state health programs (Brougher 2012). Examples include allowance for conscientious objector exemptions for members of qualified religious groups from mandatory enrollment in health coverage programs (e.g., the Amish and Medicare), presumed consent to emergency medical therapy (e.g., Jehovah's Witnesses and blood transfusions), and required licensure and underage restriction when serving sacramental psychoactive substances (e.g., Christians and ceremonial alcohol use).

Increasingly, exemptions to federal drug abuse prevention and control public health laws are being made for religious "entheogen" use practices. "Entheogen" is defined in the *Oxford English Dictionary* as "a chemical substance, typically of plant origin, that is ingested to produce a nonordinary state of consciousness for religious or spiritual purposes." It is a more neutral and nuanced alternative to the terms 'psychedelic' (mind-manifesting), 'hallucinogen' (hallucination-inducing), and 'psychotomimetic' (psychosis-mimicking), referring to drugs—psychoactive chemicals, plants, fungi, or animal secretions—"which provoke ecstasy and have traditionally been used as shamanic or religious inebriants, as well as their active principles and artificial congeners" (Ruck et al. 1979, 145). Prohibitions on drug preparation, use, and exchange under the half-century-old Comprehensive Drug Abuse Prevention and Control Act have been lifted for members of select religious groups whose use of select entheogens is now protected under enacted legislation or federal court rulings. This includes lawful recognition of the cultivation, preparation, and use of the entheogen peyote, a mescaline-containing cactus, by the Native American Church since 1993 and the entheogen ayahuasca by the Brazilian Unio de Vegetal and Santo Daime Churches since 2006. Despite recognized traditions in other countries (e.g., South Africa, Jamaica, and India), cannabis' entheogenic use has not been recognized under US law.

Aside from these exceptions, the US public health system has generally neglected the field of study concerned with the human relationship with entheogens, ignoring the possibility of healing in spaces with cannabis or other entheogens and assuming danger and high abuse potential instead. Yet, strict public health drug policies are allowing for select groups' religious practices. This begs the question: Why make exemptions only for select groups and entheogens? Spirituality is a universal, core dimension of health, irrespective of membership in any particular religious sect (Puchalski et al. 2009). Why can't respect for spiritual health and safety be universalized for all persons and all entheogen practices?

In this chapter I attempt to bridge this breach in the public health system with regard to cannabis primarily and other entheogens. In the first section, using the method of radical empiricism, I share my experience of the value of cannabis-occasioned consciousness states to help describe the space. In the second section, I explore the public health system's approach to cannabis and other entheogens from the perspective of licensed health professionals who negotiate a critical distance in engagement with the state. In the third and final section, I propose further research directions into the spiritual health value of cannabis and other entheogens in the context of an emerging fifth wave in public health focused on well-being in the face of global existential threats.

Hearing and Validating the Call

I heard the call to help develop public health safe use protections to integrate healing with cannabis and other entheogens through my own profound healing experiences with these substances. Due to the prohibitionist drug education programming of my youth, I had long dutifully avoided marijuana self-experimentation until undergoing a romantic relationship breakup as a pre-med student brought me to question this. Self-experimentation revealed an entirely undiscovered geography of therapeutic potency and potentiality. Here was a mild euphoriant that occasioned a state of mind wholly different from that produced by legally available inebriants such as alcohol, coffee, cigarettes, and energy drinks. When taken in more protected contexts, THC-rich cannabis helped me achieve flow state: a feeling of being completely absorbed in an activity—be it technical, creative, convivial, playful, or peaceful, while simultaneously performing at an optimal level (Csikszentmihalyi 1991). For someone like me who had been plagued by anxious unrest and a vocal inner critic, this simultaneously alert and relaxed flow state was integrating and liberating. Over time, I came to appreciate cannabis as a 40 million-year-old natural entheogen (Aggarwal 2018). With the smoking of virtually unprocessed, dried, resinous cannabis flowers, I experienced intentional connection with a socially foraged semi-domesticated herb that healed by helping me forget and remember. I forgot worries and negative thoughts and emotions that detracted from being fully present in the moment. I *re-membered*—or, put back together again more robustly—parts of my body, mind, and spirit, in a way they are rarely perceived. Normally, separative pathways dominate, such as when I have persisting pain in a limb or feel like my emotions are distanced. Cannabis-occasioned consciousness integration, freely chosen, helps me see things in a "cleansed" manner—I gnostically, or in a spiritually knowing way, remember that I am a human being with a finite lifespan with beautiful abilities, senses, and capacity to act for a greater purpose. Rather than the default mode, beset in possible anxiety and worry, which might tend towards social withdrawal, this mode is pro-social, engaged, and flowing. With a sensation of time slowing, there is an expansion of spatial awareness and environmental receptivity, deepening the therapeutic value of local land and seascapes. Overall this fosters an abiding sense of inner balance and inner and communal unity, and it provides relief from separation, disintegration, and emotional withdrawnness.

I similarly came to appreciate firsthand the potencies of other entheogens such as psilocybin-containing mushrooms, LSD, MDMA, DMT, *Salvia divinorum*, coca leaves, opium congeners, ayahuasca, ketamine, and powdered tobacco herbal mixtures. While I do not have space to elaborate, I experienced with several of these most profoundly ego dissolution, with all the attendant pain and challenge of sorting through long-held attachments. These occasioned a powerful healing unitive or nondualistic consciousness and a deeply felt sense of awe and reverence for life and the universe, which I returned with as my ego re-formed anew.

Like others, the insights I gained in my twenties into other-than-default modes of consciousness while exploring with cannabis and other entheogens changed my orientation towards science and medicine (Tart 1990). I find compelling the conjecture that the discovery and use of entheogens may have been the fountainhead for the development of human religion and catalyzed evolutionary developments in human consciousness (Hoffman 2006). The therapeutic relief from mental distress, promotion of well-being, and occasioning of deep insights into life and the nature of reality provided are worth understanding and sharing with others, as feasible. Given the stigma associated with cannabis and other entheogens and the limited awareness of spiritual health in medicine, I sought out validation in scientific work on other health dimensions. Learning from experts and conducting field research, I came to appreciate the state of science regarding cannabis' applications in medicine and preventative health, beyond the clinically evident medical applications for pain, nausea, and muscle spasms (Pacher and Kunos 2013). Cannabinergy, mediated by the endocannabinoid system (ECS), a homeostatic cell signaling system found throughout the body and many other organisms, validates many claims of cannabis's salutary effects. Lead scientists at the National Institutes of Health opine,

> modulating ECS activity may have therapeutic potential in almost all diseases affecting humans, including obesity/metabolic syndrome, diabetes and diabetic complications, neurodegenerative, inflammatory, cardiovascular, liver, gastrointestinal, skin diseases, pain, psychiatric disorders, cachexia, cancer, chemotherapy-induced nausea and vomiting, among many others.
>
> *(Pacher and Kunos 2013, 1918–19)*

Moreover, a recent analysis of high-quality studies of THC-rich cannabis' impact on physical health has shown periodic use correlates with measurable population-level reductions in rates of obesity, diabetes mellitus, cancers, mortality from traumatic brain injury, use of alcohol and prescription drugs, driving fatalities, and opioid overdose deaths (Clark 2017). A reduction of 989–2,511 premature deaths for each 1% of the population using cannabis was measured, and prevention of 23,500–47,500 deaths annually was projected were cannabis accessible nationwide (Clark 2017). Another recent analysis of National Vital Statistics showed a 10.8% reduction in adult male suicide rates after states liberalized their cannabis laws between 1990 and 2007 to allow medical use (Anderson, Rees, and Sabia 2014). Clearly, physical and mental public health benefits with cannabis use are scientifically valid, yet it seems ignorance and fear of its potential spiritual health benefits create a systemic breach that stymies full avail.

The Healer's Social Responsibility to Acknowledge the Breach

Licensed health professionals as public health agents have a responsibility to advocate for safe environments for all health-related behaviors. The state expects licensees to practice safely within their professional scope and creates licensing schemes to protect the public from unscrupulous individuals who may use the cover of a healing art to practice malfeasance (see Sexton Chapter 29, this volume). Licensees in turn become part of an ancient guild of healers who serve under oath with conscience and commitment, held to standards of self-regulation provided by health professional guild organizations.

Respect, protection, and value optimization for health-related behaviors with cannabis and entheogens is an important public health goal. Each licensee should articulate an educated assessment of public health policy in this area. Here is mine, having held state licenses to practice medicine and prescribe federally controlled substances for over a decade. My study of history has shown me that the drug-war status quo is a byproduct of a system of domination tied to racism and colonialism in which traditional entheogen use behaviors are disrespected and outlawed. The cannabis plant, semi-domesticated in South-Central Asia around 18,000 years ago (Duvall 2015), has been a focus of administrative bureaucracies for over a century and appears to have been brought to the attention of public health regulators by politicians and members of law enforcement.

Cannabis formally became an object of international public health concern under a UN-negotiated treaty in the 1950s, the Single Convention on Narcotic Drugs, heavily pushed by US delegates and adopted in 1961. The US enjoyed hegemonic supremacy in the wake of the Second World War, which it employed to develop and pass the treaty and two others over a 20-year period. Its inclusion (along with coca leaves and opium poppy) was pushed by Harry J. Anslinger, a former alcohol prohibition enforcer and the first director of the Federal Bureau of Narcotics. He had led a media-aided lurid and sensationalistic crusade against marijuana 25 years earlier, connecting its use to homicidal mania and racial integration fears, which culminated in the passage of the 1937 Marihuana Tax Act signed into law by President Roosevelt. This law was struck down by the Supreme Court in 1969. Despite protests from federal health scientists threatened with blacklisting, President

Nixon's administration then implemented the modern prohibition framework around marijuana and other entheogens, in line with the UN treaties. They used the scheme as a tool to suppress political dissent and funded a public health science bureaucracy that *prima facie* viewed all illegal drug use as pathological (Aggarwal 2015).

In institutional public health, fear and ignorance of cannabis' entheogenic qualities has significantly restricted its application as a preventative and ameliorative therapeutic agent in physical and mental health. These qualities are stigmatized and misconstrued as either trivial or inherently pathological by the public health establishment and the reason for its alleged danger and severely restricted accessibility. This provides cover to statutory federal law which maintains a sweeping prohibition of cannabis under the public health banner of drug abuse prevention and control. Even in locales which have state-legal access to cannabis for personal use, whether under medical authorization or not, vestiges of prohibition persist, justified as necessary to protect public health and safety. These include "carve-outs" in areas such as employment, housing, family law, road safety, the tax code, healthcare, and education, in which cannabis' legality and acceptability are ruptured or absent, imperiling one's ability to socially function and control one's health and body. These carve-outs are a manifestation of the entheogen breach in the public health system, which is likely contributing to eroding public trust in medical institutions. Gallup found in 2018 that public trust in the medical system is at 36%, unchanged for 30 years and less than half of what it was in 1974 (Keckley 2018).

Repairing the Breach: Health as Integrative

In early 2019, an influential WHO expert committee completed a critical review that called for relaxation of cannabis's prohibitive international scheduling, the first official rupture in the international treaty system regarding cannabis in over 50 years (Ghebreyesus 2019), ultimately leading to the UN's decision to remove cannabis from the most restrictive schedule in international law reserved for substances intended for complete eradication. After over 80 years of prohibition enforcement, accompanied by state-funded mass education campaigns highlighting the danger and deviancy of marijuana use, this scheme has become unpopular. Mass movements have arisen in the last several decades that have reformed local and state laws and in turn fueled shifts in public attitudes. Being 'high on marijuana' is slowly being destigmatized. A supermajority now feel that marijuana prohibition is unwarranted and medically necessary use is a fundamental right (Marijuana Majority 2019).

The shift in the present landscape allows for re-evaluation of public health understanding of the necessity and purpose of the pursuit of non-ordinary states of consciousness and enhanced sensation in general (Weil 1975). With new laws and evolving social mores, there is increased acceptance that there is something fundamental, natural, or unstoppable about the human pursuit of psychoactivation via cannabis that warrants tolerance and even curiosity or wonder. Institutional public health, through incorporating an integrative scientific understanding of health and well-being that includes mind, body, spirit, community, and environmental relationship dimensions, can broaden its prior unidimensional paradigm. An integrative public health science approach to cannabis and other entheogen use will require an openness and attunement to subjective experience and non-ordinary states of consciousness as valid sources of knowledge about health, as the privileging of ordinary state consciousness and harm-focused-only objective assessment has significantly limited scientific exploration of spiritual health.

How did institutional public health become wedded to what educator and psychologist Thomas Roberts (2019, 25) has called the "single-state fallacy" in human and natural sciences? Philosopher Arthur Buehler (2015, 325–26) has called this "cognocentrism," which posits that only the ordinary state, default "armchair" mode of consciousness, is knowledge-rich. Historically, the development of scientific inquiry in the Western tradition required a negotiation with Catholic Church authorities regarding which domains were deemed as acceptable fodder for inquiry. Known as the Cartesian split, after 16th-century French monk and philosopher Rene Descartes, the striking of this bargain by protean scientists allowed for the development of empiricism and structured inquiry into the material nature of reality. However, inquiry into the nature of soul—or spirit or consciousness—was off-limits for scientific study per the negotiated agreement with the Church, as "Care of the Soul" was reserved for the Holy Catholic Church alone. Transgression was a capital offense punishable by torture and death—the fate of many so-called heretics such as Giordano Bruno. This bounded enterprise of inquiry was still sufficiently suitable to probe the mechanics of motion, the nature of chemical reactions, the inheritance of traits in life, and other phenomena. Ultimately, after further clashes with the Church, including the trial of Galileo Galilei, and with the help of the telescope and further development of its prestige, scientific inquiry was able to interrogate geocentrism and explore freely the movement patterns of outer space celestial objects. A similar revolution with aid of entheogens has yet to occur for 'inner space' exploration.

During the Renaissance, healing arts developed and practiced by traditional healers in Europe, such as herbalism and shamanism, along with indigenous peoples' healing practices encountered by European explorers in the 'Age of Discovery,' were regularly criminalized, oppressed, or simply ignored. The demonic concept of the witch and witchcraft developed by Church authorities was the frame under which such suppression occurred. European alchemists, interested in the nature of consciousness, resisted the Cartesian split and took their work underground. In this vacuum, the birth of 'modern scientific medicine,' chronicled by Michel Foucault (2010) in *The Birth of the Clinic: An Archaeology of Medical Perception*, occurred over a period of time in France when Cartesian-split scientific inquiry was applied to the study of human disease through correlation of post-mortem pathological studies with pre-mortem observations. This was the birth of the 'clinical gaze,' in which medicine became connected with objective reduction of symptom clusters and illness presentations to tissue pathology (Sullivan 2003). In this type of medical science, there was and is no regard for subjectivity of the patient—only the gaze of the medical practitioner is seen as a warranted position from which to ascertain fact.

Out of this Cartesian-split medical science, the discipline and practice of public health was born, as a way to move clinical concerns 'upstream' in the population to prevent disease and promote health. Historians have described four waves in the development of public health, corresponding to specific concerns in given periods (Hemingway 2011). The first wave (1830–1900) had to do with civil engineering and 'the great public works period.' This arose in response to the Industrial Revolution in Northern Europe and North America, which led to conditions of overcrowding and lack of sanitation and clean water, leading to the transmission of infectious diseases. The second wave (1890–1950) was grounded in "the germ theory of disease and refinement of the scientific approach in hospitals" (Hemingway 2011, para. 1). This era corresponded with the rise of scientific rationalism in medicine, engineering, and municipalism and the development of hospitals and further specialization in medicine, in which the body was increasingly viewed as a machine divisible into discrete parts or organ systems. The third wave (1940–1980) was the "restructuring of institutions, welfare reforms, new housing, social security and the development of 'health services.'" This wave was influenced by the "materialist philosophies of Marx and Engels" that viewed health as "the compound result of the conditions of everyday life" (Hemingway 2011, para. 1–4). The fourth wave (1960–2000) had as its "dominant focus of activity the 'risk' theory of disease causation, and lifestyle issues, smoking, diet, and physical activity" as well as nascent concerns with social inequalities in health. This behaviorist focus emerged as "chronic diseases caused the majority of death and disability in the western world" (Hemingway 2011, para. 1–5).

Given the complexity of current health threats such as rising obesity, pandemics, war, violence, anxiety and depression, global climate change, environmental and ecological degradation, worsening inequality, and cycles of trauma, scholars are recognizing a fifth wave in public health cresting: an emphatic focus on well-being that centers on "a new image of what it means to be human"

(Hanlon et al. 2011, 34). In this wave, there is an emphasis on the development of an integrative public health paradigm that draws from the work of philosopher Ken Wilber. In a pair of widely cited articles, University of Glasgow Public Health Professor Phil Hanlon and colleagues described the rise of this new wave aimed at achieving the goal of enhancing well-being in the 21st century, in the face of radical and unprecedented challenges and strife (Hanlon et al. 2010, 2011). This paradigm calls for a healing of the Cartesian split that became embedded early on in public health and a return into the wheelhouse of health science and healthcare concerns related to the experience of the inner self, interiority, subjecthood, and the way that groups and collectives are experienced inter-subjectively.

In this fifth wave public health, we reintegrate the spiritually neutered foundations of science. The integrative turn in science is focused on recognition that the reductionistic Western model of scientific inquiry, especially when it comes to engagement with the biosphere, cosmos, and what it means to be human, is only one way to know and understand the world. In order to have richer inquiry, it is necessary to understand and integrate other ways of knowing, such as indigenous science (Bartlett, Marshall, and Marshall 2012). Canadian biologist Cheryl Bartlett describes integrative science emerging in the mid-1990s as a radical innovation in post-secondary science education. Her work is about fostering a new consciousness in which we "realize that we have options and alternatives as to our ways of knowing about and participating in the web of life, while realizing that science is and must always be a practical engagement with the real world" ("About the Institute" 2019). Her team champions a science inclusive of multiple perspectives, respectfully and meaningfully engaged with communities. Bartlett quotes Elder Albert Marshall of Eskasoni First Nation in Nova Scotia, who describes integrative science as a "two-eyed seeing," or

> learning to see from our one eye with the strengths of Indigenous knowledges and ways of knowing, and from our other eye with the strengths of Western (Eurocentric or mainstream) knowledges and ways of knowing . . . and learning to use both these eyes together, for the benefit of all.
>
> *("Joining Two Worlds" 2008)*

Let us now apply this integrative public health perspective towards achieving universal respect for spiritual health and well-being practices, specifically what has been dismissively called 'recreational use' of cannabis and other entheogens. At a macro level, the practice of public health through local, state, regional, national, and international health departments and agencies has yet to recognize that the two gravest threats to the long-term survival and well-being of the human species include human-activity-driven global climate system breakdown due to fossil fuel extraction and burning industries and the continued omnicidal threat of full-scale nuclear war. These threaten the survival of whole populations in staggering dimensions. What happens to the practice of public health by institutions, academicians, policy makers, and others when prevention of these grave threats becomes a central agenda item?

Such global existential issues are also present in every individual. From the time that human beings develop an awareness of our mortality, we develop existential concerns that can vary in intensity from mild to severe, depending on a variety of factors and triggers such as actual or threatened death, injury, illness, deprivation, and other trauma. In the field of hospice and palliative medicine, medical professionals are trained to diagnose and treat clinically significant existential distress associated with life-threatening or life-limiting illness. But it is fair to say, as observed by Scottish psychiatrist R. D. Laing, "life, you see, is a sexually transmitted disease and there's a 100 per cent mortality rate" (Hilmore 1985). This underscores the universality of the condition of existential stress and why spiritual health and well-being is an essential core dimension of health. Given the critical nature of socialization in mammalian neuropsychological development, existential concerns also arise in relation to crises and disturbances in social acceptance, such as ostracization, betrayal, oppression, or related pressures, traumas, or catastrophic illnesses that act as 'social death threats.' There is likely an evolutionary aspect to this as humans for millennia lived in hunter-gatherer clans, dependent on the group for basic shelter, protection, and survival. Any form of outcasting from that social protection would likely translate into death, thus triggering existential concerns. Social psychologist Ernest Becker (2007) posited that much of the social fabric of contemporary civilization is held together by collective "denial of death." In other words, individual existential concerns are mollified by being in social connection.

Given these individual and global social existential conditions, it is necessary for optimal spiritual health and well-being—a core dimension of health—that individuals be able to search for meaning and purpose. Individuals must have ongoing opportunities for *mental or spiritual consolation* and to *create again* and *renew* their spirit as they face ongoing and increasing existential concerns. All the italicized foregoing words are the definitions of the words in late Middle English and Latin from which our contemporary word "recreation" comes from. Safe recreational use of cannabis and other entheogens cannot be seen as psychopathological when the essential role recreation plays in the universal human pursuit of meaning, purpose, and renewal in the face of existential realities is understood.

Such use, which has long-standing traditional and indigenous antecedents, must be respected and protected as a matter of public health as potentially vital integrative health behaviors, even if this greater framing is not apprehended by individuals or social institutions at present. Arising from the Cartesian split, the single-state fallacy and cognocentric bias which undergird cannabis and entheogen prohibition laws and the orientation of contemporary US public health institutions are based on the flawed yet pervasive idea that all noteworthy understanding in the world is only gleaned from the ordinary rational-discursive state of mind, seen as the preferred default healthy way to be. This devalues and neglects the validity, healing potential, and tradition of entheogen-aided multistate consciousness living and places spiritual health and well-being in a blindspot. It discounts, per Buehler, the "almost limitless possibilities in the rainbow of human-consciousness" (2015, 326). An increasingly large body of literature in the last 30–40 years has substantiated the normalcy of this view of consciousness in areas such as the study of altered states, transpersonal psychology, mind-body medicine and psychiatry, the anthropology of consciousness, and the philosophy of consciousness. Like the telescope opened new vistas of understanding in astronomy and cosmology in the 17th century, a look through "the telescope of altered states" may allow public health researchers "to experience a vast inner universe" that may have profound impacts on developments in science, health, and social relations (Buehler 2015, 325–26). A great deal of further research and inquiry is needed in this area.

Conclusion

The prohibition of cannabis and other entheogens via the Controlled Substances Act in the US and similar laws globally, though adopted under the banner of public health promotion, does not further public health but rather amounts to a prohibition on societal ability to freely pursue science and discovery, promote individual and community efficacy and well-being, and fully practice the healing arts. Through adopting this spiritual health-inclusive integrative view towards individual and public health as part of the fifth wave, and by expanding the public health and spirituality nexus in the US beyond select religious groups to include all, the breach in the public health system that neglects the value and power of cannabis and entheogens can begin to be repaired by creating and protecting safe use spaces. For example, we have started to create a safe use space in a clinic in Seattle, the Advanced Integrative Medical Science Institute, that Dr. Leanna Standish and I co-founded in October 2018, which offers patients cannabis- and ketamine-assisted psychotherapy and a future home for approved MDMA, psilocybin, and ayahuasca-assisted therapy.

With a larger project of research and development, inclusive of engagement with indigenous communities and other communities, as well as institutional engagement, cannabis and other entheogen use practices can be depathologized at their core, and recreational-medical-spiritual use can be seen in unity. Their safe and maximally beneficial use can be cultivated by the public health system. They can be accepted widely for the therapeutic and well-being promoting potential they possess for all, regardless of spiritual or religious affiliation or health status.

References

"About the Institute." About | Integrative Science. Accessed September 9, 2019. www.integrativescience.ca/About/.

"About the Marijuana Majority." *Marijuana Majority*. Accessed October 4, 2019. http://marijuanamajority.com/about.php.

Aggarwal, Sunil Kumar. 2015. "Health Scientist Blacklisting and the Meaning of Marijuana in the Oval Office in the Early 1970s." *Medium*. CASP Communications, July 1. https://medium.com/@ReachCASP/health-scientist-blacklisting-and-the-meaning-of-marijuana-in-the-oval-office-in-the-early-1970s-71ea41427b49.

———. 2018. "Cannabis Fear Deconditioning: An Autobiological Marijuana Memoir of a South Asian-Oklahoman Physician-Scientist." *Journal of Ethnobiology* 38 (4): 489. https://doi.org/10.2993/0278-0771-38.4.489.

Anderson, D. Mark, Daniel I. Rees, and Joseph J. Sabia. 2014. "Medical Marijuana Laws and Suicides by Gender and Age." *American Journal of Public Health* 104 (12): 2369–76. https://doi.org/10.2105/ajph.2013.301612.

Bartlett, Cheryl, Murdena Marshall, and Albert Marshall. 2012. "Two-Eyed Seeing and Other Lessons Learned within a Co-Learning Journey of Bringing Together Indigenous and Mainstream Knowledges and Ways of Knowing." *Journal of Environmental Studies and Sciences* 2 (4): 331–40. https://doi.org/10.1007/s13412-012-0086-8.

Becker, Ernest. 2007. *The Denial of Death*. New York: Simon and Schuster.

Brougher, Cynthia. 2012. *Religious Exemptions for Mandatory Health Care Programs: A Legal Analysis*. (CRS Report No. RL34708). Congressional Research Service. www.everycrsreport.com/files/20100204_RL34708_e81657299295919d7c21b4ec6fc7bff73472e125.pdf.

Buehler, Arthur F. 2015. "Sufi Contemplation: 'Abdullah Shah's *Suluk-i Mujaddidyya*'." In *Contemplative Literature: A Comparative Sourcebook on Meditation and Contemplative Prayer*, edited by Komjathy Louis, 307–58. Albany, NY: State University of New York Press.

Chirico, Francesco. 2016. "Spiritual Well-Being in the 21st Century: It's Time to Review the Current WHO's Health Definition?" *Journal of Health and Social Sciences* 1 (1): 11–16. doi:10.19204/2016/sprt2.

Clark, Thomas M. 2017. *Cannabis Use is Associated with a Substantial Reduction in Premature Deaths in the United States*. Indiana University South Bend. Accessed August 12, 2019. https://scholarworks.iu.edu/dspace/handle/2022/21632.

Csikszentmihalyi, Mihaly. 1991. *Flow: The Psychology of Optimal Experience*. New York, NY: HarperPerennial.

Dhar, Neera et al. 2011. "Spiritual Health Scale 2011: Defining and Measuring 4 Dimension of Health." *Indian Journal of Community Medicine: Official Publication of Indian Association of Preventive & Social Medicine* 36 (4): 275–82. doi:10.4103/0970-0218.91329.

Duvall, Chris S. 2015. *Cannabis*. London: Reaktion Books.

Foucault, Michel. 2010. *The Birth of the Clinic: An Archaeology of Medical Perception*. London: Routledge.

Ghebreyesus, Tedros Adhanom. 2019. *Tedros Adhanom Ghebreyesus to António Guterres*, January 24. ECDD41. World Health Organization Director-General to United Nations Secretary-General. www.who.int/medicines/access/controlled-substances/UNSG_letter_ECDD41_recommendations_cannabis_24Jan19.pdf?ua=1.

Hanlon, P., S. Carlisle, M. Hannah, D. Reilly, and A. Lyon. 2011. "Making the Case for a 'Fifth Wave' in Public Health." *Public health* 125 (1): 30–36.

Hanlon, P., S. Carlisle, D. Reilly, A. Lyon, and M. Hannah. 2010. "Enabling Well-Being in a Time of Radical Change: Integrative Public Health for the 21st Century." *Public Health* 124 (6): 305–12. https://doi.org/10.1016/j.puhe.2010.03.014.

Hemingway, Ann. 2011. "Lifeworld-Led Care: Is It Relevant for Well-Being and the Fifth Wave of Public Health Action?" *International Journal of Qualitative Studies on Health and Well-Being* 6 (4): 10364. https://doi.org/10.3402/qhw.v6i4.10364.

Hilmore, P. 1985. "All the Secrets fit to Print: Brain Drain." *London Observer*, March 17.
Hoffman, Michael. 2006. "The Entheogen Theory of Religion and Ego Death." In *Salvia Divinorum*, Issue 4. http://egodeath.com/EntheogenTheoryOfReligion.htm.
"Joining Two Worlds." In *Science Contours: Faculty of Science Alumni Magazine. University of Alberta* 20 (2) (Fall 2008): 6–7. www.integrativescience.ca/uploads/files/Contours-UofA-2008-Integrative-Science.pdf.
Keckley, Paul. 2018. "Distrust in the U.S. Health System: Are We Paying Attention?" October 1. www.paulkeckley.com/the-keckley-report/2018/10/1/distrust-in-the-us-health-system-are-we-paying-attention.
Pacher, Pál, and George Kunos. 2013. "Modulating the Endocannabinoid System in Human Health and Disease—Successes and Failures." *FEBS Journal* 280 (9): 1918–43. doi:10.1111/febs.12260.
Puchalski, C., B. Ferrell, R. Virani, S. Otis-Green, P. Baird, J. Bull et al. 2009. "Improving the Quality of Spiritual Care as a Dimension of Palliative Care: The Report of the Consensus Conference." *Journal of Palliative Medicine* 12 (10): 885–904.
Roberts, Thomas B. 2019. *Mindapps: Multistate Theory and Tools for Mind Design*. Rochester, VT: Park Street Press.
Ruck, Carl A. P., Jeremy Bigwood, Danny Staples, Jonathan Ott, and R. Gordon Wasson. 1979. "Entheogens." *Journal of Psychedelic Drugs* 11: 145–46.
Sullivan, Mark. 2003. "The New Subjective Medicine: Taking the Patients Point of View on Health Care and Health." *Social Science & Medicine* 56 (7): 1595–604. https://doi.org/10.1016/s0277-9536(02)00159-4.
Tart, Charles T. 1990. "TASTE: The Archives of Scientists' Transcendent Experiences." www.issc-taste.org.
Weil, Andrew. 1975. *The Natural Mind*. Harmondsworth: Penguin.

9

Opioids and Substance Abuse

Cannabis as a Harm Reduction Tool

Adrianne Wilson-Poe

Conflict of Interest

Dr. Wilson-Poe is an equity interest owner in Smart Analytics LLC, which is a privately held entity with no external funding sources. Dr. Wilson-Poe is also a paid consultant and subject matter expert for Weedmaps, a technology company and online community. Neither Smart Analytics nor Weedmaps supplies monetary support or research materials to Dr. Wilson-Poe's academic research projects. Legacy Health has assessed Dr. Wilson-Poe's potential conflicts of interest and has determined that there are no conflict mitigation strategies required as of the date of this publication.

Introduction

Cannabis and opioids are both well known for their pain-relieving properties. Emerging evidence suggests that cannabis may be a critical harm reduction tool in the opioid crisis by increasing the safety of opioids, and in some cases replacing them entirely. The North American opioid overdose epidemic is an unparalleled public health crisis. Since 1979, accidental drug overdose in the United States has been increasing at an exponential rate and, alarmingly, the most profound increases in mortality are seen in the youngest generations (Jalal et al. 2018). The CDC estimates that 400,000 individuals have died from opioid overdose since 1999 (CDC 2019). In recent years, there have been concerted efforts from federal agencies, drug manufacturers, and opioid-prescribing physicians to curb opioid use and overdose. Unfortunately, measures such as abuse-deterrent formulations, prescription drug monitoring programs, revised prescription practices, and reduced drug manufacturing quotas have been largely unsuccessful in reducing opioid mortality (US Department of Justice 2018). Instead, these shifts have largely backfired, forcing opioid-dependent individuals to turn to the black market for the cheaper and more easily accessible alternative: heroin (Alpert, Powell, and Pacula 2017). In 2015, 80% of new heroin users were making the switch from prescription opioids because of cost and/or accessibility (Cicero, Ellis, and Harney 2015).

Fortunately, unlike the aforementioned interventions, promising evidence suggests that cannabis may be a powerful and efficacious tool in the alleviation of this crisis (Wiese and Wilson-Poe 2018).

DOI: 10.4324/9780429320491-9

The goal of this chapter is to provide an overview of the emerging evidence supporting the harm reduction potential of cannabis, specifically as it relates to opioid use. Despite the magnitude of the opioid crisis, the ubiquity and relative safety of cannabis render it a plausible intervention for widespread impacts on public health, yet many research questions remain. Whether the funding sources are public or private, foreign or domestic, there are numerous and diverse opportunities to characterize cannabis' potential to (1) relieve pain, either as an opioid adjunct or alternative, (2) alleviate opioid withdrawal, and (3) treat and/or prevent opioid dependence and relapse. The phytochemical diversity of cannabis and its numerous preparations present a unique challenge in fully understanding its harm reduction potential.

Background

As a preclinical and translational neuroscientist, I have been investigating the harm reduction potential of cannabis and cannabinoids for my entire adult life. Over the years, we have found that cannabinoids and opioids interact to enhance analgesia, that cannabinoids can mitigate opioid tolerance, and that pain patients readily use cannabis to substitute for opioids (Wilson, Maher, and Morgan 2008; Wilson-Poe, Lau, and Vaughan 2015; Wilson-Poe 2019). I have disseminated these findings at conferences across the globe, and developed continuing medical education curricula for pain physicians and anesthesiologists. I have also testified in state capitols about the impacts of cannabis on opioid use, and assisted Rep. Earl Blumenauer (OR) in disseminating this evidence to federal policy makers. I have served as a consultant and subject matter expert for the cannabis industry and an advisory board member for the political action committee New Approach. Thanks in large part to federal research barriers (discussed later), I have further expanded my work outside of academia through my entrepreneurial efforts by assessing the effects of "real-world" cannabis in adult-use consumers. I emphasize "real-world" cannabis here to highlight some of the barriers to conducting cannabis research within the current federal legal framework in the United States.

Historically, our scientific and medical understanding of cannabis' harm reduction potential has been most stunted by two types of research barriers: (1) insufficient funding and (2) insufficient drug supply. These obstacles, as well as additional bureaucratic hurdles, are thoroughly characterized elsewhere (NASEM 2017). Briefly, the vast majority of biomedical research funding in the United States comes from the National Institutes of Health (NIH), a federal agency. Because the federal government classifies cannabis as a Schedule I controlled substance (one with a high potential for abuse and no accepted medical use), the NIH is largely prohibited from funding research that explicitly examines the health benefits of cannabis. Most cannabis research is funded by the National Institute on Drug Abuse (NIDA), and the lion's share of these grants are still aimed at studying the negative impacts or prevention of cannabis use (NIH 2019). This funding landscape is reflective of the overarching disease prevention goals of the NIH; cannabis use has historically been categorized as an addictive disease. However, there are a handful of current studies (including my own) which essentially enter through the back door. That is, cannabis happens to be a component in the treatment or prevention of other drug abuse problems such as HIV and opioid dependence. Of course, it is plausible to obtain outside funding from non-NIH sources, such as private foundations. In some US states such as Colorado and Washington, cannabis tax dollars have been earmarked for scientific research and substance abuse treatment, although compared to the NIH, this budget is quite small; approximately $9.7 million in Washington for 2018 (Statista 2019).

The NIH as a whole has an annual research budget of approximately $35 billion, whereas NIDA's research budget is only $1 billion, which makes for an incredibly competitive funding environment with many researchers vying for a relatively small pool of money. Furthermore, for researchers who successfully secure funding, from the NIH or elsewhere, the next roadblock is the NIDA monopoly on the supply of cannabis as a research material. For almost 50 years, the University of Mississippi has held an exclusive contract with NIDA to grow and supply cannabis for research purposes. This means that both preclinical and clinical researchers are unable to study any form or source of cannabis that is not expressly provided by NIDA. This monopoly (exclusive to cannabis, no other Schedule I drugs) is particularly problematic given the lack of external validity of NIDA cannabis, which is phytochemically distinct from cannabis found in state-regulated markets (Vergara et al. 2017). Furthermore, under the current regulatory framework, Phase II trials are permitted (with NIDA-supplied cannabis), but there is no legal source for Phase III trials, which is why much of this work is taking place in Israel and Canada (Weizman et al. 2018).

Thus, in order to study the effects of "real-world" cannabis, my American colleagues and I have been obliged to get creative in navigating around the NIDA supply obstacle. For instance, investigators at the University of Colorado, Boulder, have built mobile laboratories to bring scientific instruments to cannabis-consuming research participants, rather than the typical drug study, which brings the participant into the lab (Bidwell et al. 2018). Likewise, because we are currently unable to assign non-NIDA-derived cannabis as an experimental treatment/intervention (i.e. conduct clinical trials), my colleagues and I are limited to conducting naturalistic observational studies. For example, we monitor and survey our pain patients about the types, frequency, and doses of dispensary-purchased cannabis products that they use to substitute for opioids. Furthermore, were it not for these funding and supply barriers, I would likely not be an entrepreneur. Rather, I would have simply applied for a grant to characterize the psychological and adverse side effects of adult-use, "real-world" cannabis.

Undoubtedly, NIDA-funded researchers have made significant contributions to the literature, despite constraints and the intentional emphasis on drug abuse and prevention thereof. One of the most impactful and controversial findings of NIDA-funded work in the 1970s and 80s was that cannabis use served as a "gateway" to the use of more dangerous drugs, including opioids (Yamaguchi and Kandel 1984). This seminal work by Dr. Denise Kandel has been used for decades as a rationale to uphold cannabis' status as a Schedule I controlled substance. However, more recent work has consistently refuted this hypothesis, especially in the context of opioid abuse (Reddon et al. 2018; Wiese and Wilson-Poe 2018). Importantly, and despite its 2016 refusal to reschedule cannabis, the federal Drug Enforcement Agency (DEA) acknowledges the lack of support for the gateway hypothesis (DEA 2016). An ever-growing body of evidence suggests that cannabis is not the gateway to opioid dependence, but rather an important exit strategy as either an alternative or adjunct therapy. This evidence is discussed in the following pages and falls into several distinct categories: safe and effective pain relief, alleviating opioid withdrawal, and preventing opioid dependence and relapse.

Analgesia: The First Step in Reducing Harm

No other pharmacological intervention rivals the powerful analgesic capacity of an opioid, which is precisely what makes them an ideal tool for acute, severe pain. Unfortunately, their continuous, chronic use is associated with the development of tolerance (more drug is needed to achieve the desired effect), physical dependence (the brain and body do not function properly in the absence of the drug), and other severe side effects such as abuse and lethal overdose. In 2016, the CDC estimated that more than 20% of the US population suffered from chronic pain, which highlights the scope of the need for safe and sustainable analgesic strategies that can be used for long periods of time (CDC 2018).

Humans have been using cannabis for pain relief dating back to at least 2700 BC (Abel 1980). The vast majority of patients enrolled in state-level medical cannabis programs list chronic pain as their qualifying condition (NASEM 2017). After decades of diligent research, the antinociceptive[1] properties of cannabis and its constituents have been thoroughly characterized in preclinical animal models. Both drugs produce analgesia by activating the same class of proteins (G-protein coupled receptors), on the same neurons, with the same effect on GABAergic neurotransmission[2] in the brain's descending pain pathway (Wilson-Poe, Lau, and Vaughan 2015).

Cannabinoids and opioids also exhibit synergistic analgesia when co-administered. This is a robust phenomenon that is consistent across many different cannabinoid and opioid agonists, administration routes, and species, including humans (Roberts, Gennings, and Shih 2006). Synergism inherently means that the doses of each drug required to elicit an analgesic response are lower than if the drug were used in isolation; any intervention that reduces opioid doses has obvious clinical utility. Preclinical evidence also suggests that when co-administered, cannabinoids can prevent the development of opioid tolerance (Wilson, Maher, and Morgan 2008). Taken together, these findings provide a strong rationale for adjunct cannabis during opioid administration. By enhancing the analgesic properties of opioids, cannabis appears to simultaneously support adequate pain relief while reducing opioid consumption, preventing tolerance, and preventing dose escalation. By these mechanisms, cannabis could be a powerful tool in preventing physical dependence upon opioids, thus improving their safety and reducing mortality.

In fact, when chronic pain patients are granted access to cannabis, they reduce their opioid consumption by approximately 50% (Gruber et al. 2016). This too is a robust phenomenon, which has been replicated across several research sites by various methodologies and levels of cannabis legalization (Haroutounian et al. 2016; Boehnke, Litinas, and Clauw 2016; Reiman, Welty, and Solomon 2017). Both the number of analgesic prescriptions written and overall spending in Medicare Part D (prescription drugs) is lower in states with medical cannabis laws (Liang et al. 2018; Bradford and Bradford 2016; Bradford et al. 2018). Pain patients also report that they find the side effects of cannabis more tolerable than opioids, and that, in general, they prefer cannabis to opioids (Reiman, Welty, and Solomon 2017). The opioid-sparing properties of cannabis for analgesia may at least partially contribute to the apparent ability of cannabis to reduce opioid overdose. Opioid-related hospitalizations and nonfatal overdoses are diminished in states with medical cannabis policies (Shi 2017), a phenomenon that also appears to be true for fatal overdoses. When examining data from 1999 through 2010, Bachhuber et al. (2014) demonstrated that states with medical cannabis legislation have an average of 24.8% lower annual opioid overdose mortality rates, compared to states without medical cannabis (p. 1668). These findings were subsequently validated by Columbia's School of Public Health (Kim et al. 2016), and more recent work also found that the presence of cannabis retail dispensaries is linked to fewer opioid deaths (Averett 2019). However, a recent report by Shover et al. (2019) suggests that opioid mortality (over a longer timeframe, 1999–2017) has continued to climb despite the presence of legal medical cannabis. These recent findings likely say more about the exponential growth of the overdose epidemic than they do about cannabis' impact on overdose. Interestingly, the impact of cannabis legislation does not appear to be strictly related to medical cannabis policies, as adult-use cannabis legislation is also associated with a 20%–35% reduction in annual opioid mortality (Chan 2019). This is not entirely surprising, given that 65% of adult-use (nonmedical) cannabis consumers in Colorado report using cannabis for pain relief (Bachhuber 2019).

Despite the accumulation of such promising evidence, many questions and research opportunities remain. The mechanisms underlying cannabis' ability to reduce opioid consumption are unknown but likely point to a pharmacodynamic[3] mechanism. Adjunct cannabis and cannabinoids do not alter the pharmacokinetic properties of opioids (Hurd et al. 2015; Abrams et al. 2011), and there is a large degree of translation between preclinical and clinical potentiation of analgesia. Also, although preclinical evidence suggests that cannabinoids reduce the development of opioid tolerance, this hypothesis has never been tested in humans. When feasible, randomized controlled trials (RCTs) will greatly enhance our understanding of the magnitude of the placebo effect for cannabis' analgesic and opioid-sparing properties, amongst many others.

There are also some conflicting reports, which find no evidence of opioid sparing in pain patients (Campbell et al. 2018). These conflicting findings may at least be partially attributed to the staggering phytochemical variability in cultivated varieties of cannabis (Hazekamp and Fischedick 2012). Although the analgesic properties and mechanisms of delta-9 THC are well characterized, this is only one constituent of botanical cannabis, which contains scores of other biologically active molecules with analgesic and anti-inflammatory properties. There are 114 known cannabinoids, in addition to flavonoids, terpenoids, alkaloids, ketones, and others (Brenneisen 2007). The potential for these molecules to produce potentiated benefits and buffered side effects is highly plausible (Russo 2011), yet highly variable. The chemical phenotype (chemotype) of cannabis is extremely sensitive to the environmental conditions in which it is grown. Of particular influence is the intensity and spectrum of light exposure (Hawley et al. 2018). As of this writing there was only one NIDA-funded grant examining the effect of different cannabis chemotypes on opioid use in pain patients, and even this study focuses solely on the ratio of THC to CBD (NIH 2018). Many years of rigorous research are required in order to determine the links between plant genotypes, environmental conditions, subsequent chemotypes, and resulting analgesia and opioid sparing.

Despite the extensive literature characterizing the antinociceptive properties of cannabinoids in animal models, there is shockingly sparse data about cannabis' ability to treat acute pain in humans. Until the year 2020, there was not a single published clinical study examining the efficacy of cannabis for mild-to-moderate acute pain or its efficacy to potentiate analgesia during a short course of opioids for trauma or post-operative pain. In a single-matched pilot study of patients admitted to the hospital with a traumatic injury, researchers found that in-patient administration of dronabinol (synthetic THC) was associated with a ninefold reduction in opioid consumption (Schneider-Smith et al. 2020). These results not only support the therapeutic value of cannabis for severe acute pain, but they also support the hypothesis that THC is the primary opioid-sparing component of cannabis. Herein lies what may be cannabis' greatest possible impact on public health in North America. Namely, leveraging the analgesic properties of cannabis during acute pain to prevent opioid exposure entirely, thus circumventing tolerance, dependence, and all other risks and side effects of opioids.

Harm Reduction and Withdrawal

A prominent feature of opioid dependence is the experience of withdrawal (when drug consumption is ceased), an agonizing and complex syndrome that can last for several weeks. When individuals are confronted with tolerance, the natural and often necessary response to avoid withdrawal is to escalate consumption. Dose escalation is commonly considered to be a key indicator of drug misuse, a sentiment that is confounded by insufficient analgesia. That is, even with the use of clinical tools such as the Prescription Drug Use Questionnaire, it is extremely difficult to parse out which patients are misusing medication and which simply have undertreated pain (Fishbain et al. 2008). The opioid-sparing properties of cannabis for analgesia may at least partially contribute to cannabis' apparent ability to reduce opioid overdose. However, the impact of cannabis on the nonmedical use of opioids is more nebulous.

As early as 1991 there were reports in the literature of opioid-dependent individuals using cannabis as a coping mechanism while going through self-detoxification (Gossop, Battersby, and Strang 1991). Even patients undergoing opioid replacement or medication-assisted therapy (MAT) report augmenting their regimen with cannabis when maintenance doses are not high enough to prevent withdrawal and craving (Heikman, Muhonen, and Ojanperä 2017). There is certainly a biological basis for cannabis to alleviate opioid withdrawal, given the robust evidence from cannabinoid administration in opioid-dependent animals (Lichtman et al. 2001; Scavone, Sterling, and Van Bockstaele 2013; Valverde et al. 2001). This phenomenon is at least partially mediated by the CB1 cannabinoid receptor, given that dronabinol (a synthetic analogue of THC) reduces withdrawal symptoms for patients undergoing naltrexone therapy (Bisaga et al. 2015).

The comparative efficacy of cannabis and other withdrawal medications has not been characterized, despite the fact opioid use disorder is a qualifying condition for the medical cannabis program in several US states (New York, New Jersey, and Pennsylvania at the time of publication). Supervised opioid replacement therapy (methadone and buprenorphine) is very efficacious for withdrawal symptoms. The major shortcoming of traditional MAT is not efficacy; rather, access and safety are of concern. Because methadone can cause fatal overdose, it must be administered under supervision. The highest concentration of methadone clinics is in large urban areas, leaving 47% of US counties underserved (Rosenblatt et al. 2015). Buprenorphine also carries some abuse and overdose liability, and only 3% of US physicians possess the credentials to prescribe it. Furthermore, there are strict quotas on the number of patients each licensed physician is able to serve (Sansone and Sansone 2015) and it is rarely covered by health insurance. Unlike traditional MAT, mortality and access are not a concern with cannabis. A majority of the adult population of the United States lives in a state with either recreational or medical cannabis, and fatal overdose is exceedingly rare (Politifact 2018; King and Corkery 2010). For rural America, homegrown cannabis may be not only a critical MAT, it could be the only option. For the millions of Americans who are geographically or economically unable to access opioid replacement therapy, cannabis could be a critical harm reduction tool, by alleviating withdrawal and preventing illicit opioid use.

As with analgesia, there are conflicting reports demonstrating either no effect or worsening withdrawal symptoms with cannabis use (Epstein and Preston 2015). Because participants in these studies are self-selecting cannabis cultivars, often from the black market, there is no data whatsoever with regard to which cannabis chemovars, preparations, formulations, doses, or routes of administration are the most efficacious. Most of this sparse clinical data was collected before incremental cannabis legalization in the US, when safety and potency laboratory testing became commonplace. In addition to the unknown and highly variable phytochemical makeup of pre-legalization plants, the impact of pesticides, heavy metals, mold, and other contaminants on clinical outcomes is entirely unknown.

Long-Term Recovery and Emotional Support

Opioid maintenance drugs were designed and are most efficacious for short-term use during the acute withdrawal phase. In clinical practice, they are used for great lengths of time, and for some patients, this means a lifetime of opioid dependence. Despite the high relapse rate (~50%) for both methadone and buprenorphine replacement therapy, the combination of MAT and social support remains the most efficacious relapse prevention strategy. Some studies have shown that dronabinol and intermittent and whole-plant cannabis increase MAT treatment adherence, whereas more recent studies have shown the best treatment adherence in daily cannabis users (Bagra et al. 2018). Furthermore, patients who use adjunct cannabis appear to require lower doses of buprenorphine (Socias et al. 2018), which, similar to chronic pain patients, suggests that cannabis is opioid sparing in this population.

Opioid use and misuse do not exist in a vacuum. Chronic pain and affective disorders such as depression and anxiety have a high degree of comorbidity. People with a history of substance use disorders are particularly difficult to treat; 80% of patients on MAT have had recent pain, and 37% are in chronic pain. Pain itself is a trigger for hypervigilance, catastrophizing, and self-medication through substance misuse (Garland et al. 2013). When opioid analgesics are not an option, and pain and stress converge to fuel drug craving, relapse prevention is exceedingly challenging.

Recent preclinical evidence has demonstrated a neurobiological link between bodily pain and negative affect, which at least partially explains the high degree of comorbidity of pain and disordered mood. Pain itself induces changes in the kappa opioid receptor system in the brain's reward pathway, thereby triggering dysphoria and reducing motivation (Massaly et al. 2019; Massaly, Morón, and

Al-Hasani 2016). Negative mood and anxiety are also major contributors to drug craving. There has long been a focus on developing novel opioid alternatives that produce analgesia in the absence of reinforcement or reward, but in light of this most recent evidence, this approach may not be the most prudent. Rather, mild stimulation of the reward pathway may be exactly the kind of therapy that is required to offset the pain-induced negative affect mediated by the kappa opioid system in the reward pathway. That is, if the desired outcome is not necessarily the utter erasure of somatic pain but instead quality of life with the least harm, then there is great therapeutic value in the mild euphoria and analgesia produced by THC's activation of CB1 receptors. Ironically, cannabis' ability to enhance mood is precisely the reason it has been so thoroughly studied over the decades, albeit through a drug abuse lens. The neurobiological link between the affective and somatic components of pain may be a critical turning point, inducing a paradigm shift away from the somewhat puritanical idea that medicine should not make the patient feel good.

Furthermore, recent clinical studies have demonstrated a role for cannabidiol in the prevention of opioid craving. A single oral administration of 400–800 mg CBD can prevent both drug cue-induced anxiety and craving for at least 7 days (Hurd et al. 2019). CBD is a non-intoxicating compound with a wide therapeutic window, minimal side effects and anti-inflammatory and anxiolytic properties. CBD also significantly buffers the cognitive impairment and paranoia produced by THC (Englund et al. 2013).

Combined, the data herein provide a strong rationale for cannabis-derived therapy to support the various needs of individuals in recovery from prescription and illicit opioid dependence; namely, analgesia, mood support, withdrawal alleviation, and suppression of craving. Cannabis can undoubtedly be abused and produce tolerance and withdrawal (somewhat analogous to nicotine). It also carries dose-dependent and age-dependent risks for hyperemesis, psychosis, and other psychosocial factors. Cannabis may not be risk-free, but its nonlethal side effects render it a desirable harm reduction tool.

Beyond Barriers: The Forthcoming Research Agenda

Because I am not a legal professional, it is difficult for me to speculate which imminent legislative agendas or regulatory reforms would be most effective for eliminating the research barriers necessary to fully characterize the harm reduction potential of cannabis in the opioid crisis. However, there are two overarching goals, which any and all federal reform should accomplish: (1) the entirety of the NIH research budget should be open to grant proposals that aim to study the medical utility of cannabis. This may very well require removal of cannabis from the federal list of controlled substances (de-scheduling). (2) NIDA should be removed as the mandatory and exclusive intermediary between the scientists and their research materials; a legal path for "real-world" cannabis for all research, including Phase III clinical trials, is of absolute necessity. In this post-prohibition context, research opportunities investigating cannabis' harm reduction potential are plentiful.

It stands to reason that cannabis' greatest potential impact on global health is as a first-line analgesic: entirely substituting for and preventing opioid use. Although the safety of cannabis is well known, its efficacy for acute pain in humans is poorly characterized. A short course of opioids for post-operative and severe pain is of obvious clinical utility, but the efficacy of substituted or adjunct cannabis in the post-acute phase of injury or surgical recovery is a vital line of inquiry. Likewise, the preclinical evidence demonstrating reduced tolerance and enhanced analgesia during combined opioid/cannabis administration is a phenomenon of immense clinical utility that warrants prompt investigation.

Although there are several FDA medications on the market for the treatment of opioid withdrawal symptoms, the comparative efficacy of these medications against (or adjunct with) cannabis is unknown. What little data there is about the potential for cannabis to be opioid sparing for both pain patients and those maintained on MAT warrants replication, with standardized cannabis therapy as opposed to participant-selected cannabis. Given the promising emerging evidence presented in this chapter, there is a strong rationale for concurrent measurement of mood, pain, MAT adherence, and opioid relapse, as well as a general shift toward the holistic treatment of these comorbidities with cannabis and/or CBD.

For all of the studies outlined earlier, there are of course the additional complexities of preparation, formulation, dose, and route of administration that are the most efficacious for harm reduction, as well as the underlying mechanisms. Furthermore, the long-term effects of medically relevant cannabis (as opposed to either purely intoxicating or unknown phenotypes) require rigorous characterization.

Whether future research is aimed at analgesia, opioid withdrawal, or relapse prevention, there are several commonalities that warrant attention. First, throughout the literature, "cannabis" is referred to as one intervention, essentially one drug. There are two factors to consider as we move beyond this tremendous oversimplification: (1) within-plant phytochemical diversity and (2) between-plant variability in these molecules. The former requires us to rigorously assess the "entourage effect," that is, the hypothesized clinical superiority of "full-spectrum" cannabis (with scores of biologically active ingredients), compared directly with more simplified/less chemically diverse preparations thereof (Ben-Shabat et al. 1998; Russo 2018). The latter requires unfaltering attention to the chemical phenotype of the study drug. Of particular importance is an emphasis on products or cultivars with low THC potency. Our current understanding of cannabis, particularly its long-term impacts, comes largely from studies where individuals were smoking black market cannabis, and across many illicit drug markets (including alcohol) prohibition is known to promote potency. The therapeutic value and minimized risks of legal, lower potency cannabis cultivars (ideally consumed without combustion) is a virtually untouched and immense avenue of research. Finally, the magnitude of the placebo effect of cannabis for opioid-related effects is virtually nonexistent. Randomized, placebo-controlled clinical trials will greatly enhance our understanding of the extent of the placebo effect for cannabis' harm-reducing properties, amongst many other clinical benefits.

Unrestricted by research barriers, we will be poised to make seminal contributions to the cannabis and cannabinoid literature, with immense implications for global public health. Although the harm reduction potential of cannabis is considerable, it is important that we reflect on the hard-learned lessons of the opioid crisis so as not to repeat our mistakes. We would be wise to remain steadfastly focused on safe and sustainable pain relief in the absence of drug abuse and negative socioeconomic impacts.

Notes

1 Antinociception is the process of blocking an organism's detection of noxious or painful sensations. Antinociception is different from analgesia (the relief of an unpleasant sensory and emotional experience associated with real or potential tissue damage), in that it is virtually impossible to assess "unpleasantness" in animals; it is only possible to observe an animal's behavioral response to a noxious stimulus.

2 Neurons communicate with one another in the brain using chemical messengers, known as neurotransmitters. The neurotransmitter GABA has an important role in both pain transmission (the communication of pain signals between neurons) and pain relief.

3 Pharmacodynamics is the physical interaction of a drug with its targets within the body and the physiological changes that occur as a result of this interaction. Cannabinoids do not appear to alter the absorption, distribution, metabolism, or excretion (pharmacokinetics) of opioids, which suggests they interact pharmacodynamically.

References

Abel, Ernest L. 1980. *Marihuana, The First Twelve Thousand Years*. New York: Springer Science+Business Media.

Abrams, D. I., P. Couey, S. B. Shade, M. E. Kelly, and N. L. Benowitz. 2011. "Cannabinoid-Opioid Interaction in Chronic Pain." *Clinical Pharmacology & Therapeutics* 90 (6): 844–51. doi:10.1038/clpt.2011.188.

Alpert, Abby, David Powell, and Rosalie Liccardo Pacula. 2017. "Supply-Side Drug Policy in the Presence of Substitutes: Evidence from the Introduction of Abuse-Deterrent Opioids." National Bureau of Economic Research Working Paper Series No. 23031. doi:10.3386/w23031.

Averett, S., and E. Smith. 2019. "Medical Marijuana Laws and Their Effect on Opioid Related Mortality." *Economics Bulletin* 39 (1): 347–57.

Bachhuber, M. A., J. H. Arnsten, and G. Wurm. 2019. "Use of Cannabis to Relieve Pain and Promote Sleep by Customers at an Adult Use Dispensary." *Journal of Psychoactive Drugs* Epub ahead of print. doi:10.1080/02791072.2019.1626953.

Bachhuber, M. A., Brendan Saloner, Chinazo O Cunningham, and Colleen L. Barry. 2014. "Medical Cannabis Laws and Opioid Analgesic Overdose Mortality in the United States, 1999–2010." *JAMA Internal Medicine* 174 (10): 1668–73.

Bagra, I., V. Krishnan, R. Rao, and A. Agrawal. 2018. "Does Cannabis Use Influence Opioid Outcomes and Quality of Life Among Buprenorphine Maintained Patients? A Cross-sectional, Comparative Study." *Journal of Addiction Medicine* 12 (4): 315–20. doi:10.1097/ADM.0000000000000406.

Ben-Shabat, S., E. Fride, T. Sheskin, T. Tamiri, M. H. Rhee, Z. Vogel, T. Bisogno, L. De Petrocellis, V. Di Marzo, and R. Mechoulam. 1998. "An Entourage Effect: Inactive Endogenous Fatty Acid Glycerol Esters Enhance 2-Arachidonoyl-Glycerol Cannabinoid Activity." *European Journal of Pharmacology* 353 (1): 23–31. doi:10.1016/s0014-2999(98)00392-6.

Bidwell, L. C., R. Mueller, S. L. YorkWilliams, S. Hagerty, A. D. Bryan, and K. E. Hutchison. 2018. "A Novel Observational Method for Assessing Acute Responses to Cannabis: Preliminary Validation Using Legal Market Strains." *Cannabis and Cannabinoid Research* 3 (1): 35–44. doi:10.1089/can.2017.0038.

Bisaga, Adam, Maria A. Sullivan, Andrew Glass, Kaitlyn Mishlen, Martina Pavlicova, Margaret Haney, Wilfrid N. Raby, Frances R. Levin, Kenneth M. Carpenter, and John J. Mariani. 2015. "The Effects of Dronabinol During Detoxification and the Initiation of Treatment with Extended Release Naltrexone." *Drug & Alcohol Dependence* 154: 38–45.

Boehnke, Kevin F., Evangelos Litinas, and Daniel J. Clauw. 2016. "Medical Cannabis Use is Associated with Decreased Opiate Medication Use in a Retrospective Cross-Sectional Survey of Patients with Chronic Pain." *The Journal of Pain* 17 (6): 739–44.

Bradford, A. C., and W. D. Bradford. 2016. "Medical Marijuana Laws Reduce Prescription Medication Use in Medicare Part D." *Health Aff (Millwood)* 35 (7): 1230–36. doi:10.1377/hlthaff.2015.1661.

Bradford, A. C., W. D. Bradford, Amanda Abraham, and Grace Bagwell Adams. 2018. "Association between US State Medical Cannabis Laws and Opioid Prescribing in the Medicare Part D Population." *JAMA Internal Medicine* 178 (5): 667–72.

Brenneisen, Rudolf. 2007. "Chemistry and Analysis of Phytocannabinoids and Other Cannabis Constituents." In *Marijuana and the Cannabinoids*, edited by Mahmoud A. ElSohly, 17–49. Totowa, NJ: Humana Press.

Campbell, G., W. D. Hall, A. Peacock, N. Lintzeris, R. Bruno, B. Larance, S. Nielsen, M. Cohen, G. Chan, R. P. Mattick, F. Blyth, M. Shanahan, T. Dobbins, M. Farrell, and L. Degenhardt. 2018. "Effect of Cannabis Use in People with Chronic Non-Cancer Pain Prescribed Opioids: Findings from a 4-Year Prospective Cohort Study." *Lancet Public Health* 3 (7): e341–e350. doi:10.1016/S2468-2667(18)30110-5.

CDC. 2018. "Prevalence of Chronic Pain and High-Impact Chronic Pain Among Adults—United States, 2016." Accessed June 29, 2019. www.cdc.gov/mmwr/volumes/67/wr/mm6736a2.htm.

CDC, Centers for Disease Control and Prevention. 2019. "Opioid Overdose—Understanding the Epidemic." Accessed March 25, 2019. www.cdc.gov/drugoverdose/epidemic/index.html.

Chan, N. W., J. Burkhardt, and M. Flyr. 2019. "The Effects of Recreational Marijuana Legalization and Dispensing on Opioid Mortality." *Economic Inquiry* e-pub ahead of print. doi:10.1111/ecin.12819.

Cicero, Theodore J., Matthew S. Ellis, and Jessie Harney. 2015. "Shifting Patterns of Prescription Opioid and Heroin Abuse in the United States." *New England Journal of Medicine* 373 (18): 1789–90.

DEA, Drug Enforcement Agency, Department of Justice. 2016. "Denial of Petition to Initiate Proceedings to Reschedule Marijuana." Accessed September 15, 2019. www.federalregister.gov/documents/2016/08/12/2016-17954/denial-of-petition-to-initiate-proceedings-to-reschedule-marijuana.

Englund, A., P. D. Morrison, J. Nottage, D. Hague, F. Kane, S. Bonaccorso, J. M. Stone, A. Reichenberg, R. Brenneisen, D. Holt, A. Feilding, L. Walker, R. M. Murray, and S. Kapur. 2013. "Cannabidiol Inhibits

THC-elicited Paranoid Symptoms and Hippocampal-Dependent Memory Impairment." *Journal of Psychopharmacology* 27 (1): 19–27. doi:10.1177/0269881112460109.

Epstein, David H., and Kenzie L. Preston. 2015. "No Evidence for Reduction of Opioid-Withdrawal Symptoms by Cannabis Smoking During a Methadone Dose Taper." *The American Journal on Addictions* 24 (4): 323–28.

Fishbain, D. A., B. Cole, J. Lewis, H. L. Rosomoff, and R. S. Rosomoff. 2008. "What Percentage of Chronic Nonmalignant Pain Patients Exposed to Chronic Opioid Analgesic Therapy Develop Abuse/Addiction and/or Aberrant Drug-Related Behaviors? A Structured Evidence-Based Review." *Pain Medicine* 9 (4): 444–59. doi:10.1111/j.1526-4637.2007.00370.x.

Garland, E. L., B. Froeliger, F. Zeidan, K. Partin, and M. O. Howard. 2013. "The Downward Spiral of Chronic Pain, Prescription Opioid Misuse, and Addiction: Cognitive, Affective, and Neuropsychopharmacologic Pathways." *Neuroscience & Biobehavioral Reviews* 37 (10 Pt 2): 2597–607. doi:10.1016/j.neubiorev.2013.08.006.

Gossop, Michael, Malcolm Battersby, and John Strang. 1991. "Self-Detoxification by Opiate Addicts: A Preliminary Investigation." *The British Journal of Psychiatry* 159 (2): 208–12.

Gruber, Staci A., Kelly A. Sagar, Mary K. Dahlgren, Megan T. Racine, Rosemary T. Smith, and Scott E. Lukas. 2016. "Splendor in the Grass? A Pilot Study Assessing the Impact of Medical Marijuana on Executive Function." *Frontiers in Pharmacology* 7: 355.

Haroutounian, Simon, Yael Ratz, Yehuda Ginosar, Karina Furmanov, Fayez Saifi, Ronit Meidan, and Elyad Davidson. 2016. "The Effect of Medicinal Cannabis on Pain and Quality-of-Life Outcomes in Chronic Pain: A Prospective Open-Label Study." *The Clinical Journal of Pain* 32 (12): 1036–43.

Hawley, Dave, Thomas Graham, Michael Stasiak, and Mike Dixon. 2018. "Improving Cannabis Bud Quality and Yield with Subcanopy Lighting." 53 (11): 1593. doi:10.21273/hortsci13173-18.

Hazekamp, A., and J. T. Fischedick. 2012. "Cannabis—from Cultivar to Chemovar." *Drug Testing and Analysis* 4 (7–8): 660–67. doi:10.1002/dta.407.

Heikman, Pertti Kalevi, Leea Hellevi Muhonen, and Ilkka Antero Ojanperä. 2017. "Polydrug Abuse Among Opioid Maintenance Treatment Patients is Related to Inadequate Dose of Maintenance Treatment Medicine." *BMC Psychiatry* 17 (1): 245.

Hurd, Y. L., M. Yoon, A. F. Manini, S. Hernandez, R. Olmedo, M. Ostman, and D. Jutras-Aswad. 2015. "Early Phase in the Development of Cannabidiol as a Treatment for Addiction: Opioid Relapse Takes Initial Center Stage." *Neurotherapeutics* 12 (4): 807–15. doi:10.1007/s13311-015-0373-7.

Hurd, Y. L., S. Spriggs, J. Alishayev, G. Winkel, K. Gurgov, C. Kudrich, A. M. Oprescu, and E. Salsitz. 2019. "Cannabidiol for the Reduction of Cue-Induced Craving and Anxiety in Drug-Abstinent Individuals with Heroin Use Disorder: A Double-Blind Randomized Placebo-Controlled Trial." *The American Journal of Psychiatry*: appiajp201918101191. doi:10.1176/appi.ajp.2019.18101191.

Jalal, H., J. M. Buchanich, M. S. Roberts, L. C. Balmert, K. Zhang, and D. S. Burke. 2018. "Changing Dynamics of the Drug Overdose Epidemic in the United States from 1979 through 2016." *Science* 361 (6408). doi:10.1126/science.aau1184.

Kim, J. H., J. Santaella-Tenorio, C. Mauro, J. Wrobel, M. Cerda, K. M. Keyes, D. Hasin, S. S. Martins, and G. Li. 2016. "State Medical Marijuana Laws and the Prevalence of Opioids Detected Among Fatally Injured Drivers." *American Journal of Public Health* 106 (11): 2032–37. doi:10.2105/AJPH.2016.303426.

King, L. A., and J. M. Corkery. 2010. "An Index of Fatal Toxicity for Drugs of Misuse." *Human Psychopharmacology* 25 (2): 162–66. doi:10.1002/hup.1090.

Liang, D., Y. Bao, M. Wallace, I. Grant, and Y. Shi. 2018. "Medical Cannabis Legalization and Opioid Prescriptions: Evidence on US Medicaid Enrollees during 1993–2014." *Addiction*. doi:10.1111/add.14382.

Lichtman, A. H., S. M. Sheikh, H. H. Loh, and B. R. Martin. 2001. "Opioid and Cannabinoid Modulation of Precipitated Withdrawal in Δ9-Tetrahydrocannabinol and Morphine-Dependent Mice." *Journal of Pharmacology and Experimental Therapeutics* 298 (3): 1007–14.

Massaly, N., B. A. Copits, A. R. Wilson-Poe, L. Hipolito, T. Markovic, H. J. Yoon, S. Liu, M. C. Walicki, D. L. Bhatti, S. Sirohi, A. Klaas, B. M. Walker, R. Neve, C. M. Cahill, K. I. Shoghi, R. W. th Gereau, J. G. McCall, R. Al-Hasani, M. R. Bruchas, and J. A. Moron. 2019. "Pain-Induced Negative Affect Is Mediated via Recruitment of The Nucleus Accumbens Kappa Opioid System." *Neuron*. doi:10.1016/j.neuron.2019.02.029.

Massaly, Nicolas, Jose A. Morón, and Ream Al-Hasani. 2016. "A Trigger for Opioid Misuse: Chronic Pain and Stress Dysregulate the Mesolimbic Pathway and Kappa Opioid System." *Frontiers in Neuroscience* 10: 480.

NASEM. 2017. *The Health Effects of Cannabis and Cannabinoids: The Current State of Evidence and Recommendations for Research*. Washington, DC: National Academies Press. National Academies of Sciences, Engineering, and Medicine; Health and Medicine Division; Board on Population Health and Public Health Practice; Committee on the Health Effects of Marijuana.

NIH, National Institutes of Health. 2018. "Medical Marijuana Program Participation and Changes in Controlled Substance Use." Accessed March 25, 2019. https://projectreporter.nih.gov/project_info_description.cfm?aid=9600110&icde=41905897.

———. 2019. "Research Online Reporting Tools (RePORT)." Accessed June 1, 2019. https://projectreporter.nih.gov/reporter.cfm.

Politifact. 2018. "Do a Majority of Americans Live in States with Legal Marijuana?" [Website], Last Modified April 19, 2018. Accessed August 1, 2019. www.politifact.com/california/statements/2018/apr/20/john-chiang/do-majority-americans-live-states-legal-marijuana/.

Reddon, H., K. DeBeck, M. E. Socias, H. Dong, E. Wood, J. Montaner, T. Kerr, and M. J. Milloy. 2018. "Cannabis Use is Associated with Lower Rates of Initiation of Injection Drug Use Among Street-Involved Youth: A Longitudinal Analysis." *Drug Alcohol Review* 37 (3): 421–28. doi:10.1111/dar.12667.

Reiman, Amanda, Mark Welty, and Perry Solomon. 2017. "Cannabis as a Substitute for Opioid-Based Pain Medication: Patient Self-Report." *Cannabis and Cannabinoid Research* 2 (1): 160–66.

Roberts, John D., Chris Gennings, and Margaret Shih. 2006. "Synergistic Affective Analgesic Interaction between Delta-9-Tetrahydrocannabinol and Morphine." *European Journal of Pharmacology* 530 (1–2): 54–58.

Rosenblatt, Roger A., C. Holly A. Andrilla, Mary Catlin, and Eric H. Larson. 2015. "Geographic and Specialty Distribution of US Physicians Trained to Treat Opioid Use Disorder." *The Annals of Family Medicine* 13 (1): 23–26.

Russo, E. B. 2011. "Taming THC: Potential Cannabis Synergy and Phytocannabinoid-Terpenoid Entourage Effects." *British Journal of Pharmacology* 163 (7): 1344–64. doi:10.1111/j.1476-5381.2011.01238.x.

———. 2018. "The Case for the Entourage Effect and Conventional Breeding of Clinical Cannabis: No 'Strain,' No Gain." *Frontiers in Plant Science* 9: 1969. doi:10.3389/fpls.2018.01969.

Sansone, Randy A., and Lori A. Sansone. 2015. "Buprenorphine Treatment for Narcotic Addiction: Not Without Risks." *Innovations in Clinical Neuroscience* 12 (3–4): 32.

Scavone, J. L., R. C. Sterling, and E. J. Van Bockstaele. 2013. "Cannabinoid and Opioid Interactions: Implications for Opiate Dependence and Withdrawal." *Neuroscience* 248: 637–54.

Schneider-Smith, E., K. Salottolo, C. Swartwood, C. Melvin, R. M. Madayag, and D. Bar-Or. (2020). "Matched Pilot Study Examining Cannabis-Based Dronabinol for Acute Pain Following Traumatic Injury." *Trauma Surgery & Acute Care Open* 5 (1): e000391. https://doi.org/10.1136/tsaco-2019-000391.

Shi, Yuyan. 2017. "Medical Marijuana Policies and Hospitalizations Related to Marijuana and Opioid Pain Reliever." *Drug & Alcohol Dependence* 173: 144–50.

Shover, C. L., C. S. Davis, S. C. Gordon, and K. Humphreys. 2019. "Association between Medical Cannabis Laws and Opioid Overdose Mortality Has Reversed Over Time." *Proceedings of the National Academy of Sciences of the United States of America* 116 (26): 12624–26. doi:10.1073/pnas.1903434116.

Socias, M. E., E. Wood, S. Lake, S. Nolan, N. Fairbairn, K. Hayashi, H. P. Shulha, S. Liu, T. Kerr, and M. J. Milloy. 2018. "High-Intensity Cannabis Use is Associated with Retention in Opioid Agonist Treatment: A Longitudinal Analysis." *Addiction* 113 (12): 2250–58. doi:10.1111/add.14398.

Statista. 2019. "Excise Tax Revenue of Cannabis in Washington State, United States from 2015 to 2018 (in million U.S. dollars)." Accessed July 1, 2019. www.statista.com/statistics/731917/us-washington-state-marijuana-sales-taxes/.

US Department of Justice, Drug Enforcement Agency—DEA. 2018. "Established Aggregate Production Quotas for Schedule I and II Controlled Substances and Assessment of Annual Needs for the List I Chemicals Ephedrine, Pseudoephedrine, and Phenylpropanolamine for 2019." Last Modified Friday, December 28, 2018, Accessed March 25, 2019. www.deadiversion.usdoj.gov/fed_regs/quotas/2018/fr1228.htm.

Valverde, Olga, Florence Noble, Françoise Beslot, Valérie Daugé, Marie-Claude Fournié-Zaluski, and Bernard P. Roques. 2001. "Δ9-Tetrahydrocannabinol Releases and Facilitates the Effects of Endogenous Enkephalins:

Reduction in Morphine Withdrawal Syndrome without Change in Rewarding Effect." *European Journal of Neuroscience* 13 (9): 1816–24.

Vergara, D., L. C. Bidwell, R. Gaudino, A. Torres, G. Du, T. C. Ruthenburg, K. deCesare, D. P. Land, K. E. Hutchison, and N. C. Kane. 2017. "Compromised External Validity: Federally Produced Cannabis Does Not Reflect Legal Markets." *Scientific Reports* 7: 46528. doi:10.1038/srep46528.

Weizman, L., L. Dayan, S. Brill, H. Nahman-Averbuch, T. Hendler, G. Jacob, and H. Sharon. 2018. "Cannabis Analgesia in Chronic Neuropathic Pain is Associated with Altered Brain Connectivity." *Neurology* 91 (14): e1285–e1294. doi:10.1212/WNL.0000000000006293.

Wiese, B., and A. R. Wilson-Poe. 2018. "Emerging Evidence for Cannabis' Role in Opioid Use Disorder." *Cannabis Cannabinoid Res* 3 (1): 179–89. doi:10.1089/can.2018.0022.

Wilson, Adrianne R., Lauren Maher, and Michael M. Morgan. 2008. "Repeated Cannabinoid Injections into the Rat Periaqueductal Gray Enhance Subsequent Morphine Antinociception." *Neuropharmacology* 55 (7): 1219–25.

Wilson-Poe, A. R., and A. Gries. 2019. "Efficacy, Side Effects, and Patterns of Medical Cannabis Use Among Patients with Chronic Low Back Pain." International Cannabinoid Research Conference, Bethesda, MD, June 30, 2019.

Wilson-Poe, A. R., B. K. Lau, and C. W. Vaughan. 2015. "Repeated Morphine Treatment Alters Cannabinoid Modulation of GABAergic Synaptic Transmission within the Rat Periaqueductal Grey." *British Journal of Pharmacology* 172 (2): 681–90. doi:10.1111/bph.12809.

Yamaguchi, K., and D. B. Kandel. 1984. "Patterns of Drug Use from Adolescence to Young Adulthood: III. Predictors of Progression." *American Journal of Public Health* 74 (7): 673–81. doi:10.2105/ajph.74.7.673.

10

Cannabis in Exercise and Sport

Whitney Ogle

Keywords: exercise, physical activity, sport, physiology, human performance

Introduction

Cannabis research and public health has typically been framed in terms of health and safety risks or in relation to potential benefits from medical cannabis use in medical patient populations. Indeed, surveys have shown that people are using medical cannabis to manage a variety of symptoms and health conditions (Corroon and Phillips 2018; Hazekamp et al. 2013; Lucas, Baron, and Jikomes 2019; Reinarman et al. 2011; Sexton et al. 2016; Walsh et al. 2013). But an angle of the cannabis research that has reentered the public health conversation since the emergence of legal markets is the use of cannabis in sport and during exercise. The purpose of this chapter is to summarize the history of research related to cannabis and physical activity, assess cannabis regulations in sport, and consider future directions for research on the effects of cannabis on physiological, psychological, and neuromotor control aspects of human performance.

Cannabis use has typically been associated with a "lazy stoner" archetype in popular culture (see Newhart and Dolphin Chapter 24 and Rodgers Chapter 26), so it may be counterintuitive to some to learn that some athletes consistently pair the two during training. With legalization and decriminalization of recreational cannabis becoming more common, more users are speaking openly about combining cannabis with exercise (Lev 2020; Armstrong 2018; Brand 2019; deBara 2019; Bures 2020; NORML 2015; *Emerald Magazine* 2018). Companies, hashtags, and events have been formed for the sole intention of promoting cannabis and exercise (Bonner 2018; Cannathlete 2020; Stigma Activewear 2020). There is a palpable thirst for more information about the effects of cannabis on exercise, but the current federal regulations have created such a burden on the research process that the public is filling in the gaps with anecdotes. It is clear that the public wants and needs good research to investigate the actual impacts of cannabis on exercise performance (Nguyen 2019).

DOI: 10.4324/9780429320491-10

Cannabis and Exercise

The first round of studies on the effects of cannabis on human physiology were conducted in the late 1960s to early 1980s (Weil, Zinberg, and Nelsen 1968; Manno et al. 1970; Renault et al. 1971; Schwin 1973; Tashkin et al. 1975; Peters et al. 1976; Kvålseth 1977; Maksud and Baron 1980; Tashkin, Shapiro, and Frank 1973; Steadward and Singh 1975). These studies are still cited today in part because there are not many articles in this field, but also because investigations into the effects of cannabis on heart rate, pulmonary function, mental function, and physical performance set the stage for our current understanding of cannabis and human physiology. Cannabis and human physiology research faced a lull in the 1980s and 1990s, but it has been slowly growing in the past 20 years in spite of the continued regulatory barriers to cannabis research.

In 2003, Sparling et al. provided the first evidence that endurance exercise stimulates the endocannabinoid system. They proposed that the rise in anandamide levels (which bind to CB1 receptors of the endocannabinoid system) may explain the exercise-induced analgesia and the infamous "runner's high" feeling in endurance athletes (Sparling et al. 2003). The cannabinoids found in the cannabis plant enter our systems through various methods of administration and bind to the CB1 and CB2 receptors of the endocannabinoid system. This shared pathway may explain positive responses to exercise when paired with cannabis (Gillman, Hutchison, and Bryan 2015). Learning about the location of CB1 and CB2 receptors in the endocannabinoid system, as well as the role that the endocannabinoid system plays, has already broadened our understanding and provided possible mechanisms for the role that cannabis may play in modulating human movement, exercise performance, and recovery from exercise.

In the fall of 2017, my research team at Humboldt State University started exploring the relationship between cannabis and physical activity. In a review of secondary data sources (from blogs, magazine articles, social media, etc.), we identified common reasons why people combine cannabis and exercise to build a new survey of cannabis use with exercise. As it turns out, people use cannabis with exercise for many reasons that address psychological, neuromotor, and physiological domains of performance. Lisano et al. (2019) found that people used cannabis before physical activity to manage pain, improve focus, and for relaxation. It will be important to systematically research these factors in order to determine the actual benefits of cannabis in exercise. Similarly, a recent survey of people who use cannabis before and/or after exercise found that they met official exercise recommendations and agreed that cannabis not only increased their enjoyment of and motivation for exercise but also improved their recovery after exercise (YorkWilliams et al. 2019). Growing research is revealing that people are using cannabis in conjunction with physical activity because they perceive it to contribute positively to the exercise experience (Lisano et al. 2019; YorkWilliams et al. 2019).

Preliminary results from our research reveal that people use cannabis before all kinds of exercise—from archery to waterskiing. This list includes a mixture of activities that are considered both aerobic and anaerobic, from those that require more power to those that require more precision. In addition, the timing of cannabis use related to physical activity may differ by activity (Lisano et al. 2019). Again, this highlights the need for future research into all aspects of movement and exercise. This research will also be necessary to facilitate the development of rules and regulations regarding cannabis in elite sport competitions.

Cannabis Regulations in Athletic Competition

The link between cannabis and athletics has been illuminated in multiple contexts. When looking at rates of drug and alcohol use in athletes, the research has shown that cannabis use is second to alcohol (Brisola-Santos et al. 2016; Docter et al. 2020). The rates of cannabis use in sport change depending on gender and type of activity. For example, one study found a particular pairing between cannabis and extreme "sliding" sports (such as windsurfing, skiing, snowboarding, surfing, and sailing) in athletes from a sport science university in France (Lorente, Peretti-Watel, and Grelot 2005).

But is cannabis a performance-enhancing substance? The World Anti-Doping Agency (WADA) is responsible for establishing the list of prohibited substances and methods of training in sport competitions, and cannabis is on the list of substances prohibited in competition only. This list is updated annually, with new substances added if they meet two of the following three criteria:

1. It has the potential to enhance or enhances sport performance.
2. It represents an actual or potential health risk to the athlete.
3. It violates the spirit of sport.

According to WADA, cannabis meets all three of these criteria. Generally, cannabis has the capacity to decrease anxiety in athletes prior to competition and to aid in sleep during recovery, therefore it is seen as having potential to enhance sport performance (USADA 2019; Huestis, Mazzoni, and Rabin 2011). At the same time, there may be risks to the cardiopulmonary or psychological health of athletes who use cannabis, so it represents a potential health risk to athletes (USADA 2019; Huestis, Mazzoni, and Rabin 2011). While there is sparse evidence for the first and second criteria (Docter et al. 2020), marijuana's illegal status in most countries implies that it violates the spirit of sport and is therefore prohibited in international competitions (USADA 2019).

When an athlete tests positive for cannabis, it is unclear whether they are using it for recreation or to enhance performance. Cannabis can be detected in urine weeks after use, so a positive test might reflect that an athlete used cannabis in a social environment weeks before competition (Saugy et al. 2006; Lorente, Peretti-Watel, and Grelot 2005; Huestis, Mazzoni, and Rabin 2011). This complicates our understanding of how, where, and why athletes may be using cannabis. Even though an athlete may have used cannabis socially, just as they would with alcohol, WADA has determined that a positive test for cannabis is a positive test and will discipline athletes accordingly (Huestis, Mazzoni, and Rabin 2011). Famously, in 1998, Olympic snowboarder Ross Rebagliati had to return his gold medal after testing positive for cannabis. In other sports, athletes may be suspended, fined, or ordered to attend a drug treatment program for testing positive for cannabis (Nguyen 2019; Belson 2020; Zialcita 2019).

Not all professional sports organizations uphold the WADA standards for prohibited substances, and instead each organization creates its own standards for prohibited substances and disciplinary measures. In late 2019, Major League Baseball (MLB) and the MLB Players Association agreed to changes to their drug program. In this joint statement, not only was it decided that natural cannabinoids would be removed from the MLB's list of drugs of abuse and be treated as alcohol, but that mandatory educational programs be implemented on the dangers of opioids and practical approaches to marijuana based on current scientific evidence, effective in spring 2020 (Major League Baseball Players Association 2019). They also agreed to prioritize treatment over punishment for all substance use, though the league may still punish players who break existing cannabis laws or who come to practices, meetings, or games under the influence of cannabis (Passan 2020). Meanwhile, National Football League (NFL) players sustain brain and musculoskeletal injuries at alarming rates compared to other athletes and are at high risk of opioid use and misuse (Dunne et al. 2018). After years of current and former NFL players fighting for a change in the organization's stance on cannabis use (Doctors for Cannabis Regulation 2020), it appears that the NFL is loosening its stance on cannabis as well (Belson 2020; Thompson 2021).

WADA recently decided to take cannabidiol (CBD) off the prohibited during competition list, while all other cannabinoids, including natural and synthetic tetrahydrocannabinols (THC), are still prohibited (WADA 2021). With the changes in regulations, the summer 2021 Olympics represents the first Olympic competition wherein athletes will not be penalized for using CBD. More elite athletes and national sport organizations such as USA Triathlon, CrossFit, and Ultimate Fighting Championship now have sponsorship deals with CBD companies (Futterman 2019). However, athletes are advised to use CBD products at their own risk, because some CBD products may contain more THC than labeled (USADA 2018; Vandrey et al. 2015). More research into the different effects of CBD and THC on sport performance, training, and recovery is indeed warranted so that WADA and other sport organizations can make more informed rule-making decisions regarding cannabis.

Back to the Future: Methodological Considerations for Cannabis and Kinesiology Research

While the early research on the impact of cannabis on exercise has guided our understanding and subsequently shapes current sport policies, it is important to note these studies from the late 1960s and 1970s suffered from several methodological limitations imposed by cannabis prohibition. For example, the strains used in these studies did not acknowledge a THC:CBD ratio, the studies only involved smoking as a method of administration, and the potency used was much lower than the cannabis products commercially available today. There is a clear precedent to replicate these original studies and systematically address the THC:CBD ratio, methods of administration, and dosages as they relate to different aspects of human performance.

Exercise Physiology Investigations

Athletes, trainers, coaches, and regulatory organizations wonder if cannabis use leads to changes in exercise performance. Given that people report participating in a variety of physical activities under the influence of cannabis, future research should consider the effects of cannabis on both aerobic and anaerobic exercise performance. For example, Maksud and Baron (1980) found no impairments in aerobic power and physical work capacity in men who smoked marijuana. While Steadward and Singh (1975) identified significant differences between subjects who used cannabis and the placebo and control groups in resting heart rate, blood pressure, and work on the cycle ergometer test, but no differences in lung volumes or grip strength. Smoking cannabis have also been associated with acute and subacute bronchodilation (Tashkin et al. 1975), which may affect exercise performance. It is important to acknowledge that these studies were conducted over 30 years ago, so these methods should be revisited given our current understanding of the endocannabinoid system and advances in exercise physiology research techniques.

Another aspect of exercise performance worth investigation is the role of cannabis in aiding with recovery, both in sleep and in inflammation. In 2017, the National Academies of Sciences, Engineering and Medicine conducted a comprehensive review of the recent medical literature on the therapeutic effects of cannabis and cannabinoids. They found moderate evidence for the efficacy of cannabis for addressing secondary sleep disturbances. Therefore, cannabis may help athletes recover by assisting in sleep. Cannabis may also improve recovery through the endocannabinoid's role in regulating inflammation (Gillman, Hutchison, and Bryan 2015; Ryz, Remillard, and Russo 2017).

Psychological and Psychomotor Investigations

As mentioned earlier, people report pairing cannabis with exercise for a plethora of reasons or perceived benefits. For example, we found the most common reasons people used cannabis with exercise were to increase focus/concentration, to facilitate enjoyment of exercise, to enhance mind/body/spirit connection, to stay in the zone, and to enhance body awareness.

Future research should consider these anecdotal claims in their research design: Do the perceived benefits match actual changes in performance? Cannabis may increase motivation during exercise through its effects on the endocannabinoid system (Gillman, Hutchison, and Bryan 2015; YorkWilliams et al. 2019). Cannabis may also play a role in decreasing anxiety prior to sport performance (Lorente, Peretti-Watel, and Grelot 2005), but this needs to be investigated further. Finally, research has shown cannabis impacts perception of time (Steadward and Singh 1975; O'Leary et al. 2003; Solowij 2002), so this may contribute to changes in exercise tolerance and duration. Steadward and Singh (1975) found the majority of the subjects in their research demonstrated a disruption in time perception, but the subjects denied the disturbance. O'Leary et al. (2003) then found that cannabis may accelerate the cerebellar clock, as evidenced by changes in self-paced tapping and increased blood flow to the cerebellum, particularly in chronic users.

Neuromotor Control Investigations

A change in time perception also has implications for the neuromotor control of movement, including reaction time, coordination, speed/accuracy trade-off and, ultimately, motor skill adaptation, learning, and performance. The first study to investigate reaction time was from the 1970s, where they found no differences in choice reaction time, but that cannabis affected both movement speed and accuracy in a Fitt's task (Kvålseth 1977). Both "high" and "low" potency cannabis (13% and 4% THC, respectively) has also been found to decrease performance in a tracking task and a stop reaction time task (Ramaekers et al. 2006). Research has shown deficits in auditory verbal learning, particularly in chronic users (Solowij 2002), so future investigations of the impact of cannabis on motor learning is warranted. These factors may have an impact on sport and exercise performance and should be considered in research within different sports disciplines as necessary.

Cannabinoid Profile

One of the glaring limitations of earlier research is the failure to acknowledge a THC:CBD ratio. CBD and THC have different effects on the body but may work synergistically, also known as the "entourage effect" (Piomelli and Russo 2016). Therefore, a systematic approach for investigating THC:CBD ratios is warranted to further understand the synergistic effects of these cannabinoids in humans. While the path is still not clear for researchers to do CBD-based studies, it is currently more hopeful than THC-dominant studies because hemp is now federally de-scheduled (see Silber-Coats Chapter 18, this volume). It is important to not let the excitement about CBD distract us from considering the role that THC may have in the exercise experience. Our preliminary findings suggest that people are more likely to use cannabis products with THC than CBD-only products when combining cannabis and exercise. In addition, a recent survey found that athletes who use a combination of THC and CBD showed the largest overall subjective benefit with a low risk of adverse experiences (Zeiger et al. 2019).

In addition, with the growing understanding of terpenes and other cannabinoids, we may also investigate the role that different terpenes and cannabinoid profiles have on performance (Piomelli and Russo 2016). Lisano et al. (2019) found that people reported greater use of Sativa strains before exercise and Indica strains after exercise. Therefore, it will be important to systematically test the effects that different strains of cannabis have on factors related to human performance.

Methods of Administration

There are many methods of cannabis consumption, and each method should be considered for its differential effects on human physiology. In the late 1960s, smoking "marijuana cigarettes" was recommended in studies due to its immediate effects and because it was the primary form of administration at the time (Weil, Zinberg, and Nelsen 1968). Survey data has shown that while smoking continues to be the most common method of administering THC (Hazekamp et al. 2013; Knapp et al. 2019; Spindle, Bonn-Miller, and Vandrey 2019), the most common method of administering CBD is sublingual (Corroon and Phillips 2018). Many other options are now available to consumers, and each has its advantages and disadvantages.

Inhalation of cannabis has also been found to be the most common method of consumption prior to exercise (Lisano et al. 2019). Smoking cannabis tends to elicit responses in less than five minutes and is therefore easy to self-titrate, but it may have negative long-term consequences for lung health (Russell et al. 2018). While some research has shown that vaporizing cannabis may be better for lung health (Earleywine and Barnwell 2007; Russell et al. 2018), there have been recent concerns about the use of vape pens (cartridges using cannabis oil) and lung health, particularly unregulated cartridges and in adolescents (Abeles et al. 2020; Borodovsky et al. 2017). Oral cannabis products such as edibles, tinctures, capsules, beverages, and sublingual strips may be better for pulmonary function, but they take longer to metabolize and exert a longer effect duration. There are also topical/transdermal options sold to address local symptoms (Backes 2017; Bostwick 2012).

While the early research focused on the inhalation method of administration (Weil, Zinberg, and Nelsen 1968; Tashkin, Shapiro, and Frank 1973; Tashkin et al. 1975; Manno et al. 1970), the various methods of administration currently commercially available open the door for a variety of research designs and objectives. Because the onset of effects is different for each method of delivery, it will be important to carefully and systematically investigate the impact of dosage timing and route of administration on human performance variables.

Dosages and Potencies

A recent review of pain and cannabis has identified a possible dose-dependent relationship between pain and cannabis, where some doses can relieve pain, while other doses can lead to pain hypersensitivity (Wallace et al. 2007). Therefore, it will be important to consider the percent of THC in products that subjects will be consuming. As we review older studies and make claims about the impact of cannabis on performance, we need to realize that the strains used in these studies were typically less than 5% THC (Weil, Zinberg, and Nelsen 1968; Renault et al. 1971; Manno et al. 1970; Steadward and Singh 1975; Schwin 1973). Ramaekers et al. (2006) attempted to address this problem by including two dosage groups: high potency (13% THC) and low potency (4% THC), where higher potency cannabis had more profound effects on human performance than lower potency. Because of regulatory barriers, the cannabis produced at the University of Mississippi for approved cannabis studies does not reflect the current diversity of strains that are available to the public and is, therefore, a threat to the external generalizability of such research (Vergara et al. 2017; Gillman, Hutchison, and Bryan 2015; Bidwell et al. 2018). Therefore, there is a massive gap in our scientific understanding of how cannabis products available in dispensaries affect humans.

Cannabis potency has increased over the years with many strains available commercially containing over 20% THC. In addition, THC-rich hash oil and "dabs" can contain over 50% THC (National Institute on Drug Abuse 2019). Because these products are now commercially available, the findings from earlier research are no longer relevant given the current strains and modes of ingestion. We must continue to investigate the effects of commercially available cannabis on different aspects of human performance. Researchers from the University of Colorado have proposed a path forward in using commercially available cannabis in their studies, and their model appears to be the most fruitful as regulations continue to change. In this approach, regular cannabis users are asked to use one of two legal cannabis products purchased from a local dispensary and use as they normally would before returning to the lab for testing (Bidwell et al. 2018). This novel approach will help address gaps in our knowledge of the effects of commercially available cannabis on human subjects.

Subject Profiles

As discussed in this chapter, people may be using cannabis for a variety of reasons, so the subject population should be clearly defined. For example, the anti-inflammatory effects of cannabis (Ryz, Remillard, and Russo 2017; Gillman, Hutchison, and Bryan 2015) can be studied as it relates to swelling after surgery or injury, in chronic inflammatory conditions, or in recovery from exercise. Future investigations should consider the impacts of sex and gender in cannabis research due to potential hormonal, neurochemical, or sociocultural differences on cannabis experience in humans. For example, the effects of cannabis on neurochemistry may be modulated by sex (Newman et al. 2019). In addition, future research should consider the role of cannabis in physical activity participation in the transgender and nonbinary communities, where there are currently more barriers to participation (Jones et al. 2017).

Ethical concerns immediately surface when discussing dosing naïve users. Weil (1968) acknowledged these concerns and specifically recruited subjects who were naïve to cannabis but had experience with smoking cigarettes. In subject recruitment, it will be important to make a distinction not only between naïve and experienced users but also between occasional and chronic or heavy users. Previous research has revealed that the effects of cannabis differ between long-term and short-term cannabis users (Kirk and de Wit 1999; O'Leary et al. 2003; Solowij 2002).

In future research, it will also be extremely important to control for other substances. It was at one time commonplace to specifically recruit subjects who were experienced cigarette smokers but were naïve to smoking cannabis (Weil, Zinberg, and Nelsen 1968; Renault et al. 1971; Manno et al. 1970; Schwin 1973). This was framed as a positive aspect because it meant that they all physically knew how to smoke. Depending on what aspect of cannabis and exercise science is under investigation, subject history of smoking cigarettes can be a major confounding variable.

At the same time, it is also important to control for alcohol use in study designs and subject recruitment. In one problematic example, Pearson-Dennett et al. (2017) used the operational definition of "cannabis users" so widely that the group contained people who had only used six times in their lives to those who have used over 1,000 times. In addition, the cannabis group also consumed statistically significantly more alcohol than did the control group. Given that alcohol has a detrimental effect on balance, gait, and motor control, this massive oversight blurs the lines about what really had an impact on gait in the study.

Other Considerations

When we look at the studies from the 1970s, it is important that we build upon the positive aspects of these studies. For example, Renault et al. (1971) standardized smoke administration using a spirometer to contain a fixed amount of smoke as well as an inhale-hold-exhale timing system (Renault et al. 1971). Depending on the research question, future research may call for either standardized consumption among all subjects, as a percentage of body weight, or using a numerical rating scale for subjective "highness."

Weil, Zinberg, and Nelsen (1968) specifically highlighted the importance of "set and setting" when conducting human subjects research related to cannabis consumption, where "set" refers to the subject's expectations and psychological state going into the drug experience and "setting" refers to the environmental context of use. They detailed how important it was for the subjects to be comfortable, and a simple question like, "how do you feel?" can influence the subject's experience (Weil, Zinberg, and Nelsen 1968). The University of Colorado's approach wherein subjects consume store-bought cannabis products in their own house addresses the aspect of "setting." In this approach, participants may feel more comfortable in a naturalistic versus a laboratory setting.

It is equally important to aim for the researcher to be blind to the condition so they do not influence the subjects and disrupt the "set" of the subjects. A double-blind design with cannabis is tricky because it has a very specific odor and taste. Some studies have used "portions of male hemp stalks" (Weil, Zinberg, and Nelsen 1968) while others have chemically removed the THC from the cannabis sample (Schwin 1973; Steadward and Singh 1975; Manno et al. 1970). This ensured that there were "no differences in taste, burning character, smell, or appearance" (Manno et al. 1970).

Conclusion

With the advent of legal cannabis frameworks, more and more people are using cannabis in conjunction with physical activity and sport. There is great public interest in understanding the effects of cannabis on different aspects of recreational and competitive exercise, but there is little research on the topic. Given that the regulatory barriers stunted the ability to conduct cannabis research, the opportunities for novel research into various aspects of cannabis and exercise are endless. The link between cannabis and exercise is growing in multiple contexts, from recreational physical activity to elite sports performance. There is potential to investigate different aspects of the impact of cannabis on humans performing a variety of activities. It is essential that scientists and practitioners in the realm of exercise science address the gaps in the literature so that we can inform the public. Investigations related to all aspects of kinesiology are indeed warranted to inform not only the public but also trainers, coaches, health-care providers, and sport governing bodies. Future researchers should carefully and systematically address the impacts of cannabinoid profile, methods of administration, dose and timing of the dose, and subject familiarity as they relate to different aspects of health and human performance.

References

Abeles, Michael, Stephanie Popofsky, Andy Wen, Christina Valsamis, Angela Webb, Claudia Halaby, and Melodi Pirzada. 2020. "Vaping-Associated Lung Injury Caused by Inhalation of Cannabis Oil." *Pediatric Pulmonology* 55 (1): 226–28. https://doi.org/10.1002/ppul.24579.

Armstrong, A. 2018. "5 Ways Marijuana Can Get You Excited about Fitness." *The Fresh Toast*, November 6, 2018. https://thefreshtoast.com/cannabis/5-ways-marijuana-can-get-you-excited-about-fitness/.

Backes, M. 2017. *Cannabis Pharmacy: The Practical Guide to Medical Marijuana*. New York: Black Dog & Leventhal Publishers.

Belson, K. 2020. "N.F.L. Bows to Marijuana's New Status." *The New York Times*, April 13, 2020. https://www.nytimes.com/2020/04/13/sports/football/nfl-marijuana-policy.html.

Bidwell, L. Cinnamon, Raeghan Mueller, Sophie L. YorkWilliams, Sarah Hagerty, Angela D. Bryan, and Kent E. Hutchison. 2018. "A Novel Observational Method for Assessing Acute Responses to Cannabis: Preliminary Validation Using Legal Market Strains." *Cannabis and Cannabinoid Research* 3 (1): 35–44. https://doi.org/10.1089/can.2017.0038.

Bonner, N. 2018. "The 420 Games Are Back and Bigger Than Ever." *Civilized*, 2018. https://www.civilized.life/articles/the-420-games-are-back-and-bigger-than-ever/.

Borodovsky, Jacob T., Dustin C. Lee, Benjamin S. Crosier, Joy L. Gabrielli, James D. Sargent, and Alan J. Budney. 2017. "U.S. Cannabis Legalization and Use of Vaping and Edible Products Among Youth." *Drug and Alcohol Dependence* 177 (August): 299–306. https://doi.org/10.1016/j.drugalcdep.2017.02.017.

Bostwick, J. M. 2012. "Blurred Boundaries: The Therapeutics and Politics of Medical Marijuana." *Mayo Clinic Proceedings* 87 (2): 172–86. https://doi.org/10.1016/j.mayocp.2011.10.003.

Brand, D. S. 2019. "Do's and Don'ts for Bringing Cannabis along on Your Next Hike." *Civilized*, February 15, 2019. https://www.civilized.life/articles/dos-and-donts-for-bringing-cannabis-along-on-your-next-hike/.

Brisola-Santos, M. B., J. G. de Mello e Gallinaro, F. Gil, B. Sampaio-Junior, M. C. D. Marin, A. G. de Andrade, K. P. Richter, I. D. Glick, D. A. Baltieri, and J. M. Castaldelli-Maia. 2016. "Prevalence and Correlates of Cannabis Use among Athletes-A Systematic Review: Cannabis Use Among Athletes." *The American Journal on Addictions* 25 (7): 518–28. https://doi.org/10.1111/ajad.12425.

Bures, B. 2020. "Smoking Marijuana before Exercises Can Increase Workout Productivity." *The Fresh Toast*, February 28, 2020. https://thefreshtoast.com/wellness/1-in-3-people-have-improved-workouts-after-smoking-marijuana/.

Cannathlete. 2020. "Cannathlete – Activate Yourself." 2020. cannathlete.net.

deBara, D. 2019. "Let's Get Physical: How Active People Use Cannabis to Get in the Zone." *Weedmaps.Com*, April 1, 2019. https://weedmaps.com/news/2019/04/lets-get-physical-how-active-people-use-cannabis-to-get-in-the-zone/.

Corroon, Jamie, and Joy A. Phillips. 2018. "A Cross-Sectional Study of Cannabidiol Users." *Cannabis and Cannabinoid Research* 3 (1): 152–61. https://doi.org/10.1089/can.2018.0006.

Docter, Shgufta, Moin Khan, Chetan Gohal, Bheeshma Ravi, Mohit Bhandari, Rajiv Gandhi, and Timothy Leroux. 2020. "Cannabis Use and Sport: A Systematic Review." *Sports Health: A Multidisciplinary Approach* 12 (2): 189–99. https://doi.org/10.1177/1941738120901670.

Doctors for Cannabis Regulation. 2020. "NFL Campaign: Doctors and Players for NFL Cannabis Reform." https://dfcr.org/nfl-campaign/.

Dunne, Eugene M., Catherine W. Striley, Zachary L. Mannes, Breton M. Asken, Nicole Ennis (formerly Whitehead), and Linda B. Cottler. 2018. "Reasons for Prescription Opioid Use While Playing in the National Football League as Risk Factors for Current Use and Misuse Among Former Players." *Clinical Journal of Sport Medicine*, June 1. https://doi.org/10.1097/JSM.0000000000000628.

Earleywine, Mitch, and Sara Barnwell. 2007. "Decreased Respiratory Symptoms in Cannabis Users Who Vaporize." *Harm Reduction Journal* 4 (1): 11. https://doi.org/10.1186/1477-7517-4-11.

Emerald Magazine. 2018. "The Athletics Issue," March 2018. https://theemeraldmagazine.com/wp-content/uploads/2018/02/March2018.pdf.

Futterman, M. 2019. "U.S.A. Triathlon Embraces CBD." *The New York Times*, October 20. www.nytimes.com/2019/10/20/sports/olympics/usa-triathlon-cbd.html.

Gillman, Arielle S., Kent E. Hutchison, and Angela D. Bryan. 2015. "Cannabis and Exercise Science: A Commentary on Existing Studies and Suggestions for Future Directions." *Sports Medicine* 45 (10): 1357–63. https://doi.org/10.1007/s40279-015-0362-3.

Hazekamp, Arno, Mark A. Ware, Kirsten R. Muller-Vahl, Donald Abrams, and Franjo Grotenhermen. 2013. "The Medicinal Use of Cannabis and Cannabinoids—An International Cross-Sectional Survey on Administration Forms." *Journal of Psychoactive Drugs* 45 (3): 199–210. https://doi.org/10.1080/02791072.2013.805976.

Huestis, M. A., I. Mazzoni, and O. Rabin. 2011. "Cannabis in Sport: Anti-Doping Perspective." *Sports Medicine* 41 (11): 949–66. https://doi.org/10.2165/11591430-000000000-00000.

Jones, Bethany Alice, Jon Arcelus, Walter Pierre Bouman, and Emma Haycraft. 2017. "Barriers and Facilitators of Physical Activity and Sport Participation among Young Transgender Adults Who Are Medically Transitioning." *International Journal of Transgenderism* 18 (2): 227–38. https://doi.org/10.1080/15532739.2017.1293581.

Kirk, J. M., and H. de Wit. 1999. "Responses to Oral Delta9-Tetrahydrocannabinol in Frequent and Infrequent Marijuana Users." *Pharmacology, Biochemistry, and Behavior* 63 (1): 137–42.

Knapp, Ashley A., Dustin C. Lee, Jacob T. Borodovsky, Samantha G. Auty, Joy Gabrielli, and Alan J. Budney. 2019. "Emerging Trends in Cannabis Administration Among Adolescent Cannabis Users." *Journal of Adolescent Health* 64 (4): 487–93. https://doi.org/10.1016/j.jadohealth.2018.07.012.

Kramer, Andrew, Justin Sinclair, Lara Sharpe, and Jerome Sarris. 2020. "Chronic Cannabis Consumption and Physical Exercise Performance in Healthy Adults: A Systematic Review." *Journal of Cannabis Research* 2 (1): 34. https://doi.org/10.1186/s42238-020-00037-x.

Kvålseth, T. O. 1977. "Effects of Marijuana on Human Reaction Time and Motor Control." *Perceptual and Motor Skills* 45 (3 Pt 1): 935–39. https://doi.org/10.2466/pms.1977.45.3.935.

Lev, E. 2020. "A Surprising Number of People Support Working Out Stoned." *The Growthop*, February 28, 2020. https://www.thegrowthop.com/fitness/working-out-stoned.

Lisano, Jonathon, Kristina Phillips, Jeremy Smith, Matthew Barnes, and Laura Stewart. 2019. "Patterns and Perceptions of Cannabis Use with Physical Activity." *Cannabis* 2 (2): 151–64. https://doi.org/10.26828/cannabis.2019.02.005.

Lorente, Fabrice Olivier, Patrick Peretti-Watel, and Laurent Grelot. 2005. "Cannabis Use to Enhance Sportive and Non-Sportive Performances among French Sport Students." *Addictive Behaviors* 30 (7): 1382–91. https://doi.org/10.1016/j.addbeh.2005.01.019.

Lucas, Philippe, Eric P. Baron, and Nick Jikomes. 2019. "Medical Cannabis Patterns of Use and Substitution for Opioids & Other Pharmaceutical Drugs, Alcohol, Tobacco, and Illicit Substances; Results from a Cross-Sectional Survey of Authorized Patients." *Harm Reduction Journal* 16 (1). https://doi.org/10.1186/s12954-019-0278-6.

Major League Baseball Players Association. 2019. "MLB, MLBPA Agree to Changes to Joint Drug Program." *Major League Baseball Players Association Press Release*, December 12. Accessed June 8, 2020. Major League Baseball Players Association website. www.mlbplayers.com/mlb-mlbpa-joint-drug-program.

Maksud, M. G., and A. Baron. 1980. "Physiological Response to Exercise in Chronic Cigarette and Marijuana Users." *European Journal of Applied Physiology* 43: 127–34.

Manno, J. E., G. F. Kiplinger, S. E. Haine, I. F. Bennett, and R. B. Forney. 1970. "Comparative Effects of Smoking Marihuana or Placebo on Human Motor and Mental Performance." *Clinical Pharmacology and Therapeutics* 11: 808–14.

National Institute on Drug Abuse. 2019. "A Rise in Marijuana's THC Levels." https://archives.drugabuse.gov/rise-in-marijuanas-thc-levels.

Newman, Sharlene D., Hu Cheng, Ashley Schnakenberg Martin, Ulrike Dydak, Shalmali Dharmadhikari, William Hetrick, and Brian O'Donnell. 2019. "An Investigation of Neurochemical Changes in Chronic Cannabis Users." *Frontiers in Human Neuroscience* 13 (September): 318. https://doi.org/10.3389/fnhum.2019.00318.

Nguyen, T. 2019. "Working Out with Weed." *Nature – Outlook* 572 (S14): 1–2.

NORML. 2015. "NORML Athletics." 2015. normlathletics.org.

O'Leary, Daniel S., Robert I. Block, Beth M. Turner, Julie Koeppel, Vincent A. Magnotta, Laura Boles Ponto, G. Leonard Watkins, Richard D. Hichwa, and Nancy C. Andreasen. 2003. "Marijuana Alters the Human Cerebellar Clock." *NeuroReport* 14 (8): 1145–51. https://doi.org/10.1097/00001756-200306110-00009.

Passan, Jeff. 2020. "MLB: Players Still Subject to Penalty for Using Pot." *ESPN*, February 28, 2020. https://www.espn.com/mlb/story/_/id/28804440/mlb-players-subject-penalty-using-pot.

Pearson-Dennett, V., G. Todd, R. A. Wilcox, A. P. Vogel, J. M. White, and D. Thewlis. 2017. "History of Cannabis Use is Associated with Altered Gait." *Drug and Alcohol Dependence* 178 (September): 215–22. https://doi.org/10.1016/j.drugalcdep.2017.05.017.

Peters, B. A., E. G. Lewis, R. E. Dustman, R. C. Straight, and E. C. Beck. 1976. "Sensory, Perceptual, Motor and Cognitive Functioning and Subjective Reports Following Oral Administration of Delta9-Tetrahydrocannabinol." *Psychopharmacologia* 47 (2): 141–48.

Piomelli, Daniele, and Ethan B. Russo. 2016. "The Cannabis Sativa Versus Cannabis Indica Debate: An Interview with Ethan Russo, MD." *Cannabis and Cannabinoid Research* 1 (1): 44–46. https://doi.org/10.1089/can.2015.29003.ebr.

Ramaekers, Johannes G., Gerhold Kauert, Peter van Ruitenbeek, Eef L. Theunissen, Erhard Schneider, and Manfred R. Moeller. 2006. "High-Potency Marijuana Impairs Executive Function and Inhibitory Motor Control." *Neuropsychopharmacology* 31 (10): 2296–303. https://doi.org/10.1038/sj.npp.1301068.

Reinarman, C., H. Nunberg, F. Lanthier, and T. Heddleston. 2011. "Who Are Medical Marijuana Patients? Population Characteristics from Nine California Assessment Clinics." *Journal of Psychoactive Drugs* 43 (2): 128–35. https://doi.org/10.1080/02791072.2011.587700.

Renault, P. F., C. R. Schuster, R. Heinrich, and D. X. Freeman. 1971. "Marihuana: Standardized Smoke Administration and Dose Effect Curves on Heart Rate in Humans." *Science* 174 (4009): 589–91. https://doi.org/10.1126/science.174.4009.589.

Russell, Cayley, Sergio Rueda, Robin Room, Mark Tyndall, and Benedikt Fischer. 2018. "Routes of Administration for Cannabis Use – Basic Prevalence and Related Health Outcomes: A Scoping Review and Synthesis." *International Journal of Drug Policy* 52 (February): 87–96. https://doi.org/10.1016/j.drugpo.2017.11.008.

Ryz, Natasha R., David J. Remillard, and Ethan B. Russo. 2017. "Cannabis Roots: A Traditional Therapy with Future Potential for Treating Inflammation and Pain." *Cannabis and Cannabinoid Research* 2 (1): 210–16. https://doi.org/10.1089/can.2017.0028.

Saugy, M., L. Avois, C. Saudan, N. Robinson, C. Giroud, P. Mangin, and J. Dvorak. 2006. "Cannabis and Sport." *British Journal of Sports Medicine* 40 (Suppl 1): i13–15. https://doi.org/10.1136/bjsm.2006.027607.

Schwin, Robert. 1973. "Marihuana and Tidal Volume." *JAMA: The Journal of the American Medical Association* 223 (2): 194. https://doi.org/10.1001/jama.1973.03220020060029.

Sexton, Michelle, Carrie Cuttler, John S. Finnell, and Laurie K. Mischley. 2016. "A Cross-Sectional Survey of Medical Cannabis Users: Patterns of Use and Perceived Efficacy." *Cannabis and Cannabinoid Research* 1 (1): 131–38. https://doi.org/10.1089/can.2016.0007.

Solowij, Nadia. 2002. "Cognitive Functioning of Long-Term Heavy Cannabis Users Seeking Treatment." *JAMA* 287 (9): 1123. https://doi.org/10.1001/jama.287.9.1123.

Sparling, P. B., A. Giuffrida, D. Piomelli, L. Rosskopf, and A. Dietrich. 2003. "Exercise Activates the Endocannabinoid System." *NeuroReport* 14 (17): 2209–11. https://doi.org/10.1097/00001756-200312020-00015.

Spindle, Tory R., Marcel O. Bonn-Miller, and Ryan Vandrey. 2019. "Changing Landscape of Cannabis: Novel Products, Formulations, and Methods of Administration." *Current Opinion in Psychology* 30 (December): 98–102. https://doi.org/10.1016/j.copsyc.2019.04.002.

Steadward, R. D., and M. Singh. 1975. "The Effects of Smoking Marihuana on Physical Performance." *Medicine and Science in Sports* 7 (4): 309–11.

Stigma Activewear. 2020. "Stigma Activewear." *Stigma Redefining Cannabis*. 2020. shopstigma.com.

Tashkin, D. P., B. J. Shapiro, and I. M. Frank. 1973. "Acute Pulmonary Physiologic Effects of Smoked Marijuana and Oral Δ9-Tetrahydrocannabinol in Healthy Young Men." *New England Journal of Medicine* 289 (7): 336–41. https://doi.org/10.1056/NEJM197308162890702.

Tashkin, D. P., B. J. Shapiro, Y. E. Lee, and C. E. Harper. 1975. "Effects of Smoked Marijuana in Experimentally Induced Asthma." *The American Review of Respiratory Disease* 112 (3): 377–86. https://doi.org/10.1164/arrd.1975.112.3.377.

Thompson, Jackson. 2021. "NFL Players Can Smoke Marijuana for the First Time during the Offseason and the Window Opened on 4/20." *Insider*, April 20, 2021. https://www.insider.com/nfl-players-can-smoke-marijuana-without-discipline-starting-420-2021-4.

USADA. 2018. "Athletes: 6 Things to Know About Cannabidiol." October 23. www.usada.org/spirit-of-sport/education/six-things-know-about-cannabidiol/.

———. 2019. "Marijuana FAQ." *U.S. Anti-Doping Agency*. www.usada.org/athletes/substances/marijuana-faq/.

Vandrey, Ryan, Jeffrey C. Raber, Mark E. Raber, Brad Douglass, Cameron Miller, and Marcel O. Bonn-Miller. 2015. "Cannabinoid Dose and Label Accuracy in Edible Medical Cannabis Products." *JAMA* 313 (24): 2491. https://doi.org/10.1001/jama.2015.6613.

Vergara, Daniela, L. Cinnamon Bidwell, Reggie Gaudino, Anthony Torres, Gary Du, Travis C. Ruthenburg, Kymron deCesare, Donald P. Land, Kent E. Hutchison, and Nolan C. Kane. 2017. "Compromised External Validity: Federally Produced Cannabis Does Not Reflect Legal Markets." *Scientific Reports* 7 (1): 46528. https://doi.org/10.1038/srep46528.

WADA. 2021. "World Anti-Doping Code: International Standard Prohibited List." https://www.usada.org/wp-content/uploads/wada_2021_english_prohibited_list.pdf.

Wallace, Mark, Gery Schulteis, J. Hampton Atkinson, Tanya Wolfson, Deborah Lazzaretto, Heather Bentley, Ben Gouaux, and Ian Abramson. 2007. "Dose-Dependent Effects of Smoked Cannabis on Capsaicin-Induced Pain and Hyperalgesia in Healthy Volunteers." *Anesthesiology* 107 (5): 785–96. https://doi.org/10.1097/01.anes.0000286986.92475.b7.

Walsh, Zach, Robert Callaway, Lynne Belle-Isle, Rielle Capler, Robert Kay, Philippe Lucas, and Susan Holtzman. 2013. "Cannabis for Therapeutic Purposes: Patient Characteristics, Access, and Reasons for Use." *International Journal of Drug Policy* 24 (6): 511–16. https://doi.org/10.1016/j.drugpo.2013.08.010.

Weil, A. T., N. E. Zinberg, and J. M. Nelsen. 1968. "Clinical and Psychological Effects of Marihuana in Man." *Science* 162 (3859): 1234–42. https://doi.org/10.1126/science.162.3859.1234.

YorkWilliams, Sophie L., Charleen J. Gust, Raeghan Mueller, L. Cinnamon Bidwell, Kent E. Hutchison, Arielle S. Gillman, and Angela D. Bryan. 2019. "The New Runner's High? Examining Relationships Between Cannabis Use and Exercise Behavior in States with Legalized Cannabis." *Frontiers in Public Health* 7 (April): 99. https://doi.org/10.3389/fpubh.2019.00099.

Zeiger, Joanna S., William S. Silvers, Edward M. Fleegler, and Robert S. Zeiger. 2019. "Cannabis Use in Active Athletes: Behaviors Related to Subjective Effects." Edited by Daniel Boullosa. *PLoS One* 14 (6): e0218998. https://doi.org/10.1371/journal.pone.0218998.

Zialcita, Paolo. 2019. "Major League Baseball Drops Marijuana, Adds Opioids, Cocaine to 'Drugs of Abuse' List." *National Public Radio (NPR)*, December 12, 2019. https://www.npr.org/2019/12/12/787550622/major-league-baseball-drops-marijuana-adds-opioids-cocaine-to-drugs-of-abuse-lis.

11

Utilizing Community-Based Participatory Research in Cannabis Knowledge Formation

Trecia Ehrlich

Keywords: Community-Based Participatory Research, Public Health, Epistemology, Transition

Introduction

The recent wave of cannabis legalization creates new opportunities for strengthening the epistemology of cannabis research. Given federal restrictions on cannabis research in the United States and the historical prohibition that stigmatized and criminalized those working in the cannabis economy, community-based participatory research (CBPR) provides an opportunity to formalize the knowledge created under the conditions of prohibition. This chapter explains the foundations of CBPR, the challenges in creating cannabis knowledge from a public health perspective, and the opportunities for community-based research as a methodological tool to incorporate justice and unheard voices in the process of cannabis knowledge formation. I draw on a previous study on the occupational health of cannabis farm workers to describe the possibilities for incorporating CBPR into research and the knowledge formation process.

Community-based participatory research is a research methodology that centers the voices of the researched population and improves trust between those being researched and those conducting the research. The goals of CBPR are to inform change and action by equitably incorporating the perspectives and needs of the community being researched into the research process at every turn, and for the knowledge created in the process to directly benefit the community of people being researched and serve their needs (Blumenthal 2011). Historically, CBPR has been utilized in heavily researched and often stigmatized populations, including communities of color and among people who use drugs (Damon et al. 2017). Typically, CBPR is utilized as the primary framework for a research methodology; however, this chapter will describe utilizing principles of CBPR as a part of a larger research framework.

Prior to legalization and the advent of a cannabis regulatory system, much of cannabis cultivation, possession, and wholesale occurred in remote locations within an underground illicit marketplace (August 2013). Many growers produced cannabis in remote locations to avoid detection from the law, as well as their competitors. The sale of cannabis moved through communities without the

DOI: 10.4324/9780429320491-11

formalities, like sales receipts and market data, of a regulated marketplace. Today, in the nascent stages of a national and global cannabis legalization trend, researchers, consumers, and public health practitioners yearn for a better understanding of cannabis and how it relates to a variety of disciplines. Much of the knowledge around cannabis cultivation and medicinal use has stayed within a community of cultivators who have historically had to protect themselves from the government and have had little interaction with academic institutions and/or formal research due to the illicit nature of their work. While support for legalization of adult use[1] in the United States has increased over time and in response to new legal frameworks (Pew Research Center 2015), some of the stigma around cannabis cultivation, sale, possession, and consumption still remains, which may serve as a barrier in knowledge transfer between those stigmatized due to their interaction with cannabis and the institutions seeking to learn about cannabis (Lashley 2019).

In order to advance the knowledge formation around cannabis cultivation, sale, and consumption, it is imperative for researchers to employ strategies from CBPR in order to improve trust between institutional researchers and the members of a cultural group who have been involved in the cultivation and sale of cannabis prior to its legalization. Historically, all health effects of cannabis were considered negative effects, leading much of the research conducted to exist under frameworks of misuse and abuse, or adverse cognitive effects (National Academy of Sciences 2017). As modern science has begun to acknowledge that humans have the capacity for both harmful and beneficial relationships with cannabis as it relates to health, research must evolve to engage with these parallel truths. Part of this reckoning requires bridging the gaps that exist between public health institutions and the cultivators and members of a cannabis culture who were historically alienated by messaging that was exclusive to cannabis as a health harm.

The Challenging Epistemology of Cannabis, From a Public Health Perspective

Despite being grown and used for thousands of years, the framework for how and what we know about cannabis remains unclear. When typing the word "marijuana" into a search engine of research, one can find hundreds of thousands of articles pertaining to cannabis in respect to its cultivation, chemical composition, legal framework, and beyond. However, the dominant narrative maintains that evidence surrounding cannabis is "limited" and evidence on the health effects of cannabis remains "elusive" (National Academies of Science 2017). This knowledge gap creates opportunities for the cannabis industry to create a health narrative about cannabis through advertising (Carlini 2017). While the industry utilizes health-related messaging to sell cannabis, healthcare professionals consistently report a lack of confidence in sharing the available information about cannabis with patients, citing "inadequate research" as a barrier to communicating with patients, and a desire for more education on the topic (Zylla et al. 2018).

Researchers have described the interaction between the cannabis industry and the public health community as "tense," based on the assumption that public health practitioners seek to reduce or prevent cannabis consumption, while commercial interests aim to increase it (Subritzky, Pettigrew, and Lenton 2016). However, it is worth questioning whether this tension is productive. Adults are using cannabis and therefore deserve information about safe use, harm reduction, and the plant in general, coming from a trusted source rather than a source with an economic interest to sell a product. In order to create a more productive dialogue, stakeholders must take a step back from the concept of increasing or decreasing use to look at cannabis as it relates to cultivation and the production of products, rather than cannabis solely within the context of the user's relationship to it. In order to understand more complex systems relating to how humans use cannabis in harmful or helpful ways, public health practitioners will need to engage in creating and systematizing knowledge on cannabis cultivation and manufacturing.

It is challenging to create messaging around safe use and integrating cannabis into a regulated system from a public health perspective, since many governmental and non-governmental agencies receive funding from the federal government and therefore feel limited in their capacity to produce knowledge or messaging on cannabis and health. Federal conflicts aside, it is challenging to obtain information about the cannabis plant and its effects, as much of the knowledge held around the cannabis plant was produced from within the historically illicit marketplace. Human trials on the effects of cannabis are blocked due to its status as a Schedule 1 controlled substance, and the limited amount of federally sanctioned research and cannabis created for that research can take years of processing before researchers can engage in the work (Stith and Vigil 2016).

Another challenge in creating cannabis knowledge is that all health research, not just that of cannabis, is heavily politicized, and the funding streams to create health-related research often must respond to the expectations of the funder (Dresser 2018). With cannabis, a great deal of funding comes from the National Institute on Drug Abuse (NIDA). With the word "abuse" in the name of the institute, it is clear that research funding is likely directed under the assumption of problematic use. Even if research funded by an agency like NIDA is not under the umbrella of problematic use, it is possible that consumers or people experiencing addiction will still feel stigmatized by the funder name. Cannabis research is challenged even further by its inherently interdisciplinary nature.

Modern cannabis knowledge is a unique combination of phytochemistry and cannabinoid science, biology, psychology, agriculture, plant genetics, economics, civil liberties, political science, and more. However, it is understood that interdisciplinary research is generally less successful in obtaining funding than research with a narrower scope (Bromham, Dinnage, and Hua 2016). In order to get to the heart of important questions that are more likely to receive funding, those engaging in cannabis research must stay dedicated to creating groundwork and formative literature in this burgeoning field by engaging in challenging interdisciplinary and mixed methodology research.

Despite the emergence of state-level legalization, cannabis use and cultivation continues to carry social stigma (Lau et al. 2015; Newhart and Dolphin Chapter 24, this volume). The stigmas of cannabis have also changed shape with time; the film *Reefer Madness* proclaimed the evils of marijuana and successfully stigmatized users of cannabis for decades to come (Krenzelok 2017). While this stigma remains, it has been supplemented by stigmas towards the cannabis industry; a new, corporate enterprise run by white men in suits (Zhang 2016), who are charged with corporate greed in the same way stigmas are applied to other corporate economies. This stigma may add to the tension between public health practitioners and the industry and further prevent knowledge transfer between the cannabis industry and community, and the community of public health practitioners (Hatzenbuehler, Phelan, and Link 2013). As the cannabis industry continues to grow throughout the United States, the industry will continue to grow more diverse, with some members coming from a community who participated in the historically illicit market and others coming in with little to no experience with cannabis, seeking a new economic opportunity. As the cannabis industry and community continues to evolve rapidly, it is imperative that researchers document and understand this ongoing transition and the historical process it was born from through research that engages community voices. Further, it is critical that researchers separate consumers and workers who interact with cannabis from the larger corporate interests that advertise cannabis, in order to reduce bias.

The Occupational Health of Cannabis Farm Workers: Incorporating Principles of CBPR Into Research

In 2016, I joined a research team that had been funded by the Washington State Labor and Industries Safety and Health Investment Project to identify levels of UV exposure in cannabis farm workers. All agricultural workers are at risk for sun exposure; however, researchers were curious as to how different types of indoor lighting might differentially impact worker exposure to UV radiation (see Schenker and Langer Chapter 12, this volume). In all health-related research, a major challenge to more complex study is the need for established groundwork to inform the methodology and background of the work (Dresser 2018). However, the research team understood that little formative research on the occupational health of cannabis workers had been done prior to our assessment. We had to understand and illustrate the cultivation process and distinguish outdoor and indoor grows and varying light stages used in order to design the appropriate measures of study. The need for groundwork that allowed us to understand the context that we were researching created an opportunity to incorporate principles from CBPR. We recognized that the idea of studying UV exposure was something that came from the research team, not the cannabis farm workers. While it was possible that cannabis farm workers had concerns about their exposure to UV radiation, it was also possible that this was not an issue of interest to them. Though the UV study required quantitative measurements of UV exposures, measuring bulb emissions and UV exposures measured by a wearable UV dosimeter, we chose to also collect qualitative data to identify concerns and research interests from the workers themselves.

By using principles of CBPR, we were able to collect qualitative data from cannabis farm owners and workers, collected through key informant interviews and focus groups. The focus groups and interviews were intentionally kept open-ended and adaptive in order to provide cultivators with the opportunity to engage with the topics they felt most relevant. While this information helped us understand the process of cannabis cultivation to inform the research, it also allowed us to identify the occupational health concerns coming from within the community of cultivators. Despite the research being funded to examine the UV exposures of workers, the workers themselves expressed low levels of concern about their UV exposure. The low levels of concern from the workers themselves do not negate the importance of studying UV exposure among cannabis farmworkers, but rather affirm the importance of understanding what other exposures may be worthy of research, in addition to the original research question. Workers were concerned that the respiratory and dermal allergic reactions they were having were related to components of the plant, such as plant terpenes, as well as other respiratory dusts that came off the plant. Workers and owners expressed concern about the transitioning legal landscape that they operated within. Study participants conveyed that inconsistency between state and federal laws created occupational concerns that were more sociopolitical in nature: concerns relating to crime, gender issues, emerging technologies, social stigma, cannabis use in the workplace, the capacity for investments in safety infrastructure, and modifying old habits from an illicit past (Ehrlich, Simpson, and Busch Isaksen 2019).

By highlighting the voice of cannabis cultivation workers, the majority of whom had previously worked in the illicit marketplace, we (the community and the research team in collaboration) were able to establish a knowledge base to serve as groundwork for future, focused areas of research that better speak to the needs of the community. This process allowed the research team to focus on the concerns of farm workers, rather than assumed concerns formulated by the research team, or grantors, without specific community understanding or background knowledge. Our learning suggested that doing research on what farm workers expressed as their areas of greatest concern could be more impactful, such as research relating to cannabis farm workers and their exposure to respiratory dusts or allergens. By identifying the concerns from the cultivators, we were able to examine how a workplace transitioning from an illicit to a regulated work culture created its own unique environment for worker health. This knowledge could be relevant not only in the context of cannabis, but also to other occupations, goods, or services that have transitioned from illicit to licit.

This was not exclusively community-based participatory research. However, CBPR was used as one methodological prong in an interdisciplinary, mixed-methods toolkit. The grant concept was developed by members of an institution, but the question came from the research team, not the community. As a research team, we worked with a membership-based cannabis advocacy group,

The Cannabis Alliance, to develop interview questions, create a research process and methodology, conduct data analysis, and disseminate information back to some members of the community.

In a "pure" CBPR process, the community would have been involved in developing the original research question, designing the research process, conducting the research, analyzing the data, and then disseminating the information to the larger community involved and ensuring that that information was serving them and their needs (Blumenthal 2011). We did not have the time or the resources to do "pure" CBPR work, and those seeking to conduct such a process should study the work of scholars who have carried out the process of CBPR in communities successfully for many years, as there is a wealth of material (Hacker 2013; Wallerstein 2018) dedicated to the study and process of CBPR.

That being said, it was important to us to incorporate principles of CBPR to acknowledge voices that hadn't previously been heard. In interviews and focus groups, we were frequently met with surprise by the research participants, who didn't expect people from the university to be interested in the health and safety of cannabis farm workers and didn't expect us to ask them for their expertise or opinion on the matter. Further, it was valuable to recognize these employees as members of a community or cultural group, rather than solely as members of an industry.

By acknowledging the workers as members of a community, we could create space for a shared experience based on an understanding of historical stigma and criminalization (Ehrlich, Simpson, and Busch Isaksen 2019). Additionally, it was important to distinguish workers from the greater term or label that commonly gets attached to the "cannabis industry." Employees at the farm worker level commonly identified as members of a cultural group or political movement and had lower levels of personal economic interest relative to their employers or others who are more heavily invested in the industry at large. While the cannabis industry has been increasingly associated with a "green rush" of suited investors (Wade 2015), many employees at the farm level continue to work at or near minimum wage, and therefore their intentions and power cannot be equated with narratives given to the cannabis industry at large.

Why Use CBPR to Bridge the Cannabis Knowledge Gap?

Today, much of the evidence used to discuss cannabis in mainstream media is dismissed as "anecdotal." Many researchers argue that the use of anecdotal evidence is not a valid way to inform health-related decisions and use such evidence as an argument for the need for more systematic research (Grinspoon and Bakalar 1998). However, anecdotal evidence has guided health-related decisions throughout history, informing how we eat, rear children, and more. While clinical trials and systematic data collection is an extremely important part of knowledge formation, anecdotal evidence should not be discounted. In fact, anecdotal evidence, when collected systematically in qualitative research, has the power to contribute to evidence-based public health practice, particularly in controversial or heavily debated content areas (Nagaraj 2006).

We remain in a time of transition, with a change in cannabis legal frameworks sweeping the U.S. one state at a time. We are in a fascinating moment of time to collect community voices and preserve knowledge that was created prior to the emergence of legal frameworks, as well as to document the knowledge being created as a result of the legal transition in and of itself.

By utilizing principles of community-based participatory research, researchers can collect information from the historically illicit cannabis community and the legalization process, acknowledging that this is a community that has been historically criminalized, and therefore stigmatized. It should be noted that "Utilizing Community-Based Participatory Research in Cannabis Knowledge Formation," specifically refers to "utilizing principles" of CBPR, rather than suggesting to engage fully in CBPR. This is due to the fact that pure CBPR takes several years to conduct and can be very challenging to do when research is funded by a grantor with their own research interests. While the goal of CBPR is to conduct the research most desired by the community being researched, using methods that highlight community voice and provide information back to the community, this process takes several years and is frequently challenged by the interests of whoever is funding the research. While any research team with the time and resources should most certainly try to engage in authentic CBPR, it should be acknowledged that achieving CBPR is akin to achieving nirvana; the work is never quite finished, though it still is worthy to try to follow the eightfold path. It should also be understood that this work will become harder in the future as more states legalize and the cannabis industry's composition transitions from individuals who were a part of the illicit cannabis industry and community to newcomers with less historical knowledge.

The suggested methodology of CBPR, and the research goal of systematizing anecdotal evidence, historical knowledge, or cultural transformation through qualitative research, is not simple, particularly when considering cultural distrust and the complexities of creating knowledge in a quasi-legal industry. However, if we cannot honor stigmatized voices, build bridges of cultural trust, parse out economic interests with important truths by acknowledging that even those with an economic interest may hold valuable knowledge, industry and advertisers will continue to dominate the health narrative associated with cannabis. In order to proliferate balanced cannabis knowledge that helps inform consumers, advocates, critics, and neutral bystanders alike, researchers should incorporate community voice and consider the value of CBPR as a method for advancing the knowledge base around cannabis in this unique period of time.

Note

1 The terms "retail," "adult use," and "retail adult use" are used interchangeably and intentionally in place of the term "recreational." The three aforementioned terms are used in preference of the popularly coined "recreational" cannabis to acknowledge that legalization creates a market space for a retail product directed to a consumer age group; however, the policy process cannot define the user's intentions. Customers of retail cannabis stores use the products in these stores for a variety of reasons, including but not limited to medicinal, recreational, for leisure, for sexual health, for mental health, and due to addiction/dependence. To define a retail cannabis shopper as solely a recreational consumer challenges public health and consumer autonomy.

References

August, Karen. 2013. "Women in the Marijuana Industry." *Humboldt Journal of Social Relations* 35: 89–103.

Blumenthal, Daniel. 2011. "Is Community-Based Participatory Research Possible?" *American Journal of Preventive Medicine* 40 (3): 386–89.

Bromham, Lindell, Russell Dinnage, and Xia Hua. 2016. "Interdisciplinary Research Has Consistently Lower Funding Success." *Nature* 534 (7609): 684–87.

Carlini, Beatriz. H. 2017. "Potency Increase, Product Development and Marijuana Marketing in Times of Legalization." *Addiction* 112: 2178–79.

Damon, Will, Cody Callon, Lee Wiebe, Will Small, Thomas Kerr, and Ryan McNeil. 2017. "Community-Based Participatory Research in a Heavily Researched Inner City Neighbourhood: Perspectives of People Who Use Drugs on Their Experiences as Peer Researchers." *Social Science & Medicine* 176: 85–92.

Dresser, Rebecca. 2018. "Conceptual, Structural, and Practical Challenges to Ethical Allocation of Research Funds." *The American Journal of Bioethics* 18 (11): 23–24.

Ehrlich, Trecia, C. Simpson, and T. Busch Isaksen. 2019. "Sociopolitical Externalities Impacting Worker Health in Washington State's Cannabis Industry." *Annals of Work Exposures and Health*, November 64 (7): 683–92.

Grinspoon, Lester, and James Bakalar. 1998. "The Use of Cannabis as a Mood Stabilizer in Bipolar Disorder: Anecdotal Evidence and the Need for Clinical Research." *Journal of Psychoactive Drugs* 30 (2) — Marijuana at the Millennium: Medical and Social Implications.

Hacker, Karen. 2013. *Community-Based Participatory Research*. Thousand Oaks, CA: Sage.

Hatzenbuehler, Mark, Jo Phelan, and Bruce Link. 2013. "Stigma as a Fundamental Cause of Population Health Inequalities." *American Journal of Public Health* 103 (5): 813–21.

Krenzelok, Edward. 2017. "Marijuana Legalization: A Continuing Conundrum." *American Journal of Health-System Pharmacy* 74 (22): 1843.

Lashley, Kisha, and Timothy G. Pollock. 2019. "Waiting to Inhale: Reducing Stigma in the Medical Cannabis Industry." *Administrative Science Quarterly*. https://doi.org/10.1177/0001839219851501.

Lau, Nicholas, Paloma Sales, Sheigla Averill, Fiona Murphy, and Sye-Ok Sato. 2015. "Responsible and Controlled Use: Older Cannabis Users and Harm Reduction." *International Journal of Drug Policy* 26 (8): 709–18.

Nagaraj, Anandi. 2006. "Does Qualitative Synthesis of Anecdotal Evidence with That from Scientific Research Help in Understanding Public Health Issues: A Review of Low MMR Uptake." *European Journal of Public Health* 16 (1): 85–88.

National Academies of Sciences, Engineering, and Medicine. 2017. *The Health Effects of Cannabis and Cannabinoids: The Current State of Evidence and Recommendations for Research*. Washington, DC: The National Academies Press. https://doi.org/10.17226/24625.

Pew Research Center. 2015. "In Debate Over Legalizing Marijuana, Disagreement Over Drug's Dangers." April. www.pewresearch.org/wp-content/uploads/sites/4/2015/04/04-14-15-Marijuana-release.pdf.

Stith, Sarah, and Jacob Vigil. 2016. "Federal Barriers to Cannabis Research." *Science* 352 (6290): 1182.

Subritzky, Todd, Simone Pettigrew, and Simon Lenton. 2016. "Issues in the Implementation and Evolution of the Commercial Recreational Cannabis Market in Colorado." *International Journal of Drug Policy* 27: 1–12.

Wade, Jared. 2015. "Cannabiz: The High Profits and High Risks of Legal Marijuana." *Risk Management* 62 (9) (November): 30.

Wallerstein, Nina. 2018. *Community-Based Participatory Research for Health: Advancing Social and Health Equity*. 3rd ed. San Francisco, CA: Jossey-Bass, a Wiley Brand.

Zhang, Mona. 2016. "'Suits' and 'Stoners' Are Fighting for the Soul of the Weed Industry." *Vice News*, May 16. www.vice.com/en_us/article/qbxgnd/suits-and-stoners-are-fighting-for-the-soul-of-the-weed-industry.

Zylla, Dylan, Grant Steele, Justin Eklund, Jeanne Mettner, and Tom Arneson. 2018. "Barriers to Enrollment, and Educational Needs." *Cannabis and Cannabinoid Research* 3 (1): 195–202.

12

Health and Safety of Cannabis Workers

Marc B. Schenker and Chelsea E. Langer

Keywords: agricultural workers, allergies, ergonomics, occupational health, respiratory health

Introduction

Minimal research exists regarding the occupational health and safety risks specific to cannabis cultivation and processing. Occupational health comprises "all aspects of health and safety in the workplace and has a strong focus on primary prevention of hazards" (World Health Organization 2019). Workplace hazards may lead to acute or chronic health effects, ranging from respiratory and musculoskeletal diseases to accidents and cancers (World Health Organization 2019). Safety risks, particularly in agriculture, range from a risk of falls (from ladders, trees, etc.) to electrical hazards. Work in the cannabis industry includes myriad jobs from growing and cultivating the plant to processing, manufacturing, testing, distributing, and providing security.

This chapter focuses on the agricultural aspects of the regulated cannabis industry, or the growing and cultivating of the cannabis plants. We do not address personal safety hazards or hazards of cannabis extraction facilities in this review. Little research has been done on the health hazards of cannabis cultivation, and what research does exist has primarily been done on licensed cannabis facilities, either medicinal or in states where recreational use is legal. Although there is a registry of licensed sites, researchers have noted challenges of contacting growers as well as convincing them to be forthcoming given the ambiguous legal status of cannabis (Sumner, Goldstein, and Matthews 2018).

Without an effective systematic way to sample farms or workers coupled with the quasi-legal status of the industry, it is especially difficult to conduct a rigorous scientific study on a representative population. Further, in California—and likely in other states—the small, remote locations of most outdoor facilities also affect estimates about the industry's size and workforce as well as illness and injury rates. For these and other estimates we have used the best available data, recognizing that there are often wide variations in estimates for everything related to this industry. We have also utilized case reports and small studies where appropriate to highlight potential risks to workers in the industry.

DOI: 10.4324/9780429320491-12

The legal cannabis industry in the United States is estimated to employ more than 211,000 full-time workers, with more than 64,000 jobs added in 2018 (Barcott and Whitney 2019). As described previously, this chapter will focus on employees associated with growing and cultivating cannabis; we were unable to find a published estimate of the workforce associated with the agricultural aspects of cannabis. Cannabis agricultural employees primarily fit into two categories: cultivators and trimmers. Cultivators, generally full-time employees, are responsible for caring for the plants. Trimmers, on the other hand, cut the leaves and stems from the cannabis flowers and are usually employed during the harvest season that lasts from September until December (Horizon Water and Environment 2017). This seasonality applies more to the outdoor cannabis-growing workforce, whereas indoor cultivation is associated with more year-round workers.

In California at the present time, approximately 58% of cannabis is grown in outdoor cultivation sites and only 9% in indoor facilities, with the remainder being cultivated in mixed light grows (Sumner, Goldstein, and Matthews 2018). These estimates include both regulated and nonregulated cultivation sites. Thus, the majority of cannabis workers are seasonal employees. The cannabis industry relies heavily on a migratory workforce, colloquially referred to as "trimmigrants" (Krissman 2016). In contrast to other agricultural commodities that also rely on a migrant workforce, the cannabis workforce in the United States is composed of a diverse group of people from a wide range of socioeconomic backgrounds—college students, artists, young working professionals, the homeless, migratory underage youth, and foreigners on vacation or with tourist visas (Blondell 2017; Houston 2017; Walter 2016; The Trim Camp Counselor 2014; Krissman 2016). In addition, trimming jobs are filled, in large part, by women (The Trim Camp Counselor 2014; Higgs 2016; Schirmann 2016; Walter 2016; August 2013).

After conducting a review of the existing literature to identify an emergent research agenda, we found few useful studies of the health and safety risks associated with working in the cannabis industry. There is a small literature, however, on the health effects of cannabis exposure among workers in the cannabis industry that was useful for identifying and understanding the potential health and safety hazards faced by cannabis workers.

Cannabis Industry Occupational Hazards

Allergic Effects

Although there is limited research on the causal allergens associated with *Cannabis sativa*, especially in relation to workplace exposure, increased consumption of cannabis correlates with a documented increase in IgE-mediated cannabis allergic reactions (Decuyper et al. 2017; Decuyper et al. 2015; Nayak et al. 2013). What research does exist suggests that *C. sativa* exposure through inhalation and/or ingestion can result in an allergic reaction, including respiratory symptoms, sensitization, and anaphylaxis[1] (Tessmer et al. 2012; Stokes et al. 2000). Dermal exposure from handling the plant, both before and after harvest, represents another possible route of sensitization. Skin contact exposure has been linked with allergic reaction including hives, itchy skin, and swollen or puffy eyes (Decuyper et al. 2017; Marijuana Occupational Health and Safety Work Group 2017). Two separate case reports from the United Kingdom described workers with the Forensic Science Service who had worked with cannabis plants for years and eventually developed allergic responses that appeared shortly after exposure to cannabis plants, particularly the flowers. The investigators concluded that the patients were experiencing hives in both cases (Williams, Thompstone, and Wilkinson 2008; Majmudar, Azam, and Finch 2006), as well as contact dermatitis (rash) in one (Williams, Thompstone, and Wilkinson 2008). In a recent occupational study of police workers in Belgium (Decuyper et al. 2019), 34 out of 81 participants (42%) reported respiratory and/or dermatological symptoms following occupational exposure to cannabis. In almost all cases (33 of 34, 97%) occupational exposure resulted from entering illicit cannabis plantations. However, only one subject with dermatological symptoms had a borderline basophil[2] response to cannabis. The researchers concluded that the respiratory and cutaneous symptoms were likely due to a non-immune response.[3] It is likely that the level of exposure to cannabis among law enforcement officers is lower than among trimmers or cultivators who work directly with cannabis on a daily basis.

Given the paucity of studies documenting cannabis-associated allergies as a potential occupational health hazard, more research is needed particularly to document the incidence and clinical spectrum of allergic reactions to *C. sativa* among cannabis workers.

Respiratory Effects

Mold is a common contaminant in cannabis cultivation. In fact, a study of 30 indoor cannabis growing operations in Colorado identified mold as the principal health concern (Martyny et al. 2013). Exposure to mold can result in a range of respiratory health outcomes, including wheezing, coughing, shortness of breath, and respiratory infections. In addition, endotoxin-producing bacteria may result in hypersensitivity pneumonitis (farmer's lung), chronic bronchitis, organic dust toxic syndrome, and asthma. Sensitization and allergic reaction have also been connected to microbiological exposures, including endotoxins, bacteria, and fungus—all of which can be found at cannabis cultivation sites. Further, exposures are likely higher in indoor facilities compared to outdoor grows, because workers in indoor grows will likely face higher levels of airborne pathogens than workers in outdoor plantations.

Cannabis farm workers are potentially exposed to Actinobacteria[4] as well as the cannabis plant pathogen causing gray mold, *Botrytis cinerea*, during harvesting, bud stripping, and hand trimming. A health hazards evaluation conducted by the National Institute of Occupational Safety and Health (NIOSH) in summer 2015 at an organic outdoor cannabis farm in Washington State found levels of endotoxin-producing bacterial phyla at the cannabis cultivation sites they surveyed above the recommended limits (90 EU/m^3) (NIOSH 2017; Green et al. 2018). Analysis of personal and area samples derived from the outdoor farm revealed a broad diversity of bacteria and fungi that included Gram-positive Actinobacteria as well as *B. cinerea*. Personal air samples had the highest relative abundance of *B. cinerea* (59%) compared to area-level samples from the drying room (19%), greenhouse (18%), and outdoor environment (6%) (Green et al. 2018). These results highlight potential exposure to microbiological hazards in workers that harvest, bud strip, or hand trim cannabis.

A second health hazards evaluation was conducted by NIOSH at a medicinal cannabis manufacturing facility in Minnesota in fall 2016 and spring 2017 (NIOSH 2018). Four employees had repeated personal air samples taken on two days. Although the observed endotoxin levels did not exceed the recommended limit, the authors noted a marked increase on the second sampling day, indicating that certain tasks may be associated with higher levels of endotoxin. The highest endotoxin level was observed in the grinding room (94 EU/m^3). In addition to exposure samples, 12 employees were interviewed. Three (25%) reported a stuffy nose or sinus problems within the previous four weeks that they thought was work related. Of course, these are common symptoms with many other possible explanations. Destemming, grinding, decarboxylation, and facility management were identified as possible tasks associated with higher dust levels. One employee had an abnormal lung function test but had non-occupational factors that likely contributed to a restrictive pattern. No other employees had abnormal lung function test results (NIOSH 2018).

In a Colorado study of cannabis worker health, 214 employees associated with the cannabis industry were surveyed. Of these, only 57 (27%) worked in growing/cultivating/trimming. Results were presented for all 214 workers; 36 and 34 workers reported coughing and bringing up phlegm, respectively. However, all but one smoked cigarettes and/or used cannabis daily (Walters et al. 2017;

Walters, Fisher, and Tenney 2018). It is an essential challenge of future research to disentangle possible explanatory factors.

The literature derived from the hemp industry (Zuskin et al. 1992; Zuskin, Mustajbegovic, and Schachter 1994; Zuskin et al. 1990) suggests that the relationship between cannabis microbiological exposures and worker health should be examined more closely. In a cross-sectional and subsequent follow-up study of 66 textile workers, researchers in the former Yugoslavia found high levels of byssinosis[5] (47% of women in original and follow-up studies; 64% and 68% of men in original and follow-up studies, respectively). The researchers also observed acute effects such as cough, shortness of breath, chest tightness, and throat irritation. Chronic conditions reported include (estimates were reported by gender and original versus follow-up study, range given is lowest to highest) chronic cough (50%–61%), chronic phlegm (29%–57%), chronic bronchitis (26%–57%), and sinusitis (21%–32%) (Zuskin et al. 1990; Zuskin et al. 1992; Zuskin, Mustajbegovic, and Schachter 1994). Like hemp workers, during cultivation and processing cannabis workers are exposed to the leaves, buds, sap exudate, flowers, and pollen as well as associated plant pathogens such as bacteria and fungi, suggesting similar health effects.

In general, occupational exposures in the agricultural industry are associated with numerous respiratory and dermal symptoms and diseases. In particular, agriculture workers are exposed to a variety of particulates, vapors, and fumes that can cause adverse health outcomes. These exposures can lead to increased rates of chronic obstructive pulmonary disease (COPD), asthma, asthma-like syndrome, hypersensitivity pneumonitis, interstitial lung disease, and possibly lung cancer (Nordgren and Bailey 2016; Schenker 1998). Currently, information about the likelihood and/or prevalence of these often-long-term health risks in the cannabis industry is lacking. This suggests an urgent need to study the specific health and safety risks in the cannabis industry, particularly as the emerging, legal adult-use cannabis cultivation industry takes shape, to inform regulations and guide the protection of workers.

Dermatologic Effects

A case study from Turkey described a 19-year-old male with skin redness, fluid-filled lesions, and a targetoid rash following recreational cannabis use (Ozyurt 2014). The author concluded the case study was the first publication of an erythema multiforme-like recurrent drug eruption to be associated with cannabis use. Other studies have shown that hives have occurred in forensic specialists and law enforcement officers following the handling of cannabis (Herzinger et al. 2011; Majmudar, Azam, and Finch 2006; Mayoral et al. 2008; Williams, Thompstone, and Wilkinson 2008).

In the Belgian study of police workers (Decuyper et al. 2019), eight out of 81 participants (10%) reported dermatological symptoms following occupational exposure to cannabis. Symptoms were mainly comprised of severe itching and skin redness. Of the eight individuals, none had atopic dermatitis[6] and one had asthma.[7] An additional six officers (7%) reported both respiratory and dermatological symptoms upon cannabis exposure; one (17%) had atopic dermatitis and three (50%) had asthma. The researchers concluded that a non-immune-mediated mechanism is most likely responsible for the reported symptoms.

Toxicological Effects

Cannabis cultivation sites use pesticides, rodenticides, fungicides, and insecticides (Bernstein 2017; Butsic and Brenner 2016; Migoya and Baca 2015). Exposure to pesticides can result in mild health effects from nasal congestion, respiratory difficulties, skin, eye, and throat irritation as well as more severe adverse health effects (Marijuana Occupational Health and Safety Work Group 2017). In the Colorado survey of cannabis worker health, several workers experienced a number of negative symptoms after exposure to pesticides on the job, including skin irritation (n = 33, 18%), headaches and dizziness (n = 27, 14%), and eye irritation (n = 25, 13%). In contrast, 66% of workers (n = 123) reported no symptoms after handling pesticides (Walters, Fisher, and Tenney 2018; Walters et al. 2017). Pesticides can remain after spraying, and exposure risks increase when the plants are handled extensively during the harvesting and processing activities (Cuypers et al. 2017).

Pesticides designed for safe use on marijuana represent a potentially problematic issue, as the marijuana industry continues to grow rapidly. There exists minimal science-based research regarding the safe use of pesticides for cannabis farming (Bishop 2017). Pesticides in cannabis cultivation are particularly tricky as once the Environmental Protection Agency (EPA) approves a pesticide, it is then illegal to use it in any way other than the uses specified on the label. However, as cannabis remains a Schedule I drug, pesticide use in the cannabis industry remains largely unregulated by the US EPA. The agricultural workers at greatest risk of exposure to pesticides are greenhouse workers and workers who mix, load, transport, and apply pesticides. Exposure occurs during application as well as activities during which workers come in contact with the plant. However, in some situations, exposure to pesticides can occur from accidental spills, leakages, or faulty spraying equipment. The amount of the resulting exposure for a particular activity depends on the amount of residue on foliage and on the intensity of the contact with the foliage in case of different activities. What remains on the foliage may be transferred to clothing and skin of cannabis workers during harvesting, drying, trimming, and processing.

Ergonomic Risks

Little data exist on the incidence, prevalence, or severity of musculoskeletal disorders among workers in the cannabis industry. However, in the 2015 survey of Colorado cannabis industry workers, employees identified ergonomic issues as their highest health and safety concern, with 54% (n = 101) reporting back pain, 28% (n = 53) reporting discomfort in hands/wrists/fingers, and 23% (n = 43) reporting knee pain associated with work (Walters, Fisher, and Tenney 2018, 6; Walters et al. 2017, 8). Similarly, the 2018 NIOSH report from a Minnesota medicinal cannabis facility identified ergonomic issues as a potential hazard, including one of 12 (8%) interviewed workers reporting back strain as a work-related injury, and three (25%) reporting hand or wrist pain associated with work (NIOSH 2018, 21). Further, at least one worker mentioned general ergonomic concerns with respect to work (NIOSH 2018). Although no workers reported musculoskeletal problems in the NIOSH study in Washington, the report noted that hand trimming "could increase the risk for hand, wrist, and finger musculoskeletal disorders" (NIOSH 2017). Similarly, a memorandum issued from the chief of Cal/OSHA identified repetitive strain injuries as a potential industry-related concern relevant to both indoor and outdoor cultivation sites (Cal/OSHA 2018).

Limitations

As previously noted, there are very limited data with only a few useful case studies of the health and safety risks associated with working in the cannabis industry. We have focused on the allergic, respiratory, dermatologic, toxicological, and ergonomic risks of regulated cannabis growing and processing and do not consider abusive or exploitative work conditions or other personal safety issues that may arise. We also have not addressed the safety hazards of cannabis extraction facilities, both licensed and illegal. The largest health study includes workers from all aspects of the cannabis industry, from growing and cultivating to selling in a dispensary, and reports on outcomes for all workers combined despite very different tasks and therefore very different exposures. Further, 95% of the study respondents were cannabis users (Walters, Fisher, and Tenney 2018). Future studies will need to distinguish between the effects of occupational and consumer exposures.

It is—and will be—particularly challenging to conduct a rigorous scientific study of cannabis workers given the quasi-legal status of the industry. Owners and workers are reticent about their occupation given the ambiguous legal nature of their work. In addition, research is further complicated by the lack of guidance informed by federal standards (EPA, NIOSH, Occupational Safety and Health Administration, among other agencies), which will remain a barrier as long as cannabis remains federally illegal. There are currently very little epidemiological data, and no useful prevalence or incidence studies. Further, no prospective studies exist, so the significance of a healthy worker effect and worker loss from the workforce because of health effects cannot be assessed.[8] The few studies that do exist presumably cover workers with a lower level of exposure than workers who are working directly with cannabis in the fields and/or trimming rooms. This quasi-legal status and the small, remote location of most outdoor facilities lead to widely varying estimates about the industry's size and workforce, as well as injury and illness rates. We have reviewed the best available data, recognizing the wide variations in estimates for virtually everything related to this industry.

Future Directions

In summary, the cannabis industry is a major agricultural commodity that is in the process of coming out of the darkness. There are several demonstrated or potential health and safety hazards, but little data exist on actual risk, susceptibility factors, or short- and long-term health outcomes. Additionally, cannabis workers are likely exposed to a broad diversity of plant pathogens as well as regionally abundant—and regionally dependent—microorganisms. Health studies and a focus on effective prevention are needed, with particular attention to allergic, respiratory, dermatologic, ergonomic, and toxicologic exposures. Agriculture is a known cause of diverse adverse health effects, and the rapidly growing cannabis industry is no exception. Legalization will be a positive development for attention to occupational health and safety outcomes and their prevention.

Acknowledgements

We gratefully acknowledge the work done by Jennifer TyreeHageman in conducting a literature review and compiling references for a report on the California cannabis industry. Further, we appreciate the support of the Western Center for Agricultural Health and Safety (WCAHS) at the University of California, Davis.

This publication was supported by Grant Number U54OH007550 from CDC-NIOSH. Its contents are solely the responsibility of the authors and do not necessarily represent the official views of CDC-NIOSH.

Notes

1 "Anaphylaxis: hypersensitivity (as to foreign proteins or drugs) resulting from sensitization following prior contact with the causative agent"(Merriam-Webster.com 2019a).

2 "Basophil: a type of immune cell that has granules (small particles) with enzymes that are released during allergic reactions and asthma. A basophil is a type of white blood cell and a type of granulocyte" (NCI Dictionary of Cancer Terms 2019).

3 "An allergic reaction occurs when the immune system overreacts to a harmless substance known as an allergen. The immune system protects the body from infections, viruses and diseases. In some people, substances such as pollen, certain foods, latex, mold, pet dander, dust mites or insect stings are allergens that trigger the production of antibodies called Immunoglobulin E (IgE). These antibodies travel to cells that release chemicals, causing symptoms most often in the nose, lungs, throat, sinuses, ears, lining of the stomach or on the skin" (American Academy of Allergy, Asthma & Immunology 2019a).

4 Actinobacteria, a large group of Gram-positive bacteria, are commonly found in indoor and outdoor environments, especially the soil. Studies have shown Actinobacteria are potential causative agents for respiratory and other disorders (Rintala 2011).
5 "Byssinosis: an occupational respiratory disease associated with inhalation of cotton, flax, or hemp dust and characterized initially by chest tightness, shortness of breath, and cough and eventually by irreversible lung disease"(Merriam-Webster.com 2019b).
6 "Atopic dermatitis (eczema) is a chronic or recurrent inflammatory skin disease. 'Atopic' means that there is typically a genetic tendency toward allergic disease. Atopic dermatitis usually begins in the first few years of life and is often the initial indication that a child may later develop asthma and/or allergic rhinitis (hay fever)" (AAAAI 2019b).
7 "Asthma is a chronic disease involving the airways (tubes) that carry air in and out of the lungs. These airways are inflamed in people with asthma. The inflammation makes the airways very sensitive, and the tubes often react to allergens or irritations. . . . Asthma symptoms may include wheezing, coughing, chest tightness and trouble breathing" (AAAAI 2019c).
8 The healthy worker effect in occupational epidemiology refers to the phenomenon that workers are healthier than the general population, either because unhealthy (chronically ill, disabled, etc.) people are less likely to be employed or because workers self-select out of professions if they become unwell (Li and Sung 1999).

References

American Academy of Allergy, Asthma & Immunology. 2019a. "Allergic Reaction." Accessed July 29, 2019. www.aaaai.org/conditions-and-treatments/conditions-dictionary/allergic-reaction.

———. 2019b. "Atopic Dermatitis." Accessed July 29, 2019. www.aaaai.org/conditions-and-treatments/conditions-dictionary/atopic-dermatitis-(eczema).

———. 2019c. "Asthma." Accessed July 29, 2019. www.aaaai.org/conditions-and-treatments/conditions-dictionary/Asthma.

August, Karen. 2013. "Women in the Marijuana Industry." *Humboldt Journal of Social Relations* 35: 89–103.

Barcott, B., and B. Whitney. 2019. "Leafly Special Report: Cannabis Jobs Count." Accessed August 30, 2019. https://d3atagt0rnqk7k.cloudfront.net/wp-content/uploads/2019/03/01141121/CANNABIS-JOBS-REPORT-FINAL-2.27.191.pdf.

Bernstein, Sharon. Reuters. Environment Section. 2017. "Banned Pesticides from Illegal Pot Farms Seep into California Water." September 8. Accessed July 29, 2019. www.reuters.com/article/us-usa-marijuana-environment/banned-pesticides-from-illegal-pot-farms-seep-into-california-water-idUSKCN1BJ13W.

Bishop, Jenna Hardisty. 2017. "Weeding the Garden of Pesticide Regulation: When the Marijuana Industry Goes Unchecked." *Drake Law Review* 65: 223–53.

Blondell, Amy Donovan. 2017. "Homeless Youth Labor Continuum: Working in Formal and Informal Economies from Highland Guatemala to San Francisco, California." In *Laboring and Learning*, edited by Johanna Waters, Tatek Abebe, and Tracey Skelton, 327–60. Singapore: Springer.

Butsic, Van, and Jacob C. Brenner. 2016. "Cannabis (*Cannabis sativa* or *C. indica*) Agriculture and the Environment: A Systematic, Spatially-Explicit Survey and Potential Impacts." *Environmental Research Letters* 11. doi:10.1088/1748-9326/11/4/044023.

Cal/OSHA. 2018. "Cal/OSHA Advisory Committee Findings and Recommendations on the Need to Develop Industry-Specific Regulations for Marijuana (cannabis) Establishments." State of California, Department of Industrial Relations, Division of Occupational Safety and Health.

Cuypers, Eva, Wouter Vanhove, Joachim Gotink, Arne Bonneure, Patrick Van Damme, and Jan Tytgat. 2017. "The Use of Pesticides in Belgian Illicit Indoor Cannabis Plantations." *Forensic Science International* 277: 59–65. doi:10.1016/j.forsciint.2017.05.016.

Decuyper, I. I., A. L. Van Gasse, N. Cop, V. Sabato, M. A. Faber, C. Mertens, C. H. Bridts, M. M. Hagendorens, L. De Clerck, H. P. Rihs, and D. G. Ebo. 2017. "*Cannabis Sativa* Allergy: Looking Through the Fog." *Allergy* 72: 201–6. doi:10.1111/all.13043.

Decuyper, Ine Ilona, Athina Van Gasse, Margaretha Antje Faber, Christel Mertens, Jessy Elst, Hans-Peter Rihs, Vito Sabato, Hilde Lapeere, Margo Hagendorens, Chris Bridts, Luc De Clerck, and Didier Ebo. 2019. "Occupational Cannabis Exposure and Allergy Risks." *Occupational and Environmental Medicine* 76: 78–82. doi:10.1136/oemed-2018-105302.

Decuyper, Ine Ilona, Hanne Ryckebosch, Athina L. Van Gasse, Vito Sabato, Margaretha Faber, Chris H. Bridts, and Didier G. Ebo. 2015. "Cannabis Allergy: What do We Know." *Archivum Immunologiae et Therapiae Experimentalis* 63: 327–32. doi:10.1007/s00005-0352-z.

Green, Brett J., James R. Couch, Angela R. Lemons, Nancy C. Burton, Kerton R. Victory, Ajay P. Nayak, and Donald H. Beezhold. 2018. "Microbial Hazards During Harvesting and Processing at an Outdoor United States Cannabis Farm." *Journal of Occupational and Environmental Hygiene* 15 (5): 430–40. doi:10.1080/15459624.2018.1432863.

Herzinger, T., P. Schopf, B. Przybilla, and F. Rueff. 2011. "IgE-Mediated Hypersensitivity Reactions to Cannabis in Laboratory Personnel." *International Archives of Allergy and Immunology* 156: 423–26. doi:10.1159/000324444.

Higgs, Sera. 2016. "I Spent a Season Trimming Weed in Humboldt County. This Is What It Was Like." *Matador Network*, Narrative.

Horizon Water and Environment, LLC. 2017. *CalCannabis Cultivation Licensing: Draft Program Environmental Impact Report*. Oakland, CA: California Department of Food and Agriculture.

Houston, Will. 2017. "State Seeks to Add Protections for Marijuana Farmworkers." *Eureka Times-Standard*.

Krissman, Fred. 2016. "America's Largest Cannabis Labor Market." *A Provisional Profile and Proposal for New Research*. https://hiimr.humboldt.edu/sites/default/files/hiimr/docs/MjLaborMarket.pdf: Humboldt State University, Department of Anthropology.

Li, C. Y., and F. C. Sung. 1999. "A Review of the Healthy Worker Effect in Occupational Epidemiology." *Occupational Medicine* 49 (4): 225–29.

Majmudar, V., N. A. M. Azam, and T. Finch. 2006. "Contact Urticaria to *Cannabis Sativa*." *Contact Dermatitis* 54: 127.

Marijuana Occupational Health and Safety Work Group. 2017. *Guide to Worker Safety and Health in the Marijuana Industry*. Denver, CO: Colorado Department of Public Health and Environment.

Martyny, John W., Kate A. Serrano, Joshua W. Schaeffer, and Mike V. Van Dyke. 2013. "Potential Exposures Associated with Indoor Marijuana Growing Operations." *Journal of Occupational and Environmental Hygiene* 10 (11): 622–39. doi:10.1080/15459624.2013.831986.

Mayoral, M., H. Calderon, R. Cano, and M. Lombardero. 2008. "Allergic Rhinoconjunctivitis Caused by *Cannabis Sativa* Pollen." *The Journal of Investigational Allergology and Clinical Immunology* 18: 73–74.

Merriam-Webster.com. 2019a. "Anaphylaxis." In *Merriam-Webster*. www.merriam-webster.com/dictionary/anaphylaxis.

———. 2019b. "Byssinosis." In *Merriam-Webster*. www.merriam-webster.com/dictionary/byssinosis: Merriam-Webster.com.

Migoya, David, and Ricardo Baca. 2015. "Deep Dive: Why Colorado Has Struggled to Regulate Pot Pesticides." *The Denver Post*, Business.

Nayak, Ajay P., Brett J. Green, Gordon Sussman, Noam Berlin, Hemant Lata, Suman Chandra, Mahmoud A. ElSohly, Justin M. Hettick, and Donald Beezhold. 2013. "Characterization of *Cannabis Sativa* Allergens." *Annals of Allergy, Asthma & Immunology* 111 (1): 32–37. doi:10.1016/j.anai.2013.04.018.

NCI Dictionary of Cancer Terms. 2019. "Basophil." Accessed July 29, 2019. www.cancer.gov/publications/dictionaries/cancer-terms/def/basophil.

NIOSH. 2017. *Evaluation of Potential Hazards During Harvesting and Processing Cannabis at an Outdoor Organic Farm*. Edited by J. Couch, K. Victory, B. Lowe, N. Burton, B. Green, A. Nayak, A. Lemons, and D. Beezhold. Cincinnati, OH: U.S. Department of Health and Human Services, Centers for Disease Control and Prevention, National Institute for Occupational Safety and Health, Health Hazard Evaluation Report 2015–0111–3271.

———. 2018. *Evaluation of a Medicinal Cannabis Manufacturing Facility with an Indoor and Outdoor Grow Operation*. Edited by J. Couch, D. Wiegand, G. R. Grimes, B. J. Green, A. R. Lemons, E. Glassford, L. Zwack, S. R. Jackson, and D. Beezhold. Cincinnati, OH: U.S. Department of Health and Human Services, Centers for Disease Control and Prevention, National Institute for Occupational Safety and Health, Health Hazard Evaluation Report 2016–0090–3317.

Nordgren, Tara M., and Kristina L. Bailey. 2016. "Pulmonary Health Effects of Agriculture." *Current Opinion in Pulmonary Medicine* 22 (2): 144–49. doi:10.1097/MCP.0000000000000247.

Ozyurt, Selcuk. 2014. "Cannabis-Induced Erythema Multiforme-Like Recurrent Drug Eruption." *International Journal of Dermatology* 53: e22–e23.

Rintala, Helena. 2011. "Actinobacteria in Indoor Environments: Exposures and Respiratory Health Effects." *Frontiers in Bioscience S3* (June 1): 1273–84.

Schenker, M. B., ed. 1998. "Respiratory Health Hazards in Agriculture." *American Journal of Respiratory and Critical Care Medicine* 158 (5(2)): S1–S76. doi:10.1164/ajrccm.158.supplement_1.rccm1585s1.

Schirmann, Kelly. 2016. "What It's Like to Be a 'Trim Bitch' on an Illegal Weed Farm." *Broadly Vice*.

Stokes, Jeffrey R., Rita Hartel, Linda B. Ford, and Thomas B. Casale. 2000. "Cannabis (Hemp) Positive Skin Tests and Respiratory Symptoms." *Annals of Allergy, Asthma & Immunology* 85: 238–40. doi:10.1016/S1081-1206(10)62473-8.

Sumner, Daniel A., Robin Goldstein, and William A. Matthews. 2018. "California's Nursery and Cannabis Industries." In *California Agriculture: Dimensions and Issues*, edited by P. L. Martin, R. E. Goodhue, and B. D. Wright. Accessed July 10, 2019. https://giannini.ucop.edu/publications/cal-ag-book/.

Tessmer, Ayla, Noam Berlin, Gordon Sussman, Nathan Leader, Eddie Chu Chung, and Donald Beezhold. 2012. "Hypersensitivity Reactions to Marijuana." *Annals of Allergy, Asthma & Immunology* 108: 282–84. doi:10.1016/j.anai.2012.01.008.

The Trim Camp Counselor. 2014. "Everything You Need to Know About Trim Camp (but Were Afraid to Ask)." *Reality Sandwich*.

Walter, Shoshana. 2016. "In Secretive Marijuana Industry, Whispers of Abuse and Trafficking." *Reveal News*. www.revealnews.org/article/in-secretive-marijuana-industry-whispers-of-abuse-and-trafficking/.

Walters, Kevin M., Gwenith G. Fisher, and Liliana Tenney. 2018. "An Overview of Health and Safety in the Colorado Cannabis Industry." *American Journal of Industrial Medicine*. 1–11. doi:10.1002/ajim.22834.

Walters, Kevin M., Gwenith G. Fisher, Liliana Tenney, and Kurt Kraiger. 2017. *Work and Well-Being in the Colorado Cannabis Industry*. Aurora, CO: Colorado School of Public Health.

Williams, C., J. Thompstone, and M. Wilkinson. 2008. "Work-Related Contact Urticaria to *Cannabis Sativa*." *Contact Dermatitis* 58: 62–63.

World Health Organization. 2019. "Occupational Health." Accessed July 11, 2019. www.who.int/topics/occupational_health/en/.

Zuskin, Eugenija, Bozica Kanceljak, Duska Pokrajac, E. N. Schachter, and T. J. Witek Jr. 1990. "Respiratory Symptoms and Lung Function in Hemp Workers." *British Journal of Industrial Medicine* 47: 627–32. doi:10.1136/oem.47.9.627.

Zuskin, Eugenija, Bozica Kanceljak, E. Neil Schachter, Theodore J. Witek, Saul Maayani, Satindra Goswami, Zvi Marom, and Nicholas Rienzi. 1992. "Immunological Findings in Hemp Workers." *Environmental Research* 59: 350–61. doi:10.1016/S0013-9351(05)80041-6.

Zuskin, Eugenija, Jadranka Mustajbegovic, and E. N. Schachter. 1994. "Follow-Up Study of Respiratory Function in Hemp Workers." *American Journal of Industrial Medicine* 26: 103–15. doi:10.1002/ajim.4700260109.

[illegible] 2019. [illegible] *Canadian [illegible]* 193 [illegible]

[illegible]

Section 3
Markets and Society

The creation of legal cannabis markets provides a unique opportunity to study the relationship between markets and society in a neoliberal policy landscape that tends to make little distinction between the two. Neoliberal governance prescribes market solutions for social problems, so in a sense the creation of legal markets as a solution to the problems of prohibition is a quintessential neoliberal approach to criminal justice reform. However, legal markets are embedded in thickets of regulation that substantially limit the influence of market, rather than political, forces in their creation and development. The persistence of prohibition adds even more friction to the process of rolling out cannabis capitalism as a replacement for, rather than a transition of, well-established unregulated markets that look a lot more like neoliberal free markets than strict control legal ones. The politics of legalization, so far, reflect a societal anxiety about allowing the cannabis industry to be *laissez faire* capitalist rather than strictly controlled.

That anxiety has both normative and critical dimensions when it comes to attitudes about prohibition. Normative strict control stakeholders retain prohibitionist fears about cannabis as a public health problem and a dangerous commodity, especially to children. Stakeholders who are against prohibition but critical of neoliberal capitalism as an engine of socioeconomic inequality are critical of legal cannabis market tendencies towards monopolistic corporatization. The regulatory frictions to market formation created by strict control and prohibition operating simultaneously in the landscape may be surprisingly welcome to almost any stakeholder that is not urgently seeking a return on industry investment. This includes unregulated cannabis market actors, many of whom pivoted to a virtually unregulated CBD industry opened up by the 2018 Farm Bill. The chapters in this section sketch the contours of legal cannabis market formation in the context of these dynamic and often contradictory relationships among prohibition, regulation, and market freedom.

This section begins with two chapters that consider the friction between state and federal regulations on legal cannabis market formation. In their chapter, "The Economic Impact of State Regulations and Taxes on Legal and Illegal Cannabis Markets," economists Robin S. Goldstein and Daniel A. Sumner review cannabis-specific regulatory changes in California and their influence on compliance costs and demand. In doing so, they examine how regulations compare to unregulated illicit marketplaces in influencing consumer behavior and industry practices. Designed as a natural experiment, their study compares consumer incentives to purchase from unregulated versus regulated markets. For cannabis economists, this chapter advances an innovative approach to estimating regulatory costs that may inhibit, rather than support, the broader public policy goal of establishing regulated markets.

The subsequent chapter focuses on the financial limitations related to ongoing federal prohibition, excluding U.S.-based cannabis businesses from conventional banking relationships, subjecting them to higher tax rates, and excluding them from the tax code deductions available to other legal industries. In "The Cannabis Enigma: Navigating the Inequitable Tax, Banking, and Insurance Milieu in the United States," accounting scholar Joshua Zender describes barriers to normal business practices for cannabis commerce in the United States. Arguing that cannabis entrepreneurs face discriminatory banking rules and tax codes, Zender describes the historical origins of these rules and suggests organizing business forms that provide maximum liability protection and operations flexibility. The chapter closes by articulating a research and policy agenda for cannabis scholars wrestling with the enigma of state-legal markets in the context of ongoing federal prohibition.

A critical avenue of research in regulated markets considers whether the promises of fair labor practices are actually fulfilled. In "A Labor Studies Approach to Cannabis," anthropologist Marty Otañez draws on survey data and ethnographic methods to examine the extent to which corporate social responsibility (CSR) bundled with cannabis industry philanthrocapitalism is related to a change in the lived experiences of cannabis workers. This chapter proposes a labor studies framework that centers the experiences of workers to evaluate CSR claims of fair and safe labor practices. By interviewing workers and attending industry events, Otañez disrupts the privileging of cannabis profits over adherence to labor rights. The promises of legalization are not just made by policy architects; they are also adapted by industry as a marketing strategy, and both must be critically examined rather than accepted simply because legalization is assumed to make everything better.

In the subsequent chapter, "Cannabis Corporate Social Responsibility: A Critical and Mixed-Method Approach," lawyer and MBA David Vergara joins Otañez to draw on interview data and case studies of two cannabis businesses to model a critical approach to CSR as a marketing strategy. Otañez and Vergara explore the viability of social responsibility in the context of neoliberal capitalism, as well as the limits of CSR in the cannabis space, and they call for more cannabis-focused CSR scholarship as the industry shifts from informal to formalized business relations. The authors identify the ways in which the shadows of federal prohibition undermine the capacity of cannabis corporations to engage in socially responsible business practices.

In "Consumer Activism, Sustainable Supply Chains, and the Cannabis Market," political scientist Elizabeth A. Bennett transitions this section from a critical perspective on the viability of corporate responsibility to drive ethical consumption to a critical perspective on the viability of consumer activism to develop socially responsible supply chains. Ethical purchasing is often promoted as a vehicle for consumers to address concerns about fair labor practices, environmental impacts, and product safety. In doing so, Bennett highlights both the challenges and the opportunities of ethical purchasing practices in the cannabis space. Bennett's contribution suggests a variety of rich research agendas for examining the rhetoric and reality of ethical purchasing as a form of cannabis consumer activism.

The easing of federal restrictions on hemp agriculture, discussed in the final chapter of this section, provides a glimpse into a future for the regulation of cannabis as agriculture rather than a federally prohibited commercial product. In "Zero Point Three: Current and Future Directions in the Political Economy of Medicinal Hemp," Noah Silber-Coats introduces and critically examines three intersecting phenomena: research in CBD therapeutics; how hemp has been de-linked from cannabis prohibition in the U.S. via the 2018 Farm Bill; and the emergence of hemp-derived wellness products and alternative medicines. Things are not always what they seem with prohibition's botanically problematic distinction between "hemp" and "marijuana." Silber-Coats demonstrates that these distinctions have substantial implications for policy, markets, research, and consumers.

The chapters presented in this section focus on the relationship between markets and society in a post-prohibition context utilizing a variety of methodologies and reflect a range of possible research directions. Legalization is often promoted through the promise of economic growth and related tax revenue as well as opportunities for legitimate employment.

Yet research in these areas tell us much about how the continuity of laws and anxieties associated with prohibition shape who benefits from the creation of new, strictly regulated markets, rather than transitioning historically criminalized market actors into the formal economy. Taken together, the chapters in this section map out directions for research about legal cannabis markets that are critical of tendencies towards bureaucratic central planning inspired by prohibitionist anxieties *and* the integration of cannabis into capitalist markets as usual.

13

The Economic Impact of State Regulations and Taxes on Legal and Illegal Cannabis Markets

Robin S. Goldstein and Daniel A. Sumner

Keywords: Cannabis regulation impacts, retail prices of cannabis, cannabis markets, substitution of unlicensed for licensed cannabis, regulation compliance costs

Introduction

This chapter explores the economic impacts of state-level cannabis decriminalization, regulation, licensing, and taxation on the cannabis market, using California as an empirical example. California has the longest-running legal cannabis industry in postwar America. Our analysis focuses on the cost-driven effects of the regulations and taxes that were introduced in California in 2018, including a comparison of prices at licensed vs. unlicensed retailers. Such regulatory cost assessments may help inform ongoing policy debates in the many other jurisdictions that are in the process of considering or implementing some form of legal structure for cannabis but have not yet fully regulated the industry.

We begin by noting that cannabis "legalization" is a fuzzy term. Depending on the context, legalization can mean the moment when it becomes legal to possess cannabis; when it becomes legal to buy and sell cannabis; when it becomes legal for anyone over 18 to buy cannabis with a medical prescription; when it becomes legal for any consumer over 21 to walk into a store and buy cannabis without permission; when cannabis meets government safety standards; or when cannabis sales must be licensed, reported, and taxed. For a broad discussion of the stages and definitions of cannabis legalization and decriminalization, with comparisons between different U.S. states, see Pacula and Smart (2017).

This chapter is organized into four sections. In the first section, we briefly outline the main legal and regulatory changes in its recent history. In the second section, we give three examples of regulatory costs in California: mandatory testing, operating restrictions, and taxation. In the third section, we observe some retail price trends and attrition of retailers in California before and after the regulatory changes that occurred between 2016 and 2018. In the fourth and final section, we

DOI: 10.4324/9780429320491-13

discuss the potential relevance of our observations in California to the rapidly changing cannabis markets in other U.S. jurisdictions.

Legal and Regulatory Background

Medicinal Decriminalization

California's legal medicinal cannabis industry dates back to 1996, when voters passed a state ballot initiative known as the Compassionate Use Act (Proposition 215). The Compassionate Use Act decriminalized the possession of cannabis by patients with doctor's recommendations, but did not provide much concrete protection for cannabis producers and sellers ("caregivers") from local or state law enforcement.

In 2003, the California Senate passed the Medical Marijuana Program Act (SB 420), further clarified five years later by the Brown Guidelines (Brown 2008). The Brown Guidelines provided some new protections for medicinal cannabis producers and sellers that were organized as nonprofit cooperatives or collectives while also giving more power to counties and local municipalities to establish their own rules for medicinal cannabis businesses. In some jurisdictions where cannabis trade was permitted locally, the industry thrived. Some local regulations were enforced after SB 420, but until the end of 2017, California cannabis businesses were largely unregulated at the state level, and according to state tax authorities, only 30% of their income was being reported to the state. Most businesses followed ad hoc procedures, and much of the business was done in cash.

Adult-Use Decriminalization

In November 2016, Proposition 64, a voter initiative (the Adult Use of Marijuana Act), decriminalized adult-use ("recreational" or nonmedical) cannabis for all adults 21 and over in California. Given that adult-use retailers could not legally open until January 2018 and that medicinal retailers continued to do business as usual (and enforce the requirement of an in-state doctor's recommendation) until late 2017, we neither assumed nor observed much effect of Prop 64 decriminalization in November 2016 on California's legal medicinal cannabis market. As early as 1977, the California State Office of Narcotics and Drug Abuse had concluded, in its "First Report on the Impact of California's New Marijuana Law," that "the reduction in penalties for possession of marijuana for personal use does not appear to have been a factor in people's decision to use or not use the drug" (Budman 1977, 10). Recent studies have also found little to no evidence that medicinal or adult-use cannabis decriminalization increases cannabis use among state residents (e.g. Downs, Barcott, and Corva 2019; Ammerman et al. 2015; Diep 2015; Choo et al. 2014; Lynne-Landsman, Livingston, and Wagenaar 2013; MacCoun and Reuter 2001). Given these results, we did not expect that mere decriminalization, without adult-use sale, would do much to grow the legal market in California right away (Sumner et al. 2018).

A study by RAND's Drug Policy Research Center suggests that many U.S. consumers may not even be familiar with the criminal penalties for cannabis possession in their states. According to RAND,

> [s]ubstantial fractions of the population wrongly identify the maximum penalty prevailing in their state or assert that they simply do not know what it is . . . When people are not aware of penalties, a change in penalties may not matter very much.
>
> *(RAND 2009, 1)*

This could help explain why decriminalization appears to have little impact on demand.

Regulation and Taxation

On January 1, 2018, a variety of state licensing, safety, and reporting regulations, along with a \$9.25 per ounce cultivation tax and a 15% cannabis excise tax, were all introduced in California via the Medicinal and Adult-Use Cannabis Regulation and Safety Act (SB 94). Mandatory lab testing regulations, including pesticide testing, went into effect in July 2018. By 2019, substantially all of California's new cannabis regulations and taxes were fully implemented. Although cannabis businesses were still prohibited under local laws in many counties, we assume that early-to-mid-2018 state licensing, regulation, testing, and taxation would generate a modest outward shift in aggregate cannabis demand in California, which now includes demand from people without medical recommendations, who could now walk into a store and buy cannabis from a licensed adult-use retailer, and demand from out-of-state visitors who might have previously not gone to the trouble of buying illegal cannabis.

We also assume that, to some extent, legalized cannabis represents safety to consumers (see Bennett (2018) on ethical consumerism in Portland), and that some consumers are willing to pay something extra for California's stringent testing and safety certification standards, including a more rigorous pesticide testing regime than exists for any other agricultural product in the state (Valdes-Donoso, Sumner, and Goldstein 2019). So we add another small outward demand shift for the consumer perception of safety that is generated by the 2018 regulatory changes.

Costs of Compliance With State Regulations in California: Examples From Testing, Operating Restrictions, and Taxation

The relatively swift onset of full legalization, in the context of a 22-year-old decriminalized but largely unregulated medicinal cannabis market, created an economic shock, or more precisely a set of shocks, to the market that make it useful as a natural experiment in regulatory impacts on legal and illegal markets (Sumner et al. 2018). In the remainder of this chapter, we give some concrete examples of costly 2018 regulations in California and our estimates of their associated compliance costs. In this chapter, we will give three examples of regulatory compliance costs: mandatory testing, operating restrictions, and taxation.

Mandatory Testing

As of 2019, every U.S. state with a regulated cannabis market had instituted some form of mandatory testing standards. These standards vary from state to state: For instance, in Washington, only cannabinoid potency testing is now required; whereas in Oregon and Massachusetts, like in California, pesticide testing is required. Cannabis testing can be costly when it includes certain types of pesticide and other contaminant tests that require "wet lab" technology and expensive chemical reagents.

In particular, pesticide testing can be costly. In California, minimum tolerance levels were set to levels lower than the ones for other agricultural products in the state, and early results showed high failure rates (see Valdes-Donoso, Sumner, and Goldstein 2019). State regulators exert control over per-pound testing costs by setting minimum tolerance levels for pesticides and contaminants. Tolerance levels have considerable cost impact because failed batches cannot be sold unless they are "remediated," otherwise they must be destroyed (Valdes-Donoso 2019). More tolerant standards reduce failure rates, as is widely believed to have happened in Washington State when the strictest testing standards were lifted (and prices subsequently fell). Another important lever of cost impact is the "maximum batch size" (how large a batch can be produced while only having to perform one random sampling). The relationships between failure rate, maximum batch size, and total cost per pound of retail cannabis are estimated in Table 13.1.

Table 13.1 Testing: itemized costs of cannabis testing under different rejection-rate and batch-size assumptions

Failure Rate[1]	*Max. Batch Size*	*Laboratory Cost*[1]	*Cannabis Lost*	*Remediation Cost*	*Total*
	(Pounds)	*($/pound)*	*($/pound)*	*($/pound)*	*($/pound)*
7.0%	5	$121	$83	$1	$204
7.0%	25	$28	$82	$1	$111
7.0%	50	$17	$82	$1	$99
12.5%	5	$129	$148	$1	$278
12.5%	25	$30	$148	$1	$179
12.5%	50	$18	$148	$1	$167
25.0%	5	$151	$322	$3	$476
25.0%	25	$35	$322	$3	$360
25.0%	50	$21	$322	$3	$346

Source: Valdes-Donoso, Sumner, and Goldstein (2019).

Note: Totals may not reflect sums of rows due to rounding.

1 For lab costs, in addition to those listed in Table 13.1, labs have compliance costs for surveillance, disposal, and other costs that are applied per pound tested that are $4.88 for small labs, $4.06 for medium labs, and $3.25 for large labs. The weighted average of these costs is included in the laboratory costs per pound.

Operating Restrictions

Illegal markets, by construction, have the natural advantage of not having to comply with the costly regulations and taxes that their legal counterparts do. This advantage is not only financial, but also operational. When previously unregulated cannabis businesses enter the legal market, they must retool their administrative structure, infrastructure, human resources, inventory management, storage, sales and marketing, and many other aspects of their day-to-day operations. In California, fully legal cannabis businesses must comply with security guard rules, surveillance video archival rules, GPS location and track-and-trace reporting rules, rules for waste disposal, and packaging, labeling, and many other requirements.

Some operating restrictions that are not easily quantifiable may nonetheless have considerable economic impact. For example, Tables 13.2a and 13.2b evaluate the effects of California's rule that all cannabis retailers must close to the public at 10 pm.

As shown in Table 13.2a, as of late 2016, before regulations went into effect, there were approximately 140 cannabis retailers in California operating 24 hours a day. Table 13.2b takes the hours of operation of cannabis retailers from our survey in a sub-sample of six municipalities (Los Angeles, San Francisco, San Diego, San Jose, Sacramento, and Davis) and estimates the aggregate number of opening hours that would be eliminated by the imposition of a 10 pm to 6 am curfew. We estimate that 13% of all pre-regulatory opening hours would be eliminated by the regulations.

Of course, this does not translate cleanly to a 13% reduction in the size of the legal cannabis market. In the supply and demand models used in Sumner, Goldstein, and Matthews (2018), and Sumner et al. (2018), we do not calculate the cost of hours-of-operation restrictions on a per-pound basis. Instead, we include the effect in our simulation as a shift of −2% in demand in the medicinal cannabis segment, a shift of −2% in demand in the adult-use cannabis segment, and a shift of +1.5% in demand in the illegal cannabis segment. See Sumner et al. (2018), section 6.4.6, for details.

The example of opening-hours restrictions serves to illustrate the point that there are some ways in which illegal cannabis may be *more* freely available in the marketplace than its fully legal competition. California's transition from decriminalization to full legalization had the practical effect of keeping all previously lawful late-night cannabis transactions out of the fully legal market and moving them into the illegal market.

Table 13.2a Operating restrictions: 24-hour medicinal cannabis retailers in California, 2016

	Storefront	*Delivery-Only*	*Total*
Northern California	0	11	11
Central California	1	4	15
Southern California	27	99	126
Total	28	114	142

Source: Sumner et al. (2018).

Table 13.2b Operating restrictions: number of cannabis businesses impacted by mandatory 10 pm closing rule in six California municipalities (Los Angeles, San Francisco, San Diego, San Jose, Sacramento, and Davis) upon implementation of state cannabis regulations, January 1, 2018

		Hours of Medicinal Businesses Operating as of 2016		
		Avg Closing Time	*Pct Open After 10 pm*	*Pct Open After Midnight*
City	*Obs.*			
Los Angeles	24	12:20 am	83%	33%
San Francisco	18	10:53 pm	50%	17%
San Diego	16	11:56 pm	75%	38%
San Jose	10	11:50 pm	30%	20%
Sacramento	8	11:08 pm	63%	13%
Davis	6	10:40 pm	50%	17%
Statewide averages	82	11:51 pm	63%	26%

	*Business Hours That Would Be Eliminated by a 10 pm–6 am Curfew**					
	Avg Effect on Impacted Businesses			*Effect Averaged Across All Businesses Statewide*		
City	*Lost Hrs/Day*	*Lost Hrs/Yr*	*Pct of Total Hrs**	*Lost Hrs/Day*	*Lost Hrs/Yr*	*Pct of Total Hrs**
Los Angeles	2.90	1,015	21%	2.42	846	17%
San Francisco	2.33	817	19%	1.17	408	9%
San Diego	2.75	963	20%	2.06	722	15%
San Jose	4.00	1,400	33%	1.20	420	10%
Sacramento	2.40	840	19%	1.50	525	12%
Davis	1.67	583	14%	0.83	292	7%
Statewide averages	2.71	949	20%	1.72	602	13%

* Assumes uniform statewide average opening time of 10:30 am. Lost hours calculated in a hypothetical scenario where all medicinal businesses that were operating as of 2016 were to continue operating after adult-use legalization took effect in 2018, and that all of them altered their hours to be compliant with the new 10 pm curfew.

The middle column of Table 13.3 summarizes the direct regulatory compliance costs per pound of cannabis, not including taxes, of the regulations that were proposed by the California Bureau of Cannabis Control during the 2018 rulemaking process and evaluated in Sumner et al. (2018). The leftmost column shows the estimated costs per pound of a "lower-cost alternative" package of regulations that weakens some of the security standards, and the rightmost column of Table 13.3 shows the estimated costs per pound of a "higher-security alternative" package that imposes stricter security standards.

Table 13.3 Estimated compliance costs per pound of alternative regulatory packages, California

	Lower-Cost Alternative	*Regulations*	*Higher-Security Alternative*
License fees, distribution	$4	$4	$4
License fees, microbusiness and retail	$40	$40	$40
Distribution and transport compliance, including child-resistant packaging	$46	$48	$52
Retail-delivery-methods restrictions	None	$10	$148
Other retail compliance, including surveillance video archival, track-and-trace, and other retail regulations	$25	$49	$86
Testing compliance, including cost of licenses, pre-testing, testing and remediation, labeling, plus inventory lost due to testing samples and failed tests	$235	$257	$414
Hours of operation restrictions		Not calculated on a per-pound basis	
Total compliance costs per pound	**$350**	**$408**	**$744**

Source: Sumner et al. (2018).

Notes: Numbers were rounded to the nearest $1. Cost components do not add up exactly to total costs because of rounding.

As can be seen by comparing the proposed regulations and the higher-security alternative in Table 13.4, testing rules were a major lever of potential regulatory cost variation. As we discussed previously, the maximum batch size for testing exerts a strong effect on total testing costs per pound (see Valdes-Donoso, Sumner, and Goldstein 2019).

Taxation

California state taxation at a rate of $148 per pound (before 2020) and $154 per pound (since 2020) applies to cannabis as it moves from cultivator to distributor. This tax translates to about 10% of the wholesale value of high-priced indoor-grown cannabis and as high as 50% of the price of low-priced outdoor-grown cannabis (Cannabis Benchmarks Premium Reports 2015 to 2019). Additional cultivator license fees are applied by the state, and specific taxes and fees are applied on cultivators by many local jurisdictions. California's cannabis tax laws set no upper limit on the taxes that could be charged by counties or local municipalities. A state excise tax of 15% applies to the calculated retail value determined as 160% of the wholesale value charged to retail buyers by licensed distributors. Since this tax is applied on top of taxes and fees paid at earlier marketing stages, its impact is larger than 15%. As a final stage of cannabis taxation, most cannabis businesses are also responsible for paying local taxes, which vary by jurisdiction from 3% to 10%. (Some jurisdictions do not allow cannabis businesses at all.)

Beyond cannabis-specific taxes, licensed cannabis businesses must charge and pay ordinary state sales taxes, pay employment taxes and income taxes, and incur a variety of other costs of doing legal business in California that illegal cultivators, processors, distributors, and retailers of cannabis would not be expected to pay. Across the supply chain, taxation adds costs to legal cannabis but not to illegal cannabis.

Cannabis Retailers and Retail Prices Through the Stages of Regulation and Taxation

In this section, we observe some trends in retail price ranges and attrition of retailers in the California cannabis market that we collected and analyzed at the University of California, Davis.[1] This retail price data set covers a time period between 2016 and 2018, during which the state transitioned to mandatory state-level licensing, testing, regulation, and taxation.

Beginning in October 2016, researchers collected online retail price ranges of cannabis from counties around California. We collected the minimum and maximum listed prices for three products—1/8 oz cannabis flower, 1 oz cannabis flower, and 500 mg cannabis oil—for a total of six price data points from each retailer. Prices were collected from online menus posted by the retailers themselves on Weedmaps, a popular internet cannabis portal. We collected eight rounds of price data over the 21 months from October 2016 (before adult-use decriminalization) to July 2018 (after adult-use and medicinal regulation, taxation, and mandatory testing).

Attrition From Original Panel of 542 Retailers

We begin by making some broad observations about attrition from the original October 2016 panel of retailers with listings on Weedmaps. In October 2016, the first round, we collected price ranges from 542 retailers in seven representative counties around California (Butte, Fresno, Kern, Los Angeles, Sacramento, Santa Clara, and San Diego). In the aggregate, our seven representative counties cover about half of California's total population, and the seven counties' aggregate demographics (income, racial mix, etc.) approximate the demographics of California as a whole (Goldstein, Sumner, and Fafard 2019).

In January 2017, March 2017, and August 2017, we collected price ranges from all retailers out of the original 542 that remained active on Weedmaps in each round. By August 2018, 389 (72%) of the original 542 retailers were still active, and 152 retailers (28%) were no longer active. By November 2017, as the January 2018 deadline for mandatory licensing, taxation, and regulation approached, we observed substantial attrition from the original October 2016 group of 542 retailers (with the number of retailers remaining falling to 169). On January 1, 2018, unlicensed retailers became illegal under state law (SB 94). In 2018, in addition to prices, we collected data on whether retailers had obtained temporary licenses to operate legally (Weedmaps listings include license numbers for licensed retailers, and we verified these with the official list of licenses published by the Bureau of Cannabis Control). On July 1, 2018, mandatory testing rules went into effect. We again observed substantial attrition from the original panel in the data collection period before the start of mandatory testing (May 2018). By July 2018, the number of active retailers on Weedmaps from the original October 2016 group had fallen to 74 (14% of the original 542), of which 61 were licensed and 13 were unlicensed.

Figure 13.1 shows attrition in each of the eight price data collection periods from the original panel of 542 retailers surveyed in October 2016. For the three periods in 2018, columns are split into licensed and unlicensed retailers remaining. For details on our methodology, see Goldstein, Sumner, and Fafard (2019).

Attrition rates varied substantially between counties, in part due to local laws, bans, and police crackdowns on locally noncompliant cannabis businesses in some counties and not others. The attrition shown in Figure 13.1 should not be interpreted strictly as a reflection of statewide attrition of cannabis businesses from the market. Other potential sources of bias include the possibility that some retailers removed listings from Weedmaps but continued to operate. But it is worth noting that we observed the greatest drops in the number of retailers remaining from the original group just before

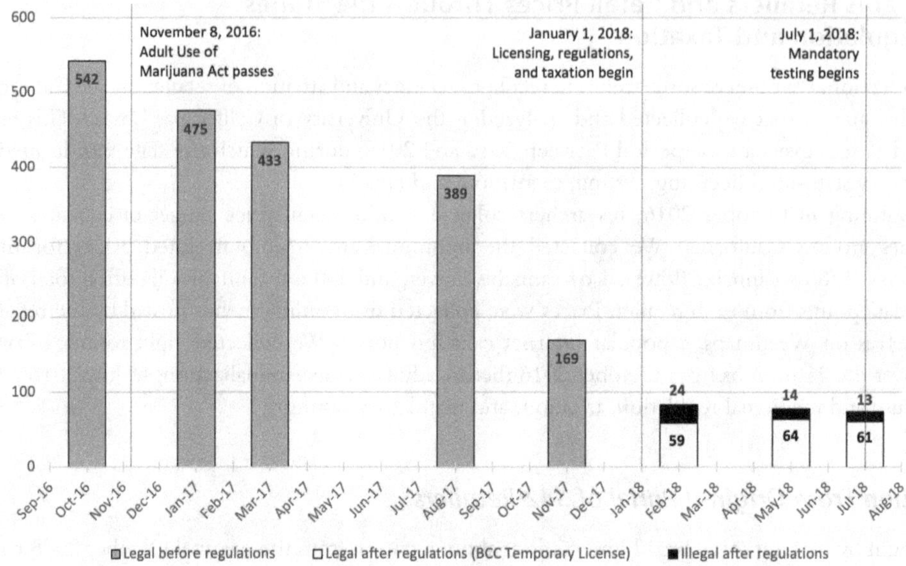

Figure 13.1 Number of retailers remaining in each data collection period from the original panel of 542 cannabis retailers in seven California counties listing prices on Weedmaps on 10/1/2016

the two most significant regulatory changes: the introduction of state and local regulations and taxes in January 2018, and the introduction of mandatory testing in July 2018.

Average Price Ranges

Figures 13.2, 13.3, and 13.4 report the average maximum and minimum (pre-tax) prices we observed in each of the three cannabis products in each of the eight rounds of price data collection. The price ranges shown are for 1 oz flower (Figure 13.2), 1/8 oz dried flower (Figure 13.3), and 500 mg oil cartridge (Figure 13.4). In order to observe differences in prices at licensed vs. unlicensed retailers, we also collected a quasi-random sample of price ranges at unlicensed retailers in 20 California counties for each of the three 2018 periods. These are shown as dotted lines in Figures 13.2, 13.3, and 13.4.

Average price ranges shown in Figures 13.2, 13.3, and 13.4 reflect the original panel of 542 retailers, with attrition, from October 2016 to August 2017. Because of the high attrition from the original panel, we supplemented the panel data by collecting a much larger set of price data from all counties in California, including retailers that had joined Weedmaps after October 2016. In November 2017, we collected price ranges from the full set of 2,521 retailers listed on Weedmaps in all of California. Beginning in November 2017, we also supplemented Weedmaps prices with prices from Leafly, a competing online cannabis portal. We found no statistically significant differences in price averages on Weedmaps vs. Leafly (Goldstein, Sumner, and Fafard 2019). For the three rounds in 2018, we collected price ranges from all *licensed* retailers in California listing prices on Weedmaps (176 retailers in February 2018, 288 in May 2018, and 270 in July 2018). In Figures 13.2, 13.3, and 13.4, price range changes in November 2017 and February 2018 should be interpreted with extreme caution in light of the bias generated by these changes to our data collection methodology.

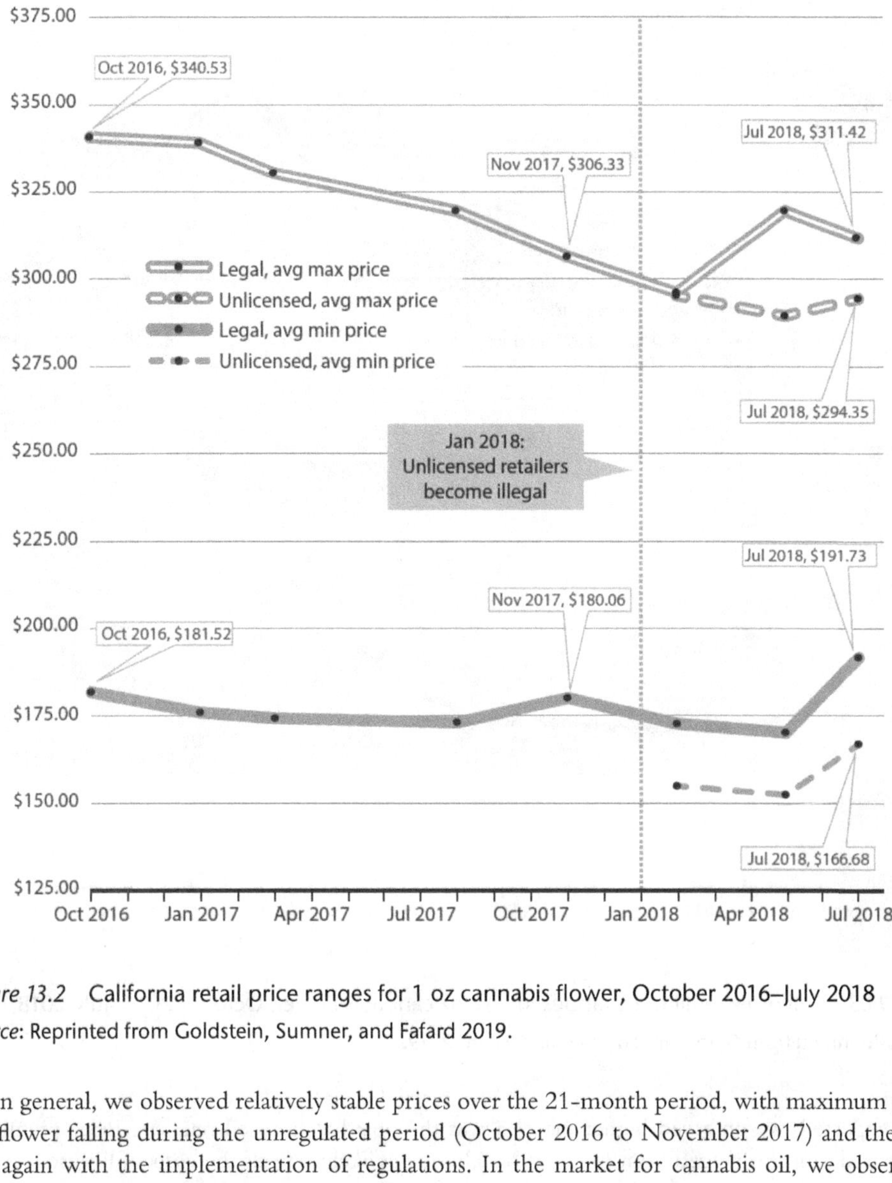

Figure 13.2 California retail price ranges for 1 oz cannabis flower, October 2016–July 2018
Source: Reprinted from Goldstein, Sumner, and Fafard 2019.

In general, we observed relatively stable prices over the 21-month period, with maximum prices for flower falling during the unregulated period (October 2016 to November 2017) and then rising again with the implementation of regulations. In the market for cannabis oil, we observed a substantial (33%) increase in maximum prices for 500 mg cartridges between November 2017 and July 2018, from an average of about $41 per cartridge to an average of about $54 per cartridge. Minimum prices, however, remained relatively stable, with the exception of increases across the board after mandatory testing began in July 2018, which is consistent with a natural response to the higher costs of testing and producing cannabis that is compliant with testing rules.

Licensed vs. Unlicensed Price Ranges

Comparisons of average price ranges at licensed vs. unlicensed retailers in February, May, and July 2018 are shown in Table 13.4.

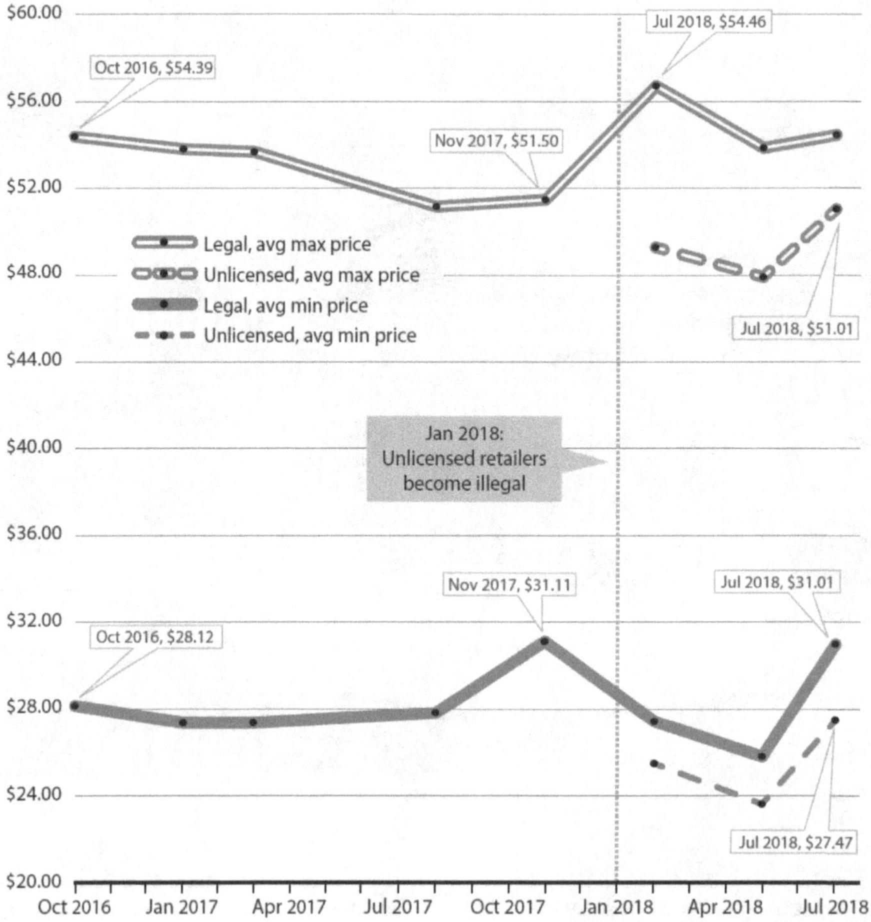

Figure 13.3 California retail price ranges for 1/8 oz cannabis flower, October 2016–July 2018

Source: Reprinted from Goldstein, Sumner, and Fafard 2019.

As expected, we observed higher prices across the board at licensed retailers. Price premiums for licensed cannabis ranged from 6% to 19%. This effect likely reflects the costs of license fees and higher regulatory and tax costs for licensed cannabis retailers.

Discussion

Before legalization and regulation, California had a decriminalized but unregulated network of medicinal cannabis retailers that were operating by their own sets of rules, largely by convention. With the introduction and refinement of legislation to regulate and tax the cannabis industry, beginning in 2015, continuing through the passage of Proposition 64 (adult-use legalization, beginning with immediate decriminalization), and culminating with the propagation of full cannabis regulations that took effect in 2018, California set up a new structure and in many ways created a new industry, as opposed to adapting an existing one to a slightly different set of rules.

Table 13.4 Legal vs. unlicensed California retail cannabis price differences, all counties, February 2018–July 2018

			Dried Flower, Average Prices			*Oil Cartridge, Average Prices*	
Data collection period	Retailers	1/8 oz min	1/8 oz max	1 oz min	1 oz max	0.5g min	0.5g max
February 2018							
Licensed[1]	176	$27.44	$56.72	$184.15	$344.59	$30.33	$49.01
Unlicensed[2]	88	$25.51	$49.25	$154.76	$295.11	$28.58	$41.78
License premium[3]		7.6%	15.2%	19.0%	16.8%	6.1%	17.3%
May 2018							
Licensed[1]	289	$25.83	$53.83	$169.90	$319.44	$31.01	$49.09
Unlicensed[2]	93	$23.61	$47.90	$152.22	$289.11	$27.60	$43.19
License premium[3]		9.4%	12.4%	11.6%	10.5%	8.5%	13.0%
July 2018							
Licensed[1]	270	$31.01	$54.46	$191.73	$311.42	$31.80	$54.07
Unlicensed[2]	89	$27.47	$51.01	$166.68	$294.35	$29.69	$44.90
License premium[3]		12.9%	6.8%	15.0%	5.8%	7.1%	13.7%

Source: Retail price data collected by researchers from Weedmaps. Table reprinted from Goldstein, Sumner, and Fafard (2019).

1 Prices listed by retailers active in each data collection round that had obtained temporary licenses from the Bureau of Cannabis Control to operate legally at the time of the data collection round.

2 Prices from a representative sample of unlicensed retailers in 20 counties around California (Alameda, Contra Costa, Los Angeles, Marin, Mendocino, Orange, Riverside, Sacramento, Santa Clara, San Bernardino, San Diego, San Francisco, San Luis Obispo, Santa Cruz, Shasta, Solano, Sonoma, Stanislaus, Tulare, and Yolo). The 20-county unlicensed sample was collected by arbitrarily selecting several retailers that appeared in the first page of Weedmaps search results from each of these counties, in approximate proportion to their relative populations. We collected the 20-county unlicensed sample separately for the purposes of this comparison, and only in the three 2018 data collection rounds. The 20-county unlicensed sample aims to be representative of the whole state, and is unrelated to the original October 2016 sample with attrition or the seven-county sample shown in Tables 13.2 and 13.3. Differences between licensed and unlicensed prices in the original October 2016 sample, with attrition, are also shown in Table 13.3; however, because of unequal attrition in the seven original counties, licensed-unlicensed differences in Table 13.3 are more likely to be biased. We thus calculate percentage license premiums only in Table 13.4.

3 Calculated as (licensed – unlicensed) / unlicensed.

At the end of 2017, preexisting medicinal cannabis retailers had to choose between one of three options: first, entering the new legal system, engaging with the licensing process on both the local and state levels, and following all the new regulations; second, going underground as illegal sellers; or third, exiting the cannabis business entirely.

Meanwhile, longtime cannabis-consuming customers of the pre-existing medicinal retailers faced a binary choice in January 2018: to continue buying from their preferred outlet, thus migrating from the legal to the illegal market; or, instead, to take their business to a new retailer in the legal system, where the customer might not be known by name or get the products the customer was used to buying. Since adult-use decriminalization in November 2016, California consumers have faced no penalties for buying from an illegal seller. California consumers have no *punitive* incentive to buy from a licensed retailer. However, as we mentioned earlier, some consumers are likely to *prefer* legal cannabis to illegal, all other things being equal, because of the perception that it is safer or more effective.

The 33% increase in maximum prices for cartridges between November 2017 and July 2018 reflects an increase in what was already the most expensive product category as measured by price per gram of pure THC equivalent (Sumner, Goldstein, and Matthews 2018). This effect may have been generated in part by increasing prices for existing products and in part by the introduction of

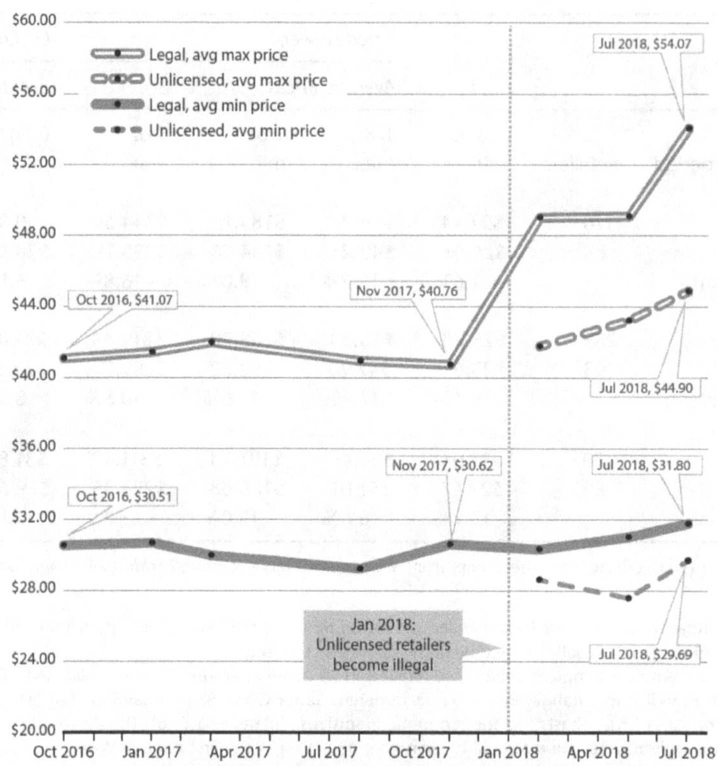

Figure 13.4 California retail price ranges for 500 mg cannabis oil cartridges, October 2016–July 2018
Source: Reprinted from Goldstein, Sumner, and Fafard 2019.

new higher-end cartridge products introduced at higher price points than legacy products. The legal market may provide a fertile ground for the growth of a new high-end segment that did not exist in the pre-regulatory environment, perhaps catering to an older and wealthier audience of consumers that might not have participated in the medicinal market.

Nonetheless, in 2018, California's first year of licensing, taxation, and regulation, cannabis tax revenues were below many of the projections from the state government and outside analysts. The smaller-than-expected legal market for cannabis in California in 2018 might be attributable to consumer substitution of illegal cannabis for legal cannabis given the costs of regulations, and an overall compounded tax rate in the neighborhood of 40% on legal cannabis (including cultivation, excise, sales, and local cannabis taxes).

Some of the market challenges in California's first year of full legalization probably resulted from fleeting short-term effects. For instance, a larger-than-usual cannabis supply might have ended up in the illegal market after a "grandfather clause" exempting preexisting cannabis inventory from testing standards expired in July 2018. This effect might even have drawn new consumers into the illegal market just as the legal market was getting off its feet. We note that two of the first three U.S. states to legalize cannabis—Colorado and Oregon—eventually cut state cannabis taxes. The Tax Foundation reports, "Colorado concluded with strong evidence that its 30 percent tax rate did not sufficiently reduce the black market" (Scarboro 2017).

The potential market impacts of taxes and regulations suggests that policy makers could benefit from economic evidence and careful analysis of substitution between legal and illegal cannabis. The impacts of illegal cannabis markets are hard to measure and incorporate into practical policy analysis, but state policy makers who understand the potential resilience of illegal markets would be better equipped to face challenges presented by the legalization of cannabis.

The biggest obstacle on the road to understanding substitution between legal and illegal markets at the different stages of regulation is the lack of reliable price and quantity data from the illegal cannabis marketplace. We hope that data on illegal prices and quantities may soon emerge, in whatever form, to help economists better observe the impacts of regulations and taxes on the legal and illegal markets.

Note

1 The research we discuss was partially funded by the California Bureau of Cannabis Control.

References

Ammerman, S., S. Ryan, and W. P. Adelman. 2015. "The Impact of Marijuana Policies on Youth: Clinical, Research, and Legal Update." *Pediatrics* 135 (3).

Bennett, E. A. 2018. "Extending Ethical Consumerism Theory to Semi-Legal Sectors: Insights from Recreational Cannabis." *Agriculture and Human Values* 35 (2): 295–317.

Brown, J. 2008. *Guidelines for Security and Non-Diversion of Marijuana Grown for Medical Use.* Memo from California Attorney General Jerry Brown (the "Brown Guidelines").

Budman, K. B. 1977. *A First Report on the Impact of California's New Marijuana Law* (SB 95). Sacramento: California State Office of Narcotics and Drug Abuse.

Cannabis Benchmarks Premium Reports. 2015 to 2019. https://reports.cannabisbenchmarks.com/.

Choo, E. K., M. Benz, N. Zaller, O. Warren, K. L. Rising, and K. J. McConnell. 2014. "The Impact of State Medical Marijuana Legislation on Adolescent Marijuana Use." *Journal of Adolescent Health* 55 (2): 160–66.

Diep, F. 2015. "The Science of Decriminalizing Drugs." *Popular Science.* www.popsci.com/science-decriminalize-legalize-drugs-marijuana-weed.

Downs, D., B. Barcott, and F. Corva. 2019. "Special Report: Debunking Dispensary Myths." *Leafly Literature Review.* http://leafly.com.

Goldstein, R., D. Sumner, and A. Fafard. 2019. "Retail Cannabis Prices in California Through the Stages of Legalization, Regulation, and Taxation." *California Agriculture* 73 (3–4): 136–45.

Lynne-Landsman, S. D., M. D. Livingston, and A. C. Wagenaar. 2013. "Effects of State Medical Marijuana Laws on Adolescent Marijuana Use." *American Journal of Public Health* 103 (8): 1500–6.

MacCoun, R., and P. Reuter. 2001. "Evaluating Alternative Cannabis Regimes." *British Journal of Psychiatry* 178 (2): 123–28.

Pacula, R. L., and R. Smart. 2017. "Medical Marijuana and Marijuana Legalization." *Annual Review of Clinical Psychology* 13: 397–419.

RAND. 2009. "Drug Policy Research Center (DPRC) Insights." www.rand.org/well-being/justice-policy/centers/dprc/newsletter/2009/12.html.

Scarboro, M. 2017. "How High Are Marijuana Taxes in Your State?" *The Tax Foundation.* https://taxfoundation.org/marijuana-taxes-state/.

Sumner, D. A., R. Goldstein, W. Matthews and O. Sambucci. 2020. "Cannabis in California." Chapter 13 in *California Agriculture: Dimensions and Issues*, 2nd Ed. P. L. Martin, R. E. Goodhue, and B. D. Wright, Eds. Giannini Foundation Information Series 20–01: 281–300. https://giannini.ucop.edu/publications/cal-ag-book/.

Sumner, D., R. Goldstein, W. Matthews, Y. Pan, H. Lee, and J. Lapsley. 2018. "Standardized Regulatory Impact Analysis, Medicinal and Adult-Use Cannnabis Regulation and Safety Act, Including Appendix." *Prepared for the California Bureau of Cannabis Control by the University of California Agricultural Issues Center and submitted to the California Department of Finance.* www.dof.ca.gov/Forecasting/Economics/Major_Regulations/Major_Regulations_Table/documents/DCA_Cannabis_SRIA_2018.pdf.

Valdes-Donoso, P., D. Sumner, and R. Goldstein. (2020). "Costs of Cannabis Testing Compliance: Assessing Mandatory Testing in the California Cannabis Market." *PLoS One* 15 (4): e0232041.

14

The Cannabis Enigma

Navigating the Inequitable Tax, Banking, and Insurance Milieu in the United States

Joshua Zender

Keywords: Cannabis, taxation, banking, accounting, insurance

Introduction

The purpose of this chapter is to expose scholars to key restraints imposed upon the cannabis sector. In this discussion, the cannabis industry is narrowly defined as state licensed legal cultivators, producers, manufacturers, distributors, and retailers of recreational cannabis. While many of the points raised may also apply to medicinal and industrial hemp activities, this segment of the industry is not the focus of the chapter. With an interdisciplinary perspective in mind, this content will be especially relevant to business, legal, economic, and public policy scholars. Three essential research questions are explored:

- Do existing tax policies unfairly target the cannabis sector?
- Does the sector have equal access to banking products and services?
- Is the industry subject to excessive indirect costs associated with doing business?

This work identifies the obstacles that currently limit cannabis entrepreneurs across the country. The first part of the chapter explores specific examples of inequitable tax treatment of cannabis-related business activities in the United States. The discussion is expanded to include the spillover effect of such policies within the financial services sector and how these practices have further stigmatized the industry when seeking business insurance, as well as other critical support services. These research findings are significant in that high taxes, inequitable banking access, and other onerous indirect costs may lead to unintended and undesirable policy outcomes (Jensen and Roussell 2016, 98–99). For instance, existing economic policies may lead to higher rates of noncompliance with respect to business licensing and highlights how a new policy approach can be persuasively justified (Doussard 2019, 83–90). The chapter closes by postulating that the easing of restrictions imposed at a federal level will promote market development. Recent legislative initiatives show great promise for shaping a more equitable and accessible cannabis marketplace for stakeholders. An appreciation

 DOI: 10.4324/9780429320491-14

for this complex tax and regulatory landscape will help one navigate future business, economic, or tax policy research in this field.

The Political Economy of Cannabis Taxation

At the time of this publication, 90% of U.S. states had legalized medical use of cannabidiol (CBD), over half of states permitted medicinal marijuana use, and one-fourth of states allowed adults to use cannabis on a recreational basis. In essence, over three-fourths of Americans now live in states where some form of cannabis commerce is permitted (National Cannabis Industry Association 2020). Furthermore, the policy landscape is quickly evolving towards greater acceptance of the substance. Dadayan notes the number of states expected to decriminalize cannabis production and consumption is only expected to grow (2019, 748). Despite states demonstrating widespread tolerance of cannabis, existing taxation policies remain punitive and have severely constrained this burgeoning market. As the cannabis marketplace is expected to grow to $25 billion or higher by 2025 (Song 2018), establishing a fair and equitable taxation system of the industry is paramount. In many respects, the failure to adapt to the changing times is incentivizing many businesses and consumers to continue to participate in the illicit market (Dadayan 2019, 748). Further, existing tax laws and related fiscal regulations are likely leading to a suboptimal level of tax revenue collection at all levels of government in that a substantial amount of unlicensed cannabis continues to penetrate the marketplace (Sambucci, Sumner and Goldstein 2020, 1–62).

Given U.S. Congress' leading role in designing tax systems and ability to influence tax policy afforded under the Commerce Clause, legal scholars argue the institution is in the best position to unravel the more convoluted aspects of the federal cannabis taxation system. However, divided government has resulted in a limited appetite to engage in such an undertaking in past years. With Democrates seizing control of both chambers of Congress and the White House in the election cycle of 2020, there was renewed optimism that cannabis reforms are forthcoming. With that said, the extent to which President Biden will support proposed policy changes remains in doubt at the time of this writing.

Meanwhile, there is far more certainty surrounding tax policy at the state and local level. We know cannabis trade activities are subjected to multiple levels of taxation, including but not limited to income, property, permitting fees, sales, and excise taxes. Excise taxes serve the role of not only raising revenues, but also attempting to curb use of controlled substances. This practice is described by some as being Pigouvian as the tax seeks to recover costs to society that are not included in the normal market price of the substance. In essence, this is an attempt to recapture the negative externalities made to innocent bystanders. Oglesby explores another possibility of cannabis taxation: no tax at all. This could be accomplished through a public monopoly whereby all cannabis sales occur exclusively through state-owned stores and no production-based taxes are imposed elsewhere within the supply chain (2011, 53–54).

The fact that methods of applying cannabis excise taxes vary significantly from state to state highlights the various tax schema options available to policy makers under an entrepreneurial model. In California, as one example, cannabis is subject to excise tax surcharges at different stages of the supply chain, from harvest to the over-the-counter sale of the product at a retail establishment (Tax Guide for Cannabis Businesses, n.d., para. 4). For instance, assume a California retailer purchases two pounds of cannabis buds for sale in their retail storefront. Let's say an unrelated wholesale supplier charges $2,400 for the product and $600 in distribution fees. Additionally, the retailer intends to mark up the product by 30%. Under this scenario, the supplier is required to withhold $585 in excise taxes; in essence, 15% of the average market price of $3,900.

Similarly, Washington and Colorado, like California, impose a multitiered sales tax (Vaida 2015, 762). In Alaska, marijuana is taxed based on production weight (Vaida 2015, 764). With so many different methods of taxation being applied, cannabis has become the "most ubiquitous form of drug taxation in the United States" (Vaida 2015, 766). Table 14.1 from the Tax Foundation reflects a sample of state recreational cannabis sales and excise tax rates by largest regional markets in the United States.

How did the tax code evolve around this substance? The precedent to tax cannabis was officially established on October 1, 1937, with the enactment of the Marihuana Tax Act. The measure was the first national effort to criminalize individual possession and sale of marijuana for private citizens. Ironically, medicinal use of marijuana and the import of industrial hemp would remain legal; however, the 1937 Act created a costly taxation system that significantly curbed the size of the overall cannabis market. For instance, the law imposed a special occupational excise tax of $1 per ounce on registered dealers and a transfer tax of $100 per ounce for any unregistered dealer transaction (Marihuana Tax Act 1937, Sec. 7). The 1937 Act would eventually be overturned by the Supreme Court in 1969 on the grounds that private citizens would have to "self-incriminate" in order to comply with the law enforcement inspections, thereby violating the Fifth Amendment of the constitution (Leary vs. US 1969). Nonetheless, Congress quickly acted to close the gap in cannabis regulation by passing the Controlled Substances Act (CSA) Title II in 1970 that introduced strict controls on marijuana cultivation, possession, and distribution (Dadayan 2019, 745–47).

While the revised CSA of 1970 that regulated hallucinogens and other pharmaceuticals served as the federal "re-prohibition" of domestic cannabis use, federal tax policy would be leveraged to severely limit supply. One form of discrimination against the industry manifests itself in the definition of gross income established through the primary federal tax authorities. Official sources of the tax law are created through statutory authority of the Congress, judicial precedent set by U.S. tax courts and courts of appeals, and Treasury and Internal Revenue Service (IRS) pronouncements. In the case of all business sales, the Internal Revenue Code (IRC) defines "gross income as all income from whatever source derived."[1] Under the court precedent established prior to the enactment of the CSA of 1970, monies derived from the cultivation or distribution of cannabis are not considered excluded income sources (James 1961). For all practical purposes, this means that all income, regardless of being derived from the sale of legal or illegal substances, is subject to federal income tax. Despite uniformly assessing income tax, a series of court cases have established a precedent of precluding the cannabis industry from business deductions related to "all ordinary and necessary business expenses" traditionally utilized to reduce business income tax burdens[2] (CHAMP 2007).

Remarkably, discriminatory tax policies were not always present in the tax code system. In 1981, the Tax Court allowed an illegal business to recover the cost of controlled substances and deduct certain business expenses like a traditional business could. Under this precedent, a street-level drug dealer was permitted to deduct various costs, such as telephone costs, transportation, etc., associated with their illegal enterprise (Edmondson 1981). Congress was not happy with this ruling, and

Table 14.1 Cannabis sales and excise tax rates

State	*Tax Rates*
Alaska	$50/oz
California	15% excise tax; $9.25/oz flowers; $2.75/oz leaves
Colorado	15% excise tax; 15% sales tax
Massachusetts	10.75% excise tax
Nevada	15% excise tax; 10% sales tax
Oregon	17% sales tax
Washington	37% sales tax

Source: Cammenga (2019)

within one year action was undertaken to close a perceived loophole by reversing the precedent established under the Edmondson. In 1982, Congress updated the tax code to include a provision, known as IRC 280E, that would not allow individuals to deduct business expenses related to the sale of controlled substances[3]; however, the measure did not explicitly exclude cost of goods sold (COGS) or inventory costs. While Congress enacted IRC Section 263A in 1986, greater clarity was offered around what constituted "allowable" inventory costs as direct costs of property purchased or produced and the proper share of indirect costs allocable in whole or part to that property (US Tax Code, 26 U.S.C. §263A(a)(2)). When technical corrections were made to IRC Section 263A about specific nondeductible costs, Congress remained silent about excluding IRC section 280E costs. Although cannabis was not specifically contemplated at the time, these "bright line standards" would be applied in future years to establish judicial standard.

The *Olive* case (2012), as one example, established official precedent that while other business deductions were exempt, an adjustment for COGS would be permitted. In this case, the court upheld the decision that the taxpayer may deduct cost of goods sold for business, noting in footnote 2, "COGS is subtracted from gross receipts in determining taxpayer's gross income." Ultimately, the final ruling tilted in the IRS's favor as the court found the taxpayer, Vaper Room Herbal, had failed to substantiate allowable costs. The Rupp (2012) precedent would further operationalize the standard by offering nine factors for determining the appropriate eligibility of deductible expenses and establishing that business activities must be separated.[4]

Tax court rulings have effectively established a precedent that cannabis-related businesses are permitted to deduct costs directly used in the cultivation or manufacturing process, as well as partially deduct indirect production costs, but not other common costs associated with running a business. In other words, product cost items, also known as cost of goods sold, can be adjusted from gross income; but most selling, administrative, investing, and financing expenses cannot be deducted.[5] In the case of a retail business, a cannabis-related storefront can charge off the cost of the purchase of merchandise, transportation costs to bring the product into inventory, and a portion of other necessary service charges incurred in acquiring the goods, but cannot deduct general overhead like most other traditional businesses can.[6] This discriminatory taxation practice, a holdover from keeping CSA Schedule I substances like cannabis intact, has led some involved in the cannabis trade to circumvent paying federal income tax by avoiding the proper licensure process altogether (ABA 2019, 4–5).

Tax Preferences and Business Structure Considerations

Outside of IRC 280E, cannabis operations can be singled out within the tax code system through other less visible means. For instance, when Congress introduced the new Opportunity Zone tax incentive established in 2017 that sought to focus capital investments within underserved communities, specific organizations were excluded. Businesses that engaged in vices, such as horseracing and gambling facilities, were ineligible to take advantage of the tax credit (Internal Revenue Service "Opportunity Zones," 2020b). Although cannabis businesses were not specifically excluded, President Trump's treasury secretary, Stephen Mnuchin, opined that he did not think cannabis businesses should receive these benefits because of disparate federal and state laws (Blake 2019). As interpretations made by public officials in effect become administrative rules, this action has led most tax professionals to generally advise their clients to avoid utilizing this benefit when establishing a tax position.

In 2019, the Treasury also denied the tax-exempt status of an organization that provided financial assistance to medical cannabis patients. Even though the organization did not "touch" the plant or reimburse patients directly for the cost of their medicine, the Treasury opined, "the organization advocated for and engaged in activities that contravene federal law by assisting persons engaged in illegal activities" (Mill 2019). Thus, the precedent of excluding cannabis operators from economic tax incentives had been established.

One key factor that can affect tax burden is the choice of business form, such as sole proprietorship, partnership, or corporation. When business owners initially set up their enterprise, business structures are dictated by a number of different factors, including but not limited to the number of owners, concern for limiting personal liability, extent to which owners wish to freely control business management activities, tolerance for paying organizational filing costs, and need to raise outside capital. In essence, differences in the formalities of these entities establishes the legal rights and responsibilities bestowed on the owner of the enterprise. In the next section, a brief outline of the pros and cons of various business structures from a tax and a non-tax perspective will be explored.

As an emerging industry consisting of largely small to medium enterprises, most cannabis organizations are sole proprietors, partnerships, or S corporations. According to IRS Number of Returns by Business Form (2013) data, over 72% of all business tax filers are classified as sole proprietorships, making it the most likely business structure for a cannabis entrepreneur to initially set up. Under this business structure, owners face unlimited liability. In essence, if business debts are not paid, creditors are likely to seize personal assets of the business owner, such as their residential home and vehicles. Although easy and cheap to set up, this form of business would not be ideal for a cannabis entrepreneur who seeks to limit personal liability. By the very nature of this business form, the owner is unable to raise equity from outside investors.

As evidenced by state licensing data, cannabis businesses are far more likely to be formed as a state-authorized partnership or corporation. Partnerships, as a general rule, offer business owners greater personal liability protections in the event of ordinary negligence. Unlike the sole proprietorship model, this business form offers an ability to cultivate equity from multiple parties. Further, the model offers attractive pass-through tax benefits in that partnership income is taxed only once based on the owner's tax basis. This represents the carrying value at a given point in time, measured as the initial tax basis (cost plus capital improvements less depreciation and amortization). However, entrepreneurs wishing to raise money from any prospective investor will likely lean towards a corporate business structure. In fact, 13% of business tax filers across all industries utilize the S corporation business model.[7]

Like a partnership, S-corps have the benefit of similar pass-through tax treatment. This business model is ideal for cannabis cultivators and manufacturers because the activity is not subject to "double taxation." This term describes the tax reality of C corps, which are subject to two layers of taxation: a tax on corporate business income and a tax at the individual level based on the amount of the dividend distribution to respective investors. While S corporations offer some limitations of personal liability, the extent of limited liability can be deceptive because

> bankers and other creditors often want assurance that the debts are secured by personally guaranteeing loans (e.g., securitizing the loan with their homes, cars or other personal assets) . . . therefore, shareholders of closely held corporations often have only partial limited personal liability.
>
> *(Murphy and Higgins 2020, 13–7)*

The most profitable businesses within the United States, such as Fortune 500 companies, are C corporations. These are legal enterprises in which the owners are taxed separately from the entity. As a separate statutory entity, a C corporation can enter into contracts in its own name, own property, and be sued. Once an entity incorporates, this gives the unit a separate legal identity (aka "corporate personhood") that has attributes of limited liability, unlimited life, free transferability of ownership, and centralized management. These entities often are ideal as "multistate" operations given their general administrative capacity. Given the ability to secure higher amounts of capital under the provisions of state law, C corps are an ideal business form for cannabis retailers who may seek to franchise their operations. The major disadvantage of this business structure is the costs associated with incorporating and the fact the corporation is subject to double taxation. In essence, business owners must pay a special corporate income tax rate and are also taxed on dividend distributions at an individual level (this phenomenon is described as "double taxation"). Despite this disadvantage, most large cannabis businesses will elect to incorporate if they seek the ability to raise capital from outside investors (Roberts and Daar 2020, para 5).

> As the cannabis industry keeps pushing forward, more companies are moving to list their stock on a major U.S. exchange like the NYSE or NASDAQ as C-corps. However, the club remains relatively small . . . fewer than 25 companies at the beginning of 2020.
>
> *(Benzinga Cannabis 2020)*

Depending on the corporate form a cannabis entrepreneur elects to undertake, this can have a significant impact on their overall tax liability. For instance, the Tax Cuts and Jobs Act of 2017 established a new lower income rate of 21% for C corporations or publicly traded enterprises. In an effort to benefit privately held companies, Congress also established a Section 199A tax relief provision to promote more tax fairness for S corps, partnerships, and other pass-through business structures that would otherwise be subject to a 29.6% business income tax rate. The Section 199A deduction is taken on the owner's personal income tax return rather than on the entity's tax return. Section 199A effectively allows a portion of the cannabis-owner deduction to be increased because 280E increases the QBI (qualified business income); thus, the 20% deduction (Internal Revenue Service "QBI," 2020c). This provision of the tax code enables pass-through enterprises to take advantage of a generous tax deduction.

Unequal Banking Rights

Access to conventional banking solutions is essential to any liquid and efficiently run business enterprise. Unlike any other industries, the cannabis sector is largely excluded from these financial services due to the federal prohibition discussed previously. Banks and credit unions alike are hesitant to serve the industry as they fear sanctions, such as losing access to Federal Deposit Insurance Corporation (FDIC) or National Credit Union Administration (NCUA) insurance. These two programs offer federally backed insurance up to $250,000 per depositor, per insured bank, for each account of ownership category. Non-cannabis business owners would be unlikely to do business with a bank unable to offer this form of insurance. Just as cannabis entrepreneurs are vulnerable to conflicting state and federal laws, financial institutions lack any form of protection from prosecution of state-sanctioned cannabis organizations they might serve. As evidenced by the FDIC/NCUA insurance limitations, existing laws encourage financial institutions to be risk averse, and consequently the vast majority of banks are not accepting cannabis clients (Crabb 2019, 1–4). In fact, more than 99% of all U.S. financial institutions view such dealings to be taboo and are unwilling to establish banking relationships with the industry (Webster 2018, 38). In many respects, we see the intersection between the federal prohibition and existing cultural stigmas as demonstrated by a reluctance of the banking sector to service the industry.

Further complicating matters is the fact the Financial Crimes Enforcement Network (FinCEN), a unit of the U.S. Treasury established to analyze financial transactions for fraud, has issued guidance discouraging financial institutions from serving the cannabis industry (Sparks 2018, 41–42). The bureau periodically issues guidance to clarify issues related to FinCEN regulations 31 CFR Chapter X. While some FinCEN guidance is reasonable in nature and important for detecting fraud and money laundering, many best practices unfairly target the cannabis sector. For instance, the rapid movement of funds, increased participation of third-party suppliers, and significant outside investment activities are all identified as red flags according to FinCEN guidance (Suspicious Activity Report 2012). In most business schools, students are taught such signs to be leading indicators of healthy business activity. As such, a traditional business would likely be rewarded with access to a wider suite of banking services if these trends were to persist. However, in the cannabis sector, such activity is likely to jeopardize an otherwise positive banking relationship between the bank and the client.

FinCEN guidelines and related banking laws also create costly barriers for financial institutions electing to serve the cannabis industry. For example, the Money Laundering Control Act of 1986 prohibits transacting funds originating from specified unlawful activity. The Bank Secrecy Act of 1970 requires financial institutions to assist U.S. government agencies, such as the FBI, in detecting and preventing money laundering (Bank Secrecy Act 1970). Any person who deposits more than $10,000 in cash must be reported to the Treasury by the bank. In order to comply with these various laws, financial institutions incur significant compliance costs (Peterson 2019, 20). Cannabis clients are monitored regularly, even to the extent of social media account activity (Webster 2018, 38). Despite having a rapidly expanding industry with a plethora of investment opportunities in real estate, non-cannabis-related raw materials, equipment, hardware, and technology, many banks are electing to deny the cannabis industry access to the basic financial solutions that ordinary businesses are allowed to utilize due to the risk and cost burden (Dullum 2019, 17). For instance, access to basic checking account services, electronic fund transfers, credit card services, and basic business loans are severely restricted within the cannabis sector.

Availability of credit represents another essential feature of any healthy business. For many small to medium-sized enterprises (SMEs), Small Business Administration (SBA) lending represents an important source of loan financing. The value of having access to this market became most evident in 2020 when the global coronavirus pandemic wreaked havoc on economic activity. During the crisis, C corporations generally maintained sufficient liquidity levels to continue operations, whereas many SMEs were forced to temporarily or permanently close. Unemployment levels soared while many businesses deemed "nonessential" were forced to temporarily close their doors. Although most state jurisdictions allowed medical cannabis dispensaries to remain open as essential businesses (Glasser, Regne, and Emanuelson 2020), the industry was nonetheless deemed ineligible to apply for SBA emergency funding provisions afforded under the $2 trillion Coronavirus Aid, Relief and Economic Security (CARES) Act and subsequent stimulus bills. Notable small business relief provisions under CARES included the Paycheck Protection Plan (PPP) designed to provide cash-flow assistance for employers to maintain payroll through a loan with no fees, requiring no collateral, and a six-month deferral on loan payments. An attractive provision of the relief program was debt forgiveness for business that maintained payroll (in essence, converting the terms from a loan to a government grant). CARES also provided Emergency Economic Injury Grants and Loans up to $2 million to help small businesses weather the crisis (S.3548 "CARES Act" 2020). Despite the cannabis industry being particularly vulnerable to COVID-19 transmissions given the labor-intensive nature of the work and the fact that employees are only allowed to engage in cash-only transactions, existing banking laws and regulations left the industry with limited emergency relief provisions that were otherwise made available to most other small businesses impacted by the crisis. This is an acute example of limiting normal payroll protections and other emergency short financing afforded to other industries.

Other Excess Indirect Costs Levied on Cannabis Operations

Given limited resources to enforce all violations under federal law, the U.S. Department of Justice has prioritized enforcement activities, such as preventing access to cannabis by minors, curbing criminal and gang-related activities, and restricting interstate trade of the substance, to name a few federal priorities regardless of state laws (Cole 2013, para 3). Ultimately, the choice of a Department of Justice official to file charges against an individual or organization comes down to prosecutorial discretion.[8] These actions open the door to arbitrary administrative discretion, thereby creating a high degree of uncertainty among market participants. In essence, breeding a culture of fear for stakeholders participating in the cannabis sector.

Engaging a professional to navigate these legal complexities presents its own set of challenges. Legal and accounting professionals encounter ethical dilemmas when representing clients who are complying with state statute but violating federal law (Fucile 2015, 34–40). For instance, accountants are not granted the same confidential privileges as attorneys (Arthur Young 1984, para 27). In fact, accountants are granted very limited privilege regarding taxpayer communications with their return preparers under IRS rules.[9] As such, there is general reluctance within the accounting profession to serve cannabis clients (Brus 2018). In the absence of this professional support, the cannabis industry encounters challenges to complying with complex IRS regulations (Hood 2019, 2–3).

Outside of potentially high legal and accounting expenses resulting from a limited supply of experts willing to serve the industry (due to cultural stigma and legal liability), cannabis operators are also faced with overcoming other administrative hurdles. Without access to modern banking services, the industry is forced to operate almost exclusively on a cash basis. Cannabis organizations are unable to utilize emerging technologies, such as accounting software, that are often linked to banking databases. For example, a notable feature of QuickBooks accounting software is the ability to link the system to one's banking account, which expedites the otherwise tedious bank reconciliation process. Further, some organizations are forced to outsource administrative functions to third-party management holding companies, essentially promoting a "shell game" in that monies are passed through cannabis operators to seemingly unrelated professional service organizations through less than transparent means.

Given limited access to these services, cannabis enterprises must pay a premium for "work-around" solutions relating to on-boarding employees, workplace insurance, and payroll services. Work sites are often deemed to be less safe than traditional agricultural or manufacturing sites. As a consequence, a major cost of operation includes not only higher overhead associated with workplace accident prevention and litigation fees (roughly $200,000 per incident), but also the price of paying a risk mitigation premium for general business liability insurance (Elliot, Kersting, and Salver 2019, 19–25). In order to operate as a legitimate business and in some cases to comply with state licensing laws, cannabis operators are required to carry umbrella liability policy insurance with coverages exceeding one million dollars or more. However, many are reluctant to do so out of fear that confidential information obtained by insurance agencies may be retrieved by government officials (Sacirbey 2018, para 5–6).

Further, insurance companies often require cannabis operators to pay steeper rates for inferior insurance coverage, which some might describe as coverage that does not actually address anything that a business would need coverage for. Often, policy riders limit exposure for the insurance company deep within legal documents in a nontransparent manner. According to Bench (2020), examples of such limiting provisions specific to the cannabis industry include but are not limited to the policy not covering seeds, seedlings, vegetative plants, flowering plants, or harvested material that are not yet finished stock; failure to cover workers compensation for business owners and volunteers; and exclusions around nutraceutical substances, such as essential oils, and vaporizing devices. By identifying more risk factors, insurance companies can more easily justify charging higher rates from their cannabis clients (Bench 2020, para 10).

While much attention of this chapter has focused on excess costs imposed on cannabis operations, there are also adverse public externalities arising from the existing regulatory model. As one example, challenges are created for tax agents charged with auditing a cash-basis industry. When conducting tax audits, agents will seek to verify sources of all income, methods used to comply with IRC 280E, bookkeeping, recordkeeping, and accounting systems (Internal Revenue Service "Small Business Self-Employed Recordkeeping," 2019). In a traditional business, much of this information would be readily accessible using accounting software and bank ledgers; however, this is often not the case for a cannabis operation as they have been excluded from the banking sector. As a consequence, the tax agent must closely scrutinize the methods used to manage cash, access to cash, cash safeguards, etc., costing the government agency more time, energy, and labor costs when conducting a review or audit.

Movement Towards a New Future

Public choice theory promotes the idea that individuals seek to live in states and communities that are aligned with their own policy preferences. In order to promote healthy economies, our federalist system must offer flexibility to allow particular communities the space to adopt their own unique laws and tax structures. Eliminating conflicting economic and regulatory policy in many cases improves markets, and breaking down traditional bureaucratic controls can lead to innovations (Ostrom 1989, 42–48). Further, the promotion of open transactions represents an important check on bureaucratic control and abuse (Tullock 1965, 34–75) with the goal of ultimately improving overall market conditions (Weimer and Vining 2005, 185–186). Eliminating fraud and tax evasion would be a "win-win" for the industry and government alike. Based on the experience of other countries like Canada, such environments appear to not only promote business profitability, but also lead to desirable outcomes for society as a whole, such as higher government tax collection rates and ability to fund education, public health, and other important government services (Sen and Wyonch 2018, 1–23).

High tax rates and limited tax deductions for the cannabis industry, as well as significant barriers to forming partnerships with financial institutions, represent major obstacles to market development. Although current tax provisions, banking laws, and other industry rules have led to undesirable outcomes for the cannabis industry, recent initiatives within Congress signal future directions away from exclusionary policies. Multiple bills introduced in the Senate and House would normalize regulatory activities of the cannabis industry. For instance, bills alive at the time of this writing with cannabis-related reforms include H.R. 6800 The Heroes Act, H.R. 6602 Emergency Cannabis Small Business Health and Safety Act, H.R. 2843 Marijuana Freedom and Opportunity Act, and H.R. 3884 Marijuana Opportunity Reinvestment and Expungement Act. Reclassifying cannabis as a non-CSA Schedule I substance would result in the immediate eradication of the undesirable effects of IRC 280E, as well as banking and insurance restrictions that place the industry at a strategic disadvantage (Peckenpaugh 2019, 11).

Another important development for academic researchers to monitor will be the House Financial Services Committee–proposed Secure and Fair Enforcement Banking (SAFE) Act (or similar evolving laws), introduced at the time of this writing, which would exempt banks and credit unions from federal prosecution for providing services to state-authorized cannabis businesses. The SAFE Act H.R. 1595 and S. 1200 would prohibit federal regulators from terminating FDIC/NCUA deposit insurance. Under the proposed measure, banks would need to follow certain due diligence compliance and reporting requirements before accepting a cannabis client. Further, track and trace requirements focused on inventory recordkeeping and movement of cannabis and related products through the commercial supply chain would still apply. Nonetheless, the bill represents a more rational and measured approach to serving this population than under current law (H.R. 1595 2019). These actions, as well as recent passage of the 2018 Farm Bill that eased regulations on commercial hemp (as discussed in Chapter 18), represent a positive sign, as previous court rulings have clearly ruled that the aforementioned conflicts involving medicinal and recreational use of cannabis must be addressed by Congress, not the judiciary (Olive vs IRS 2012, 24).

Recommendations for Future Research

Although the federalization of cannabis regulation seems increasingly likely at some future period, states will continue to serve as policy laboratories for experimenting with cannabis-related economic and regulatory frameworks. Federal restrictions have been cited as a significant obstacle towards achieving a thriving cannabis market (Munoz 2014, 715–26). Until a fundamental shift in federal policy occurs, state-level research will remain ground zero for most economic impact research. Scholars may benefit from closely following legislative initiatives that seek to remove the cultural stigma that is currently tied to the industry by normalizing the taxation and other regulations imposed on the industry. In essence, can tax reforms bring more participants into the regulated cannabis market, as opposed to unregulated black markets, as modeled under public choice theory? As one example, if the Section 280E "ordinary and reasonable business expense" restriction is lifted, there will be an immediate demand for understanding the extent to which this tax policy change will impact both business profitability and government tax revenue raising capabilities. As present banking and insurance restrictions are gradually eased, a study of the effect of transactional efficiency and effectiveness will be warranted. Additional changes in federal law will encourage research evaluating the economic cost-benefit associated with such action. Individuals wishing to examine this topic in greater depth are encouraged to closely monitor tax court opinions, as well as Congressional tax code reforms, which are likely to be the first signs to telegraph a shifting political landscape.

Notes

1 United States Tax Code, 26 U.S.C. §61(a).
2 United States Tax Code, 26 U.S.C. §162(a).
3 United States Tax Code, 26 U.S.C. §280(e).
4 Nine factors include (1) Are undertakings conducted at the same place? (2) Are the undertakings part of a taxpayer's efforts to find sources of revenue from his or her land? (3) Were the undertakings formed as separate activities? (4) Did one undertaking benefit from the other? (5) Did the taxpayer use one undertaking to advertise the other? (6) To what extent did the undertakings share management? (7) To what degree did one caretaker oversee the assets of both undertakings? (8) Did the taxpayers use the same accountant for the undertakings? (9) To what degree did the undertakings share books and records?
5 IRM §1.471.11, citing the Internal Revenue Code.
6 IRM §1.471.3, citing the Internal Revenue Code.
7 IRS 2013c data indicates 5% of all business tax filers are incorporated.
8 United States v. Batchelder, 442 U.S. 114, 125 (1979). Paragraph 4.
9 IRM §1.7525.1, citing the Internal Revenue Code.

References

American Bankers Association. 2019. "The Public Benefits of Banking Cannabis Businesses." Accessed July 19, 2019. www.aba.com/advocacy/policy-analysis/public-benefits-banking-cannabis-businesses.

Arthur Young & Co v. United States. 1984. United States Supreme Court.

Bank Secrecy Act. 1970, 31 U.S.C. §5318(g).

Bench, Jonathan. 2020. "Anatomy of a Cannabis Insurance Policy: Exclusions." *Cannabis Business Executive*. Accessed March 3, 2020. www.cannabisbusinessexecutive.com/2020/02/anatomy-of-a-cannabis-insurance-policy-exclusions/?utm_source=CBE+Master+List&utm_campaign=de22314fc0-CBE+Policy+%26+Legal-Issue-160-Feb-13–2020-V2&utm_medium=email&utm_term=0_1f64189714-de22314fc0–264270197.

Benzinga Cannabis. 2020. "A Complete List of NYSE and NASDAQ-Listed Cannabis Companies." Accessed April 22, 2020. www.benzinga.com/markets/cannabis/20/04/12591805/a-complete-list-of-nyse-and-nasdaq-listed-cannabis-companies.

Blake, Andrew. 2019. "Treasury Secretary Declines to Weigh in on Conflict Between Federal, State Laws." *Washington Times*. Accessed 15, 2019. www.washingtontimes.com/news/2019/mar/15/treasury-unable-to-advise-on-marijuana-issues-unle/.

Brus, Brian. 2018. "Accountants Await Guidelines for Medical Marijuana." *Journal Record* 10: 1–3.

Cammenga, Janelle. 2019. "How High Are Taxes on Recreational Marijuana in Your State?" *Tax Foundation*. Accessed April 24, 2019. https://taxfoundation.org/2019-recreational-marijuana-taxes/.

CHAMP—Californians Helping to Alleviate Medical Problems, Inc. v. IRS Commissioner. 2007. United States Tax Court.

Cole, James. 2013. *Guidance Regarding Marijuana Enforcement*. Washington, DC: Department of Justice.

Crabb, John. 2019. "Lack of Regulatory Clarity in Hemp and Marijuana Industry Still Hindering Bankability." *International Financial Law Review* 11: 1–4.

Dadayan, Lucy. 2019. "States' Addiction to Sins: Sin Tax Fallacy." *Tax Journal* 72 (4): 723–54.

Doussard, Marc. 2019. "The Other Green Jobs: Legal Marijuana and the Promise of Consumption-Driven Economic Development." *Journal of Planning Education and Research* 39 (1): 79–92.

Dullum, Justin. 2019. "Bankers of Cannabis Industry Gain Tech Tool." *Northwestern Financial Review* 204 (5): 17–17.

Edmondson v. IRS Commissioner. 1981. United States Tax Court.

Elliott, Teressa, Lee Kersting, and Robert Salver. 2019. "The Legalization of Marijuana: Tax Issues and Costs to Employers." *Journal of Management Policy and Practice* 20 (1): 15–25.

Fucile, Mark. 2015. "The Intersection of Professional Duties and Federal Law as States Decriminalize Marijuana." *The Professional Lawyer* 25 (1): 34–40.

Glasser, Nathiel, Anatasia Regne, and Eric Emanuelson. 2020. "Medical Marijuana Deemed 'Essential' During COVID-19 Pandemic." *The National Law Review*. Accessed April 16, 2020. www.natlawreview.com/article/medical-marijuana-deemed-essential-during-covid-19-pandemic.

Hood, Daniel. 2019. "Cannabis: A Major New Opportunity for Accountants." *Accounting Today* 33 (1): 1–8.

H.R. 1595 — Secure and Fair Enforcement Banking Act of 2019, 116th Congress (2019–2020). www.congress.gov/bill/116th-congress/house-bill/1595/text.

Internal Revenue Service. 2019. "Small Business Self-Employed Recordkeeping." Accessed November 15, 2019. www.irs.gov/businesses/small-businesses-self-employed/recordkeeping.

———. 2020a. "Number of Returns, Total Receipts, Business Receipts, Net Income (Less Deficit), Net Income, and Deficit by Form of Business Tax Years 1980–2013." Internal Revenue Service. Accessed March 4, 2020. www.irs.gov/statistics/soi-tax-stats-integrated-business-data.

———. 2020b. "Opportunity Zones Frequently Asked Questions." Accessed January 14, 2020. www.irs.gov/newsroom/opportunity-zones-frequently-asked-questions.

———. 2020c. "Qualified Business Income Deduction." Accessed January 16, 2020. www.irs.gov/newsroom/qualified-business-income-deduction.

James v. United States. 1961. United States Supreme Court.

Jensen, Eric L., and Aaron Roussell. 2016. "Field Observations of the Developing Legal Recreational Cannabis Economy in Washington State." *International Journal of Drug Policy* 33: 96–101.

Leary v. United States. 1969. United States Supreme Court.

Mill, Karl. 2019. "Warning for Cannabis-Related Charities (And Others): IRS Applies Legality Doctrine in Denial 201917008." *Alder & Colvin*. Accessed May 1, 2019. www.adlercolvin.com/blog/2019/05/01/warning-for-cannabis-related-charities-and-others-irs-applies-legality-doctrine-in-denial-201917008/.

Money Laundering Control Act of 1986, 18 U.S.C. §§1956(a)(1) and 1957(a).

Munoz, Adam. 2014. "Blunt the Violence: How Legal Marijuana Regulation in the United States Can Help End the Cartel Violence in Mexico." *Seattle Journal for Social Justice* 13 (2): 691–729.

Murphy, Kevin, and Mark Higgins. 2020. *Concepts in Federal Taxation*. Boston, MA: Cengage.

Oglesby, Pat. 2011. "Laws to Tax Marijuana (How to Tax It)." *State Tax Notes* 59 (4): 1–56.

Olive v. IRS Commissioner. 2012. United States Tax Court.

Ostrom, Vincent. 1989. *The Intellectual Crisis in American Public Administration*. Tuscaloosa, AL: University of Alabama Press.

Peckenpaugh, Douglas. 2019. "Cannabis Banking Seeks Clarity." *Food Engineering* 2 (1): 10–11.
Peterson, Ann. 2019. "The Painstaking Work Behind Cannabis Banking." *Credit Union Magazine* 85 (2): 10–20.
National Cannabis Industry Association. 2020. "Resource Map: State by State Marijuana Policies." Accessed January 25, 2020. https://thecannabisindustry.org/ncia-news-resources/state-by-state-policies/.
Roberts, Scott, and Alexander Daar. 2020. "Cannabis Business: Selecting the Best Corporate Structure." *Scott Roberts Law (blog)*. Accessed March 4, 2020. https://scottrobertslaw.com/cannabis-business-selecting-the-best-corporate-structure/.
Rupp v. IRS Commissioner. 2012. United States Tax Court.
Schaffer Library of Drug Policy. "Marihuana Tax Act of 1937." Accessed March 2, 2020. www.druglibrary.org/schaffer/hemp/taxact/mjtaxact.htm.
S.3548 — Coronavirus Aid, Relief and Economic Security (CARES) Act of 2020, 116th Congress (2019–2020). www.congress.gov/bill/116th-congress/senate-bill/3548/text?q=product+update.
Sacirbey, Omar. 2018. "Finding Right Insurance Is Key to Any Marijuana Company's Business Plan." *Marijuana Business Daily*.
Sambucci, Olena, Daniel Sumner, and Robin Goldstein. 2020. "Effect of Taxes and Costly Regulations on the Licensed and Unlicensed Cannabis Markets." *Working Paper*, 1–62.
Sen, Anindya, and Rosalie Wyonch. 2018. "Cannabis Countdown: Estimating the Size of Illegal Markets and Lost Tax Revenue Post-Legalization." *Commentary—C.D. Howe Institute* 523: 1–25.
Song, Bertie. 2018. "U.S. Legal Cannabis Market to Grow to $25 Billion by 2025." *New Frontier Data*.
Sparks, Evan. 2018. "The Cannabis Conundrum." *ABA Banking Journal* 110 (4): 41–42.
"Suspicious Activity Report." 2012. Financial Crimes Enforcement Network, Washington, DC.
"Tax Guide for Cannabis Businesses." California Department of Tax and Fee Administration. Accessed February 2, 2020. www.cdtfa.ca.gov/industry/cannabis.htm.
Tullock, Gordon. 1965. *The Politics of Bureaucracy*. Washington, DC: Public Affairs Press.
Vaida, Jeremy. 2015. "The Altered State of American Drug Taxes." *The Tax Lawyer* 68 (4): 761–93.
Webster, Alaina. 2018. "The Highs and Lows of Marijuana Banking." *Bank News* 118 (10): 38–38.
Weimer, David, and Vining, Aidan. 2005. *Policy Analysis*. Upper Saddle River, NJ: Prentice Hall.

15

A Labor Studies Approach to Cannabis

Marty Otañez

Keywords: labor rights, trade unions, corporate cannabis, transnational cannabis capitalist class, anthropology

Introduction

What are workers saying about occupational risks, wage disparities, and working conditions in an emergent legal cannabis industry increasingly shaped by corporate ownership structures? I present a labor studies approach to cannabis, illustrating a mixed-methods framework that constructs corporate-driven cannabis labor politics and low-wage cannabis workers as relational political economy subjects. Centering cannabis workers in a transnational capitalist class analysis (Sklair 2002), defined later, comprises a labor-centric framework designed to intervene in the cannabis political economy and counter the dominant cannabis culture that puts profit-making above the recognition of labor rights standards. This adds a "C" to TCC: transnational cannabis capitalist class. The labor studies approach featured in the discussion provides an alternative to methods that privilege top-down data sources and study sites.

In 2016, I administered a survey questionnaire about health concerns and labor rights to nineteen cannabis employees in the Denver Metro Area as part of a University of Colorado Denver research project called "Air Monitoring by Settle Plate in Mold-Filled Occupational Environments." A portion of the results is presented in this chapter. Recruitment strategies included social media platforms such as Facebook and Reddit as well as snowball sampling using new and existing contacts. I invited respondents, at the end of the survey, to participate in a videotaped thirty-minute interview based on themes in the survey as part of my web-based television show called "Getting High on Anthropology," which plays on Denver Open Media.

Additional study methods included participant observation at over fifteen cannabis-related events like job fairs, industry conferences, and health and safety workshops, as well as informal conversations with over 150 industry stakeholders in the legal cannabis industry in Colorado and elsewhere. These procedures, experiences, and interview findings inform the labor studies approach presented in this chapter.

DOI: 10.4324/9780429320491-15

The discussion begins with a focus on workers' experiences in Colorado's legal cannabis industry. Next, I present a review of cannabis worker-related literature and discuss the transnational cannabis capitalist class as it relates to labor politics in the cannabis political economy. In the closing sections, I address trade unionism and the role of labor peace agreements in spaces where workers seek to assert labor rights and companies protect their profits. My labor studies approach constitutes a relational political economy in research, by highlighting the precarity of cannabis work against celebratory narratives of corporate cannabis social responsibility common in neoliberal TCC discourse.

The Transnational Cannabis Capitalist Class

TCCC refers to the consumerist culture marketed by financial elites who expand the commercialization of cannabis on the global level. TCCC is my contribution to cannabis-focused labor studies by integrating cannabis in the transnational capitalist class concept introduced by sociologist Leslie Sklair (2002). According to Sklair, the transnational capitalist class appears to be acting like a global ruling class in some areas, and this class is associated with "the profit-driven culture-ideology of consumerism" that is a key feature of the globalized capitalist system (168). I extend Sklair's transnational capitalist class concept to include cannabis and describe the main factions of TCCC: stakeholders who own and control cannabis companies with an international focus (corporate faction), globalizing politicians and officials at the state level (state faction), globalizing professionals (technical faction), and merchants and media (consumerist faction) (Sklair 2002, 160). A recent example of TCCC and its interest to consolidate its class power at the global level and normalize corporate cannabis is the meeting of cannabis executives such as Bruce Linton, former CEO of Canopy Growth in Canada, and former politicians such as Ehud Barak, chairman of InterCure cannabis company and former prime minister of Israel, who gathered to discuss the cannabis sector at the World Economic Forum, an international organization for public-private cooperation in Davos, Switzerland (Bloomberg TV 2019).

I apply TCCC to the cannabis space to address the increasing class power of cannabis elites that influences the laboring lives of cannabis workers. As in other corporate sectors, cannabis brands often seek to add value to products by marketing them as produced in a socially responsible fashion (fair trade, organic, union-made, dolphin-friendly, and so forth). In doing so, they seek to tap into segments of the market that align their individual consumption preferences with some element of public interest. This approach includes, but is not limited to, the concept of ethical consumerism critically examined by Bennett in this volume. Members of the corporate cannabis class advance the culture-ideology of consumerism to create and meet the needs of a range of stakeholders at corporate and global levels (Sklair 2016).

Cannabis elites invoke consumer culture and legitimize class power by branding their products with social justice causes, but this may distract from other problematic social relationships in the supply chain such as maintaining workplaces that may be harmful to employees. Otañez and Vergara (this volume) show that cannabis companies integrate labor politics and environmental issues in corporate social responsibility (CSR) schemes. Companies engage in CSR as a marketing ploy to "greenwash" their prime directive to grow shareholder value. I use "greenwash" here to mean the practice of using social justice causes for branding purposes rather than strong interventions to bring about social change. This may include, for example, the dissemination of disinformation to present an environmentally responsible image to the public, rather than respect worker's rights. A labor studies approach places cannabis workers' voices at the center of analysis, disrupting TCCC promotion of CSR as a marketing strategy.

Cannabis elites at the center of the TCCC concept who pay lip service to public interest in an attempt to maximize shareholder value operate at the global financial level. Twelve of the largest cannabis companies in the USA, overall, at the time of this writing, are valued at more than $14 billion

(Borchardt 2019). Three of the largest cannabis companies (Canopy Growth Corporation, Aurora Cannabis, and Aphria) have a combined valuation of more than $22 billion (Young 2018). Forecasters suggest that spending in the legalized cannabis sector at the global level is expected to grow from $16 billion in 2019 to $31 billion in 2022 (Arcview Group 2019), and by 2027, spending in the global cannabis sector will reach $57 billion (Arcview Group 2018). The corporate-owned cannabis sector, in both North America and around the globe, is a force that influences cannabis worker's lives, their wages, and the strategies they deploy to secure protections for labor rights.

TCCC applied to the corporatization of cannabis markets points to a new area of study in the labor approach to cannabis. The rise of corporate cannabis means that the legal cannabis industry has entered corporate modernity. This requires that critiques of transnational corporate modernity be extended to the cannabis industry. Worker-centered labor studies are the starting point for the foundational critique of transnational corporate modernity (see Benson and Kirsch 2018 as an example). A pro-worker approach in legalized cannabis spaces may help to raise the bar for corporate accountability and push respect for labor rights as a precondition for cannabis industry investment (Athreya and Campbell 2013). The promise of occupational health and wellness is one critical element of safeguarding the rights of cannabis workers.

The Plight of Workers in Cannabis Production

Cannabis workplaces, comprised of both cultivation centers and dispensaries, have a number of potential health hazards. Hazards that trimmers and cultivators may experience include exposure to mold, allergens, CO_2, CO, pesticides/fungicides, cuts, and ergonomically harmful workspaces (Colorado Department of Public Health and Environment 2017; Walters, Fisher, and Tenney 2018). Endotoxins and mycotoxins are found in mold (Carroll 2017). Powdery mildew (PM) is a common mold that grows in white and gray powdery patches on cannabis leaves (Douglas and Sullivan 2013; Cranshaw 2013), contributing to chronic allergies for cannabis workers (Adelman 2013) and skin rashes (Majmudar, Azam, and Finch 2006), pulmonary histoplasmosis (Ramirez 1990), and respiratory illnesses for law enforcement officers who interact with unlicensed cannabis grows (Martyny et al. 2013).

The US Occupational Health and Safety Administration (OSHA) conducted a study of health and safety issues in a Minnesota cannabis company with indoor and outdoor cultivation facilities in 2016 and 2017. OSHA documented a number of issues, including moderate job stress due to heavy workload, safety concerns related to working with high-pressure carbon dioxide, exit doors needing a badge to unlock for egress, ergonomics, working with large amounts of solvents, concerns about having to perform tasks that are not part of their job description, and allergic, irritant, and musculoskeletal symptoms (Couch et al. 2018).

OSHA conducted a different study of an outdoor farm using organic agricultural practices in Washington State in 2015 and reported that cannabis trimmers "have exposure to highly repetitive work . . . which increases workers' risk for musculoskeletal disorders" (Victory 2018, 259). Schenker and Langer (Chapter 12) provide a systematic review of current literature focused on cannabis workers' health and safety.

In addition to navigating workplace safety hazards, cannabis labor is characterized by income inequality that mirrors other corporate industries. Labor markets in the post-prohibition context tend to be mostly low-wage jobs. Details of cannabis wage issues are available in the industry-produced report "Cannabis Jobs Count" (Barcott and Whitney 2019). Authors of the report state that the total number of full-time jobs in the cannabis industry in the US is 211,000. The number jumps up to 296,000 when jobs in the indirect and ancillary industries are counted (Barcott and Whitney 2019). The average hourly wage for trimmers, who devote their labor to manicuring and preparing harvested weed for cannabis stores, is $12.50, with some earning as high as $14.50 per hour (Barcott and Whitney 2019) while budtenders earn an average hourly rate of $13.75 (Barcott and

Whitney 2019). The average wage for trimmers is below the living wage rate of $12.95 required for a single employee in Denver (Denver Labor Law 2018) and below the floor of $15.00 that Denver mayor Michael Hancock approved for city workers in March 2019 (Denver Business Journal 2019). A trimmer receiving an average annual salary of $29,667 would need to work 17.8 years to earn the $529,090 that a cannabis executive earns in a year (Cowee 2019). Trimmers and other workers experience pressure on wages due to the rate of increase of living expenses that is three times the rate of wage increases (Denver Labor Law 2018). This occurs in an industry expanding at a phenomenal rate at the national and global levels.

Workers' Experiences in the Colorado Cannabis Industry

Workers' voices are insufficiently featured in literature on worker's health and safety. This section showcases interview responses from cannabis workers in Colorado as a central component of a labor studies approach to cannabis.

One day before I interviewed Daniel in the fall of 2016, he spoke with state senators at the capitol in Denver to provide a worker's perspective on pesticide use, exposure to powdery mildew, and other health risks of cannabis production. He accompanied labor organizers with the United Food and Commercial Workers International Union (UFCW) at the state house who were supporting the movement for rules to ensure that certified investigators, not cannabis company representatives, select samples of cannabis needed for state pesticide testing requirements. When asked about his safety issue concerns, he stated that PM is one of the biggest problems threatening worker health and "that most of the companies are not doing a damn thing about it."

Daniel worked several years trimming cannabis and was part of a team of contracted workers. He described trimming as devalued service. When he first started trimming a few years earlier, Daniel earned $20 an hour, but after cannabis legalization in Colorado in 2014 and an influx of people to the state to work in cannabis, he witnessed a growth in the number of individuals who accepted $10 an hour. Bosses informed Daniel that if he refused the lower wage, there were five people willing to step in and take his place. While I've been unable to determine if Daniel's experience with wage devaluation is part of a broader pattern in the legalized corporate cannabis sector, his experience shows the uncertainty of cannabis work.

Daniel is HIV positive, with a compromised immune system, making him acutely aware of PM and other health risks in cannabis workplaces. According to Daniel, exposure to PM triggers an itchy throat, headaches, itchy skin, and red bumps on exposed body surfaces. Except for headaches, symptoms identified by Daniel are consistent with case reports in the clinical literature (Colorado Department of Public Health and Environment 2017). Deep cleaning in the shower after work and washing infected clothes are ways to address the PM problem. "But the breathing issues are pretty constant, and they linger for quite a while." Daniel recounted PM as a health risk and companies' intransigence to address PM:

> The one guy that I know [who went] to a hospital, you know, he fell to the ground and started having seizures [at work] because he couldn't breathe and things were happening because the powdery mildew was so bad . . . The doctors did say that it was related to the working conditions . . . I wouldn't work for certain clients in this industry because after three years of visiting them at random, nothing has changed. It's like they are concerned with profit most of the time . . . Most of the average consumers walking in [to retail stores] don't know what [PM] is and they just see this product and "Oh, that looks like extra crystals" and [companies] sell it because they, you know, think people are stupid . . . [Trimmers and I] joke like it's going to be called trimmer lung [in the future] because of all the chemicals and powdery mildew, bugs. We just don't know. There's no research. There's no data. There's no long-term study. We know

> what it can potentially do. We just, we don't have proof yet. Until somebody dies, until somebody has such a severe issue where it forces a change, there's not much, not much, we can do.

I interviewed Jessica in 2016. She was a grow lead in a cannabis facility in one of Colorado's largest cannabis companies. Earlier, she completed her bachelor's degree with a focus on the music business from the University of Colorado Denver. Growing up, Jessica's mom had non-cannabis houseplants and an outdoor garden. Her home environment contributed to her passion for cannabis. Jessica's love for pesticide-free home gardening partly explains her concern about the lack of regulations for pesticides in the cannabis industry. When she first entered the industry in 2014, Jessica realized that few or no regulations existed to limit worker exposure to pesticides. Protective clothing wasn't even required, and according to Jessica, the application of Eagle 20 was the key method of pest control. Applied on a weekly basis, Eagle 20 killed everything, including spiders and flies, except the plants. In 2015, the Colorado Department of Agriculture (DoA) adopted Pesticide Applicators' Act rules pertaining to pesticide use in cannabis production, which included a DoA list of pesticides allowed for use on cannabis (Colorado Department of Agriculture 2015). DoA listed Eagle 20 as a banned pesticide, and several large cannabis companies had thousands of plants confiscated due to the application of Eagle 20 and other banned pesticides beginning in 2015 (Mitchell 2015). Jessica indicated that the changes in pesticide regulations for cannabis companies that promoted organic alternatives to toxic chemicals enhance the health of workers, consumers, and plants.

When I met with Scott in fall 2016, he indicated that he had several years of experience in cannabis jobs, mostly working for himself doing trim work, leading a crew of trimmers, and doing some consultancy work for cannabis companies in Colorado. According to Scott, PM is the biggest concern for workers in the cannabis sector. PM is linked to skin rashes and respiratory problems such as bronchitis. He invoked the term "green lung" to describe how individuals working in trim rooms for over ten hours a day, five to six days a week, are exposed to relatively high concentrations of mold and mildew. He equates mold spores to glass, that, when inhaled, create respiratory problems. "Green lung," while qualitatively different from work in extractive industries, is functionally equivalent to black lung experienced by coal miners who inhaled coal dust without proper safety protections, insofar as they are known industry-caused ailments (Smith 1981). Scott recalled an experience during one of his trim jobs in a large grow house where there was an excessive number of spores:

> I started noticing that my breathing was becoming worse and worse. I started having a lot of mucus problems and, you know, there's always congestion and I was constantly coughing all the time . . . I don't smoke cigarettes. It was not hard to figure out where it was coming from.

Unionization is one remedy proposed by Scott to address workplaces filled with powdery mildew and other occupational hazards. He indicated that his support for unions is due to low wages and that a union could help address the safety issues. A union campaign, according to Scott, "is not about punishing owners or asking for three-hour lunches or four weeks of vacation." Instead, he wishes to receive pay so that he can feed himself and pay his bills on time. Through a union, the problem of PM and other health risks might be addressed. Scott is hopeful that state legislators will put "laws into place that will, you know, protect the workers and not just the owners."

Findings from interviews with Scott and other cannabis workers reveal concerns about occupational health in a sector where transnational cannabis capitalist class members foster consumer culture. Workers express dissatisfaction with exposure to pesticides and powdery mildew in cannabis workplaces. They support unionization and put faith in legislators who may increase parity in power relations between workers and owners. However, TCCC interests, to get people to consume cannabis products and services, appear to trump workers' desires for improved occupational health and union representation. Cannabis elites that expand consumer culture and TCCC power by sponsoring industry conferences and professional meetings may at the same time be obstructing workers' efforts to advance their own interests through representative groups such as labor unions. Conferences and meetings are social milieus where discourses about corporate cannabis are created and normalized, with dominant industry actors participating in a process of TCCC formation that typically exclude workers and workers' concerns. Evaluating the development of TCCC class power through industry conferences and meetings is beyond the scope of this study. The concept of TCCC, in the labor studies approach to cannabis, provides researchers with an analytical tool to examine workers' responses to cannabis elites. For example, "Cannabis Workers Rising," which is addressed in the next section.

"Cannabis Workers Rising"

In 2010, UFCW established its "Cannabis Workers Rising" campaign (United Food and Commercial Workers International Union 2016), and in May 2021 UFCW represents the interests of over 10,000 cannabis workers (Tegethoff 2021) in 15 states in the US, including Washington, DC (United Food and Commercial Workers International Union 2019a). Membership in the cannabis union represents about .01% of the total UFCW membership of 1.3 million in 2019 (United Food and Commercial Workers International Union 2019b). The organization has legally binding contracts that involve cannabis labor in California, Colorado, Delaware, Illinois, Maryland, Massachusetts, Minnesota, Nevada, New Mexico, New Jersey, New York, Oregon, Pennsylvania, Rhode Island, Washington, and Washington, DC. Details on labor contracts discussed later are sourced from UFCW Local 770 in Los Angeles (United Food and Commercial Workers International Union 2018), one of the largest and most active cannabis labor unions in North America.

Labor contracts provide guaranteed working conditions, such as wages, hours of work, and employee benefits. Additional components include a dispute resolution process and paid time off for illness, holidays, and vacations. Contracts define respect and ensure fairness at workplaces. Labor contracts contribute to a safe working environment, company stability, and productivity. In union workplaces, in states where cannabis is legal, contracts lift standards for the businesses. Colorado experienced one of the first UFCW organizing campaigns in 2011, but the campaign lost traction when employers who previously partnered with UFCW over cannabis legalization withdrew support after the passage of a dispensary ban in Fort Collins in 2011 (Warner 2017). Though I've been unable to determine if the ban was seen as the reason for withdrawing support for unionization, union-related developments in the cannabis sector demonstrate the limits of top-down unionization efforts and the challenges of organizing low-wage workers in the age of TCCC dominance.

Labor peace agreements (LPAs), which codify that employers will not obstruct workers' rights and unions will refrain from job actions such as strikes, create a path to cannabis trade unionism, employee protections, and healthful workplaces. LPAs exist in Arkansas, California, Georgia, Hawaii, Illinois, New Jersey, New Mexico, New York, Ohio, Oregon, Pennsylvania, Rhode Island, and Washington. In 2016, the California Bureau of Cannabis Control issued Regulation 16 C.C. R § 5600(20), requiring applicants for any licensed facility with twenty or more employees to enter into and abide by LPAs. *Marijuana Business Daily* (Smith 2019) reported that applicants for medical cannabis business licenses in New York are required to sign an LPA with a union, and that legislators integrated LPA provisions in draft adult-use bills in New York and New Jersey in 2019.

Los Angeles (Los Angeles Department of Cannabis Regulation 2017) and San Francisco (San Francisco Office of Cannabis 2018) passed regulations that state LPAs must be established with companies that have ten or more employees. In spring of 2019, UFCW Local 7 in Denver promoted LPAs through legislative advocacy in Colorado. Randy Tiffey, director of organizing with UFCW Local 7, stated that formidable obstacles to LPA-related language in draft legislation exist in the form of lobbyists from VS (Vicente Sederberg) Strategies, the Marijuana Industry Group, Sewald Hanfling

Public Affairs, and Young Public Affairs, as well as from cannabis companies such as Native Roots, Medicine Man, LivWell, and Green Solution (Tiffey 2019).

Colorado Secretary of State records for fiscal year 2018–19 show that lobbyists associated with these companies earned revenues from cannabis companies and their ancillary groups totaling $656,263 in January–March 2019 (Colorado Secretary of State 2019) and, in 2018, the amount for the year was $918,517. The behavior of cannabis companies that oppose LPAs and engage in anti-union practices is a key feature of transnational cannabis capitalist class labor politics.

Conclusion

As cannabis employees voice their concerns with workplace issues while companies and their lobbyists obstruct labor unionism, company executives seek to optimize their profits in these legalized cannabis environments. To challenge the anti-labor and anti-union sensibilities in the cannabis industry, a labor studies approach is used to unpack the relational political economy comprised of corporate-driven labor politics and low-wage cannabis workers. There are little to no signs that transnational cannabis capitalist class members in Colorado and elsewhere will abandon their anti-labor sensibilities. Corporate cannabis makes claims of job creation when the actual jobs tend to be low wage and workers experience precarity in cannabis production. Neoliberal-friendly cannabis companies promote narratives that celebrate their contributions to market success and social equity, for example, in cannabis spaces. Simultaneously, employees at the ground level desire workplace protections and their fair share of cannabis earnings.

The findings and discussion presented in this chapter are relevant for labor scholars focusing on the cannabis space. A worker-based approach places at its core voices and experiences of trimmers and other cannabis employees. Too often, studies rely on surveys that abstract from lived experience to report on individuals and their laboring lives (Freire 1996). Collecting and sharing stories about workers and their concerns provide a more nuanced analysis of key industry actors who tend to be overlooked because of the power and influence of corporate class members. In the process, scholars need to counter stereotypes of wageworkers as lacking knowledge about workplace health issues and of workers who do not desire labor unions.

Voices of workers can be juxtaposed with findings from workers' legitimate complaints of unsafe workplaces and unfair labor practices in different government departments to show how what cannabis companies *say* they do contrasts with what they *actually* do. It may be important to ask companies that make claims of equity as part of CSR schemes to make public the money companies spend on these schemes. Funds can be compared to cost savings of cannabis companies that prefer to pay for responsibility projects rather than pay living wages to workers.

Readers who apply the TCCC concept discussed in this chapter could examine the extent to which consumers desire cannabis products made by workers who receive living wages and are unionized. Researchers may analyze different segments of TCCC and their relationships with government officials and labor unionists and determine the influence of industry funding on campaigns for labor peace agreements in states where cannabis is legal. Research on alternatives to TCCC include making space for non-shareholder ownership to counter cannabis capitalist structures (Cooperative Cannabis Company 2019; Ranis 2019). Future researchers might use the framework presented in this chapter to conceptualize cannabis corporations as sites of occupational health hazards (Otañez 2019), places of labor exploitation, and relational spaces to build alternatives to corporate cannabis.

Acknowledgement

The University of Colorado Denver Office of Research Services provided funds for this research project.

References

Adelman, Alisha. 2013. "Gender Dynamics and Social Relations of Production in Humboldt's Marijuana Industry." Master's Thesis, Humboldt State University, Arcata, CA.

Arcview Group. 2018. "The Road Map to a $57 Billion Worldwide Market." Accessed March 1, 2019. https://arcviewgroup.com.

———. 2019. "Worldwide Legal Cannabis Spending Hits $12.2 Billion in 2018, Projected to Grow 38% to $16.9 Billion in 2019." *GlobeNewswire News Room*. Accessed April 15, 2019. www.globenewswire.com/news-release/2019/01/15/1691880/0/en/NEW-REPORT-Worldwide-Legal-Cannabis-Spending-Hits-12–2-Billion-in-2018-projected-to-Grow-38-to-16–9-Billion-in-2019.html.

Athreya, Bama, and Brian Campbell. 2013. "No Access to Justice: The Failure of Ethical Labeling and Certification Systems for Worker Rights." In *Workers' Rights and Labor Compliance in Global Supply Chains: Is a Social Label the Answer?* edited by Jennifer Bair, Marsha Dickson, and Doug Miller, 226–44. New York: Routledge.

Barcott, Bruce, and Beau Whitney. 2019. *Cannabis Jobs Count*. Seattle: Leafly. Accessed June 1, 2019. www.leafly.com/news/industry/legal-cannabis-jobs-report-2019.

Benson, Peter, and Stuart Kirsch. 2018. "Capitalist Corporation, the." In *The International Encyclopedia of Anthropology*, edited by Hilary Callan, 1–9. Oxford: John Wiley and Sons.

Bloomberg TV. *Cannabis Meets the Business Elite in Davos*. New York. Accessed May 15, 2019. www.bloomberg.com/news/videos/2019-01-23/cannabis-meets-the-business-elite-in-davos-video.

Borchardt, Debra. 2019. "The Cannabis Industry's Top 12 U.S. Multi-State Operators." *Green Market Report*. Accessed March 15, 2019. www.greenmarketreport.com/the-cannabis-industrys-top-12-u-s-multi-state-operators.

Carroll, M. 2017. "How to Tell If Your Weed Is Moldy?" *AllBud*. Accessed January 23, 2019. www.allbud.com/learn/story/how-tell-if-your-weed-moldy.

Colorado Department of Agriculture. 2015. *Pesticide Applicators' Act*.

Colorado Department of Public Health and Environment. 2017. *Guide to Worker Safety and Health in the Marijuana Industry*. Denver, CO: Colorado Department of Public Health and Environment.

Colorado Secretary of State. 2019. "Online Lobbyist System." Online Lobbyist System. Accessed October 8, 2019. www.sos.state.co.us/lobby/Home.do.

Cooperative Cannabis Company. 2019. *Chicago Cannabis Company*. Accessed November 7, 2019. www.chicannaco.com/pages/cooperative-cannabis-company.

Couch, James, Douglas Wiegand, George Grimes, Brett Green, Angela Lemons, Eric Glassford, Leonard Zwack, Stephen Jackson, and Donald Beezhold. 2018. "Evaluation of a Medicinal Cannabis Manufacturing Facility with an Indoor and Outdoor Grow Operation." U.S. Department of Health and Human Services, Public Health Service, Centers for Disease Control and Prevention, National Institute for Occupational Safety and Health. Cincinnati, OH.

Cowee, Maggie. 2019. "How They Compare: A Look at How Cannabis Industry Salaries Stack Up Against Those in Traditional Sectors." *Marijuana Business Magazine*.

Cranshaw, Whitney. 2013. *Pest Management of Indoor-Grown Medical Marijuana in Colorado*. Fort Collins, CO: Bug Books.

Denver Business Journal. 2019. "Separate Minimum Wage Hike Measures for Colorado, Denver Take Significant Steps." *Denver Business Journal*. Accessed May 3, 2019. www.bizjournals.com/denver/news/2019/03/15/denvers-minimum-wage-hike-signed-into-law-colorado.html.

Denver Labor Law. 2018. "What Is Considered a Living Wage in Colorado?" *Denver Labor Law* (blog). Accessed June 6, 2019. https://denverlaborlaw.com/2018/08/06/what-is-considered-a-living-wage-in-colorado.

Douglas, Janet, and Richard Sullivan. 2013. "The Role of Child Protection in Cannabis Grow Operations." *International Journal of Drug Policy* 24 (5): 445–48.

Freire, Paolo. 1996. *Pedagogy of the Oppressed* (revised). New York: Continuum.

Los Angeles Department of Cannabis Regulation. 2017. *Los Angeles Municipal Code. 104.11(I)*.

Majmudar, V., N. A. M. Azam, and T. Finch. 2006. "Contact Urticaria to Cannabis Sativa." *Contact Dermatitis* 54 (2): 127–27.

Martyny, John, Kate Serrano, Joshua Schaeffer, and Mike van Dyke. 2013. "Potential Exposures Associated with Indoor Marijuana Growing Operations." *Journal of Occupational and Environmental Hygiene* 10 (11): 622–39.

Mitchell, Thomas. 2015. "Denver Investigated 10 Pot Grows for Use of Banned Pesticides, Holds Plants." *Westword*. Accessed May 22, 2019. www.westword.com/news/denver-investigated-10-pot-grows-for-use-of-banned-pesticides-holds-plants-6654706.

Otañez, M. 2019. "The Cannabis Industry as an Occupational Hazard." *Hemp Connoisseur Magazine*. Accessed October 16, 2019. www.hcmagazine.com/the-cannabis-industry-as-an-occupational-hazard.

Ramirez, J. 1990. "Acute Pulmonary Histoplasmosis: Newly Recognized Hazard of Marijuana Plant Hunters." *American Journal of Medicine* 88 (5N).

Ranis, Peter. 2019. "Worker Cooperatives: The Default Alternative to Predatory United States Capitalism." *Socialism and Democracy* 33 (1): 112–40.

San Francisco Office of Cannabis. 2018. "1609(b)(12) Labor Peace Agreement." Office of Cannabis.

Sklair, Leslie. 2002. "The Transnational Capitalist Class and Global Politics: Deconstructing the Corporate-State Connection." *International Political Science Review* 23 (2): 159–74.

———. 2016. "The Transnational Capitalist Class, Social Movements, and Alternatives to Capitalist Globalization." *International Critical Thought* 6 (3): 329–41.

Smith, Barbara Ellen. 1981. "Black Lung: The Social Production of Disease." *International Journal of Health Services* 11 (3): 343–59.

Smith, Jeff. 2019. "What Are the Business Implications of Labor Peace Agreements for the Cannabis Industry?" *Marijuana Business Daily*. Accessed July 1, 2019. https://mjbizdaily.com/business-implications-of-labor-peace-agreements-for-the-cannabis-industry.

Tegethoff, Eric. 2021. "Unionization Efforts Leave Cannabis Growers Behind, But Change Could Be Coming." *Cannabis News Wire*. Accessed April 27, 2021. https://cannabiswire.com/2021/04/26/unionization-efforts-leave-cannabis-growers-behind-but-change-could-be-coming.

Tiffey, Randy. 2019. "Labor Peace Agreements." *Email Communication*, March 15.

United Food and Commercial Workers International Union. 2016. "Cannabis." Accessed June 19, 2019. www.ufcw.org/cannabis-workers.

———. 2018. "Growing a Cannabis Workers Movement." Accessed December 21, 2018. www.ufcw770.org/cannabis.

———. 2019a. "Consumer and Worker Protections Must Be Top Priority for Northeast Governors in Cannabis Framework." Accessed November 29, 2019. www.ufcw.org/2019/11/25/protections.

———. 2019b. "About: The United Food and Commercial Workers International Union." Accessed July 13, 2019. www.ufcw.org/about.

Victory, Kerton R. 2018. "Notes from the Field: Occupational Hazards Associated with Harvesting and Processing Cannabis, Washington, 2015–2016." *MMWR. Morbidity and Mortality Weekly Report* 67.

Walters, Kevin M., Gwenith G. Fisher, and Liliana Tenney. 2018. "An Overview of Health and Safety in the Colorado Cannabis Industry." *American Journal of Industrial Medicine* 61 (6): 451–61.

Warner, Joel. 2017. "Unionizing Efforts in Colorado's Cannabis Industry Got Nipped in the Bud." *Westword*. Accessed January 20, 2017. www.westword.com/news/unionizing-efforts-in-colorados-cannabis-industry-got-nipped-in-the-bud-9575515.

Young, David. 2018. "Big Cannabis Is Rising High." *Matters of Substance* 29 (3): 14–17.

16

Cannabis Corporate Social Responsibility

A Critical and Mixed-Method Approach

Marty Otañez and David Vergara

Keywords: Corporate social responsibility, cannabis legalization, greenwashing, qualitative research, content analysis

Introduction

Corporate social responsibility (CSR) is a disputed term with inconsistent definitions. The European Commission defines it as "a concept whereby companies integrate social and environmental concerns in their business operations and in their interaction with their stakeholders on a voluntary basis" (European Commission 2001, 6). Brooks and Dunn (2018, 509) understand CSR as the degree to which an organization takes the interests of stakeholders into account and acts according to them. In modern media outlets, CSR, sustainability, and ESG (environmental, social, and governance) are used interchangeably to describe the same concept of corporate engagement, whereby the terms differ only regarding the metrics used to measure companies' performance (Kell 2014; Chadwick 2013; npower Business Solutions 2019).

The most prominent critique of the CSR concept stems from a neoliberal perspective, spearheaded by Milton Friedman's shareholder theory. According to this perspective, businesses have no other social responsibilities aside from delivering profit to their shareholders (Friedman 1970, 6). A strict implementation of this theory rejects any notion of CSR since it sees no role of society in business obligations. Other critical anti-neoliberal researchers, as well as consumers, tend to invoke the term *greenwashing* to describe a company's efforts to promote inflated positive beliefs about its environmental performance (Lyon and Montgomery 2015). Even though we recognize that critiques of CSR come from different angles, we also acknowledge its momentum and increasing visibility within current social and business landscapes. Our aim is to examine how (and if) the CSR idea plays out and interacts with the flourishing cannabis industry.

Critical CSR literatures such as Cai, Jo, and Pan (2012) as well as Lindorff, Prior Jonson, and McGuire (2012) have examined "controversial" industries such as alcohol or tobacco but have not focused on cannabis. Critics are suspicious of the motives behind corporate social behavior in controversial industries, with the World Health Organization (WHO) even describing the possibility of CSR in the tobacco industry as an "inherent contradiction" (World Health Organization 2004).

DOI: 10.4324/9780429320491-16

Others claim that CSR is only "window dressing"—an attempt to whitewash questionable business practices and improve a business' perception amongst consumers but with no real intent of acting for the benefit of society or the environment (Palazzo and Richter 2005).

Viewed from a historical perspective, this critique could also apply to cannabis. In the past, market actors operating outside the law were virtually invisible, engaging in nontransparent and questionable practices in order to produce, market, and sell their products. The foundations of the existing legal cannabis sector were partially built on a pattern of informal sector business practices for which CSR principles were logistically incompatible or very difficult to translate into the formal sector. With legalization, cannabis enterprises become legible, providing opportunities to assess emerging CSR practices and initiatives. Marc Ross, a CSR private sector consultant with a focus on cannabis, recognizes four areas of CSR: communication engagement, strategic philanthropy, sustainability, and employee engagement (Lit and Lucid Podcast 2019). The latter area refers to cannabis companies providing a living wage, ensuring that workers have a say in workplace issues, and allowing people time off and paying them for CSR-related volunteer work (Lit and Lucid Podcast 2019). Cannabis companies that portray themselves as responsible corporate citizens weaken their CSR claims when companies obstruct employee rights and trade unionism.

The expansion and diversification of the cannabis market raises important ethical questions that are yet to be addressed. Considering the perceived danger cannabis represents, there is a need to implement sustainable strategies to produce, market, and distribute the products in a responsible manner and prevent public health problems similar to those of the tobacco and alcohol industries. Despite this need, there is a significant research gap concerning CSR, since the academic scholarship places no focus on cannabis. We address this gap by contributing an evidence-based research approach and addressing CSR in the cannabis industry from an academic perspective. Our examination is meant to be an incentive for cannabis corporations to implement CSR strategies that go beyond mere marketing ploys. We aim to achieve relevance by critically approaching our methodology and showing how it can be improved. This way, our findings can be useful for a wide range of academics from diverse fields looking to perform research in the cannabis space.

In each section, we apply an auto-ethnographic approach and situate ourselves in the study of cannabis workers and CSR. We discuss in-depth interviews from Vergara's work focused on CSR activities in the cannabis sector and the content analysis approach in two case studies from Otañez's study of workplace practices and CSR schemes. We conclude by suggesting wider implications of our work and future research directions in the post-prohibition context. Our goal is to advance a critical research agenda about cannabis CSR as necessary to push cannabis corporations to use CSR, and not just as a marketing ploy and greenwashing.

Can the Cannabis Industry Develop Best Practices in the Pursuit of Corporate Social Responsibility?

While attending business school at the University of East London, Vergara became interested in business ethics and CSR. Simultaneously, Germany, his country of residence at the time, legalized medicinal cannabis in spring 2017. Aware of the significant economic potential of this industry in Europe and North America, Vergara embarked on a master's thesis project to explore how, and if, the idea of socially responsible corporate behavior was compatible with the cannabis industry. The question guiding the study was *Which best business practices can a company in the cannabis industry adopt to achieve CSR?* Colorado seemed an ideal place to perform research, since it was one of the first states to legalize market relationships and therefore provides an important example to investigate the consequences of specific cannabis policy choices (Subritzky, Lenton, and Pettigrew 2016, 511–13). Since answering his research question required insight exclusive to business insiders, Vergara conducted semi-structured, in-depth interviews with industry experts in Colorado and included Otañez (co-author) as one of his interviewees. Vergara identified a sample of 13 experts in the Denver and Boulder regions of Colorado using purposive sampling.

Vergara's methodology combined deductive and inductive research strategies and integrated different research paradigms. Following this dual approach, his research was divided into two phases. In the hypothesis-building portion (phase 1) of his project, Vergara used insights and information gathered from the existing literature to develop research questions in the form of best business practices. In the research portion (phase 2) of the project, Vergara's study process consisted of testing the hypotheses elaborated in the first phase by conducting qualitative research with experts in the Colorado cannabis industry. Vergara's approach was based on an interpretivist paradigm, which implements naturalistic methods—such as interviews—in which the researcher operates within a natural research context in order to access meaning and gain in-depth understanding (Lincoln, Lynham, and Guba 2011, 105; Saunders, Lewis, and Thornhill 2012, 163). Following this logic, the research was designed to be conducted in the study participant's natural environment, and a special emphasis was placed on context and individual experience. To achieve this, Vergara elaborated several open-ended questions and then compiled an interview guide. Next, he modified the questions depending on the insight gained from previous interviews and on the individual experience of each participant.

Vergara's research generated mixed results, and he was not able to obtain a definitive answer to his research question. Findings showed the cannabis sector in Colorado as a hyperlocal, differentiated, and highly fragmented industry with no distinguishable trends or common characteristics. Consequently, no general standards or blanket statements of "good behavior" could be made regarding the industry as a whole. Participants in Vergara's research described regulatory divergences from state to state, and between counties and cities. Participants addressed traditional scales of regulatory composition, while missing others such as nation and state, and states and cities. They discussed subsectors of the industry: medicinal, recreational, and hemp, each with different environmental and social factors that require different CSR standards. Several methods of consumption were highlighted by study participants: smoking, edibles, dabbing, and vaping. Dabbing was noted as a concern because consumers may inhale dangerously high amounts of THC and handle flammable, toxic chemicals (Meehan-Atrash, Luo, and Strongin 2017, 6112). Also, study participants acknowledged the irregular landscape of cannabis in Colorado and avoided making blanket statements describing cannabis businesses as a collective.

Vergara concluded that Colorado's cannabis industry may still be too immature to produce definitive answers or that the state may not be the best example when it comes to providing applicable business practices for the implementation of cannabis-related CSR. Additionally, his research in this state provided an example of how inconsistent and divergent the landscape is and how the dichotomy between ongoing federal illegality and state experiments in legalization adds a layer of complexity that can hinder the emergence of cannabis-specific CSR "best practices."

Cannabis is still federally listed as a Schedule I drug. Because of this, clinical research requires a DEA license and approval from the FDA and the National Institute on Drug Abuse, all of which are federal agencies. In practice, such permissions are rarely granted. Without scientific research, no objective observations about the benefits and risks of cannabis can be made, and businesses cannot be transparent and will eventually fail to educate consumers and the public. Vergara's interview participants largely viewed federal illegality as a hindrance for business operations. In particular, the tax structure was regarded as a primary obstacle for the free development of businesses. Cannabis businesses not only pay 15% retail tax and 2.9% sales tax at the state level in Colorado (Colorado Department of Revenue 2019; Livni 2017), but also they are required to pay federal taxes, even though they are considered illegal by the US government. At the same time, and due to a clause in the Internal Revenue Code (USC 280E), cannabis businesses are forbidden from deducting ordinary expenses from gross income associated with the trafficking of Schedule I substances (National Cannabis Industry Association 2015). As a result, businesses in the sector pay taxes on their gross profit instead of their operating profit, so that their tax rates exceed those in regular industries, even if they have comparable costs.

An analysis of Vergara's findings suggests that although the cannabis industry might have reached legality at the state level, it still operates in a gray market due to federal restraints. As long as federal illegality collides with state legality, cannabis will be associated with the underground. This undermines any efforts of bringing the industry out of the shadows and reaching any form of transparency. Also, as long as the plant is federally scheduled, organizations will not fulfill societal expectations and will not reach legitimacy. In the post-prohibition context, in which cannabis is formally incorporated into the landscape of corporate modernity, corporations that are able to implement substantial and effective CSR policies that go beyond marketing ploys or greenwashing might be able to achieve a level of corporate citizenship that parallel industries, such as the alcohol and tobacco industries, have never reached.

Similarly, no general CSR standard could be applied to the emergent industry, since it is dependent on the subsector or even on the consumption method. For example, cannabis edibles are considered especially risky because of their delayed effect after consumption and the lack of standards in potency (Grinspoon 2019). Also, edibles represent an increased risk for children because of their appealing commercial presentation (e.g. candy, baked goods) that can lead to unintentional poisoning (Ghosh et al. 2015). For these reasons, different and perhaps higher responsibility standards regarding standardization, packaging, and labeling should apply to producers of edibles. On the other hand, a cannabis producer with relatively large indoor cultivation facilities should have a higher commitment towards environmental sustainability than should a hemp farmer with outdoor crops because of the high amount of energy required to maintain artificial lighting and dehumidification devices. The indoor cannabis producer should therefore deploy more adequate and appropriate CSR strategies geared towards securing a higher environmental sustainability standard.

The Cases of Cannabis Companies Native Roots and Have a Heart

In 2014, Otañez started an exploratory study focused on cannabis workers and industry practices in Colorado. He conducted videotaped interviews with six study participants and administered a survey to 19 individuals employed in the cannabis sector to document workers' health and safety concerns. His goal was to contrast experiences of cannabis workers with cannabis companies' efforts to portray themselves as responsible corporate citizens. Content analysis of the videotaped interviews with employees in Colorado's cannabis sector as well as company web pages, news stories, and documents from government agencies was used to identify and discuss details of Native Roots and Have a Heart cannabis companies engaged in practices to portray themselves as good corporate citizens. Search terms included "Native Roots," "corporate social responsibility," and "community engagement." Searches via the online University of Colorado Denver library, including Google Scholar and Nexis Uni, an electronic database with news, business, and legal sources, occurred between August 2018 and March 2019. Findings obtained through online searches were combined with details of the broader context of cannabis in Colorado collected by Otañez beginning in 2014. The Native Roots case was developed using company web pages, news stories, and documents from government agencies with rules pertaining to the cannabis sector, such as the Occupational Safety and Health Administration (OSHA), and the Colorado Department of Agriculture (CDA).

Established in Denver in 2010, Native Roots has the highest number of cannabis licenses in the state, operating 20 dispensaries and two cultivation facilities in Colorado. It employs over 600 individuals, and the workforce is expected to increase by a couple of thousand in the next few years (DeMuro and Holmgren 2018). The company produces 30,000 pounds of cannabis annually, mostly in its Denver-based "mothership" facility with 200,000 square feet, one of the largest grow houses in the world (Amercanex International Exchange 2018).

Native Roots administers CSR activities through the Native Roots Foundation (Cannabis Business Executive 2017), a nonprofit group established in February 2017. Beginning in 2017, Native Roots clocked over 450 company-wide community service hours annually and "tens of thousands of philanthropic contributions to nonprofit organizations" (Cannabis Trade Federation 2019). Recent examples of its CSR initiatives are a $25,000 donation to the Chanda Plan Foundation (Denver Business Journal 2018), a Colorado-based organization that provides funding for healthcare services to people with physical disabilities, and sponsorship of the Cannabis Sustainability Symposium in Denver that brings together experts in cannabis-related environmental practices.

Native Roots' CSR activities are suspect, however, because of its track record in workplace safety and labor-related violations. The case of Native Roots highlights the tension between social responsibility initiatives and worker safety issues. Records for the period 2014–2019 obtained by Otañez through the Federal Freedom of Information Act and Colorado Open Records Act show that 83 separate complaints across five agencies against Native Roots exist in the files of the National Labor Relations Board, OSHA, the Colorado Marijuana Enforcement Division, CDA, and Denver's Excise and License division. The number of cases against Native Roots appears to be relatively high, but additional research is needed to compare this with cases against over 1,600 licensed cannabis companies in Colorado. The case of Native Roots and complaints against it are resources to explore the extent that what the company says it does through CSR schemes contrasts with what it actually does in the workplace.

In one particular violation, Sebastian (a pseudonym), a former employee of Native Roots, submitted a complaint to the US Environmental Protection Agency (EPA) on April 4, 2017:

> While clearing out a reservoir used to store pesticide applications, I collected 17 gallons of the pesticide *Rinsate* together in four 5-gallon buckets with lids and labeled them for proper disposal. That day I was reprimanded and told that I was to dump *Rinsate* down the drain because it cost too much to pay for proper disposal. I refused and was threatened with my job for insubordination.

On April 11, the EPA forwarded Sebastian's message to CDA. From April 2017 to August 2018, CDA inspectors investigated Native Roots, interviewing nine employees and collecting 18 residue samples from drains in its main facility. CDA concluded that Native Roots violated the Pesticide Applicators' Act and failed to comply with the requirements of the federal Worker Protection Standards. Native Roots used the pesticide "Hydrogen Peroxide 30% Solution" not registered with CDA on cannabis to control powdery mildew. It used the pesticide EverGreen in a manner inconsistent with labeling requirements. CDA issued a written warning on August 8, 2018, allowing the company to remedy the violation before issuing a civil penalty.

Going deeper into CDA documents provides a fuller picture of Native Roots' response to Sebastian's complaint. On April 13, 2017, CDA inspector Burnett conducted a second in-person interview with Sebastian. Handwritten notes in the document, with the heading "Taylor Burnett's notes," showed that "Native Roots is offering $2,500 to stop (OSHA) investigation." The "$2,500" from Native Roots is not mentioned in other CDA documents. "Investigation" refers to a complaint Sebastian submitted to OSHA on April 12, 2017. The note suggests that Native Roots wanted to persuade Sebastian with a financial payment to withdraw his OSHA complaint. OSHA documents show that Sebastian's case closed on May 8, 2017. This indicates that the alleged complaint conditions did not exist or that the conditions did not actually create a serious hazard or a violation of an OSHA standard.

"Native Roots is offering $2,500 to stop (OSHA) investigation" is an example of companies that obstruct workers' rights while portraying themselves as good corporate citizens. Sebastian's experience with Native Roots is an example of strategies companies use to intimidate workers who raise workplace concerns. The example's power stems from how the note weakens industry claims of CSR and demonstrates that genuine CSR requires unobstructed labor rights in cannabis workplaces.

Have a Heart is presented as a second case study to illustrate CSR claims in the cannabis industry, highlighting how labor politics are worked into the mix. The back cover of the industry magazine *Cannabis Now* (February/March 2019 issue) displayed an advertisement from Have a Heart, a cannabis company with dispensaries in Washington State, Oregon, Iowa, and California. The ad header states, "We give 2% of our earnings back to charity, supporting union membership, living wages, community service and sustainable economic values." In August 2018, the company signed a collective bargaining agreement (CBA) with the United Food and Commercial Workers International Union (UFCW) Local 367, making it Washington's first contract covering wage and non-wage issues for 134 cannabis workers in five dispensaries (Seattle Times 2018).

Have a Heart with its unionized shops as well as its workers are in a position to benefit from the passage of Washington State Senate Bill (SB) 6393, "An act relating to cannabis industry workplace standards" (Senate Bill Report SB 6393 2020). The bill creates a point system where the adoption of practices such as employee benefits equates to point values used to renew the license of a cannabis producer, processor, retailer, or transportation company. The second draft of SB 6393 (PSSB 6393 Conway Tan S-5642.2 2020) presents a point system of cannabis licensing with 25 points awarded to applicants "establishing and having in effect an agreement with a labor organization to remain neutral or to work with or provide information to the labor organization for the purposes of unionizing employees" and 40 points for "having in effect a collective bargaining agreement covering the licensee's employees." The bill does not apply to licensees that averaged 20 or fewer full-time equivalent employees in the 12 months prior to the licensee's application for renewal.

In a public hearing on SB 6393 on January 23, 2020, 24 individuals provided oral testimony (Senate Labor and Commerce Committee 2020). Fourteen of the individuals supported the bill, including UFCW legislative director LaQuita Honeysucker. In Honeysucker's testimony, she indicated that labor peace agreements in other states where cannabis is legal "have been good for the health and safety of workers . . . and ensure quality jobs. That means well-paid, safe and family sustaining jobs." Two employees with Have a Heart voiced their support for the bill. Other bill supporters at the hearing pointed out that the rules will not require unionization and collective bargaining agreements and that employers will be obligated to remain neutral. The emerging rules will grant Have a Heart with two extra retail licenses beyond the five licenses that are available for any one licensee in Washington State. Arguments against SB 6393 were framed around potential closure of small businesses, anticipated job losses, and a scoring system disproportionately weighted towards labor-related peace agreements and union rights.

Have a Heart's display of support for cannabis labor unionism illustrates the political deployment of labor politics to gain market advantage by aligning company values with notions of workplace democracy and economic equity. The case study reflects an analysis of the politics of creating workplace standards legislation with an outcome of a draft bill to award points to licensee applicants with certain pro-worker and pro-union provisions. Additional research is needed to examine the ways that multistate operators like Have a Heart benefit from UFCW-supported legislation and how labor-related corporate responsibility schemes influence the livelihoods of cannabis workers.

On the surface, the actions of Have a Heart, its employees, and UFCW seem consistent with the cannabis sector's origins in counterculture and concerns for social justice. The lived realities of workers featured in this analysis present a complex picture. Situating workers in the center of critical studies of cannabis CSR schemes requires a deeper understanding of the overlapping and contradictory alliances that exist among company representatives, union leaders, and employees. Cannabis workers experience workplace violations, occupational risks, and anti-union employers as companies administer community engagement schemes that address a range of social justice issues, excluding workplace protections and labor rights. The economic power of companies that exploit workers shows that the corporate-owned cannabis sector in North America and globally is a force that influences cannabis worker livelihoods, wages, and occupational health concerns. The cases of Have a Heart and Native Roots show that further research is needed to interrogate CSR claims and determine the extent that responsibility initiatives are more than just marketing schemes.

CSR Research Conclusions and Directions in the Post-Prohibition Context

In a hyperlocal industry such as cannabis, particularities in geography, legality, and regulation play a fundamental role in academic research. Each cannabis market has its own singularities that must be considered by researchers. Reliance on a single methodology, such as in-depth interviews or content analysis, might not be the optimal approach for studying CSR in this context. Rather, as researchers dive deeper into the field of legalized cannabis, a constructive step is to apply a critical and mixed-methods approach to capture changes in regulatory environments and CSR practices. Research methods should depend on and be adapted to specific cannabis environments, such as at the state and federal levels and within medicinal and recreational industries, and even consider different consumption methods such as edibles and dabbing. Given the many environments in the current cannabis space, researchers should not limit themselves to only one methodology when engaging in CSR studies. Also, the methods they employ should be malleable and flexible, and they must be constantly revised and updated in order to keep up with the industry's ongoing development. As long as cannabis legality in the US remains inconsistent, for example, qualitative and quantitative research will continue to provide only partial snapshots of individual experiences and contexts of local market industry players.

An uneven market landscape leads to a high degree of uncertainty for all stakeholders. One basic requirement for the effective implementation of CSR is a relatively mature industry with homogenized structures. Even though the research described in this chapter generated uncertain results, it still provides valuable lessons that can be gradually carried out by market actors as the cannabis space develops. With approaching potential federal legalization of medicinal and adult-use cannabis markets in the US (Malandrakis and MacGuill 2019), corporate cannabis proponents in a hyperlocalized and highly diverse industry should effectively develop and implement CSR components such as standardization, regulation, accountability, transparency, and education focused on science. The path to CSR may include strategies targeting implementation, including defining general standards of responsibility, replacing plastic packaging with hemp alternatives, reducing barriers of access to cannabis medicine for patients, guaranteeing equal treatment of employees, and implementing labor standards. Along the way, cannabis corporations might be able to construct a solid CSR foundation, so that they can be evaluated critically. The extent that cannabis companies move beyond CSR as a marketing ploy and greenwashing is uncertain, though examples of perceived responsibility in the alcohol and tobacco industries may be within reach of corporate cannabis.

We are cautiously optimistic about any genuine cannabis-related CSR. Industry leaders make claims of CSR by "going beyond compliance," "demonstrating maturity and responsibility," and "exceeding existing requirements" without any specific business details to back them up. Calls for "self-regulation" among cannabis executives suggests that companies want to govern themselves and continue to put corporate profits over people. In the meantime, genuine CSR means cannabis companies respect worker's rights and do not obstruct employees who seek through a labor union to negotiate better wages, benefits, and working conditions in their workplace.

Ultimately, acknowledgement of the CSR–worker's rights nexus and the industry's heterogeneity should lead to a more differentiated research approach. To generate more exact results, individual CSR policies within a particular business, which concentrates on certain products and within a precise industry subsector, need to be examined. Also, future research should embrace a mixed-methods approach, combining qualitative aims based on interviews to gain industry insights and quantitative ones based on standardized surveys to reflect consumer and cannabis labor perspectives. Stories of cannabis in Colorado are still being formed, and these stories may serve as examples of regulatory frameworks and CSR initiatives emerging in other cannabis spaces. A comparative approach and one that examines workplace issues as part of genuine CSR behavior might help scholars determine the extent that cannabis companies act ethically and transparently in the post-prohibition context.

Acknowledgement

The University of Colorado Denver Office of Research Services provided funds for Otañez's research featured in this chapter.

References

Amercanex International Exchange. 2018. "Josh Ginsberg Joins Amercanex as Strategic Industry Consultant." March 9. https://amercanex.com/josh-ginsberg-joins-amercanex-as-strategic-industry-consultant.

Brooks, Leonard J., and Paul Dunn. 2018. *Business and Professional Ethics for Directors, Executives & Accountants*. 8th ed. Boston, MA: Cengage Learning.

Cai, Ye, Hoje Jo, and Carrie Pan. 2012. "Doing Well While Doing Bad? CSR in Controversial Industry Sectors." *Journal of Business Ethics* 108 (4): 467–80. https://doi-org.aurarialibrary.idm.oclc.org/10.1007/s10551-011-1103-7.

Cannabis Business Executive. 2017. "The Season of Giving Cannabis Business Alliance Members Support Communities in Need This Holiday Season and All Year Long." *Cannabis Business Executive*. www.cannabisbusinessexecutive.com/2017/12/season-giving-cannabis-business-alliance-members-support-communities-need-holiday-season-year-long.

Cannabis Trade Federation. 2019. "Founding Board Members." *Cannabis Trade Federation*. www.cannabistradefederation.com/founding-board-members.

Chadwick, Peter. 2013. "Understanding the ESG/CSR Value Chain—IEDP." *IEDP—Developing Leaders*. March 22. www.iedp.com/articles/understanding-the-esgcsr-value-chain.

Colorado Department of Revenue. 2019. "Marijuana Taxes." *Colorado Official State Web Portal*. www.colorado.gov/pacific/tax/marijuana-taxes-file.

DeMuro, Catherine, and Hannah Holmgren. 2018. "Christine Hodgdon from Native Roots." www.buzzsprout.com/213418/844521-episode-1-christine-hodgdon-from-native-roots.

Denver Business Journal. 2018. "Good Works: Cannabis Company Donates Big Money to Charity." *Denver Business Journal*. www.bizjournals.com/denver/news/2018/08/01/good-works-cannabis-company-donates-big-money.html.

European Commission. 2001. "Green Paper Promoting a European Framework for Corporate Social Responsibility." www.eea.europa.eu/policy-documents/com-2001-366-final-green.

Friedman, Milton. 1970. "The Social Responsibility of Business Is to Increase Its Profits." *The New York Times Magazine*, September 13.

Ghosh, Tista S., Michael Van Dyke, Ali Maffey, Elizabeth Whitley, Dana Erpelding, and Larry Wolk. 2015. "Medical Marijuana's Public Health Lessons—Implications for Retail Marijuana in Colorado." *New England Journal of Medicine* 372 (11): 991–93. doi:10.1056/NEJMp1500043.

Grinspoon, Peter. 2019. "Cannabis Is Medicine—Don't Make It Taste Good." *Harvard Health Blog*, May 6. www.health.harvard.edu/blog/cannabis-is-medicine-dont-make-it-taste-good-2019060516764?utm_campaign=shareaholic&fbclid=IwAR3sm6yDUW5oG6cW3H2uLHCDVoe7o5lym8Ti4Wdgfm2Vz5KSv7OZK-D6AsE.

Kell, Georg. 2014. "Five Trends That Show Corporate Responsibility Is Here to Stay." *The Guardian*, August 13, sec. Guardian Sustainable Business. www.theguardian.com/sustainable-business/blog/five-trends-corporate-social-responsbility-global-movement.

Lincoln, Yvonna S., Susan A. Lynham, and Egon G. Guba. 2011. "Paradigmatic Controversies, Contradictions, and Emerging Confluences, Revisited." In *The SAGE Handbook of Qualitative Research*, edited by Norman K. Denzin and Yvonna S. Lincoln. 4th ed., 97–128. Thousand Oaks: Sage.

Lindorff, Margaret, Elizabeth Prior Jonson, and Linda McGuire. 2012. "Strategic Corporate Social Responsibility in Controversial Industry Sectors: The Social Value of Harm Minimisation." *Journal of Business Ethics* 110 (4): 457–67. https://doi-org.aurarialibrary.idm.oclc.org/10.1007/s10551-012-1493-1.

Lit & Lucid Podcast. 2019. "Corporate Responsibility in Cannabis Featuring Marc Ross of Needle Consultants." *Lit & Lucid Podcast (Blog)*, February 12. https://litlucidpodcast.com/corporate-responsibility-cannabis.

Livni, Ephrat. 2017. "Marijuana Businesses Pay Super High Taxes to the US Government." *Quartz*, April 20. https://qz.com/963873/marijuana-businesses-pay-super-high-taxes-to-the-us-government.

Lyon, Thomas P., and A. Wren Montgomery. 2015. "The Means and End of Greenwash." *Organization & Environment* 28 (2): 223–49. https://doi.org/10.1177/1086026615575332.

Malandrakis, Spiros, and Shane MacGuill. 2019. *Cannabis Legalisation: How It Will Disrupt the Future*. London: Euromonitor International.

Meehan-Atrash, Jiries, Wentai Luo, and Robert M. Strongin. 2017. "Toxicant Formation in Dabbing: The Terpene Story." *ACS Omega* 2 (9): 6112–17.

National Cannabis Industry Association. 2015. "Internal Revenue Code Section 280E: Creating an Impossible Situation for Legitimate Businesses." https://thecannabisindustry.org/uploads/2015-280E-White-Paper.pdf.

npower Business Solutions. 2019. "Why ESG Is Replacing CSR—and What This Means to Your Business." April 19. www.npower.com/business-solutions/blog/2019/04/26/why-esg-is-replacing-csr-and-what-this-means-to-your-business.

Palazzo, Guido, and Ulf Richter. 2005. "CSR Business as Usual? The Case of the Tobacco Industry." *Journal of Business Ethics* 61 (4): 387–401. https://doi-org.aurarialibrary.idm.oclc.org/10.1007/s10551-005-7444-3.

PSSB 6393 Conway Tan S-5642.2. 2020.

Saunders, M. N. K, Philip Lewis, and Adrian Thornhill. 2012. *Research Methods for Business Students*. 6th ed. Harlow and New York: Pearson.

Seattle Times. 2018. "Marijuana Retailer Is the State's First to Unionize." *Seattle Times*, August 24, 2019. www.seattletimes.com/business/retail/marijuana-retailer-is-the-states-first-to-unionize.

Senate Bill Report SB 6393: An Act Relating to Cannabis Industry Workplace Standards. 2020.

Senate Labor and Commerce Committee. 2020. *Public Hearing: SB 6393 (Proposed Sub), SB 6057, SB 6033, SB 6269, SB 6188*. Seattle, Washington. www.tvw.org/watch/?eventID=2020011246.

Subritzky, Todd, Simon Lenton, and Simone Pettigrew. 2016. "Legal Cannabis Industry Adopting Strategies of the Tobacco Industry." *Drug and Alcohol Review* 35 (5): 511–13. doi:10.1111/dar.12459.

World Health Organization. 2004. "Tobacco Industry and Corporate Social Responsibility . . . an Inherent Contradiction." https://escholarship.org/uc/item/6kf7q7v9.

17

Consumer Activism, Sustainable Supply Chains, and the Cannabis Market

Elizabeth A. Bennett

Keywords: political consumerism, sustainability, voluntary certifications, supply chains, fair trade

Ethical Consumerism

"Ethical consumerism" refers to the leveraging of purchasing power to support or oppose a particular group, country, cause, or outcome (see Boström, Micheletti, and Oosterveer 2018). "Voting with your dollar" is a form of collective action in which individual actions aggregate to form a larger movement with significant effects (Bossy 2014). Although ethical consumerism is not new—boycotts were used in the anti-slavery movement of the late 1800s, for example—over the past two decades it has become an increasingly popular response to free-market policies and globalized supply chains (Bartley et al. 2015).

Ethical consumerism takes many forms. *Ethical purchasing* leverages boycotts, brand loyalty, and ethical labeling to reward particular modes of production; *lifestyle politics*, such as voluntary simplicity, time banks, tiny houses, and freeganism, challenge mainstream consumerism (see Haenfler, Johnson, and Jones 2012); and *culture jamming*—when guerilla billboard takeovers and ad busting pushes the public to reconsider their own consumption habits (see Lekakis 2017). People engage in ethical consumerism for various (and often overlapping) reasons such as altruistic commitments, expressing moral identity, and bolstering cultural capital (Brown 2013).

This chapter describes ethical consumerism in the context of the US and Canadian cannabis markets. Are consumers purchasing organic, fair trade, or sustainably produced cannabis? If so, how? If not, why? The chapter is organized into 11 sections as follows: methods; legalization and regulation; labor and environmental issues; organic, fair trade, and sustainability standards; lifestyle politics and legalization; ethical purchasing; consumer demand; ethical labeling; new cannabis certifications; and opportunities, challenges, and recommendations for a more ethical cannabis market.

Data and Methods

A proliferating interdisciplinary literature examines ethical consumerism in agri-food, textiles, handicrafts, forest products, and (to a lesser extent) mining/extraction, electronics, investment, and

 DOI: 10.4324/9780429320491-17

tourism (Raynolds and Bennett 2015). Very few studies examine semi-legal contexts[1] such as boycotting mafia-supportive businesses (Forno 2015) or advocating sex workers' rights (Stryker and Pennington 2014). This chapter is largely based on the author's own mixed-methods research, taking place over three years, from 2015 to 2018, mostly in the Pacific Northwest of the United States (Bennett 2017, 2018, 2019). Data were gathered through a survey and semi-structured interviews with cannabis supply chain actors, policy advocates, community organizers, and budtenders at over half (64) of the dispensaries in Portland, Oregon; participant-observation at over a dozen relevant meetings, events, and conferences; over 100 hours of pro bono consulting work with two ethical purchasing start-ups; interviews with the founders of all nine sustainability certification programs; analysis of 48 relevant articles from five news outlets; and a review of relevant academic literature.

Cannabis Legalization and Regulation in the United States and Canada

Like most countries, the United States and Canada are signatories to the three principal treaties that identify cannabis as a controlled (illegal) substance.[2] They are unique, however, in that they are at the forefront of legalization and the heart of the industry: they produce and consume a substantial amount of cannabis, and most Canadians and Americans support full legalization and believe consumption is socially acceptable (see Bennett 2017).

In the United States, cannabis is illegal at the federal level, and those engaged in the industry can be prosecuted. However, individual states have been using voter referenda to legalize medicinal cannabis since 1996 (California) and to legalize adult cannabis since 2012 (Colorado and Washington). As of early 2019, more than a third of states have legalized medicinal cannabis and ten states (plus the capital District of Columbia) have legalized adult-use cannabis, though many have not yet developed the regulatory frameworks required to facilitate legal sales. Each state regulates its market differently. However, all require growers to obtain a license and comply with regulations such as quantity of plants, pesticide testing, theft prevention, and sales accounting. Likewise, all dispensaries must be licensed and follow regulations related to purchasing protocols, customer age restrictions, and purchase limits. It is prohibited to transport cannabis across state boundaries, even between two states in which possession is legal.

In Canada, medical cannabis has been federally legal since 1999. Consumers were permitted to grow a small number of plants ("home grow") or designate someone to grow on their behalf, creating an industry of small cannabis farms. In 2014, however, Health Canada shifted policies to support a supply chain that more closely resembled synthetic pharmaceuticals. Large commercial operations were licensed and home grows prohibited. As a result, cannabis production quickly became dominated by a small number of large-scale firms able to finance compliance with costly regulations. In 2015, Canadians elected Justin Trudeau, a pro-legalization prime minister, and in 2017 the Cannabis Act was introduced. By 2018 regulations came into force, legalizing the production, sale, and consumption of cannabis for adult use. Under the Cannabis Act, Health Canada continues to regulate production. It has now established slightly different standards for large-scale and micro producers. Provinces regulate cannabis sales. Some permit privately owned dispensaries, while others limit sales to government-operated stores or websites. It is legal to transport cannabis across provincial borders, but not between the United States and Canada. In both countries, the black market persists.

Labor and Environmental Issues in Cannabis

Labor advocates argue that US and Canadian policies are inadequate for protecting workers in many industries. US farm workers, for example, are excluded from key labor protections, such as the right to collective bargaining, even though farm work is one of the most dangerous occupations.[3] In both countries, farming relies heavily on migrant workers—some national, others foreign—whose complaints about unsafe housing, poor sanitation, inadequate access to nutritious food, and sexual harassment in the fields is too often met with threats of deportation, termination of employment, and abuse (Otero and Preibisch 2015; PAN 2010; FJ 2015). For these reasons, many ethical consumerism initiatives aim to improve protections for workers.

Cannabis workers are also exploited and abused. Trimmers (the workers who process the harvested plant), especially women, have experienced sexual harassment, assault, discrimination, unsafe housing, mandatory overtime, and pervasive wage theft. Some have experienced or been threatened with acts of violence or been held hostage to improve productivity and silence dissent. Many choose not to report incidents for fear of legal consequences to themselves. This contributes to the persistence of workplace abuse (August 2013; Krissman 2016; Schirmann 2016).

Similar to labor standards, environmental regulations often fall short of protecting natural resources and the ecosystem. Like all agricultural crops, cannabis has the potential to generate adverse environmental consequences. Three issues of concern are energy, water, and inputs. Cannabis uses energy to heat/cool air, dehumidify, ventilate, pump water, heat water, and provide light for indoor grows.[4] Some growers pump CO_2 into grow houses, improperly dispose of bulbs containing neurotoxins, or damage ecosystems by clearing land, building terraces, and diverting streams, at times on public land. Especially in drier environments, cannabis is a relatively water-intensive crop (Mills 2012; O'Hare, Sanchez, and Alstone 2013; Bauer et al. 2015; Carah et al. 2015).

Pesticide misuse and overuse has drawn much attention because of the risks to workers, consumers, and the environment (Voelker and Holmes 2015). Although Canada and legalized US states have banned specific pesticides, enforcement is weak. In 2015, Oregon became the first state to mandate testing for adult-use products. In Canada, unless a grower has a history of using banned substances, inspectors spot-check for residue. It is not uncommon for contaminated products—with high residue levels of legal pesticides or evidence of chemicals unfit for consumption—to be sold on the legal market (Crombie 2015a; Robertson 2017).

Organic, Fair Labor, and Sustainability Standards in the United States and Canada

Concerns about state-based regulation have given rise to the organic, fair labor, and sustainability movements, which aim to improve social and environmental outcomes by creating and enforcing alternative standards.

The organic movement originated with farmers in the 1960s. Canada and the US began investing in research around 1980, committed to organic development in 1990, and published national organic standards around 2000. Today, the US Department of Agriculture oversees the National Organic Program (USDA/NOP), and the Canadian Food Inspection Agency oversees the Canada Organic Regime (CFIA/COR). Both require third-party audits to verify compliance, and since 2009, they recognize each other's systems as equivalent. Consumer demand has surged over the past decade. In 2016, 43% of Americans said someone in their household had purchased organic products "several times" in the past week, and 57% of Canadians report buying organic products weekly (Pew 2016; Mackinnon 2013).

The contemporary fair trade movement emerged after WWII, when Americans and Western Europeans provided market access to handicraft producers in developing and war-torn countries. This process was scaled up in subsequent decades through nonprofit mail-order catalogues and "world shops," such as Ten Thousand Villages. In the 1990s, several fair trade brands emerged, and the international nongovernmental organization (NGO) Fairtrade International rolled out a widely recognized global label that conventional (non-fair trade) companies could use to communicate that some inputs were purchased according to fair trade standards (e.g., minimum price, no child labor). Supply and demand of fair trade goods has grown rapidly, with the International Fairtrade label regulating the working conditions of more than 1.5 million farmers and workers. In wealthier countries, fair trade initiatives are sometimes referred to as "fair labor" or "domestic fair trade." In the United States and Canada, the Domestic Fair Trade Association and the Worker Driven Social Responsibility Network are at the forefront of this movement (Raynolds and Bennett 2015).

Often drawing on the principles of organic and fair trade labeling, sustainability certification programs have emerged to promote both social and environmental responsibility in a variety of sectors. The Eco Label Index shows rapid proliferation of sustainability labels. Around 2000, the ISEAL Alliance was established to codify best practices and accredit sustainability programs that adopt them. Research on sustainability and fair trade labeling suggests that labels managed by NGOs and civil society groups are more likely to adopt inclusive governance practices, rigorous standards, and credible verification. It also shows that competition among sustainability labels can create a "race to the bottom" as certification programs lower standards to attract more companies. Today, consumers face "label fatigue"—the inability to learn about each label they face and adjudicate among seemingly similar programs. Thus, watchdog and advocacy organizations play an important role in monitoring labels and publicizing comparative studies (Auld 2014; Bartley et al. 2015).[5]

Lifestyle Politics as Legalization Advocacy

Before the recent wave of legalization, ethical consumerism largely took the form of lifestyle politics. People used their everyday consumption habits, leisure activities, modes of speech, and dress to challenge mainstream thinking about cannabis culture. The objective was to "normalize" cannabis consumption—and thus make it more challenging to sustain its prohibition—by highlighting that adult cannabis consumption is common, can occur in moderation, may address health issues, and does not preclude productivity or healthfulness (Erickson and Hathaway 2010; Hathaway, Comeau, and Erickson 2011).[6]

Ethical consumers purchased and displayed clothing, flags, doormats, and other goods featuring the cannabis leaf. Record shop owners proudly displayed pipes, bongs, and other paraphernalia in street-facing windows and point-of-purchase display cases. Celebrities, CEOs, and politicians "went public" about their own consumption. Thousands of people celebrated the unofficial US cannabis holiday of April 20th by consuming publicly—on college campuses, in parks, in front of capitol buildings, and even outside the White House. These activities reframed prohibition as antiquated and anti-social, turning the stigma against cannabis consumers on its head (Bennett 2018; Dioun 2018).

Post-Legalization Emergence of Ethical Purchasing

Legalization shifted the contours of political consumerism. First, in an uncoordinated effort, an ad hoc "buy legal" campaign emerged, highlighting the links between illegal cannabis, non-state armed conflict, border violence, and labor exploitation. Advocates compared black market cannabis to "blood diamonds" and asked, "How can you go and be very particular about buying only fair trade coffee and then go home and smoke dope that was produced by women who were being gang raped and kidnapped and murdered and all of that?" (Brekke 2015).

Second, the cannabis community shifted focus from legalization to regulatory debates. Growers, trimmers, distributors, and other supply-side actors, who were previously unable to disclose their roles in and perspectives about the industry, began developing a public presence. They voiced social and environmental concerns and shared information about their supply chains and sustainable production practices. In jurisdictions where the legal market was flooded with competing growers and dispensaries, ethical attributes also became a mode of differentiation. As described in the following sections, these changes generated consumer demand for ethical products and the development of cannabis-specific certification programs (Bennett 2018).

Consumer Demand for Ethical Products

A survey of dispensaries in Portland, Oregon (US), suggests that cannabis consumers are interested in ethical products. About 30% of dispensaries reported that consumers frequently requested environmentally friendly or socially responsible products and 50% reported occasional queries. Requests were more frequent in high-end dispensaries and in wealthier, White, and educated neighborhoods, which is consistent with demographic trends for other products (Bennett 2017). The study also identified several potential constraints to demand. First, people accustomed to purchasing illegally may not be in the habit of requesting supply chain information. Research shows that ingrained habits can interfere with adopting ethical purchasing practices for new products, even among consumers committed to ethical purchasing in other categories (Lyon, Ailshire, and Sehon 2014). Second, studies show that consumers "earmark" certain types of products as more (or less) important for ethical shopping than others. For example, coffee is more commonly earmarked than consumer electronics (Wheale and Hinton 2007). Several interviewees said that combining a "seedy" product with a "wholesome" practice feels uncomfortably paradoxical, and suggested organic cannabis would be as strange as Portland's vegan strip clubs would. Third, qualitative data suggested that consumers mistakenly assume that the sector's heavy regulation includes rigorous social and environmental standards, making ethical certifications unnecessary. Fourth, many Americans and Canadians (including several industry leaders interviewed) are ignorant about labor exploitation within their borders and believe fair trade is unnecessary for domestic goods (Guthman and Brown 2016). Finally, stereotypes about cannabis as a "natural drug" grown by "earth-loving hippies" may wrongly assuage consumers' concerns about sustainable production.

In other sectors, marketing materials and retail employees typically play a key role in framing ethical issues. In cannabis, these educational opportunities were often underutilized. For example, materials advertising the 2018 Cultivation Classic, a cannabis competition for "ethically-grown product free of pesticides," failed to explain the risks associated with conventional methods. Similarly, "eco" product packaging does little to educate consumers. Interviews suggest that people working in cannabis are reticent to critique an industry they have long defended, even if doing so would promote their objectives. Although budtenders can dramatically influence consumer choice, they have not proved to be a reliable source of information. In the Portland study, only 20% of dispensaries provided accurate information on social and environmental issues. The other 80% gave slightly inaccurate or significantly misinformed information. Incorrect information (such as all cannabis being organic, a myth propagated by 10% of dispensaries) can inhibit ethical purchasing in the sector (Bennett 2017).

Extending Organic, Fair Trade, and Sustainability Labels to Cannabis

Although the US and Canadian national organic labeling programs are somewhat similar, their approaches to cannabis labeling differ greatly. In Canada, small medical growers have been certified since 2003. In 2014, after Health Canada authorized large commercial operations, the CFIA/COR developed organic-specific standards. Shortly after, ECOCERT, an accredited auditor, certified the first large operation. In the United States, however, the USDA will not create a standard for a federally illegal substance. According to several organic auditors, growers have inquired about organic certification since the late 1990s. In the absence of a formal program, unofficial claims proliferated, and by 2015 a journalist asserted, "Walk into any marijuana dispensary in Portland, and you'll see jars of dried marijuana flowers and containers of marijuana concentrates labeled as organic" (Crombie

2015b). She found many growers were ill informed about organic methods. Lab tests revealed levels of pesticide residue above the threshold safe for consumption and exposed the use of chemicals—such as roach killer—not intended for human consumption (Crombie 2015a). Similarly, the Portland study found that although 86% of dispensaries offered an "ethical" product, 16% did not know why it was ethical and 64% said they simply trusted growers to "do the right thing."

Although there are several fair labor and sustainability certifications in Canada and the United States, none extend their programs to include cannabis. Although producers have reached out to express interest, the organizations fear that collaboration with the cannabis sector will jeopardize support from consumers or donors (Bennett 2017).

New Cannabis Certification Programs

In the United States and Canada, about a dozen standards-setting organizations have emerged to certify cannabis as "ethical."[7] While most voluntary certifications were established by nonprofits or business associations, cannabis labels were founded by individual entrepreneurs motivated to professionalize the sector; improve health, safety, or environmental regulations; bolster credibility of organic claims; or help growers differentiate their products. Clean Green, the first and most well-known certification program for cannabis, has captured much more of the market than have the other certification programs. Most cannabis certifications have standards for soil, energy, and water, and all are more focused on environmental issues than fair labor. Some are owner-operated, while more formal boards or multi-stakeholder advisory systems govern others. None of the certifications have successfully adopted best practices for ethical standards, such as a nonprofit structure, governance that minimizes conflicts of interest, third-party audits, publicly available standards, and processes that include workers in decision-making. Overall, sustainability certifications for cannabis are underdeveloped, are vulnerable, and lack credibility.

A 2018 study argues that these challenges are largely attributed to the lack of support cannabis certification programs have received from existing certifications, philanthropic organizations, consumer movement organizations, and individuals with relevant expertise. Without mentoring, training, financial support, and reputational incentives, cannabis certification programs are unlikely to engage in a "race to the top." Instead, they focus to stay afloat, move quickly, and increase market share. Experts can help by identifying front-runners, investing in them, and publicly recognizing their rigorous work (Bennett 2019).

Opportunities, Challenges, and Recommendations

The legalization of cannabis provides a special opportunity to apply lessons from other sectors and improve on their disappointing social and environmental results. Accordingly, activists have rallied around the idea of making cannabis "the first" to achieve a number of goals, such as proportional representation of women in leadership and prioritizing racial justice.

Several features of the cannabis sector make it particularly well suited for ethical consumerism. First, because cannabis is sold in a limited number of highly regulated retail spaces (or, in Canada, on websites), the consumer experience can be carefully crafted, regulated, and analyzed. Consumers are required, in most places, to interact with budtenders, providing an opportunity for point of purchase education. Budtenders are required (in most places) to keep detailed purchasing records, enabling dispensaries to track information about consumer habits. Market research firms have already developed sophisticated tools for understanding the cannabis consumer. Second, because cannabis is increasingly sold as "edibles," consumers accustomed to ethical purchasing of food may have an easier time earmarking cannabis for ethical consumption. Third, and related, as the markets for organic, fair trade, and biodynamic beer, wine, and liquor continue to grow, consumers may be better equipped to consider the supply chains behind adult consumption products. Finally, because many consumers are actively learning about new products and techniques for consuming cannabis and accessing research about the potential effects of cannabis, they may be more likely to access and internalize educational materials for it than for products with which they already feel familiar.

Ethical consumerism in cannabis also faces many challenges, although there are clear ways in which these can be overcome. First, budtenders, one of the key sources of consumer information, are often not knowledgeable about social and environmental issues or ethical products. The responsibility for providing consumers with accurate information rests not only on budtenders but also on the dispensaries that train them, the growers and processors that supply them, and the policy makers that regulate them. Budtenders should be required to earn credentials from an accredited provider. Second, there is very little information about what might be lost if consumers do not act responsibly. Industry actors need to be more forthcoming about the social and environmental impacts of cannabis cultivation and legalization. By highlighting concerns and educating the public, they motivate consumers to leverage their purchasing power. Third, sustainability advocates within the cannabis sector need support from experts from other industries. Cannabis organizations and businesses should bring environmental and labor advocates to key decision-making tables. Likewise, organizations with relevant expertise should offer their support to the new industry. Media can contribute by highlighting the positive contributions that non-cannabis leaders make in the sector and (more broadly) work to undermine the stigmas that discourage participation. These small shifts—informing budtenders, discussing social and environmental issues, and collaborating with experts—could generate meaningful impacts on ethical consumerism and, thus, communities and the environment.

Notes

1 "Semi-legal" refers to sectors in which consumption, production, and transaction activities all occur both legally and illegally, with many actors moving between legal and illegal markets or operating in both at the same time (Bennett 2017).
2 1961 Single Convention on Narcotic Drugs, 1971 Convention on Psychotropic Substances, and 1988 Convention Against Illicit Traffic in Narcotic Drugs and Psychotropic Substances.
3 Each year, about one in 100 US agricultural workers experiences acute pesticide poisoning (PAN 2010).
4 In some places, it is illegal to grow outdoors.
5 See, for example, the "International Guide to Fair Trade Labels."
6 "Normalization," in this context, refers to widespread acceptance, marked by easier access, higher consumption rates, and greater tolerance from non-consumers (Parker, Williams, and Aldridge 2002).
7 Including, in the United States: Cannabis Certification Council (CCC), Certified Kind, Clean Green, EnviroCan, Foundation of Cannabis Unified Standards (FOCUS), Patient Focused Certification (PFC), Resource Innovation Initiative (RII), Oregon Sungrown Certified, and The Cannabis Conservancy (TCC); and in Canada: National Institute for Cannabis Health and Education (CannabisWise).

References

August, Karen. 2013. "Women in the Marijuana Industry." *Humboldt Journal of Social Relations* 35: 89–103.

Auld, Graeme. 2014. *Constructing Private Governance: The Rise and Evolution of Forest, Coffee, and Fisheries Certification*. New Haven, CT: Yale University Press.

Bartley, Tim, Sebastian Koos, Hiram Samel, Gustavo Setrini, and Nik Summers. 2015. *Looking Behind the Label: Global Industries and the Conscientious Consumer*. Bloomington, IN: Indiana University Press.

Bauer, Scott, Jennifer Olson, Adam Cockrill, Michael Van Hattem, Linda Miller, Margaret Tauzer, and Gordon Leppig. 2015. "Impacts of Surface Water Diversions for Marijuana Cultivation on Aquatic Habitat in Four Northwestern California Watersheds." *PLoS One* 10 (3): 1–25.

Bennett, Elizabeth A. 2017. "Extending Ethical Consumerism Theory to Semi-Legal Sectors: Insights from Recreational Cannabis." *Agriculture and Human Values* 35 (2): 295–317.

———. 2018. "Prohibition, Legalization, and Political Consumerism: Insights from the US and Canadian Cannabis Markets." In *The Oxford Handbook of Political Consumerism*, edited by Magnus Boström, Michele Micheletti, and Peter Oosterveer. Oxford: Oxford University Press.

———. 2019. "Passing on Pot: When Environmental Organizations Disengage from Political Consumerism in Highly Stigmatized Sectors." *Environmental Politics* published online August 25.

Bossy, Sophie. 2014. "The Utopias of Political Consumerism: The Search of Alternatives to Mass Consumption." *Journal of Consumer Culture* 14 (2): 179–98.

Boström, Magnus, Michele Micheletti, and Peter Oosterveer. 2018. *The Oxford Handbook of Political Consumerism*. London: Oxford University Press.

Brekke, Kira. 2015. "'The Cartel' Author Don Winslow: It's Very Possible You're Smoking 'Blood Weed'." *Huffington Post*, July 17.

Brown, Keith. 2013. *Buying into Fair Trade: Culture, Morality and Consumption*. New York: New York University Press.

Carah, Jennifer K., Jeanette K. Howard, Sally E. Thompson, Anne G. Short Gianotti, Scott D. Bauer, Stephanie M. Carlson, David N. Dralle, et al. 2015. "High Time for Conservation: Adding the Environment to the Debate on Marijuana Liberalization." *BioScience* 65 (8): 822–29.

Crombie, Noelle. 2015a. "A Tainted High." *The Oregonian*, June 11.

———. 2015b. "Pot Buyers: Pretend 'Organic' Means?" *The Oregonian*, June 17.

Dioun, Cyrus. 2018. "Negotiating Moral Boundaries: Social Movements and the Strategic (Re)Definition of the Medical in Cannabis Markets." *Research in the Sociology of Organizations* 56: 53–82.

Erickson, Patricia G., and Andrew D. Hathaway. 2010. "Normalization and Harm Reduction: Research Avenues and Policy Agendas." *International Journal of Drug Policy* 21 (2): 137–39.

FJ (Farmworker Justice). 2015. "US Department of Labor Enforcement in Agriculture: More Must Be Done to Protect Farmworkers Despite Recent Improvements."

Forno, Francesca. 2015. "Bringing Together Scattered and Localized Actors: Political Consumerism as a Tool for Self-Organizing Anti-Mafia Communities." *International Journal of Consumer Studies* 39 (5): 535–43.

Guthman, Julie, and Sandy Brown. 2016. "I Will Never Eat Another Strawberry Again: The Biopolitics of Consumer-Citizenship in the Fight Against Methyl Iodide in California." *Agriculture and Human Values* 33 (3): 575–85.

Haenfler, Ross, Brett Johnson, and Ellis Jones. 2012. "Lifestyle Movements: Exploring the Intersection of Lifestyle and Social Movements." *Social Movement Studies* 11 (1): 1–20.

Hathaway, Andrew D., Natalie C. Comeau, and Patricia G. Erickson. 2011. "Cannabis Normalization and Stigma: Contemporary Practices of Moral Regulation." *Criminology and Criminal Justice* 11 (5): 451–69.

Krissman, Fred. 2016. "America's Largest Cannabis Labor Market." Humboldt State University Working Paper.

Lekakis, Eleftheria J. 2017. "Culture Jamming and Brandalism for the Environment: The Logic of Appropriation." *Popular Communication* 15 (4): 311–27.

Lyon, Sarah, Sara Ailshire, and Alexadra Sehon. 2014. "Fair Trade Consumption and the Limits to Solidarity." *Human Organization* 73 (2): 141–52.

MacKinnon, Shauna. 2013. "The National Organic Market: Growth, Trends, & Opportunities, 2013." Canada Organic Trade Association. https://ota.com/sites/default/files/indexed_files/COTA_NationalOrganicMarket Summary.pdf.

Mills, Evan. 2012. "The Carbon Footprint of Indoor *Cannabis* Production." *Energy Policy* 46: 58–67.

O'Hare, M., Daniel L. Sanchez, and Peter Alstone. 2013. "Environmental Risks and Opportunities in Cannabis Cultivation." *BOTEC Analysis Corporation*. Project #430–5d. Accessed March 7, 2017. https://lcb.wa.gov/publications/Marijuana/SEPA/BOTEC_Whitepaper_Final.pdf.

Otero, Gerardo, and Kerry Preibisch. 2015. "Citizenship and Precarious Labour in Canadian Agriculture." *Canadian Centre for Policy Alternatives: BC Office*. www.policyalternatives.ca/sites/default/files/uploads/publications/BC Office/2015/11/CCPA-BC_CitizenshipPrecariousLabourCdnAgri_web.pdf.

PAN AP (Pesticide Action Network Asia Pacific). 2010. "Communities in Peril: Global Report on Health Impacts of Pesticide Use in Agriculture." http://paninternational.org/wp-content/uploads/2013/12/PAN-Global-Report-communities-peril.pdf.

Parker, Howard, Lisa Williams, and Judith Aldridge. 2002. "The Normalization of 'Sensible' Recreational Drug Use: Further Evidence from the North West England Longitudinal Study." *Sociology* 36 (4): 941–64.

Pew Research Center. 2016. "Survey Questionnaire and Topline." *Pew Research Center's American Trends Panel.* http://assets.pewresearch.org/wp-content/uploads/sites/14/2017/02/01171104/PS_2017.02.02_vaccines_TOPLINE.pdf.

Raynolds, Laura T., and Elizabeth A. Bennett, eds. 2015. *The Handbook of Research on Fair Trade.* London: Edward Elgar.

Robertson, Grant. 2017. "Medical Marijuana; Ottawa Clamps Down on Growers." *The Globe and Mail,* February 10.

Schirmann, Kelly. 2016. "What It's Like to Be a 'Trim Bitch' on an Illegal Weed Farm." *Vice,* August 2. Accessed January 2, 2019. https://broadly.vice.com/en_us/article/what-its-like-to-be-a-trim-bitch-on-an-illegal-weed-farm-women-in-cannabis.

Stryker, Kitty, and Louise Pennington. 2014. "Can Porn Be Ethical?" *New Internationalist* March 2, 2014. https://newint.org/sections/argument/2014/03/01/argument-can-porn-be-ethical.

Voelker, Rodger, and Mowgli Holmes. 2015. "Pesticide Use on Cannabis." *White Paper, Cannabis Safety Institute.* https://cannabissafetyinstitute.org/wp-content/uploads/2015/06/CSI-Pesticides-White-Paper.pdf.

Wheale, Peter, and David Hinton. 2007. "Ethical Consumers in Search of Markets." *Business Strategy and the Environment* 16 (4): 302–15.

18

Zero Point Three

Current and Future Directions in the Political Economy of Medicinal Hemp

Noah Silber-Coats

Keywords: medicinal hemp, cannabinoids, agricultural policy, agrarian studies, legalization/illegalization

Introduction

Following passage of the 2018 Farm Bill in the U.S. Congress, media outlets touted the purported legalization of hemp (Lopez 2018). The declaration that "hemp is legal," however, fails to fully capture the complexity of the situation. Exactly what hemp is and the instances in which it can be considered legal both remain highly contested. This chapter unpacks the changing definition of hemp, situating recent developments within the history of cannabis prohibition, biomedical research, and an emerging quasi-legal market for hemp-derived alternative medicine and "wellness" products containing CBD (cannabidiol).

Hemp grown for CBD is quite different from the fiber and seed crop long understood as hemp. These new cultivars, which are being bred from "drug-type" progenitors, have expanded the definition of hemp. As a result, a better label for these plants might be "medicinal hemp" (Richmond and Clarke 2019).

The challenge of stabilizing the gene that determines whether cannabis will synthesize either the intoxicating Δ9-THC or the medicinally promising but little understood CBD—as well as the potential for plants to express these genes differently in response to environmental conditions[1]—creates a taxonomic mismatch between cannabis biology and newly redefined legal categories. Under federal law, cannabis that stays under the 0.3% THC[2] threshold is a legal commodity called "hemp" regulated by the Department of Agriculture (USDA), but a crop that exceeds this limit is a Schedule I controlled substance regulated by the Drug Enforcement Administration (DEA).

This puts the lie to the "legal" side of the equation—medicinal hemp is legal as long as it remains "hemp." The regulatory frameworks being constructed around hemp in the U.S. are concerned with measuring and eliminating THC—that is, they are driven by a prohibitionist focus on the arbitrary threshold of 0.3%.[3] And while commerce in medicinal hemp is growing fast—a recent survey of herbal supplement sales in the U.S. reports that CBD now makes up a greater share of this multi-billion dollar market than any other product (Smith et al. 2019)—a protracted struggle between

DOI: 10.4324/9780429320491-18

and within federal and state-level agencies in the U.S. over the legality of CBD consumer products continues to play out.

The central argument of this chapter is that the congressional mandate to treat hemp as a legal crop and commodity has provided stimulus to medicinal cannabis markets that are beyond the reach of regulated marijuana markets being constructed at the state level and that are as yet subject to little federal oversight. Paradoxically, "legalization" has allowed medicinal hemp products to circulate in a largely unregulated market.

As the market for medicinal hemp takes off, this chapter seeks to chart a course for the political economy of this phenomenon. After briefly expanding on the challenge of cannabis terminology and taxonomy, it provides a history of chemistry and pharmaceutical research with CBD. The following section situates hemp within prohibition policies and then explains the emergence of medicinal hemp as a legal crop. The chapter turns next to the geography of hemp production in the aftermath of the 2018 Farm Bill, drawing on ongoing research in Oregon. The final section outlines a set of key issues and proposes three areas in which social scientists might contribute to shaping these conversations.

What Is "Hemp"?

The botanical nomenclature of the genus *Cannabis* is convoluted, with debates continuing for more than two centuries.[4] In search of clarity, some authors have found it more illuminating to categorize the plant according to its intended use. These categories match well, if imperfectly, with taxonomies based on plant morphology, genetic, or chemical analysis.

Following Clark and Merlin (2013), there have historically been four broad types of cannabis. Populations isolated in the eastern Himalayan foothills during the last ice age contained the genetic code to synthesize Δ9-THC, while those in the Caucasus of western Eurasia lacked this feature. The latter group diffused into Europe and central Asia, where plants were selected for fiber and seed production. They term this group "narrow-leaf hemp."

The Himalayan population, which they call "narrow-leaf drug-type," was selected mainly for its intoxicating properties. A separate population of a different lineage flourished in the mountains of Afghanistan, the "broad-leaf drug-type." A fourth group, "broad-leaf hemp," was selected for fiber and food use across northeast Asia but is more closely related to the drug-type South Asian varieties than the western hemp.

Beginning in the 19th century, but especially since the 1960s, these categories have blurred. Outlaw cannabis "strainhunters" searched for promising genetic lines of both the narrow- and broad-leaf drug-types (vernacularly known as "sativa" and "indica," respectively) (Duvall 2016). These have become so widely interbred that they are best considered one group (ibid.; McPartland 2018). Following the Second World War, East Asian hemp cultivars were introduced into the European gene pool, so these too are best conceptualized as one category. "The present-day genetic distinction," according to Clarke and Merlin (2013, 402), "is essentially 'dope vs. rope.'"

High-CBD cannabis upends this taxonomy. By selecting for the CBD-synthesizing gene, lineages of drug-type cannabis have been repositioned relative to the "dope" category. In the scope of a legal definition concerned only with THC, these plants are grouped with fiber-food cannabis as "hemp." Because of this new twist, Clarke and Merlin's schema becomes unwieldy. We may continue to refer to fiber and seed cultivars as hemp, but how shall we distinguish this new "hemp" which is in fact the offspring of drug-type cannabis? Studies examining the phytochemistry of cannabis have suggested that plants with the CBD synthesizing gene "switched on" and the THC gene "off" could be described as "Type III/non-drug" (de Meijer et al. 1992; see Oregon CBD 2020). However, these schemes never considered that CBD would become a desired trait—its presence was merely an aide in differentiating fiber-seed hemp from drug-type cannabis (Small and Cronquist 1973).

Following these existing taxonomies, then, would result in a paradoxical term like "non-drug drug-type" cannabis. Richmond and Clarke (2019) gloss this more simply as "medicinal hemp," which this chapter adopts with some reservation. Rather than affirming or disputing the medicinal nature of various compounds found in cannabis, I suggest that the question of what these substances *are* ought not to be foreclosed: Is CBD medicinal? In what form, for what purposes, at what dose? If so, how widely available should it be? Is it a "necessary nutrient"[5] to be widely consumed, a drug to be carefully administered, or something else entirely (Hazekamp 2018)? The next section situates this unsettled debate in the context of chemical and pharmacological research on CBD.

Cannabinoid Chemistry and Pharmaceutical Research

Efforts to identify the psychoactive component of cannabis date to 19th-century Europe where the emerging discipline of chemistry collided with interest in the psychotropic fruits of colonial conquest—opium, coca, and "Indian hemp" (Mills 2003). In 1896, a group at Cambridge isolated a "resinous phenol" they called cannabinol or CBN (Mechoulam and Hanuš 2000). Building on this work six decades later, Israeli chemists described the structures of both Δ9-THC and CBD, identifying the former as the principal intoxicant in cannabis (Mechoulam and Shvo 1963). But identifying a molecule is not the same as understanding its physiological effects or how it achieves them. It was not until the 1980s that a group at St. Louis University led by Allyn Howlett identified a neurotransmitter in rat brains to which cannabinoids bind—the first breakthrough in the endocannabinoid system, now known to exist in all vertebrates (Elphick 2012).

Researchers then sought molecules produced endogenously within animal brains that stimulate these sensors. The Israeli group discovered and named the first of these—anandamide—which acts similarly to THC, creating a sense of euphoria as it binds to endocannabinoid receptors (Mechoulam and Hanuš 2000). Later research identified additional receptors linked to the immune system. These "tiny vibrating scanners perpetually primed to pick up biochemical cues" appear to regulate functions including pain, inflammation, appetite, bowel function, sleep, immune cell production, hormones, and mood (M. Lee 2012, 210).

Studies of the effects of CBD on non-human subjects suggest that it can work as an anti-oxidant, anti-psychotic, anti-anxiety, anti-inflammatory, anti-nausea, stimulant *or* sedative (with dose-dependent effects little understood). It *may* combat the pathologies of disorders like Alzheimer's, benefit diabetes patients, and support bone growth (Izzo et al. 2009). Such a wide profile of potential applications might have sparked a flurry of medical research, if not for a patent on CBD filed in 2003 by researchers at the National Institutes of Health. Despite the ostensible purpose of making the patent available for private sector research, it was licensed to only one company—New York–based Kannalife Sciences, Inc.—beginning in 2011 (Walker 2016).

With U.S. research limited, it is not entirely surprising that the first cannabinoid-based drug to receive FDA approval was developed in the U.K. GW Pharmaceuticals, which went public in 2001 and whose shareholders include a suite of wealth management and private equity firms (Kollewe 2011), markets two prescription drugs made from cannabis. Sativex, which contains both THC and CBD, is approved in the UK and around 25 other countries (U.S. approval pending) to treat symptoms of multiple sclerosis. Epidiolex, which is indicated to treat certain rare seizure disorders with only CBD as an active ingredient, became the first cannabis-derived drug to receive FDA approval in 2018. As GW works to roll out additional cannabinoid medications, its financial disclosures indicate operational losses but a steadily growing market cap as investors anticipate eventual gains of distribution deals with pharmaceutical giants like Bayer and Novartis (GW Pharmaceuticals 2011, 2019).

The increasingly wide availability of CBD products may appear to make a farce of GW's *de jure* monopoly, but the high price of these medications indicates that there are significant rents to be captured through this biopharmaceutical business model. Backed by strict quality controls and dosing recommendations derived from clinical trials, this model allows GW to claim a monopoly on physician-recommended CBD, for which Epidiolex patients (or their insurers) are billed $32,500 annually (Wood 2018).

Placing Hemp in Prohibition

Hemp (fiber/seed cannabis) was widely cultivated in the British American colonies of the 18th century, driven by the need of the Royal Navy for sailcloth and ship-rigging rope. U.S. hemp revivalists frequently reference its cultivation on the estates of George Washington and Thomas Jefferson as evidence of the plants' potential to consummate American greatness, though the role of enslaved workers is predictably ignored in these narratives (Bourrie 2003; Ventura 2016; Robinson 1996).[6]

Although production was already waning by the turn of the 20th century, hemp production plummeted following the Marihuana Tax Act of 1937, which required growers of any cannabis to hold a federal permit and pay a tax on their harvest. On the one hand, anti-"*marihuana*" propaganda constructed it as a dangerous drug, distinct from hemp. On the other hand, the difficulty in distinguishing harmful drug from legitimate crop effectively subsumed hemp into the former category, resulting in a restriction on all cannabis.[7]

During World War II, Congress subsidized hemp to stimulate production of fiber for naval cordage, which had of late been made from jute imported from plantations in parts of Southeast Asia under Japanese control.[8] But with the tax restored after the war, hemp fiber production declined again from a peak of 150 million pounds in 1943 to zero by the late 1950s (Johnson 2018, 12).

The blanket cannabis ban intensified under the Controlled Substances Act of 1970 (CSA), which listed "all parts of the plant *Cannabis sativa L.* Whether growing or not" under Schedule I—substances which have "no currently accepted medical use in the United States, a lack of accepted safety for use under medical supervision, and a high potential for abuse."

In the 1990s, some national governments loosened restrictions on hemp, made possible by the exemption of food and fiber uses of cannabis in the 1961 U.N. Single Convention on Narcotic Drugs. Advocates in Canada and the E.U. successfully lobbied for government-licensed production, while China's hemp crop[9]—licensed and otherwise—is now the world's largest (Chen 2017; Schluttenhofer and Yuan 2017; Small and Marcus 2002). In the U.S., however, the DEA firmly maintained its prohibitionist stance towards all cannabis, as enshrined in the Schedule of Controlled Substances.

Given this, efforts to distinguish "hemp" from "marijuana" in the U.S. shifted to agricultural policy. While several states passed laws allowing hemp production throughout the 1990s, changes at the federal level—which the states would need before acting on their plans—moved more slowly. A bipartisan group in Congress led by Ron Paul (R-TX) first introduced the Industrial Hemp Farming Act (IHFA) in 2005, which failed then and in subsequent sessions. It was not until 2014 that an amendment to the Farm Bill allowed for hemp "pilot programs" overseen by state departments of agriculture or research institutions (Johnson 2018). This has since been supplanted by the 2018 Farm Bill, to which a version of the IHFA—championed by senators from Kentucky and Oregon—was attached as an amendment. Under this framework, states (as well as tribes and territories) may submit plans to the USDA detailing licensing requirements, THC testing, and procedures for enforcing violations. As of this writing, 43 states[10] have approved such a plan, with market watchers predicting that the remaining seven will allow the crop by 2020 (Hemp Benchmarks 2019).

Since the USDA declined to respond to state and tribal plans while it underwent an internal rule-making process in 2019, those states that developed a hemp program were directed to operate under the guidance of the 2014 Farm Bill. The new interim rule—released on October 31, 2019, and in effect for the following two years[11]—significantly narrows the scope of what will be considered a legal hemp crop by mandating testing procedures that may make compliance with the 0.3% THC rule difficult for high-CBD hemp growers. Perhaps more than the details[12] of this policy, though, it is worth underscoring the singular focus on control of THC that motivates these guidelines. A naïve reader of this document wondering why the Hemp Production Program is so narrowly focused on this question will at last learn on the seventeenth page, "Because cannabis plants with a THC level higher than 0.3 are marijuana and on the Federal controlled substances list, ensuring that hemp produced under this program is not marijuana is of national significance" (Agricultural Marketing Service 2019, 58538).

While the 2018 Farm Bill allows production of cannabis under the 0.3% THC threshold, the FDA maintains that although "CBD seems to be everywhere," it is illegal to market as a "dietary supplement" or with "drug claims" (FDA 2019). These definitions have important implications: Though herbal dietary supplements are subject to considerably less oversight than pharmaceutical drugs—for instance, pre-market testing for safety is virtually unheard of—such products are still subject to numerous regulations and FDA enforcement actions (Brown 2017).

The possibility of treating ingestible CBD products as a food or dietary supplement—which the agency is considering following a public hearing in May 2019—is further complicated by its approval of Epidiolex as a prescription-only pharmaceutical. The question before the FDA now is whether to exercise its authority to grant an exception for the use of a pharmaceutical ingredient in food or dietary supplements.[13]

Though no new policy has yet been announced as a result of the May hearing, in a recent speech an FDA commissioner highlighted "serious concerns about issues like harmful contaminants such as pesticides, heavy metals, or other drugs like THC," noting that such issues "[put] the public at risk, and we are making it a significant enforcement priority for FDA" (Schiller 2019). States seeking to comply with FDA guidelines, including California and Washington, have recently banned the sale of ingestible CBD outside of licensed marijuana dispensaries (Herron 2019).[14]

While the 2018 Farm Bill marks a watershed in U.S. cannabis policy, the medicinal hemp phenomenon can also be traced to California's medical marijuana movement and market. To maximize returns in a high-risk venture, breeders operating in this gray market developed cannabis plants with dense clusters of high-THC flowers. When commercial labs first opened to serve medical dispensaries in 2008, they pinpointed plants displaying the high-CBD trait that had nearly been bred out of the gene pool. Nonprofit organizations Project CBD and the Society of Cannabis Clinicians formed the center of a movement promoting non-intoxicating cannabinoids as alternative medicine (Gardner 2009, 2010; Project CBD n.d.; Rendon 2012, 174).

Public awareness spiked in 2013 following the release of CNN's television documentary *Weed*, in which Dr. Sanjay Gupta narrates the story of Charlotte Figi, a Colorado child suffering from Dravet syndrome (a form of epilepsy), who showed remarkable improvement after her parents began treating her with CBD oil they made from cannabis purchased at a state-licensed marijuana dispensary (Gupta 2013). As this history suggests, and as the following discussion highlights, the medicinal hemp markets now booming originated in THC-centric cannabis commodity chains.

Emerging Geographies of U.S. Hemp Production

Even as the USDA scrambled to catch up to its mandate in the 2018 Farm Bill, production of medicinal hemp skyrocketed in 2019. The geography of this crop is fast changing, with production currently concentrated in four states: Colorado, Oregon, Kentucky, and Montana (Hemp Benchmarks June 2019).

In each of these contexts, hemp agriculture is shaped by regional agrarian structures that will provide fertile ground for further comparative research. In Montana's great plains, farmers are sowing extensive fields of hemp with CBD content typically under 5% (Hemp Benchmarks April 2019; Hathaway 2019). Kentucky lawmakers have been instrumental in promoting hemp as an alternative cash crop for tobacco growers facing a declining market (K. Lee 2019). Illustrative of the tension between legal and illegal cannabis crops in this context, the Kentucky Department of Agriculture maintains a list of approved varieties, which include medicinal hemp strains like "Special Sauce," while also flagging prohibited and "varieties of concern" that have exceeded the 0.3% threshold.

In contrast to these states, where high-THC cannabis is prohibited or restricted, Colorado has fostered medicinal hemp alongside legalization of "recreational marijuana." Colorado's Department of Agriculture was the first to launch a hemp seed certification program, testing for 0.3% compliance across the state's eco-regions (Nichols 2017). Though reliable figures on the capacity to produce cannabinoid extracts from medicinal hemp biomass are not available, anecdotal reports point to Colorado as a leader in this area as well (Mitchell 2019).

Production of medicinal hemp in California, where interest in CBD first emerged a decade ago, seems to be limited in 2019. The state's agriculture department approved a hemp plan in May, but several counties maintain restrictions on cultivation—including the "Emerald Triangle" of the north coast long known for cannabis, and the agricultural powerhouses of the Central Valley (Thorne 2019).

But while the Emerald Triangle typically refers to Humboldt, Mendocino, and Trinity Counties of Northern California, cannabis growers in southern Oregon insist this region is the Triangle's northern tip. Sheltered from coastal fog by the Siskiyou Mountains and somewhat insulated from the domestic drug war being waged in California under the Campaign Against Marijuana Planting (Corva 2014), a highly productive outdoor cannabis sector has taken shape here.

When Oregon voters passed Measure 91 legalizing recreational marijuana in 2014, southern Oregon already had a long history in cannabis production. Along with Northern California, back-to-the-landers began cultivating the plant here in the 1960s (Brown 1995). Oregon's early adoption of medical marijuana in 1998 led to a proliferation of small farms—over 30,000 grow sites were registered across the state in 2015 (Oregon Health Authority 2015). Following Measure 91, Oregon sought to bring these growers into the licensed recreational system—where plants would be tracked and revenue taxed—and to restrict market access for those who were unable or refused to transition.

Legalization of hemp in Oregon actually dates to 2009, well before the recreational marijuana law. The Oregon Department of Agriculture (ODA), however, did not move forward with issuing hemp permits until launching a pilot program under the 2014 Farm Bill guidelines. Even when this program began with only 13 permits in 2015, it was the subject of controversy in the state capitol, where a bill imposing a hemp moratorium narrowly failed in the senate (Sliwosky 2015). Marijuana growers advocated for this policy, seeing hemp as a material threat—a broad acreage sown with cannabis is likely to contain male plants that many fear could pollinate female flowers, causing cannabinoid content to plummet as these molecules are metabolized in the process of producing seeds. In 2017, when Douglas County attempted to impose a hemp moratorium (in this case motivated by a general anti-cannabis stance), the ODA insisted that it *would* approve licenses in the county and that such local restrictions violate the state's Right to Farm law (Perkowski 2017). Though this attracted little notice at the time, it cemented ODA's reversal from reluctant regulator to industry champion.

As investment flowed into production for the recreational marijuana market, the fall harvests in 2017 and 2018 brought a glut of cannabis (Oregon Liquor Control Commission 2019). Growers report that the farm-gate price fell from a one-time high of $3,000/lb to as low as $200 (author interviews; Stangle and Sheperd 2018). This meant that those who had transitioned into the new market faced both additional costs and reduced revenue, while those who did not transition had no outlet other than black markets.

Against this background, medicinal hemp has emerged as an alternative for many experienced growers. One producer licensed for Oregon's recreational marijuana market reported shifting 85% of production to high-CBD strains, which growers and brokers say are fetching upwards of $1,000/lb for "top-shelf" smokable flower. The plants grown for this purpose emphasize many of the same characteristics desired by marijuana consumers, other than THC—as one medicinal hemp broker put it, "terpy, super-stacked, frosty buds."[15] Another broker described his market as "I can't believe it's not marijuana."

Several sources with experience in both the black market and the licensed recreational market have suggested that some "hemp" growers are using their ODA permit as cover to grow high-THC plants that still command higher prices on the East Coast, though the extent of this is unknown. And while some raise concerns about marijuana masquerading as hemp in the field, the inverse is also raising alarms—actors in the black market have suggested that hemp is being pawned off on pot dealers as high-THC cannabis.[16]

Data from the ODA indicate over 60,000 acres registered for hemp production across the state in 2019, 13,000 of which are in the southern counties of Jackson and Josephine. These counties also record over three million square feet of greenhouse cultivation, about 40% of the statewide total. While one company accounts for over a third of this, the majority of the over 200 greenhouse growers have registered 5,000 square feet or less. The sudden appearance of so many small-scale "greenhouses" likely reflects planting of medicinal hemp in the tarp-covered hoop houses that many growers here use to force-flower cannabis on a shortened production timeline by using the "light deprivation" technique.[17]

With "hemp" the most extensively cultivated crop in Jackson County as of 2019 (Rubin 2019), these ventures are not limited to those with cannabis experience. To take one example, the owner of a specialty grocery store who planted medicinal hemp for the first time in 2018 grew 100 acres on land leased at $1,000/acre in 2019. He estimates the total cost—including rent, field preparation, drip irrigation, and seeds—at around $25,000/acre with revenue forecast at over $200,000/acre.

These wide margins drove significant land use change in the Rogue Valley in 2019, as would-be hemp planters rushed to lease fallow land, hay fields, and even pear orchards from landowners eager for extra income. Many of these are small relative to the hemp fields of other regions—ODA records show the median acreage for southern Oregon at 6.4, often divided between multiple fields.[18] But even such relatively limited production is untethered to the limitations of licensed THC cannabis, where both cultivation space and the legal market are restricted. With these restrictions removed, several entities are investing in production, as well as facilities, to dry, store, and extract cannabinoids from large volumes of medicinal hemp. However, local interviews indicate that the capacity for processing this year's crop is far behind production.

While it is too early to identify the winners and losers of this boom, it is apparent that medicinal hemp will continue to be the focus of a scramble for capital accumulation. In the following section, I propose three areas in which social science scholars will be well positioned to provide insights to interpret and shape this phenomenon.

Future Directions for the Political Economy of Medicinal Hemp

This concluding section outlines several areas for future inquiry into developing medicinal hemp markets. The first subsection draws lessons from agrarian political economy and commodity studies to point toward processes that tend to subordinate farmers to the exigencies of capital. This is not meant to be predictive of any predetermined outcome but rather suggestive of possibilities. The second subsection returns to the definitional challenge, calling for continued exploration of the actual practice of determining what counts as hemp—decisions which have far-reaching consequences for defining the boundary between legal and illegal markets and the profits to be derived from them. The third part turns to consumption—an area that has been underrepresented in this largely production-focused chapter. As CBD becomes ever more widely available, there is an urgent need for work that critically interrogates the interplay of profit motive, discourses and practices of alternative medicine, and individual decisions to consume this cannabinoid.

First the Seed, Then the Shelf

Agrarian political economy suggests that farming typically offers low returns that drive capital up- and downstream of production (Mann 1990; Friedmann 1978; Page 1996). While medicinal hemp may offer multimillion-dollar profits to early adopters, prices may soon fall with rising production. As margins tighten, efforts to capture value will likely focus on enclosing genetic resources (upstream) and on processing and retail (downstream).

Efforts to "improve" and claim ownership of plant genetics are central to the commodification of farming (Kloppenburg 2005). The recent consolidation of seed production and ownership of genetic resources as intellectual property by agrochemical firms illustrates the direction that such developments may take (Howard 2015).

So far, key actors in the medicinal hemp seed industry appear to be former "outlaw" cannabis breeders who have shifted their efforts to developing low-THC/high-CBD cultivars. What direction will cannabis breeding and ownership of genetics take as land grant universities and corporate agrichemical/seed giants enter this arena? Already, unique partnerships are emerging in this area, as evidenced by a recent $1 million donation from Oregon CBD—a company founded by self-taught black-market cannabis breeders—to support the Global Hemp Innovation Center at Oregon State University (Plaven 2019).

Efforts to enclose cannabis genetics are already underway, including a patent recently awarded to New West Genetics of Colorado for "industrial hemp cannabis cultivars and seeds with stable cannabinoid profiles."[19] Following the ways in which value circulates around the seed will be an important area for future research. Moreover, scholars might seek to foster initiatives that support equitable access to genetic resources through open-source breeding (Luby et al. 2015).[20]

Sinking investment into manufacturing processes that convert crops into uniform outputs is another way in which capital extracts value from agriculture (Goodman, Sorj, and Wilkinson 1987; Fitzsimmons 1986). Since most agricultural commodity chains are buyer driven (Gereffi, Korzenievicz, and Korzenievicz 1994; Bair 2009), there is every reason to expect that medicinal hemp may follow a similar trend. Along the lines of Burch and Lawrence's (2013) labeling of grocery retailers as "masters of the food system," who will emerge as the "masters of the CBD system"?

The transformation of CBD from an alternative medicine promoted by word of mouth to a mass-marketed consumer good is perhaps best illustrated by Charlotte's Web, the Colorado company that gained notoriety with CNN's *Weed* in 2013. The self-proclaimed "#1 brand by market share," now traded on the Toronto Stock Exchange, predicts that the future of the CBD market is in retail chain stores. Positioning itself for growth in this area, the company boasts of a CPG (consumer packaged goods) team of executives formerly employed by corporations like Proctor and Gamble, Kellogg's, and Coca-Cola (Charlotte's Web 2019).

In other ways, too, legalized medicinal hemp is colliding with practices common in agriculture that redistribute risk and create new opportunities for speculation. Scholars who view markets as embedded in social processes (Polanyi 2001 [1944]) will find hemp to be a fruitful arena to explore the practices of "economists in the wild" (Çalışkan and Callon 2010) working to establish commodity futures and other links to financial capital (see Cronon 1991; Freidberg 2017).

Another practice emerging for the first time in cannabis is contract farming. In these arrangements, a contractor supplies inputs, dictates production practices, and buys the crop at a set price. Contract farming—which became widespread throughout global food chains beginning in the 1990s—is notorious for converting growers into "little more than propertied laborers" in constantly intensifying production systems (Little and Watts 1994, 34; Narotzky 2016). Such critiques notwithstanding, a Colorado hemp company called Garden Om is promising "ethical contract farming." As cannabis contract farming becomes better established, researchers could evaluate its varied forms and outcomes.

"What Is Hemp?" Revisited: Defining and Translating Standards

Because the same cannabis plant may now be seen by the state as either an agricultural commodity whose commerce is protected[21] or a dangerous drug that must be destroyed, the rules for testing and verifying the legality of crops will continue to be highly contested.

How exactly "0.3% THC" will be defined[22] and enforced is a thorny question that could be illuminated by multisited ethnographic work that draws on the field of science, technology, and society (STS) to follow the formation and translation of standards across regulatory agencies, laboratories, and cannabis fields (see for instance Latour 2005; Bijker 2001; Mutersbaugh 2005). The USDA interim rule complicates rather than resolves this question. As the guidelines state, "the issue of providing assurance as to proper testing" will continue to be negotiated through formation of standards, and possibly a hemp-specific Laboratory Approval Program[23] (Agricultural Marketing Service 2019, 58525).

The contrast between legal definitions of "marijuana" and "hemp" and the material realities of cannabis will also play out in spatial conflicts over cultivation of different varieties and the flow of genes between them. For producers of cannabis flower, pollination can ruin a crop by causing the plants to produce seed, thereby lowering cannabinoid content. With extensive cultivation of medicinal hemp, the possibility of a rogue male plant pollinating nearby crops becomes increasingly likely. Such conflicts will be most acute in regions with both legalized outdoor or greenhouse "marijuana" cultivation and an emerging "hemp" sector (e.g. parts of Oregon, Colorado, and California).

The CBD-Consuming Subject

Another area begging for additional exploration is the consumption of non-intoxicating cannabinoids. We lack even basic information about the geographic distribution and demographics of CBD users. As market makers predict that U.S. CBD sales could grow to anywhere from $6 to $22 billion in the coming years (Johnson 2019), we might ask: Who is consuming CBD? How and why do individuals become CBD-consuming subjects? How is this consumption co-produced by marketing strategies? And in what ways are these subjectivities shaped by gendered, racialized, and classed notions of wellness and self-care?

Such an approach to CBD could be a valuable contribution to critical discussions of wellness (Kirkland 2014). The marketing of CBD for pet health[24] could likewise be analyzed through the lens of "critical pet studies" that considers the intertwining of affective devotion to animals with practices and spaces of consumption and commodification (Nast 2006a, 2006b).

There are complex ethico-political issues to be explored in this area. On the one hand, CBD may provide real health benefits for patients whose needs are not being met through conventional means. On the other hand, this challenge to medical expertise has also created an opening for "unscrupulous actors peddling crooked, corrupt, and contaminated products" (Gupta 2019). As scholarship on this topic continues to grow, it will hopefully shed light on the tensions inherent in negotiating the status of hemp and CBD.

Notes

1 For instance, THC levels have been shown to increase with greater exposure to UV-B radiation at higher altitudes (Lydon, Teramura, and Coffman 1987).

2 The complete definition from the 2018 Farm Bill reads as follows:

> the plant *Cannabis sativa* L. and any part of that plant, including the seeds thereof and all derivatives, extracts, cannabinoids, isomers, acids, salts, and salts of isomers, whether growing or not, with a delta-9 tetrahydrocannabinol concentration of not more than 0.3 percent on a dry weight basis.

3 0.3% THC is used in the definition of hemp in the U.S. and Canada, as well as China. The European Union uses a 0.2% threshold, though industry groups are clamoring for an increase to 0.3% (see https://eiha.org/cap-reform/). Switzerland, which is not part of the EU, has adopted a 1% threshold (Zobel 2019). Rules in Australia vary by state, with 0.35% and 1% adopted in different jurisdictions (Hemptoday, August 26, 2018). In Latin America, Uruguay—the first country to legalize and regulate "recreational" cannabis—defines "non-psychoactive" cannabis as less than 1% THC and regulates this crop separately from marijuana. Colombia, which regulates hemp under the umbrella of medical marijuana, also uses 1% THC as a threshold across which a different set of rules apply. Other Latin American nations that have recently implemented legalized medical marijuana (Argentina, Chile, Peru, Ecuador, and Costa Rica) appear to follow Colombia's approach to regulating medicinal cannabis as one category with minor distinctions based on THC content. For instance, in Costa Rica, recently proposed legislation would create separate regulatory structures for medicinal cannabis (THC *and/or* CBD) and food/fiber cannabis, rather than using THC content as a determinant (Thompson 2019).

4 A fuller account of the botanical taxonomy of *Cannabis* is not possible here. Suffice to say, this is a debate that encompasses seminal figures in botany and ethnobotany from the 18th to the 20th century, including Linnaeus, Lamarck, Vavilov, and Shultes (Duvall 2015). Competing positions in this debate are presently represented by Robert Clarke and John McPartland (see Clarke and Merlin 2013; McPartland 2018).

5 Exhemplary Life (www.exhemplarylife.com/about-us) is not alone in making such claims.

6 A much less well-known hemp economy, also underpinned by slave labor, flourished in the missions of Spanish California around the turn of the 19th century (Mosk 1939).

7 On this history of this act, see Earleywine (2002) and Hashim (2017).

8 The 1942 film *Hemp for Victory* produced by the USDA (whose existence was later denied by the government [Robinson 1996, 161]) has provided further fodder for the "patriotic hemp" narrative. The original film can now be seen at www.youtube.com/watch?v=d3rolyiTPr0

9 Although China is the clear global leader in fiber hemp, Chinese CBD is also widely available. Chinese e-commerce site Ali Baba advertises pure CBD isolate in the range of $5,000–$7,000 per kilogram. Any future studies on Chinese hemp/CBD exports and their relationship to newly forming domestic hemp economies would be most welcome.

10 The adoption of hemp plans by tribal entities is less easily indexed, though one case may be emblematic of conflicts between tribal, federal, and state authority to come. The Flandreau Santee Sioux Tribe, whose territory is located within South Dakota (which has no hemp program), has sued the USDA for refusing to approve the tribe's plan. A federal district court ruled against the tribe, saying that the USDA is not obligated to act until its own rule-making process is complete (Kelly Drye and Warren LLP 2019).

11 However, states with a program under the 2014 Farm Bill may choose to continue their program under this authority through 2021. For an approximate idea of which states this includes, see Nichols (2017). In fall 2021, USDA will issue its revised final rule, and by 2022 all states/tribes/territories will be mandated to operate under these guidelines (Agricultural Marketing Service 2019).

12 Significant provisions in the interim rule include requiring that labs conducting THC tests must be registered with the DEA. There is no obvious way to even identify such labs, and industry participants in Oregon have said they know of only one. In addition, testing protocols call for taking the top two inches of flowering tops—which have the highest cannabinoid content. Current rules in Oregon test the top eight inches, while the study that originated the 0.3% figure tested "vigorous young leaves" (Small and Cronquist 1976). The rule does provide flexibility for test results that slightly exceed 0.3%, requiring that lab reports include a confidence interval—a result over 0.3% but within the margin of error will be considered compliant. It also specifies that a noncompliant crop up to 0.5% will be destroyed, but its owner would not be considered to have committed a "negligent violation."

13 Such an exception is usually reserved for substances that were marketed before they were ever approved or studied as drugs. Even though the first clinical trial for Epidiolex began in 2013—several years after CBD was first marketed in California—the FDA has determined that an exception will not be made in this way. The "notice-and-comment" rulemaking process, of which the May 2019 hearing was a part, is a separate channel which *could* result in an exception (Schiller 2019).

14 For a state-by-state guide to CBD retail laws in 2019, see https://plantpeople.co/cbd-legal-states/

15 "Terpy" refers to volatile aromatic oils called terpenes; "stacked" means dense or "chunky" flowers; "frosty" refers to the trichomes (tiny glandular hairs) that coat the flowers, where the highest concentration of cannabinoids is to be found.

16 See @theblacklistxyz on Instagram, October 16, 2019: "the drought is coming . . . it'll be catastrophic . . . watch out for hemp buds disguised as THC buds."

17 See the Instagram account @541pineapplewellness for an example of intensively cultivated "[light] dep hemp."
18 As a point of comparison, mean acreage for Montana hemp growers in 2019 was 217 (Rose 2019).
19 Patent number US 2019/0230882.
20 See the recent controversy over the now-defunct Open Cannabis Project and its relationship plant breeding firm Phylos for a cautionary note on undertaking such work (Hymes 2019).
21 The 2018 Farm Bill directs sub-federal entities not to interfere in interstate hemp commerce. In the meantime, high-profile seizures of hemp shipments have taken place in Idaho, Kansas, and Oklahoma.
22 Cannabinoid content increases throughout the plant's life cycle and varies within different parts of the plant and throughout a population. The wording of the Farm Bill applies the 0.3% standard to concentrates and extracts as well, meaning that a legal plant can be used to produce an illegal extract. Finally, different testing methods produce different results. See Kight (2018).
23 On LAPs see www.ams.usda.gov/services/lab-testing/lab-approval
24 You can now buy CBD for your pet from Willie Nelson, just one of many companies in what one market research firm predicts will grow to $1.7 billion in consumer spending by 2023 (Schau 2019; www.willies-rescue.com).

References

Agricultural Marketing Service. 2019. "Establishment of a Domestic Hemp Production Program." *Federal Register* 84 (211): 58522–64.

Bair, Jennifer, ed. 2009. *Frontiers of Commodity Chain Research*. Stanford, CA: Stanford University Press.

Bijker, W. 2001. "Sociohistorical Technology Studies." In *Handbook of Science and Technology Studies*, edited by S. Jasanoff, G. Markel, J. Peterson, and T. Pinch, 229–56. Sage.

Brown, Amy Christine. 2017. "An Overview of Herb and Dietary Supplement Efficacy, Safety and Government Regulations in the United States with Suggested Improvements. Part 1 of 5 Series." *Food and Chemical Toxicology* 107 (September): 449–71. https://doi.org/10.1016/j.fct.2016.11.001.

Brown, Beverly A. 1995. *In Timber Country: Working People's Stories of Environmental Conflict and Urban Flight*. Philadelphia: Temple University Press.

Bourrie, M. 2003. *Hemp: A Short History of the Most Misunderstood Plant and Its Uses and Abuses*. Richmond Hill, ON: Firefly Books.

Burch, David, and Geoffrey Lawrence. 2013. "Financialization in Agri-Food Supply Chains: Private Equity and the Transformation of the Retail Sector." *Agriculture and Human Values* 30 (2): 247–58.

Çalışkan, Koray, and Michel Callon. 2010. "Economization, Part 2: A Research Programme for the Study of Markets." *Economy and Society* 39 (1): 1–32.

Charlotte's Web. 2019. "*Investor Presentation: Building a Global CPG Company*." October. https://s22.q4cdn.com/636117063/files/doc_presentations/2019/09/CWEB_Oct2_2019-Canaccord-Presentation-Print.pdf.

Chen, Stephen. 2017. "Green Gold: How China Quietly Grew into a Cannabis Superpower." *South China Morning Post*, August 17. Accessed September 18, 2019. www.scmp.com/news/china/society/article/2108347/green-gold-how-china-quietly-grew-cannabis-superpower.

Clarke, Robert Connell, and Mark David Merlin. 2013. *Cannabis: Evolution and Ethnobotany*. Berkeley: University of California Press.

Corva, Dominic. 2014. "Requiem for a CAMP: The Life and Death of a Domestic U.S. Drug War Institution." *International Journal of Drug Policy* 25 (1): 71–80.

Cronon, W. 1991. *Nature's Metropolis: Chicago and the Great West*. New York, NY: WW Norton & Company.

de Meijer, E. P. M. de, H. J. van der Kamp, and F. A. van Eeuwijk. 1992. "Characterisation of Cannabis Accessions with Regard to Cannabinoid Content in Relation to Other Plant Characters." *Euphytica* 62 (3): 187–200.

Drye, Kelly, and Warren LLP. 2019. "Court Rules Indian Tribe Cannot Regulate Hemp Production (Yet)." *JDSupra*, June 19, 2019. Accessed May 2, 2021. https://www.jdsupra.com/legalnews/court-rules-indian-tribe-cannot-91549/.

Duvall, Chris S. 2015. *Cannabis*. London: Reaktion Books.

———. 2016. "Drug Laws, Bioprospecting and the Agricultural Heritage of *Cannabis* in Africa." *Space and Polity* 20 (1): 10–25.

Earleywine, M. 2002. *Understanding Marijuana: A New Look at the Scientific Evidence.* Oxford: Oxford University Press.

Elphick, Maurice R. 2012. "The Evolution and Comparative Neurobiology of Endocannabinoid Signalling." *Philosophical Transactions: Biological Sciences* 367 (1607): 3201–15.

FitzSimmons, Margaret. 1986. "The New Industrial Agriculture: The Regional Integration of Specialty Crop Production." *Economic Geography* 62 (4): 334.

Food and Drug Administration. 2019. "*What You Need to Know (And What We're Working to Find Out) About Products Containing Cannabis or Cannabis-Derived Compounds, Including CBD.*" Accessed July 17, 2019. www.fda.gov/consumers/consumer-updates/what-you-need-know-and-what-were-working-find-out-about-products-containing-cannabis-or-cannabis.

Freidberg, Susanne. 2017. "Trading in the Secretive Commodity." *Economy and Society* 46 (3–4): 499–521.

Friedmann, Harriet. 1978. "World Market, State, and Family Farm: Social Bases of Household Production in the Era of Wage Labor." *Comparative Studies in Society and History* 20 (4): 545–86.

Gardner, Fred. 2009. "CBD-rich Cultivars Becoming Available to Patients as Lab Starts Testing MJ for Pathogens and Cannabinoids." *O'Shaughnessy's: The Journal of Cannabis in Clinical Practice* (Summer). www.beyondthc.org.

———. 2010. "Doctors to Study Effectiveness of CBD." *O'Shaughnessy's: The Journal of Cannabis in Clinical Practice* (Summer). www.beyondthc.org.

Gereffi, G., M. Korzenievicz, and R. P. Korzenievicz. 1994. "Introduction: Global Commodity Chains." In *Commodity Chains and Global Capitalism*, edited by G. Gereffi and M. Korzeniewicz, 1–14. Westport, CT: Praeger Publishers.

Goodman, D., B. Sorj, and J. Wilkinson. 1987. *From Farming to Biotechnology: A Theory of Agro-Industrial Development.* New York: Basil Blackwell.

Gupta, S. 2013. "Why I Changed My Mind on Weed." *CNN*, August 8. Accessed September 30, 2019. www.cnn.com/2013/08/08/health/gupta-changed-mind-marijuana/index.html.

———. 2019. "Dr. Sanjay Gupta on Medical Marijuana: We Are in an Age of Wisdom, but also an Age of Foolishness." *CNN*, October 11. Accessed October 16, 2019. www.cnn.com/2019/09/27/health/weed-5-cbd-craze-gupta/index.html.

GW Pharmaceuticals. 2011. "GW Signs Exclusive License Agreement to Commercialise Sativex in Australia, Asia, Middle-East and Africa." *Press Release*, Accessed August 19, 2019. https://web.archive.org/web/20120731031422/http://gwpharm.com/GW%20Signs%20Exclusive%20Licence%20Agreement%20to%20Commercialise%20Sativex%20in%20Australia%20Asia%20Middle%20East%20and%20Africa.aspx.

———. 2019. "Annual General Meeting, June 13, 2019." (presentation). Accessed August 19, 2019. http://ir.gwpharm.com/static-files/0dbd227a-910f-470f-95a5-fc8d02e48604.

Hathaway, Joel. 2019. "The New Faces of Hemp: Traditional ag bets big in Montana." *Hemp*, February 11. https://thehempmag.com/2019/02/traditional-agriculture-montana-hemp/.

Hashim, N. O. 2017. *Hemp and the Global Economy: The Rise of Labor, Innovation, and Trade.* Lanham, MD: Lexington Books.

Hazekamp, Arno. 2018. "The Trouble with CBD Oil." *Medical Cannabis and Cannabinoids* 1 (1): 65–72. https://doi.org/10.1159/000489287.

Hemp Benchmarks. 2019. "U.S. Wholesale Hemp Price Benchmarks." June. www.hempbenchmarks.com.

Hemptoday. 2018. "Australian State Cites Job Creation in Raising THC Limit to a Full 1%." *Hemptoday.net*, August 26. Accessed November 8, 2019. https://hemptoday.net/wa-raises-thc-limit/.

Herron, Elise. 2019. "After Washington State Ban, Oregon Becomes the Last West Coast State Where Consumers Can Buy CBD-Infused Food and Beverages." *Willamette Week*, August 29, 2019. Accessed April 29, 2021. https://www.wweek.com/news/2019/08/29/after-washington-state-ban-oregon-becomes-the-last-west-coast-state-where-consumers-can-buy-cbd-infused-food-and-beverages/.

Howard, Philip H. 2015. "Intellectual Property and Consolidation in the Seed Industry." *Crop Science* 55: 1–7.

Hymes, Tom. 2019. "The Phylos Affair." *Future Cannabis Project*, May 2019. http://futurecannabisproject.org/2019/05/phylos-breeding-genetics-patents-ip-cannabis/.

Izzo, Angelo A., Francesca Borrelli, Raffaele Capasso, Vincenzo Di Marzo, and Raphael Mechoulam. 2009. "Non-Psychotropic Plant Cannabinoids: New Therapeutic Opportunities from an Ancient Herb." *Trends in Pharmacological Sciences* 30 (10): 515–27.

Johnson, Reneé. 2018. "Hemp as an Agricultural Commodity." *Congressional Research Service*. Accessed April 29, 2021. https://fas.org/sgp/crs/misc/RL32725.pdf.

———. 2019. "Hemp-Dervied Cannabidiol (CBD) and Related Hemp Extracts." *Congressional Research Service: In Focus*, June 21, 2019. Accessed May 2, 2021. https://crsreports.congress.gov/product/pdf/IF/IF10391.

Kight, Rod. 2018. "Hemp Testing 101: Analytical Testing Protocols Explained and Evaluated." *Kight on Cannabis*, December 3. Accessed October 16, 2019. https://cannabusiness.law/hemp-testing-101-analytical-testing-protocols-explained-and-evaluated/.

Kirkland, A. 2014. "What Is Wellness Now?" *Journal of Health Politics, Policy and Law* 39 (5): 957–70.

Kloppenburg, Jack Ralph. 2005. *First the Seed: The Political Economy of Plant Biotechnology*. Madison: University of Wisconsin Press.

Kollewe, Julia. 2011. "The Man Who Secretly (and Legally) Grows 20 Tonnes of Cannabis a Year." *The Guardian*, April 16, 2011. Accessed April 29, 2021. https://www.theguardian.com/business/2011/apr/17/gw-pharmaceuticals-justin-gover-cannabis-sativex-multiple-sclerosis.

Latour, Bruno. 2005. *Reassembling the Social-an Introduction to Actor-Network-Theory*. New York: Oxford University Press.

Lee, Kurtis. 2019. "Must Reads: As Tobacco Sales Dry Up, Kentucky Farmers Look to the State's 'Original Crop'—Hemp." *Los Angeles Times*, February 12, 2019. Accessed April 29, 2021. https://www.latimes.com/nation/la-na-kentucky-hemp-farmers-20190212-story.html.

Lee, Martin A. 2012. *Smoke Signals: A Social History of Marijuana-Medical, Recreational and Scientific*. New York, NY: Scribner.

Little, Peter D., and Michael Watts, eds. 1994. *Living Under Contract: Contract Farming and Agrarian Transformation in Sub-Saharan Africa*. Madison: University of Wisconsin Press.

Lopez, German. 2018. "Trump and Congress Just Legalized Hemp." *Vox*, December 20, 2018. Accessed April 29, 2021. https://www.vox.com/policy-and-politics/2018/12/12/18136408/hemp-marijuana-legalization-trump-congress-farm-bill.

Lydon, John, Alan H. Teramura, and C. Benjamin Coffman. 1987. "UV-B Radiation Effects on Photosynthesis, Growth and Cannabinoid Production of Two Cannabis Sativa Chemotypes." *Photochemistry and Photobiology* 46 (2): 201–6.

Luby, Claire H., Jack Kloppenburg, Thomas E. Michaels, and Irwin L. Goldman. 2015. "Enhancing Freedom to Operate for Plant Breeders and Farmers Through Open Source Plant Breeding." *Crop Science* 55 (6): 2481.

Mann, Susan. 1990. *Agrarian Capitalism in Theory and Practice*. Chapel Hill: UNC Press Books.

McPartland, John M. 2018. "Cannabis Systematics at the Levels of Family, Genus, and Species." *Cannabis and Cannabinoid Research* 3 (1): 203–12.

Mechoulam, Raphael, and Lumír Hanuš. 2000. "A Historical Overview of Chemical Research on Cannabinoids." *Chemistry and Physics of Lipids* 108 (1–2): 1–13.

Mechoulam, Raphael, and Y. Shvo. 1963. "Hashish—I: The Structure of Cannabidiol." *Tetrahedron* 19 (12): 2073–78.

Mills, James H. 2003. *Cannabis Britannica: Empire, Trade, and Prohibition 1800–1928*. Oxford: Oxford University Press.

Mitchell, Thomas. 2019. "Nation's Largest Hemp Processing Plant Opens in Colorado." *Westword*, August 29, 2019. Accessed April 29, 2021. https://www.westword.com/marijuana/nations-largest-hemp-processing-plant-opens-in-colorado-11464777.

Mosk, Sanford. 1939. "Subsidized Hemp Production in Spanish California." *Agricultural History* 13 (4): 171–75.

Mutersbaugh, Tad. 2005. "Fighting Standards with Standards: Harmonization, Rents, and Social Accountability in Certified Agrofood Networks." *Environment and Planning A* 37 (11): 2033–51.

Narotzky, Susana. 2016. "Where Have All the Peasants Gone?" *Annual Review of Anthropology* 45 (1): 301–18.

Nast, Heidi J. 2006a. "Loving. . . . Whatever: Alienation, Neoliberalism and Pet-Love in the Twenty-First Century." *ACME: An International Journal for Critical Geographies* 5 (2): 300–27.

———. 2006b. "Critical Pet Studies?" *Antipode* 38 (5): 894.

Nichols, Kristen. 2017. "Hemp Report: Top 10 U.S. States." *Hemp Industry Daily*. www.hempindustrydaily.com.

Oregon CBD. 2020. "0.3% THC." *Oregon CBD Blog*, November 24, 2020. Accessed April 29, 2021. https://oregoncbdseeds.com/farmerresources/?post=03-thc.

Oregon Health Authority. 2015. "The Oregon Medical Marijuana Program Statistical Snapshot January, 2015." Accessed April 29, 2021. https://www.oregon.gov/oha/PH/DISEASESCONDITIONS/CHRONICDISEASE/MEDICALMARIJUANAPROGRAM/Documents/ed-materials/OMMP%20Statistic%20Snapshot%20-%2001-2015%20Final_3.pdf.

Oregon Liquor Control Commission. 2019. "2019 Recreational Marijuana Supply and Demand Legislative Report." Accessed April 29, 2021. https://www.oregon.gov/olcc/marijuana/Documents/Bulletins/2019%20Supply%20and%20Demand%20Legislative%20Report%20FINAL%20for%20Publication(PDFA).pdf.

Page, Brian. 1996. "Across the Great Divide: Agriculture and Industrial Geography." *Economic Geography* 72 (4): 376–97.

Perkowski, Mateusz. 2017. "ODA: 'Right to Farm' Law Protects Hemp Growers." *Capital Press*. September 20. Accessed October 16, 2019. www.capitalpress.com/state/oregon/oda-right-to-farm-law-protects-hemp-growers/article_96cbc9ff-1abb-53d8-a3ea-b6f7f527b6a9.html.

Plaven, George. 2019. "OSU Receives $1M Donation to Study Hemp Genetics." *Capital Press*, October 1. www.capitalpress.com/ag_sectors/research/osu-receives-m-donation-to-study-hemp-genetics/article_9371ed40-e470-11e9-b5d6–27d828500945.html.

Polanyi, Karl. 2001 (1944). *The Great Transformation: The Political and Economic Origins of Our Time*. Boston, MA: Beacon Press.

Project CBD. n.d. "About Project CBD." Accessed April 29, 2021. https://www.projectcbd.org/about-pcbd.

Rendon, Jim. 2012. *Super-Charged: How Outlaws, Hippies, and Scientists Reinvented Marijuana*. Portland, OR: Timber Press.

Richmond, M., and R. Clarke. 2019. "The Challenges of Seeded vs. Seedless Cannabis." *Cannabis Business Times*, September. Accessed September 18, 2019. www.cannabisbusinesstimes.com/article/seeded-seedless-cannabis-hemp-fiber-seed-oil-cbd-needs/.

Robinson, Rowan. 1996. *The Great Book of Hemp: The Complete Guide to the Environmental, Commercial, and Medicinal Uses of the World's Most Extraordinary Plant*. New York: Inner Traditions/Bear&Co.

Rose, Morgan. 2019. "2019 a Huge Year for Montana Hemp." *The Prairie Star*, October 25. Accessed November 15, 2019. www.agupdate.com/theprairiestar/news/crop/a-huge-year-for-montana-hemp/article_70779b0c-f4e5-11e9-86c9-578280cb1889.html.

Rubin, Alicia. "Oregon's Agricultural Landscape Shifts as Hemp Surpasses Pears and Grapes." *KDRV*, December 11, 2019. Accessed April 29, 2021. https://www.kdrv.com/content/news/Oregons-agricultural-landscape-shifts-as-hemp-surpasses-pears-and-grapes-566093951.html.

Schau, Jamie. 2019. "Projections: Pet CBD Marches Toward the Mainstream." *Cannabis Business Times*, August. Accessed September 18, 2019. www.cannabisbusinesstimes.com/article/pet-cbd-products-treats-mainstream/.

Schiller, Lowell. 2019. "Remarks by Lowell Schiller, JD at the Council for Responsible Nutrition Conference—11/7/2019." *Speeches by FDA Officials*. Accessed November 14, 2019. www.fda.gov/news-events/speeches-fda-officials/remarks-lowell-schiller-jd-council-responsible-nutrition-conference-1172019-11072019.

Schluttenhofer, Craig, and Ling Yuan. 2017. "Challenges Towards Revitalizing Hemp: A Multifaceted Crop." *Trends in Plant Science* 22 (11): 917–29.

Sliwosky, Vince. 2015. "Oregon Hemp: Onward!" *Canna Law Blog*, July 12, 2015. Accessed April 29, 2021. https://harrisbricken.com/cannalawblog/oregon-hemp-onward/.

Small, Ernest, and Arthur Cronquist. 1976. "A Practical and Natural Taxonomy for Cannabis." *Tazxon* 25 (4): 405–35.

Small, Ernest, and David Marcus. 2002. "Hemp: A New Crop with New Uses for North America." *Trends in New Crops and New Uses*, 284–326.

Smith, Tyler, Michelle Gillespie, Veronica Eckl, Jake Knepper, and Claire Morton Reynolds. 2019. "Herbal Supplement Sales in US Increase by 9.4% in 2018." *HerbalGram: The Journal of the American Council* 123 (2019): 62–73.

Stangle, Matt, and Katie Sheperd. 2018. "Oregon Grew More Cannabis Than Customers Can Smoke. Now Shops and Farmers Are Left With Mountains of Unwanted Bud." *Willamette Week*, April 18, 2018. Accessed April 29, 2021. https://www.wweek.com/news/2018/04/18/oregon-grew-more-cannabis-than-customers-can-smoke-now-shops-and-farmers-are-left-with-mountains-of-unwanted-bud/.

Thompson, Roy. 2019. "Medical and Industrial Cannabis Production in Costa Rica." *JD Supra*, June 18. Accessed November 8, 2019. www.jdsupra.com/legalnews/medical-and-industrial-cannabis-30452/.

Thorne, Griffen. 2019. "Breaking News: California Opens Up for Commercial Hemp Cultivation." *Canna Law Blog*, May 1. www.cannalawblog.com/breaking-news-california-opens-up-for-commercial-hemp-cultivation/.

Ventura, Jesse. 2016. *Jesse Ventura's Marijuana Manifesto: How Lies, Corruption, and Propaganda Kept Cannabis Illegal*. New York: Skyhorse Publishing.

Walker, Alicia. 2016. "Patent No. 6,630,507: Why the U.S. Government Holds a Patent on Cannabis Plant Compounds." *The Denver Post*, August 28. www.denverpost.com/2016/08/28/what-is-marijuana-patent-6630507/.

Wood, Sam. 2018. "First Marijuana-derived Prescription Drug Will Cost $32,500 a Year." *The Philadelphia Inquirer*, August 9, 2018. Accessed April 29, 2021. https://www.inquirer.com/philly/business/cannabis/epidiolex-marijuana-derived-drug-gw-pharmaceuticals-sativex-cbd-20180809.html.

Zobel, Frank. 2019. "Cannabis Regulation in Europe: Country Report Switzerland." *Transnational Institute Country Report*, February. www.tni.org/files/publication-downloads/cr_swiss_27032019.pdf.

Section 4
Ecology and the Environment

Like public health and market regulation, legal cannabis regulation is advertised as beneficial to another policy landscape, in this case the environment. Legalization promises to address environmental impacts of unregulated cannabis cultivation, similar to claims that it will improve public health outcomes and raise revenue from previously untaxed informal sector markets. This promise of legal cannabis environmental regulation is limited by its complex relationship with strict control policies as well as ongoing prohibition. First, strict control policies tend to favor fewer and larger scale licenses over many decentralized ones, because they are easier to regulate, not because they necessarily create fewer environmental impacts. Second, the continuity of places and people who are prohibited from engaging in regulated market activity, especially in conditions of economic crisis, continues to stimulate prohibition market activity that may or may not be environmentally impactful, depending on the sustainability of their practices. Beyond these two challenges, the promise of legal cannabis environmental regulation is limited by the effectiveness of environmental regulation *at large* to address "normal" impacts associated with industrial agriculture and manufacturing.

This section focusing on Ecology and the Environment thus shares two types of post-prohibition analyses with the prior section addressing Markets and Society. First, dynamics that entangle prohibition laws and policies with legal ones limit the effectiveness of regulations to address unregulated sector environmental impacts. And second, legal cannabis environmental regulations reveal limits to the effectiveness of broader environmental regulations to address the impacts of other legal industrial activities, especially with respect to pesticide use, water, and energy consumption. The former is an environmental problem related to the continuity of prohibition in the legal landscape, while the latter is a systemic problem related to other systemic problems produced by industrial capitalism. These relational analyses are not limited to considerations of environmental impacts, however. Cannabis cultivators unnecessary shape and are shaped by other relationships to land and identity, as the last two chapters in this section show.

In "Industrializing Cannabis? Socio-Ecological Implications of Legalization and Regulation in California," Dillis and colleagues, an interdisciplinary team from the University of California Berkeley Cannabis Research Center that has published extensively on the environmental impacts of unregulated cultivation in California, now ask: How will cannabis production and associated environmental impacts change in regulated landscapes? The way production is regulated is an open political question for them, as they draw on extensive fieldwork from prior publications to define and critique the politics of environmental regulation for "normal" industrial agriculture. The research agendas they call for support a reorientation of environmental policies to support small-scale, low-impact production in California as part of a wider reformation of industrial agriculture. Varieties of environmental regulation pertaining to legal cannabis could be far more effective if they are complemented by varieties of market regulation that promote sustainability in farming practices at large.

In "The Environmental Impact of Cannabis Liberalization: Lessons From California," environmental sociologist Anthony Silvaggio catalogues unintended environmental impacts incentivized by the ebb and flow of prohibition policing in California, during the "liberalizing" transition between 1996 and 2018 and the emergence of legal regulation in California. He draws on unstructured interviews and archival content analysis to investigate how policing functioned historically as informal environmental regulation. Silvaggio's work highlights the ongoing importance of researching how new forms of environmental policing intersect with regulations and policies to reproduce predictable spaces and subjects of environmental damage, including industrial impacts in nontraditional production areas. His work encourages research agendas about environmental impacts that identify their structural causes, rather than simply the outcome of criminal intent.

In 2012, energy and climate change scientist Evan Mills published the first research paper examining the carbon footprint of indoor cannabis cultivation. In "Energy Use by the Indoor Cannabis Industry: Inconvenient Truths for Producers, Consumers, and Policy Makers" Mills and cannabis industry consultant Scott Zeramby significantly update the scope and importance of that previous work. The update provides a comprehensive critique of legal cannabis environmental regulation, which they see as decoupled from policies of market creation and implementation. The authors provide researchers with a deep grounding in technical aspects of environmental impacts across the supply chain, although they are most intensively focused here on indoor production. Mills and Zeramby's comprehensive research provides solid direction for technical research, but they also raise the urgency of such research for policy makers to take action before big money interests capture environmental regulation completely.

In "Two Rural Industries Intersecting Over Time: Cannabis Production and Ecological Restoration in the Mattole Valley, California, USA," forestry scholars Erin Clover Kelly and Marisa Lia Formosa examine the emergence of the restoration sector in southern Humboldt County from its earliest cannabis producers, countercultural "new settlers" seeking freedom from postwar industrial modernity. Their case study, derived from semi-structured interviews with local restoration actors, suggests that Mattole Valley hippies created two economic development livelihoods, cannabis production and forest restoration, that became increasingly in tension over time as cannabis commercialized and restoration professionalized as a rural nonprofit industry. Kelly and Formosa suggest that further rural development research be developed in other areas where cannabis production and environmental restoration intersect and on other sectors that intersect with cannabis production. Their work points researchers towards considering the co-evolution of cannabis livelihoods and environmental stewardship. This is an ontology in which cannabis is more than a potential environmental impact, more than an engine of economic growth: it has been and may yet be a catalyst for the formation of ecocultural identity (see Milstein and Sotomayer 2020).

In the concluding chapter of our section, "Cannabis Seed in the Rif Region of Morocco: The Commodification of Nature and the Construction of a Contested International Market," sociologist Kenza Afsahi also points towards research agendas that consider ecologies of cannabis production at the intersection of cultural, environmental, and economic studies. She draws on ethnographic fieldwork to study socio-ecological transformations wrought by a rapidly globalizing seed market in Morocco's traditional cannabis cultivation region, the Rif. Her chapter is a case study in applying insights from an established interdisciplinary research field, critical development studies, to the cannabis research landscape. She investigates the transformation of cultivation practices through the replacement and hybridization of traditional landrace genetics by seeds created for global markets by transnational seed breeders. Afsahi's work provides another, international angle on the social problems that may be created when cannabis emerges from prohibition, only to find itself embedded in problems familiar to scholars of neoliberal modernity.

The chapters in this section map out critical directions for researching cannabis as a subject of environment and ecology, encompassing a broad range of possible interdisciplinary fields. In the age of climate change, environmental protection is of critical importance. But environmental protection is also a political discourse, useful for demonizing "unregulated" cannabis cultivation at large. Unregulated cannabis cultivation is the outcome of often very different cultural attitudes and practices towards the environment, as is regulated agriculture in society. These cultural attitudes informally regulate—or not—how sustainable those practices can be. As with the rest of the legal economy, more research is needed on formal (bureaucratic) and informal (cultural) methods of regulating legal cannabis environments because one without the other is clearly not enough.

Reference

Milstein, Tema, and Jose Castro-Sotomayer, eds. 2020. *The Routledge Handbook of Ecocultural Identity*. London: Routledge.

19

Industrializing Cannabis?

Socio-Ecological Implications of Legalization and Regulation in California

Christopher Dillis, Michael Polson, Hekia Bodwitch, Jennifer Carah, Mary E. Power, and Nathan F. Sayre

Keywords: marijuana, agriculture, industrialization, formalization, socio-ecology

Introduction

One of the major features of cannabis legalization is its attention to matters of production. In California, the nation's largest cannabis producer (Rea 2015), this is a departure from earlier waves of decriminalization and medicalization, which liberalized consumption and distribution yet left cultivation largely unregulated. With the new shift in regulation toward cultivation itself, new questions are emerging: How will patterns of cannabis production and associated environmental impacts change as the sector becomes visible, regulated, and taxed? Will legalization result in the *industrialization* of cannabis production, following the example of US agriculture in general (Magdoff, Foster, and Buttel 2000)? Or can a different model emerge, one that fosters substantive sustainability for ecosystems, farmers, and producer communities?

Focusing on California, we briefly review the characteristics of industrialized agriculture in general. We then consider the environmental impacts of cannabis production, pre- and post-legalization, as well as the policy factors that shape them. With early evidence that industrialization is already under way in regions of California far from the traditional epicenter of cannabis production, we contemplate what industrialized cannabis agriculture might entail for socio-ecological dynamics in the future. We conclude by discussing obstacles to research and the urgent need for interdisciplinary, mixed-methods collaboration, particularly in the period *prior* to full industrialization and its likely impacts on ecology, industrial structure, and regulation.

Industrial Agriculture

Conventional industrial agriculture in the US displays a number of recognizable characteristics. First, industrial agriculture is *capitalist* agriculture: commercially oriented and profit motivated. This is especially true for California agriculture, which never witnessed any significant history of

DOI: 10.4324/9780429320491-19

family-scale or "yeoman" farming (Walker 2004). Second, relations among farms are characterized by *competition* to increase market share and return on investment by lowering costs and increasing productivity. Thus, third, industrial agriculture displays a drive to achieve greater *economies of scale* through the development and application of technologies in every dimension of production. Prominent among these are biotechnologies to improve seeds through selective breeding and genetic engineering (Kloppenburg 2004); mechanization to reduce labor per unit output, in the field and in processing, storage, and distribution (Olmsted and Rhode 1988; Valdés 1994); chemical pesticides to manage insects, weeds, diseases, and other pests (Duncan 1996; Romero 2016); application of organic and especially synthetic fertilizers to augment and replenish soil nutrients (Smil 2001); irrigation in areas of limited or irregular rainfall, drawing on groundwater resources and/or large (often public) investments in dams, aqueducts, and canals (Reisner 1986; Worster 1992); and scientific research and development, both publicly and privately funded, to accelerate innovation in all of the aforementioned arenas. California has long been at the forefront in all of these technological frontiers, reflecting its unusually diverse, productive, and profitable agricultural sector.

Acting together, these traits enable and perpetuate a set of complex dynamics that are widely, if unevenly, evident across the agricultural systems of the US and much of the developed world[1] and increasingly evident in the developing world as well (Galt 2014). Market competition in agriculture, as compared with other sectors, tends to be particularly severe due to the large number of farms, their geographical dispersion, limited options for product differentiation, and the perishability of many crops, which inhibits farmers' ability to choose when to sell. Pronounced consolidation among downstream buyers and processors of farm outputs, especially in recent decades, exacerbates these forces further (Hauter 2012). And as a primary component of real wages, the production of cheaper consumption goods is structurally advantageous to capital in general. On farm, the pressure to reduce labor costs is intense, leading to chronic—and often violent—struggles with farm laborers in sectors where mechanization has not (yet) made inroads, including large portions of California's major agricultural regions (McWilliams 1939; Mitchell 1996; Olmsted 2015; Wells 1996). Meanwhile, the imperative to invest in the latest technologies to keep up with ever-increasing productivity induces heavy reliance on credit, even as the aggregate result is chronic production surpluses, which depress prices and narrow profit margins further (Cochrane 2003; Dudley 2000; Henderson 1998). Each boom and bust cycle in market prices thus results in a wave of foreclosures and farmland consolidation (Graddy-Lovelace 2019). In the US, the average farm size increased throughout the 20th century, while mid-sized farms declined and reliance on off-farm income increased for most farm households (Fitchen 1991).

These dynamics give rise to two additional features of industrial agriculture that are particularly relevant to cannabis in California today, as legalization releases producers from the need to hide their operations in remote locations. The first is the tendency toward geographical differentiation, as farmers seek to match the crops they grow to the characteristics of specific places and locations—the soils, hydrology, climatic conditions, water supplies, and access to markets for labor, inputs and outputs, etc. (Walker 2004). Differentiation can manifest at various scales depending on biophysical variation, from large regions such as the Corn and Wheat Belts of the Midwest to micro-regional specialization in California's Central Coast. With micro-regional specialization in the cannabis industry comes the potential for product differentiation via branding to enhance demand for products from particular regions (e.g. through an accredited appellation system). The second relevant feature of industrial agriculture is a chronic tendency, under the pressure of market competition, to overexploit the ecological resources available at any given site, through extensification (e.g. farming "fencerow to fencerow" to maximize the area under production) and intensification (planting more densely, applying excessive quantities of fertilizers or pesticides, or gradually depleting groundwater supplies) (Kloppenburg 2004; Graddy-Lovelace 2019). State processes to govern cannabis production and trade may also create incentives for cannabis farmers to extensify and intensify production to transform the scale, location, and environmental impacts of industry dynamics.

Socio-Ecological Dynamics of Cannabis Prior to Legalization

Until 1996, cannabis production in California occurred outside of legal systems. In 1996, California voters approved the Compassionate Use Act (CUA), decriminalizing use and cultivation of cannabis for medical purposes (State of California 1996). The state implemented the CUA in 2004 legislation[2] but did not thoroughly address cultivation (Butsic et al. 2018), leaving cities and counties to create and enforce guidelines individually and, thereby, unevenly (Short-Gianotti et al. 2017). Illegal under federal law, production in California remained quasi-legal (Carah et al. 2015; Short-Gianotti et al. 2017). Federal enforcement efforts to eradicate cannabis production continued throughout this period for California farms, medical and otherwise, though it increasingly prioritized larger grows, especially ecologically impactful ones on public lands (Corva 2014; Polson 2019). In 2015, California passed a package of bills comprehensively regulating medical cannabis production, distribution, and use, known as the Medical Cannabis Regulation and Safety Act (MCRSA) (State of California 2016a). In 2016, California voters passed the Adult Use of Marijuana Act (AUMA), which legalized adult recreational use and production of cannabis (State of California 2016b), and regulation of recreational production began in January 2018.

Though cannabis cultivation has a long history in the US (Weisheit 2011), countercultural migrants initiated more widespread production in the late 1960s (Potter, Bouchard, and Decorte 2013; Raphael 1985). In line with "back-to-the-land" ethics (and in contrast to California's industrial agricultural dynamics), cannabis cultivation in Northern California at that time was primarily small, off-grid, without chemical inputs, and for non-market consumption. After adopting new horticultural techniques, acquiring seeds suited to US latitudes, and building consumer circuits, cultivators began producing more regularly for markets. Prices steadily increased through the early 1980s but spiked with the intensification of governmental eradication programs (Corva 2014; Leeper 1990; Polson 2018; Weisheit 2011).

Under full-throttle prohibition, rewards for cultivation incentivized risk-taking and more intensive, profit-focused, environmentally impactful production practices (Corva 2014), such as indoor growing, "trespass" and public land cultivation, and increased violation of informal community norms around environmental care (McCubbrey 2007; Polson 2019). Farm siting focused on secrecy to avoid enforcement action, directing cultivation to remote, rural watersheds on both public and private lands where plants were generally grown outdoors and sometimes associated with unpermitted water diversion, native vegetation clearing, pollution from pesticides and herbicides, or trash dumping associated with informal residences for temporary cultivator-guards (Butsic and Brenner 2016; Carah et al. 2015; Gabriel et al. 2012; Gabriel et al. 2013; Thompson et al. 2014; Wang, Butsic, and Brenner 2017). These locations, many of which were concentrated on California's North Coast (particularly Humboldt, Mendocino, and Trinity Counties), overlap with areas of high conservation value, such as forested watersheds (Wang, Butsic, and Brenner 2017) that harbor rare or US Endangered Species Act–listed species like coho salmon, steelhead trout, and Pacific fisher (Butsic et al. 2018; Gabriel et al. 2012).

Fear of detection placed informal limits on farm size, especially on private property where plants could be tied to owners and property seizure and arrest was a real threat (Polson 2019). Further, price inflation due to prohibition (Raphael 2012) allowed some farmers to experiment with labor-intensive, ecologically conscious growing methods, including permacultural, organic, and pesticide-free techniques. Informal self-regulation on private lands also took place during this time, where some farmers abided by local norms surrounding farm size, location, and cultivation techniques to reduce incidence of detection by or conflict with neighbors (Anders 1990; McCubbrey 2007; Polson 2019; Raphael 1985).

The allowance of medical cannabis cultivation after 1996 affected production dynamics. Legal-medical protections, particularly physician recommendations, made it less risky to cultivate, thus fueling an expansion of the number of (patient-)cultivators. Collective gardens enabled multiple patients to grow in one site rather than many or, conversely, for single growers to cultivate for multiple patients and distribute through medical dispensaries and collectives, thus increasing garden size. "Reasonable compensation" (State of California 2003) for medically designated cultivators made medical cultivation economically viable and, for some, made it possible to resist pressures to expand scale. Pressure to produce "medical-grade" cannabis, especially with the growing utilization of quality and safety testing, discouraged use of pesticides and encouraged organic inputs, though agricultural practices were far from uniform (Polson 2019). All this said, there was significant mixing between medical and underground market production during this time period (Short-Gianotti et al. 2017). Often, this meant cultivators used medical recommendations to produce large amounts of cannabis, only a portion of which (if any at all) would go to verified patients, thus alleviating pressure to produce medical-grade product.

Between 2008 and 2010, garden sizes increased, often to 99 plants, the limit at which federal minimum sentencing guidelines activated—an increase at least partly attributable to the *Kelly* decision, which struck down California's efforts to limit plant numbers (Schwab and Butsic 2017). Expanded production placed downward pressure on prices, resulting in price instability that only increased between 2012 and 2016. Characterized as a "green rush," farmers began producing significantly more cannabis in even larger gardens, possibly in anticipation of full legalization and relatively less enforcement (Butsic et al. 2018). For example, between 2012 and 2016 in Humboldt and Mendocino Counties, the number of cannabis farms increased by 56%, the number of plants increased by 183%, and the total area under cultivation increased by 91%, with significant expansion happening in environmentally sensitive areas such as those on steep slopes or near creeks with salmon and steelhead (Butsic et al. 2018). These environmental transformations were a primary focus of state cultivation regulations and county ordinances passed since 2015 (Polson 2019).

In 2015, the state first began targeted regulatory programs of cultivation in Northern California, but comprehensive statewide regulation of production was not implemented until 2018 (Butsic et al. 2018). Prior to 2018, the first farms seeking to enter a regulated cannabis industry in Northern California remained relatively small, largely due to county ordinances that restricted size (e.g. HGA 2010). With implementation of adult-use regulations in 2018, a statewide licensing program implemented by the California Department of Food and Agriculture opened opportunities for localities to develop cannabis ordinances and welcome—or ban—a new regulated cannabis industry.

Socio-Ecological Dynamics of Cannabis Since Legalization

By early 2019, industrial-scale commercial cannabis appears to have arrived in California. A cursory review of cultivation license data from the California Department of Food and Agriculture (CDFA) shows that large-scale operations have already been proposed or initiated in counties representing new frontiers for the cannabis industry (CDFA 2019) (Figure 19.1(A)). The emergence of these farms may have environmental implications, both directly through their local impacts and indirectly as competitors for smaller operations on the North Coast.

In some respects, cannabis cultivation regulations are substantially stricter than are requirements for traditional agriculture. These regulations include mandatory summer water diversion forbearance (State of California 2019a), extensive site maintenance standards, exclusive use of organic amendments, and mandatory product testing with certified laboratories (State of California 2019b). Local regulations, such as zoning restrictions, are highly variable in requirements between jurisdictions and

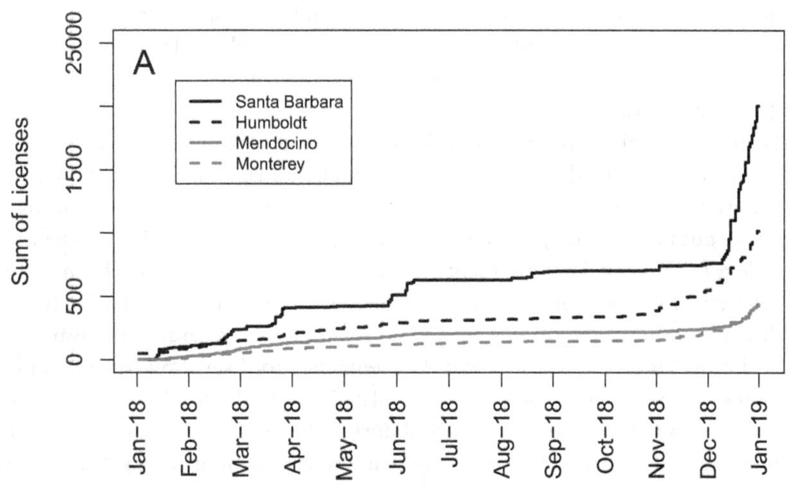

Figure 19.1(A) California Department of Food and Agriculture Cultivation Licenses by County—2018

Cumulative sum of cultivation licenses issued by the California Department of Food and Agriculture in 2018 for the top four counties in licenses issued. Data are restricted to temporary licenses that remained active as of January 2019, excluding specialty and cottage-scale license types.

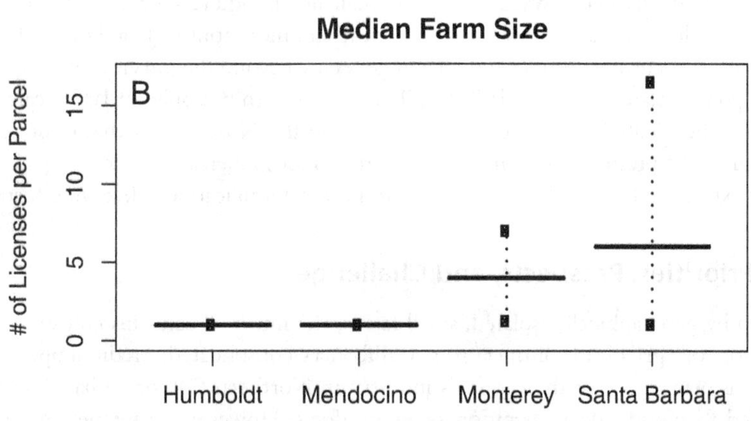

Figure 19.1(B) Typical number of cultivation licenses per parcel, California—2019

Size of cultivation area is limited for a single license, but the number of licenses per parcel is not. Bars depict median values and dashed lines represent the interquartile range (25th–75th percentile).

likely play a significant role in siting decisions for legal and illicit growers in the state (Polson and Petersen-Rockney 2019). In traditional cannabis-producing communities, adherence to new production criteria can require overhaul of existing operations, limit new development, and also incentivize noncompliance (Bodwitch et al. 2019; Polson and Petersen-Rockney 2019). The remote and rugged terrain that once attracted illicit cultivation in attempts to avoid detection may now hinder the ability of farms in these areas to comply with environmental regulatory standards and ultimately become licensed. Multiple environmental permits may be required in order to obtain a CDFA cultivation license if growing outdoors or in greenhouses, and the fees and information requirements may represent significant hurdles to some farmers (Bodwitch et al. 2019).

Initial evidence indicates the first wave of regulated, industrial-scale cannabis has largely begun not in the historical epicenter of Northern California but in the hills and isolated valleys of the Central Coast. Although select counties in the Central Valley have allowed a token number of large cannabis farms (as many as five to ten times larger than their North Coast counterparts; CDFA 2019), licenses for farms of equivalent size have been issued en masse in counties such as Santa Barbara and Monterey (Figure 19.1(A)). In these areas, it is not yet clear if large-scale cannabis farms will more commonly repurpose existing infrastructure (e.g. abandoned facilities from the former cut-flower industry) or stake out new territory farther from existing agriculture and closer to natural spaces.

Understanding the potential environmental impacts of industrialized cannabis requires knowing where and why extensification or intensification occurs, the patterns of natural resource use, and how these dynamics relate to regulatory mandates. For example, regarding the issue of water, the legacy of illegal cannabis cultivation sites and their tendency to divert from streams and springs has led to these sources of water becoming tightly regulated within the legal cannabis industry. In particular, extraction from these sources is prohibited during the growing season, and farms that rely on them must either instead collect and store this water in the off season or use an alternative source. For the majority of regulated cannabis farms, the choice has been to use well water, and this is already the most common source for irrigation (Dillis et al. 2019). Given the hurdle of developing sufficient storage, especially at increasingly larger farm sizes, the use of wells will likely increase in frequency (Dillis et al. 2019b). While the story of groundwater depletion in California is common knowledge (Reisner 1986; Scanlon et al. 2012), the use of wells by commercial cannabis farms is fundamentally different, given their tendency to occur outside of large aquifer basins (Butsic et al. 2018). Such wells that are located adjacent to watercourses, in small alluvial aquifers, or in fractured bedrock have the potential to reduce crucial stream flow during the summer months (Konikow and Leake 2014), although this topic is currently understudied and generally beyond the purview of current California groundwater policy (State of California 2014). This is a concern not only for large-scale farms in the new frontier of the Central Coast, but also for farms on the North Coast that must compete with these operations. The pressure on farms on the North Coast to increase size to compete, while using groundwater extraction to comply, has latent environmental implications, deserving further research.

Research Priorities, Prospects, and Challenges

Characterized by geographically isolated, small farms, the informal cannabis cultivation sector represented a form of agriculture distinct from California's consolidated, credit-supported industrial model. The historic legacy of the cannabis industry in Northern California has differentiated this region and led to worldwide recognition of its products. However, remoteness has now isolated traditional cultivation regions from an emerging legal supply chain and new markets, while obligating farms to navigate high regulatory costs associated with operating in environmentally sensitive locations. How farmers in these remote watersheds respond holds importance for the future of the cannabis industry and its socio-ecological dynamics. Formation of grower cooperatives (allowed at small scales under statewide regulations), appellation systems, caps on farm size and license consolidation (which the state government has not implemented), or a return to medical provisioning collectives (which the state terminated in 2019) may provide tools to overcome steep start-up and licensing costs for small farmers. Due to ongoing federal prohibition, farmers do not have access to traditional supports such as bank loans or crop insurance and instead must rely on private capital, limiting engagement in legal markets by many smaller farmers. Paradoxically, if barriers to capital are reduced, it may invite institutional investment and accelerate further industrial consolidation and upscaling.

More research is needed to understand the socio-ecological dynamics that underpin changes in cannabis cultivation in California and beyond. California's statewide legalization opens some research pathways through regulatory databases, harmonization among institutions and jurisdictions, and new funding mechanisms. Yet, federal prohibition still creates a "quasi-legal challenge" for robust research (Short-Gianotti et al. 2017), with consequences for effective policymaking and environmental health (Carah et al. 2015). Federal prohibition can inhibit institutional funding (since many research and agricultural extension institutions receive federal funds) (Wilson et al. 2019), discourage participation of informants in studies (Short-Gianotti et al. 2017), lead to suspicion of researchers by potential study participants (Polson and Petersen-Rockney 2019), create difficulty for institutional review boards and researchers to estimate and mitigate risks for human subjects, and create asymmetries in data collection and knowledge types. High numbers of producers operating outside of regulatory systems impede the ability for comprehensive and representative studies and projects limited to only "compliant" producers and cannot account for the total socio-ecological dynamics of cultivation. With a lack of robust research, resulting policies cannot be driven by direct research on cannabis, may impair social equity in the transition of informal producers to formal markets (Kelly and Peluso 2015; Putzel et al. 2015), and complicate implementation of strategies to govern common environmental resources (Ostrom 1990). Further, policies that incentivize industrial consolidation and eliminate small producers may have environmental consequences (Guthman 2004; Vásquez-León 1998).

Among cannabis producers, decisions about production can alter ecological and hydrological conditions, requiring attention not just to stream flows, pest management, indicator species, and wildlife movement patterns, but also to the social calculus of decision-making. Analyses of production decisions necessitate the development of qualitative research methods to understand how policy formations, social norms, knowledge access, and enforcement practices, among other variables, shape production practices across different kinds of ecologies and regions. In particular, many farmers are electing to avoid compliance (Bodwitch et al. 2019). Factors influencing noncompliance may derive from prohibition (e.g. distrust or fear of officials) or may only emerge post-legalization (e.g. concern that compliance costs will make it impossible to earn a living; negative interactions with regulatory officials) (Bodwitch et al. 2019). Understanding the perspectives of noncompliant farmers is crucial to researching the social and ecological dynamics of cannabis production. Equally important is a qualitative, political-economic understanding of how and why policies take particular forms in certain jurisdictions at certain times. Which interests and groups are most and least influential in forming policy? Who bears the consequences and rewards of the resulting regulatory regimes?

Rapid transformations in cannabis policy are corresponding to the emergence of new scales, practices, and ecological consequences of cannabis cultivation. Lessons from other legal forms of agriculture suggest that increased market pressures may lead to industrialization, extensification and/or intensification, and increased reliance on credit fueled by debt. Siting patterns described here indicate that all three may already be trending upward in California since legalization of production for recreational use. As changes rapidly occur, research is urgently needed to understand the relations between regulatory change, farm size, location, environmental outcomes, and the geographical distributions of benefits and impacts. Such analyses will aid policymakers' ability to govern and farmers' capacities to participate in this newly regulated industry. If done with an eye toward equitable and just outcomes, it may also point the way toward a cannabis agriculture that incorporates and learns from the lessons and failures of industrialized agricultural production.

Notes

1 Meaning the Organisation for Economic Co-operation and Development (OECD) countries, often glossed as the First World or the Global North.

2 This eight-year gap in legislative implementation can be attributed to legislative fears of federal reprisal, though there were also many forces opposed to implementation altogether.

References

Anders, J. 1990. *Beyond Counterculture: The Community of Mateel.* Pullman, WA: Washington State University Press.

Bodwitch, H., J. Carah, K. M. Daane, C. Getz, T. Grantham, G. Hickey, and S. Wilson. 2019. "Growers Say Cannabis Legalization Excludes Small Growers, Supports Illicit Markets, Undermines Local Economies." *California Agriculture* 73 (3–4): 177–84. https://doi.org/10.3733/ca.2019a0018.

Butsic, V., and J. C. Brenner. 2016. "Cannabis (*Cannabis sativa* or *C. indica*) Agriculture and the Environment: A Systematic, Spatially-Explicit Survey and Potential Impacts." *Environmental Research Letters* 11: 044023.

Butsic, V., J. K. Carah, M. Baumann, C. Stephens, and J. C. Brenner. 2018. "The Emergence of Cannabis Agriculture Frontiers as Environmental Threats." *Environmental Research Letters* 13: 124017.

California Department of Food and Agriculture. 2019. *CalCannabis Licensing Data.* https://cannabis.ca.gov/check_a_license/.

Carah, J. K., J. K. Howard, S. E. Thompson, A. G. Short-Gianotti, S. D. Bauer, S. M. Carlson, D. N. Dralle, M. W. Gabriel, L. L. Hulette, B. J. Johnson, C. A. Knight, S. J. Kupferberg, S. L. Martin, R. L. Naylor, and M. E. Power. 2015. "High Time for Conservation: Adding the Environment to the Debate on Marijuana Liberalization." *Bioscience* 65: 822–29.

Cochrane, W. W. 2003. *The Curse of American Agricultural Abundance.* Lincoln and London: University of Nebraska Press.

Corva, D. 2014. "Requiem for a CAMP: The Life and Death of a Domestic US Drug War Institution." *International Journal of Drug Policy* 25: 71–80.

Dillis, C. R., T. E. Grantham, C. McIntee, B. McFadin, and K. V. Grady. 2019. "Watering the Emerald Triangle: Irrigation Sources Used by Cannabis Cultivation in Northern California." *California Agriculture* 73 (3): 146–53.

Dillis, C., C. McIntee, V. Butsic, L. Le, K. Grady, and T. Grantham. 2020. "Water Storage and Irrigation Practices for Cannabis Drive Seasonal Patterns of Water Extraction and Use in Northern California." *Journal of Environmental Management* 272: 110955.

Dudley, K. M. 2000. *Debt and Dispossession.* Chicago, IL: University of Chicago Press.

Duncan, C. A. M. 1996. *The Centrality of Agriculture.* Montreal and Kingston: McGill-Queen's University Press.

Fitchen, J. M. 1991. *Endangered Spaces, Enduring Places: Change, Identity, and Survival in Rural America.* Boulder, CO: Westview Press, Inc.

Gabriel, M. W., G. M. Wengert, J. M. Higley, S. Krogen, W. Sargent, and D. L. Clifford. 2013. "Silent Forests? Rodenticides on Illegal Marijuana Crops Harm Wildlife." *Wildlife Professional* 7: 46–50.

Gabriel, M. W., L. W. Woods, R. Poppenga, R. A. Sweitzer, C. Thompson, S. M. Matthews, J. M. Higley, S. M. Keller, K. Purcell, R. H. Barrett, G. M. Wengert, B. N. Sacks, and D. L. Clifford. 2012. "Anticoagulant Rodenticides on Our Public and Community Lands: Spatial Distribution of Exposure and Poisoning of a Rare Forest Carnivore." *PLoS One* 7 (7): p.e40163. doi:10.1371/journal.pone.0040163.

Galt, R. E. 2014. *Food Systems in an Unequal World.* Tucson: University of Arizona Press.

Graddy-Lovelace, G. 2019. "U.S. Farm Policy as Fraught Populism: Tracing the Scalar Tensions of Nationalist Agricultural Governance." *Annals of the American Association of Geographers.* doi:10.1080/24694452.2018.1551722.

Guthman, J. 2004. *Agrarian Dreams.* Berkeley: University of California Press.

Hauter, W. 2012. *Foodopoly.* New York: New Press.

Henderson, G. L. 1998. *California and the Fictions of Capital.* New York: Oxford University Press.

HGA [Humboldt Growers Association]. 2010. *Humboldt County Outdoor Medical Cannabis Ordinance Draft.* http://library.humboldt.edu/humco/holdings/HGA2.pdf.

Kelly, A. B., and N. L. Peluso. 2015. "Frontiers of Commodification: State Lands and Their Formalization." *Society & Natural Resources* 28 (5): 473–95.

Kloppenburg Jr, J. R. 2004. *First the Seed.* 2nd ed. Madison: University of Wisconsin Press.

Konikow, L. F., and S. A. Leake. 2014. "Depletion and Capture: Revisiting 'the Source of Water Derived from Wells'." *Groundwater* 52: 100–11.

Leeper, J. S. 1990. "Humboldt County: Its Role in the Emerald Triangle." *California Geographer* 30: 93–109.

Magdoff, F., J. B. Foster, and F. H. Buttel. 2000. *Hungry for Profit.* New York: Monthly Review Press.

McCubbrey, J. P. 2007. "Impacts of Illicit-drug Policy on Community Cohesion: A Case Study of the Campaign Against Marijuana Planting in Southern Humboldt County, California." Doctoral dissertation, Western Institute for Social Research, Berkeley.

McWilliams, C. 1939. *Factories in the Field*. Boston: Little, Brown and Co.

Mitchell, D. 1996. *The Lie of the Land*. Minneapolis: University of Minnesota Press.

Olmsted, A., and P. Rhode. 1988. "An Overview of California Agricultural Mechanization, 1870–1930." *Agricultural History* 62 (3): 86–112.

Olmsted, K. S. 2015. *Right Out of California*. New York: The New Press.

Ostrom, E. 1990. *Governing the Commons: The Evolution of Institutions for Collective Action*. Cambridge: Cambridge University Press.

Polson, M. 2018. "Marketing Marijuana: Prohibition, Medicalisation and the Commodity." In *Economy, Crime and Wrong in a Neoliberal Era*, edited by James Carrier. New York: Berghahn Books.

———. 2019. "Making Marijuana an Environmental Issue: Prohibition, Pollution, and Policy." *Environment and Planning E: Nature and Space*. doi:10.1177/2514848619834847.

Polson, M., and M. Petersen-Rockney. 2019. "Cannabis Farmers or Criminals? Enforcement-First Approaches Fuel Disparity and Hinder Regulation." *California Agriculture* 73 (3–4): 185–93. https://doi.org/10.3733/ca.2019a0017.

Potter, G. R., M. Bouchard, and T. Decorte. 2013. *The Globalization of Cannabis Cultivation. World Wide Weed: Global Trends in Cannabis Cultivation and Its Control*, 1–20. Farnham, England: Ashgate Publishing.

Putzel, L., A. B. Kelly, P. O. Cerutti, and Y. Artati. 2015. "Formalization as Development in Land and Natural Resource Policy." *Society & Natural Resources* 28 (5): 453–72.

Raphael, R. 1985. *Cash Crop: An American Dream*. Caspar, CA: Ridge Times Press.

———. 2012. "Green Gold and the American Way." In *West of Eden: Communes and Utopia in Northern California*, edited by I. Boal, J. Stone, M. Watts, and C. Winslow, 187–98. Oakland, CA: PM Press.

Rea, P. 2015. *The State of Legal Marijuana Markets*. 3rd ed. Oakland, CA: Arcview Market Research.

Reisner, M. 1986. *Cadillac Desert*. New York: Penguin.

Romero, A. M. 2016. "Commercializing Chemical Warfare: Citrus, Cyanide, and an Endless War." *Agriculture and Human Values* 33: 3–26.

Scanlon, B. R., C. C. Faunt, L. Longuevergne, R. C. Reedy, W. M. Alley, V. L. McGuire, and P. B. McMahon. 2012. "Groundwater Depletion and Sustainability of Irrigation in the US High Plains and Central Valley." *PNAS* 109 (24): 9320–25.

Schwab, B., and V. A. Butsic. 2017. "Green Acres? Cannabis Agriculture and Rural Land Values in Northern California." Agricultural & Applied Economics Association Annual Meeting, Chicago, Illinois.

Short-Gianotti, A. G., J. Harrower, G. Baird, and S. Sepaniak. 2017. "The Quasi-Legal Challenge: Assessing and Governing the Environmental Impacts of Cannabis Cultivation in the North Coastal Basin of California." *Land Use Policy* 61: 126–34.

Smil, V. 2001. *Enriching the Earth*. Cambridge and London: MIT Press.

State of California. 1996. Compassionate Use Act of 1996, California Health and Safety Code §11362.5 et seq.

———. 2003. Senate Bill 420.

———. 2014. Sustainable Groundwater Management Act.

———. 2016a. Medical Cannabis Regulation and Safety Act.

———. 2016b. Adult Use of Marijuana Act.

———. 2019a. State Water Resources Control Board. Cannabis Cultivation Policy.

———. 2019b. California Code of Regulations Title 3. Food and Agriculture Division 8. Cannabis Cultivation Chapter 1. Cannabis Cultivation Program.

Thompson, C., R. Sweitzer, M. Gabriel, K. Purcell, R. Barrett, and R. Poppenga. 2014. "Impacts of Rodenticide and Insecticide Toxicants from Marijuana Cultivation Sites on Fisher Survival Rates in the Sierra National Forest, California." *Conservation Letters* 7: 91–102.

Valdés, D. N. 1994. "Machine Politics in California Agriculture, 1945–1990s." *Pacific Historical Review* 63 (2): 203–24.

Vásquez-León, M. 1998. "Neoliberalism, Environmentalism, and Scientific Knowledge: Re-defining Natural Resource Use Rights in Mexico." In *States and Illegal Practices*, edited by J. M. Heyman, 233–60. Oxford, UK: Berg Publishers.

Walker, R. 2004. *The Conquest of Bread*. New York: The New Press.

Wang, I. J., V. Butsic, and J. C. Brenner. 2017. "Cannabis, an Emerging Agricultural Crop, Leads to Deforestation and Fragmentation." *Frontiers in Ecology and the Environment* 15: 495–501.

Weisheit, R. A. 2011. "Cannabis Cultivation in the United States." *World Wide Weed: Global Trends in Cannabis Cultivation and Its Control*: 145–62.

Wells, M. 1996. *Strawberry Fields*. Ithaca, NY: Cornell University Press.

Wilson, H., H. Bodwitch, J. Carah, K. Daane, C. Getz, T. Grantham, and V. Butsic. 2019. "First Known Survey of Cannabis Production Practices in California." *California Agriculture* 73 (3): 119–127.

Worster, D. 1992. *Rivers of Empire*. Oxford and New York: Oxford University Press.

20

The Environmental Impact of Cannabis Liberalization

Lessons From California

Anthony Silvaggio

Keywords: cannabis, prohibition, environment, policy, California

Introduction

This chapter examines California's 20-year experiment with cannabis liberalization under federal prohibition, focusing on the unintended environmental consequences of cannabis policy. To understand the impact of cannabis liberalization (1996–2018) on the environment, I examine trends in cultivation practices before and after key policy changes at the state and federal levels. While the policy trade-offs between economic growth, public health and safety, and environmental protections have been central to cannabis policy debates, this study describes how liberalization efforts have facilitated and encouraged decades of environmental harms, leading to significant impacts on forests, fish, wildlife, and the atmosphere. I close the chapter by outlining a set of policy recommendations that regulators should consider that could better reduce and mitigate the environmental harms associated with cannabis cultivation. The specific policy changes examined are the following:

- *Legalization of medical marijuana (Proposition 215, 1996)*
- *Liberalization of the medical marijuana law (Senate Bill 420, 2003)*
- *Legalization of recreational marijuana (Proposition 64, 2016)*
- *State Cannabis Licensing Authorities Proposed Regulations (2018)*

While there has been a large body of research devoted to the economic (Kilmer 2014; Dills, Goffard, and Miron 2016; Caulkins and Pacula 2006; Miron 2010), public health (Keith et al. 2015; Chapkis and Webb 2008), and public safety outcomes (Shepard and Blackley 2007; Austin 2005) of cannabis legalization, only recently have policy makers and cannabis scholars given attention to the environmental impacts of the cannabis industry. These concerns have focused mostly on the environmental harms to public lands and the impacts of cannabis cultivation on fish (Bauer et al. 2015), wildlife (Gabriel et al. 2012), water (O'Hare, Sanchez, and Alstone 2013), and forests (Koch et al. 2016). In policy debates, it is generally assumed that the environmental impacts associated with cannabis cultivation will be reduced through cannabis liberalization and regulation. In this chapter,

DOI: 10.4324/9780429320491-20

I question these assumptions and build on the work of social scientists who have highlighted some of the unintended environmental consequences of cannabis prohibitionist policies (Silvaggio 2012, 2018; Corva 2014, 2018; Miller and Silvaggio 2018). I draw on data gathered from semi-structured interviews with cannabis cultivators, legalization advocates, law enforcement, natural resource managers, cannabis regulators, and environmentalists, as well as secondary sources to understand the sociopolitical context that shaped the development of cannabis policy and the related environmental outcomes.

A Brief Environmental History of the (Pre-Liberalization) Cannabis Industry in California

The cannabis industry in Northern California emerged during the back-to-the-land movement of the late 1960s, when mostly well-educated whites left the city to set up homesteads in the remote counties of Northern California where land was abundant and cheap (Anders 1990). This counterculture brought with them a distrust of authority, a desire to be close to the land, and an appreciation of the cannabis plant. They settled in remote valleys and cultivated small patches of cannabis, primarily for personal use. At the time, there was little domestic production of cannabis, with the majority of cannabis consumed in the US coming from Mexico (Raphael 1985). In 1971, the Nixon administration declared a "War on Drugs" and attempted to stem the flow of cannabis through increased interdiction efforts at the border and the creation of the controversial "paraquat" herbicide eradication program.[1] While these policing efforts reduced cannabis imports from Mexico, it did little to control the supply of cannabis coming into the United States from other countries. Rather than restrict supply of cannabis in the US, the industry simply reoriented the supply chain to access cannabis from other countries (Corva 2014). Domestically, the federal government's drug war efforts helped to shift cannabis production to Northern California's "Emerald Triangle," triggering the first "green rush" of cannabis entrepreneurs to the region hoping to cash in on the emerging cottage industry (Raphael 1985; Raskin 2012).[2] Although the Nixon administration had succeeded in classifying cannabis as a Schedule 1 narcotic, defined as having no accepted medical use and a high potential for abuse, the administration's policies were ineffective in reducing domestic consumption and production, with the wholesale price of cannabis rising to $2,000 a pound by 1980 (Corva 2014). The environmental impacts of the domestic cannabis industry at this time were negligible, but this was short lived as a result of strict federal drug laws and increased state funding for domestic cannabis eradication efforts that began in the 1980s.

The Comprehensive Crime Control Act

Prior to 1980, back-to-the-landers were able to cultivate cannabis with little fear of arrest, as cannabis policing was almost nonexistent in the region. The scale of the industry and the cultivation practices during these early days reflected the ecological values of the "new settlers" and posed little risk to the environment (Bosk 2000). The election of Ronald Reagan in 1980, however, marked the launch of a new, more aggressive drug policy regime with his administration passing the 1984 Comprehensive Crime Control Act, which established new mandatory minimums for drug offenses and granted authorities the right to seize the property of suspected cannabis cultivators without a trial (Lee 2012). While asset forfeitures for cannabis cultivation generated over $26 million during the first five years of enforcement, this did not come without environmental costs (CAMP 1990). These policy changes led to a number of unintended environmental consequences that were not present during the 1970s. Cultivators, attempting to avoid these new criminal sanctions, began shifting their operations off of their private homesteads and into more remote areas on public land and private timber estates, clearing forests, diverting water, and polluting watersheds with fertilizers and pesticides (Campaign Against Marijuana Planting Annual Report 1983, 1985, 1990; Gabriel et al. 2012). This increased policing of cannabis agriculture directly incentivized the development of ecologically destructive agricultural practices in the cannabis industry.

Campaign Against Marijuana Planting (CAMP)

In 1983, California governor George Deukmejian established the cannabis eradication program known as Campaign Against Marijuana Planting (CAMP). This was a coordinated effort between federal, state, and local law enforcement to eradicate cannabis cultivation in the Emerald Triangle. Using fixed-wing aircraft and helicopters to spot cannabis plantations from the air, CAMP conducted large-scale military style raids on cannabis communities in the region for over two decades. Flying mainly during the harvest months, plant eradications rose annually with the program claiming to have eradicated the majority of the cannabis crop in some areas in Northern California (Campaign Against Marijuana Planting Annual Report 1985). Not surprisingly, the increased risks associated with this aggressive surveillance of cannabis communities helped push the price of cannabis to over $3,000 a pound.[3] CAMP's activities led to a geographical dispersion of the industry, with outdoor cultivation spreading to other counties in California and onto public lands (Corva 2014).

Cultivators also innovated by moving production indoors, often times employing large industrial diesel generators to power their operations. This "off the grid" indoor growing method allowed cultivators to conceal their crops from aerial surveillance and offered the opportunity for multiple harvests annually. "Diesel doping" became a popular cultivation technique throughout the 1980s and 1990s, but it came at a high price to the environment (Corva 2014). Placed close to creeks and waterways to conceal the noise, the move to "off the grid" industrial diesel generators required the delivery and storage of thousands of gallons of fuel annually to cannabis farms throughout the Emerald Triangle. Diesel and oil spills from leaky tanks and unattended generators were commonplace, at times contaminating local water supplies for aquatic and human communities (Gurnon 2005).

The environmental impacts of this new cultivation method included the pollution of water, soil, and air. This shift to indoor cannabis cultivation was an adaptation to increased policing and represented a direct industry response to the eradication policies of the 1980s. The move to indoor thus marked a shift away from the ecologically benign outdoor practices of the back-to-the-landers and instead towards more negative environmental consequences for the fragile ecosystems that had been devastated by decades of resource extraction by the logging, mining, and fishing industries (Raphael 1985; Harris 1997; House 1999). By the mid-1990s, cannabis cultivation continued to expand, with public lands trespass grows, off-the-grid diesel doping, and outdoor cultivation the dominant forms of cannabis agriculture in the region.[4]

Cannabis Liberalization

Proposition 215, Legalization of Medical Marijuana (1996)

In 1996, California became the first in the United States to legalize medical cannabis by passing Proposition 215, the California Compassionate Use Act. This legislative victory marked a watershed moment for legalization advocates, complicating the prohibitionist efforts of federal authorities. While the act provided cultivators and medical patients a justification and legal defense for growing and possessing cannabis in California, it provided no real guidance for cultivators or state regulators concerning the scale of production or enforcement. Additionally, Proposition 215 did not outline which medical conditions could be treated with cannabis and set no limits on the number of plants or possession amounts. With little threat of arrest and prices upwards of $4,000 a pound, this liberalization policy led to a second wave of "green rushers" to the Emerald Triangle, who set up large-scale industrial cannabis farms all over the region.[5]

The legalization of medical cannabis also led to the expansion of indoor operations that required enormous amounts of energy (Mills 2012) and water (O'Hare, Sanchez, and Alstone 2013). With legal protections awarded to cultivators, this became the standard cultivation method in semi-rural towns and cities throughout the region (McKinley 2008). Law enforcement reported the growth of large-scale indoor cannabis operations in residential neighborhoods, with some areas reporting double-digit spikes in electricity consumption (Sims 2015). Outdoor, the failure of federal and state authorities to come to agreement on cannabis policy resulted in a fragmented policy regime that created the perfect conditions for environmental abuses to flourish, with cultivators free to divert water, build roads, and illegally clear forests and vegetation to expand their operations. By the end of the decade, with no regulatory or state-level licensing system in place and no rules regarding who could grow and distribute cannabis, large-scale indoor and outdoor cannabis enterprises dominated the region.

Senate Bill 420: Liberalization of the Medical Marijuana Law (2003)

In 2003, Senate Bill 420 was passed, addressing a number of legal ambiguities of Proposition 215 regarding cultivation and distribution. Although it did not establish a statewide regulatory system, it clarified the scope of Proposition 215, allowing local governments the freedom to establish their own regulations on cultivation. The bill also established a voluntary patient registry and made cannabis collectives legal, allowing medical patients the right to either grow their own or become a member of a collective that would provide them with cannabis. Counties in the Emerald Triangle opted for the most liberal regulations in the state, creating the regulatory conditions that led to a "Wild West" for cannabis growers in the region. Spurred on by prices that spiked to over $4,000 a pound, cultivators increased the square footage of their operations, employing new agricultural practices such as light deprivation, a mix of indoor/outdoor techniques where for a short time early in the season lights and heaters are utilized, usually powered by diesel generators.[6] This technique allowed cultivators multiple outdoor crops, as well as an early harvest that would fetch a higher price than they would get later in the harvest season when the market was saturated. This adaptation commonly required additional natural resource inputs (land and water) and energy (fossil fuels), putting increased pressure on ecosystems with cultivators clearing additional forests and vegetation for greenhouse expansion and diverting vast amounts of water from sensitive fish habitat for longer periods. Within a decade, large-scale outdoor grow sites (> 100 plants) with multiple greenhouses and full-sun plants numbered in the thousands in the watersheds of the Emerald Triangle. Department of Fish and Wildlife investigations mapping one watershed estimated that cannabis cultivation combined to use over 18 million gallons of water that accounted for over 50% of the stream flow during the driest part of the summer (Bauer et al. 2015, 13). Natural resource managers found that cannabis operations had completely dewatered streams that contained endangered salmon and steelhead populations already compromised by multiple years of drought. Left with few resources and absent any clear policy guidance, law enforcement and land managers had little success enforcing environmental and land management regulations on the overwhelming number of large-scale grows in the region, with California becoming the main supply source for cannabis consumed in the United States (Northern California High Intensity Drug Trafficking Area Drug Market Analysis 2011).

The increase in awareness of environmental impacts by land managers and the public became an important driver of efforts to regulate the cannabis industry.[7] In 2015, the California legislature passed a series of bills that for the first time regulated medical cannabis. Assembly Bill 266, Assembly Bill 243, and Senate Bill 643 created the Medical Cannabis Regulation and Safety Act (MCRSA), giving regulatory power to three government agencies, with the California Department of Consumer Affairs regulating retail sales, distribution, and testing; the California Department of Public Health regulating manufacturing; and the California Department of Food and Agriculture regulating cultivation. Included in MCRSA were important environmental protections that restricted the use of pesticides in production and put limits on the size of both indoor and outdoor cultivation, essentially banning large-scale commercial medical cannabis agriculture.[8] For the first time in two decades, the state outlined environmental protections by establishing detailed guidelines on water diversions and discharges, pesticides, product testing, and health and safety rules to mitigate the environmental problems associated with cannabis cultivation.

Proposition 64, Legalization of Recreational Cannabis (2016)

In 2016, California voters passed Proposition 64, the Adult Use of Marijuana Act (AUMA), legalizing recreational cannabis.[9] Heralded by legalization activists and policy makers as the environmental gold standard of cannabis legislation, the measure allocated funding for conservation, restoration, and enforcement of environmental laws. A number of very important environmental protections were written into AUMA to address environmental concerns. State regulations mandated unprecedented environmental assessments as well as permits for every type of cannabis commerce, accompanied by heavy fines for noncompliance. It contained severe restrictions on pesticide use in cultivation, established low pesticide tolerances in cannabis products, and required rigorous testing for other contaminants that could be harmful to cannabis consumers. Additionally, it required that licensees provide evidence that they are in compliance with the California Environmental Quality Act (CEQA), the Clean Water Act, as well as other existing water quality control laws and wastewater discharge permits.[10]

More controversial to small cultivators and natural resource managers was AUMA's removal of the cultivation cap, which limited the size of farms to one acre. Rather than keep in place the acreage cap outlined under MCRSA, AUMA removed it but gave small-scale growers a five-year head start in the regulated market by forbidding licenses for cannabis farms larger than one acre until 2023. Interestingly, small farmers revealed a hopeful optimism regarding the five-year window of protection offered by the state, which incentivized some cultivators to enter the regulated market (Houston 2017).

In June 2017, the California State Legislature passed Senate Bill 94, merging MCRSA with AUMA into one bill, creating the Medicinal and Adult-Use Cannabis Regulation and Safety Act (MAUCRSA). This bill provided a unified regulatory framework to govern both medicinal and adult-use cannabis in California, establishing the following three licensing authorities:[11]

- Bureau of Cannabis Control (Department of Consumer Affairs), which oversees the licensing of testing laboratories, retailers, distributors, and microbusinesses.
- CalCannabis Cultivation Licensing (Department of Food and Agriculture), which manages the track and trace system, and licenses cultivation.
- Manufactured Cannabis Safety Branch (Department of Public Health), which licenses manufacturers of cannabis products.

There are two important environmental policy implications to note regarding MAUCRSA. First, while MCRSA placed limits on the number of licenses one company could hold, MAUCRSA permits companies to hold multiple licenses, thereby opening up the opportunity for vertical integration and the potential for large corporations to dominate the industry. Rather than encourage small-scale specialization, the policy has produced economic challenges for new small businesses who want to enter the industry and for existing small growers who now have to compete with larger well-capitalized companies (Allen 2018a). The second, and more significant, environmental policy change under MAUCRSA is scale. The hopes of small farmers getting a five-year head start on big cannabis were dashed on the eve of legalization when the Department of Food and Agriculture released a series of temporary rule changes that allowed unlimited small cultivation licenses for individual companies. This policy change essentially removed the five-year moratorium on large-scale cultivation, contradicting the state's Final Environmental Impact Report, allowing those with enough capital to buy as many licenses as they desired.[12]

Well-resourced companies were able to purchase, or "stack," unlimited small cultivator licenses, which removed economic protections for small cultivators trying to enter into the regulated market.[13] Legislators in the Emerald Triangle predicted that removing the cap on the number of licenses would "crush the livelihood of small family farmers" (Garofoli 2017). As of this writing, state licensing data (2018) bears out this claim with a handful of companies holding hundreds of cultivator licenses (McVey 2018; Kaskey 2018).[14] While the state issued over 8,000 permits to cultivate cannabis in 2018, 729 were awarded to just five companies. In short, the combination of these two policy changes further complicates efforts to reduce the environmental impacts of cannabis cultivation by encouraging cultivators to expand operations, increasing their demands on environmental resources.

Post-Prohibition Environmental Challenges

Although the environmental impact of cannabis liberalization will not be clear for several years, next I outline a number of significant policy challenges that will need to be addressed to effectively reduce and mitigate the environmental harms associated with cannabis legalization.

Regulatory Fees and Taxation

In the first six months of legalization, California has struggled to reign in the unregulated market and bring growers into the regulatory environment. While an accurate assessment of data on compliance is difficult to determine at this time, the cannabis industry estimates that of the over 60,000 cannabis cultivators in California, less than 10% have made the transition to the legal market, with about half driven back to the unregulated market by the new rules (Allen 2018a). Small-scale cultivators point to the complexity of the new rules and the costs of state/local licensing and compliance fees as substantial barriers, leaving only those with the financial resources—who in the past have been some of the most egregious violators of environmental laws—access to the regulated market.

Another problem identified as a barrier to entry by small-scale cultivators is the regressive tax levied on cultivation. Cultivators, regardless of size, must pay an excise tax of 15%, as well as state cultivation taxes of $9.25 per ounce of flower and $2.75 per ounce of leaves they sell. Municipal taxes are added to that, which can range from $1 to $25 dollars per square foot of cultivation. Not only is this an economic burden for small family farmers, the cultivation and square-footage taxes encourage growers to expand their operations and change their cultivation methods to achieve more harvests annually through outdoor, indoor, and mixed light methods, thus increasing demands on water, forests, and the energy grid. Thus, the current tax model incentivizes large-scale cultivation while discouraging sustainable practices such as crop rotation practiced by small farmers.

Local Bans

While the state sets the minimum licensing standards under MAUCRSA, many local government agencies have been more restrictive in permitting commercial cannabis activities in their communities, effectively locking out growers who practice environmental sustainability. As many local governments lack the expertise and resources needed to draft and enforce cannabis regulations, many have opted to ban cannabis businesses altogether. NIMBY (Not in My Back Yard) zoning practices, such as odor abatement, have been commonly applied to prohibit otherwise compliant and permittable cannabis businesses in many municipalities. As a result, cannabis businesses are not permitted in over 70% of jurisdictions in California, driving thousands of cultivators back into the unregulated market where there is no environmental oversight (Allen 2018b). While the use of Google Earth and other mapping technologies has facilitated surveillance and environmental enforcement of non-permitted cultivation, their deployment has forced outdoor cultivators to return to the "dirty" indoor cultivation methods (with diesel generators) to avoid detection, creating another set of environmental problems.

Energy Use and Greenhouse Gas (GHG)

One of the most important environmental impacts of the legal cannabis industry might be its carbon footprint, if indoor, greenhouse, and mixed light production are allowed to dominate. According to Mills (2012), indoor cannabis agriculture *prior to legalization* was estimated at 3% percent of the state's electricity consumption, the equivalent to the electricity consumption of one million California homes. State licensing data shows that over half of all the licensed recreational cannabis cultivators in the state are engaged in indoor or mixed light operations, with both relying heavily on the electric grid (Staggs 2018).[15] Pacific Gas & Electric's decision to extend its agricultural energy rate to commercial cannabis businesses will also facilitate the expansion of indoor/mixed light production and increase electricity demands.[16] This complicates efforts of communities throughout the state who have developed climate action plans and clean energy goals to reduce their regional carbon emissions (Arthur 2017). As the leading supplier of cannabis in the nation, the tax revenues generated will not reflect the true climate costs of the carbon footprint of the legal cannabis industry, which is certain to have detrimental impacts on the environment and public health in coming years.

Packaging

Along with the old environmental problems of illegal water diversions, forest degradation, and pesticide use, liberalization has mandated a new kind of pollution in the form of packaging, the bulk of which is not recycled (Eichner 2018). Child-resistant packaging, the centerpiece of MAUCRSA, requires that all cannabis goods be prepackaged prior to distribution and placed into an additional secondary package at the time of sale. While the environmental impact of these packaging requirements will not be known for some time, it is thought to be substantial with plastic packaging and the nonrecyclable waste from vape pens and oil cartridges likely to result in more waste in California's landfills.[17] With over $2.5 billion in sales in 2018, the cannabis industry in California produces well over one million units of single-use plastic packaging waste per year (Arcview Market Research and BDS Analytics 2019; Black 2018).[18]

Policy Recommendations

As the overall environmental impacts of MAUCRSA will not be clear for several years, further policy reforms will be necessary to more effectively protect the environment. In developing these reforms, policy makers must do a better job reducing the barriers to entry, incentivizing ecologically sustainable agriculture, and setting stronger waste management standards for the industry. There is a desperate need for data collection and analysis on the impacts of cultivation practices and size of the industry on the environment to give policy makers and natural resource managers a better understanding of the ecological footprint of the industry. Given the current lack of empirical data on the environmental costs associated with cannabis cultivation, state legislators should consider reinstating the acreage cap (one acre maximum) and applying a moratorium on all Type 5 (no acreage limits) permits. Expanding cannabis cultivation in a state that has been estimated to have produced over 13 million pounds of cannabis in 2017, five times more than the 2.5 million pounds it consumed, is certain to lead to significant impacts on water, fish, and wildlife and merits a revision of the cultivation cap (Allen 2018a). To further incentivize entry into the regulated market, policy makers should eliminate the cultivation and square footage tax entirely. Not only is this tax a substantial economic burden for small family farmers, the cultivation and square-footage taxes are disincentives to compliance and are anti-ecological, encouraging growers to expand their operations and change their cultivation methods to achieve more harvests annually, thus increasing demands on water, forests, and the energy grid.

There is also a significant need to broaden participation in policymaking beyond the voices of large industry advocates to include small cultivators and environmental scientists who have been left out of initial state and local decision-making concerning the development of cannabis regulations. Important environmental voices and advocates for strong environmental policies have been denied appointments on influential state cannabis boards and regulatory advisory commissions. Of the 22 members appointed to the California Cannabis Advisory Committee, over half represent economic interests, with none having any environmental science expertise.[19] While the full extent of the cannabis industry's lobbying activities are hard to measure, the number of registered cannabis lobbyists in Washington has increased substantially from only one lobbyist in 2014 to 80 in 2019.[20] The national cannabis lobby, which spent more than $3.7 million (2019) lobbying policy makers, will continue to use its financial and political capital to pressure regulatory agencies to relax environmental protections such as pesticide tolerances and other regulations that impact profitability (Miller 2018; Reklaitis 2019).[21] For example, the National Cannabis Industry Association has lobbied the Environmental Protection Agency to amend federal regulations to allow pesticide use in the cannabis industry.[22] To ensure that the environment and public health is adequately safeguarded, policy makers will also need to develop stronger environmental regulations regarding industry carbon emissions and energy consumption. While the long-term goal should be a net-zero emissions industry, state and local governments must take concrete steps to significantly reduce the industry's CO_2 emissions by incentivizing energy conservation through a carbon tax and tax credits for cultivators who significantly reduce their ecological footprint.

Conclusions

While there is no doubt that cannabis agriculture has produced environmental problems, these are problems associated with social and environmental policies that have facilitated and rewarded poor environmental practices in the cannabis industry. Contrary to the claims of prohibitionist drug warriors, it is not simply unscrupulous cannabis cultivators but regulatory policies that have had an adverse effect on the environment. This is a result of over two decades of poorly drafted cannabis policy that has disincentivized participation in regulated markets and incentivized the development of ecologically destructive agricultural practices.

Twenty-five years into the liberalization of cannabis in California, the illicit market continues to dwarf the legal cannabis market. In light of policy efforts to reign in unpermitted cannabis cultivators, it seems safe to assume that continuing an approach that relies on negative incentives to bring cultivators into the regulated market will continue to prove unsuccessful. At this point, the state must engage in a comprehensive review of the cannabis regulatory system and policy impacts on cultivators to figure out which approaches to compliance are working and which are not. The current approach, which favors highly capitalized corporations and incentivizes industrial-scale agriculture, puts at a disadvantage small-scale farmers who practice sustainable agriculture. In order to adequately address the unintended environmental impacts, it is critical for regulators to move away from the use of negative incentives that are characteristic of prohibition and create policies with positive rewards that incentivize ecological sustainability and encourage entry into the regulated market.

Notes

1 See Riding (1978), Jones (1985), and Potter, Gaines, and Holbrook (1990) for assessments of the effectiveness of the herbicide program.

2 California's Emerald Triangle refers to the three largest cannabis-producing counties in the United States: Humboldt County, Mendocino County, and Trinity County.

3 As Reuter (1983) notes, criminal sanctions associated with federal prohibition act as a price support by inflating the cost of cannabis production, manufacturing, and distribution.

4 Throughout the region, plant eradications rose from a low of 47,841 in 1983 to a high of 337,927 in 1996, with an average of 25,000 plants removed from public land annually. www.drugscience.org/Archive/bcr2/DCESP.html

5 Eradication numbers on private land doubled in the years following the passage of Proposition 215, with 2.5 million eradicated from 1997 to 2000, to 6.4 million in the years 2001–2004. Public lands also saw an increase over the same period from 646,943 (1997–2000) to 1.7 million (2001–2004). Source: NDIC 2009.

6 Keegan (2016) provides an analysis of the environmental and physiological effects of light pollution from "mixed light" cannabis cultivation.

7 From 2010 to 2014, public symposiums and scholarly research on cannabis and the environment helped to raise awareness about the environmental impacts of cannabis agriculture. Notable was the *Earth Day Symposium on Marijuana and the Environment* (2013) at Humboldt State University, which brought together cannabis cultivators, policy makers, land managers, tribal leaders, academics, law enforcement, and environmental organizations to examine environmental issues associated with the cannabis industry.

8 Outdoor cultivation was capped at one acre for outdoor (Type 3 license), while the maximum for indoor was 22,000 square feet (Type 3A/3B licenses).

9 The full text of Proposition 64 is available at https://leginfo.legislature.ca.gov/faces/codes_displayexpandedbranch.xhtml?tocCode=BPC&division=10.&title=&part=&chapter=&article

10 The California Porter-Cologne Water Quality Control Act and the federal Clean Water Act are two existing laws that may also apply to cultivation.

11 For a comprehensive list of state regulatory agencies and responsibilities see https://leginfo.legislature.ca.gov/faces/billTextClient.xhtml?bill_id=201720180SB94

12 www.cdfa.ca.gov/calcannabis/PEIR.html

13 In January 2018, the California Growers Alliance (CGA), a cannabis industry trade association representing small and medium-size cultivators, filed a lawsuit against the California Department of Food and Agriculture over the rule changes. Source: https://www.sacbee.com/news/california/california-weed/article196400149.html

14 Source: California Department of Food and Agriculture (2018).

15 Indoor and mixed light accounted for over 58% of all temporary recreational cultivation licenses in 2018. Source: California Department of Food and Agriculture.

16 In states like Colorado, where the majority of legal cannabis is produced indoors, surging electricity consumption has taxed the electrical grids with over 4% of Denver's total electricity devoted to cannabis (Hood 2018).

17 Ward (2018) reports that the packaging for one gram of cannabis concentrate can weigh as much as 30 times as much as the product.

18 One Northern California cannabis company reported adding over 100,000 plastic joint packaging tubes into the waste stream each month (Ruskin 2019).

19 This has also been the case with Oregon www.oregon.gov/olcc/marijuana/Documents/CEBP/CEBP_Roster.pdf

20 www.opensecrets.org/federal-lobbying/industries/summary?cycle=2019&id=N09

21 In the case of Colorado, pesticide regulators complained that the industry was "the biggest challenge" to stronger pesticide regulations in the state (Migoya 2015).

22 See the National Cannabis Industry Association's white paper, "Overcoming Federal Obstacles to the Sensible Use of Pesticides on Cannabis" https://thecannabisindustry.org/wp-content/uploads/2018/08/NCIA-Pesticides-white-paper_v2r2_Final.pdf

References

Allen, Hezekiah. 2018a. "The Transition to Legal Cannabis." 14th Annual Schaub Memorial Lecture, Humboldt State University, March 26.

———. 2018b. "California's Cannabis Supply Chain Panel." Meadowlands Cannabis Conference. Camp Navarro, Mendocino, CA. June 16.

Anders, Gentry. 1990. *Beyond Counterculture*. Pullman: Washington State University Press.

Arcview Market Research and BDS Analytics. 2019. *The State of Legal Marijuana Markets*. 6th ed. Accessed May 4, 2021. https://bdsa.com/wp-content/uploads/2019/07/2019_Update_20190409.pdf.

Arthur, Damon. 2017. "PG&E Gives Marijuana Growers Ag Electricity Rates." *Record Searchlight*, March 1. Accessed March 29, 2017. www.redding.com/story/news/2017/03/01/pge-gives-marijuana-growers-break/98611352/.

Austin, James. 2005. *Rethinking Consequences of Decriminalizing Marijuana*. Washington, DC: The JFA Institute.

Bauer, Scott, Jennifer Olson, Adam Cockrill, Michael van Hattem, Linda Miller, Margaret Tauzer, and Gordon Leppig. 2015. "Impacts of Surface Water Diversions for Marijuana Cultivation on Aquatic Habitat in Four Northwestern California Watersheds." *PLoS One* 10 (9): e0137935. www.ncbi.nlm.nih.gov/pmc/articles/PMC4364984/.

Black, Lester. 2018. "Will New Pot Packaging Rules Make California's Weed Less Green?" *Emerald Report*, March 18. Accessed May 21, 2018. www.emeraldreport.com/will-new-pot-packaging-rules-make-californias-weed-less-green/.

Bosk, Beth Robinson. 2000. *The New Settler Interviews*. White River Junction, VT: Chelsea Green.

Campaign Against Marijuana Planting Annual Report. 1983. "Archived by Humboldt State University Special Collections." http://library.humboldt.edu/humco/holdings/CAMP/CAMP1985.pdf.

———. 1985. "Archived by Humboldt State University Special Collections." http://library.humboldt.edu/humco/holdings/CAMP/CAMP1985.pdf.

———. 1990. "Archived by Humboldt State University Special Collections." http://library.humboldt.edu/humco/holdings/CAMP/CAMP1990.pdf.

Caulkins, Jonathan P., and Rosalie L. Pacula. 2006. "Marijuana Markets: Inferences from Reports by the Household Population." *Journal of Drug Issues* 36 (1): 173–20.

Chapkis, Wendy, and Richard J. Webb. 2008. *Dying to Get High: Marijuana as Medicine*. New York: New York University Press.

Corva, Dominic. 2014. "Requiem for a CAMP: The Life and Death of a Domestic U.S. Drug War Institution." *International Journal of Drug Policy* 25 (1): 71–80.

———. 2018. *Rethinking the Nature of Cannabis and Social Policy in the Context of Post-Prohibition*. Sustainable Futures Speaker Series. Arcata, CA: Humboldt State University, April 19.

Dills, Angela, Sietse Goffard, and Jeffrey Miron. 2016. *Dose of Reality: The Effect of State Marijuana Legalizations*. Cato Institute Policy Analysis no. 799, September 16. www.cato.org/publications/policy-analysis/dose-reality-effect-state-marijuana-legalizations.

Eichner, James. 2018. "The Cannabis Industry Has A Plastic Problem." *Cannabis Compliance and Packaging Magazine*, February 22. Accessed May 12, 2018. https://cannabiscomplianceandpackaging.com/2018/02/22/cannabis-industry-plastic-problem/.

Gabriel, M. W., L. W. Woods, R. Poppenga, R. A. Sweitzer, C. Thompson, S. M. Matthews, J. M. Higley, S. M. Keller, K. Purcell, R. H. Barrett, G. M. Wengert, B. N. Sacks, and D. L. Clifford. 2012. "Anticoagulant Rodenticides on Our Public and Community Lands: Spatial Distribution of Exposure and Poisoning of a Rare Forest Carnivore." *PLoS One* 7 (7): e40163. www.iercecology.org/wp-content/uploads/2012/07/Gabriel_et_al_2012.

Garofoli, Joe. 2017. "Smaller Growers Say Regulators Reneged on Pot Plot Ownership." *San Francisco Chronicle*, December 10. Accessed March 21, 2018. www.sfchronicle.com/politics/article/Smaller-growers-say-regulators-reneged-on-pot-12420404.php.

Gurnon, Emily. 2005. "Environmental Scourge of 'Diesel Dope': KMUD Forum Seeks to Educate Public." *North Coast Journal*. Accessed December 15, 2017. www.northcoastjournal.com/021005/news0210.html.

Harris, David. 1997. *The Last Stand: The War Between Wall Street and Main Street Over California's Ancient Redwoods*. San Francisco, CA: Sierra Club Books.

Hood, Grace. 2018. "Nearly 4 Percent of Denver's Electricity Is Now Devoted To Marijuana." *Colorado Public Radio*, February 19. Accessed June 10, 2018. www.cpr.org/news/story/nearly-4-percent-of-denver-s-electricity-is-now-devoted-to-marijuana.

House, Freeman. 1999. *Totem Salmon. Life Lesson From Another Species*. Boston, MA: Beacon Press.

Houston, Jim. 2017. "Wood, McGuire Call for One-Acre Cap on Cannabis Cultivation." *Eureka Times Standard*, December 6. Accessed December 7, 2017. www.times-standard.com/article/NJ/20171206/NEWS/171209892.

Jones, Roberta. 1985. "U.S. Revives Plan to Kill Marijuana with Paraquat." *Los Angeles Times*, July 28. Accessed June 2, 2014. http://articles.latimes.com/1985-07-28/news/mn-5386_1_marijuana-eradication.

Kaskey, Jack. 2018. "California's Weed Black Market Ramps Back Up." *Bloomberg News*, June 28. Accessed June 12, 2018. www.bloomberg.com/news/articles/2018-06-28/california-pot-industry-at-reckoning-as-new-rules-upend-market.

Keegan, Kyle. 2016. "In Defense of the Stars: The Use of 'Mixed-Light' Greenhouses is Changing Our Night Skies and May Be Altering Our Nocturnal Ecology." *Redheaded Blackbelt*. Accessed June 10, 2018. http://kymkemp.com/2016/06/02/in-defense-of-the-stars-the-use-of-mixed-light-greenhouses-is-changing-our-night-skies-and-may-be-altering-our-environments/.

Keith, D. R., C. L. Hart, M. P. McNeil, R. Silver, and R. D. Goodwin. 2015. "Frequent Marijuana Use, Binge Drinking and Mental Health Problems Among Undergraduates." *The American Journal on Addictions* 24: 499–506.

Kilmer, Beau. 2014. "Policy Designs for Cannabis Legalization: Starting with the Eight P's." *The American Journal of Drug and Alcohol Abuse* 40 (4): 259–61.

Koch, Frank, Jeffrey P. Prestemon, Geoffrey H. Donovan, Everett A. Hinkley, and John M. Chase. 2016. "Predicting Cannabis Cultivation on National Forests Using a Rational Choice Framework." *Ecological Economics* 129: 161–71.

Lee, Martin. 2012. *Smoke Signals: A Social History of Marijuana—Medical, Recreational, and Scientific*. New York: Scribner.

McKinley, Jesse. 2008. "Marijuana Hotbed Retreats on Medicinal Use." *The New York Times*, June 9. Accessed May 12, 2018. www.nytimes.com/2008/06/09/us/09pot.html?hp.

McVey, Eli. 2018. "Chart: Handful of Growers Hold Hundreds of Cultivation Licenses in California's Legal Marijuana Market." *Marijuana Business Daily*, June 18. Accessed June 21, 2018. https://mjbizdaily.com/chart-handful-growers-hold-hundreds-cultivation-licenses-california-legal-marijuana-market/.

Migoya, David. 2015. "Colorado Yields to Marijuana Industry Pressure on Pesticides." *Denver Post*, October 3. Accessed May 13, 2018. www.denverpost.com/2015/10/03/colorado-yields-to-marijuana-industry-pressure-on-pesticides/.

Miller, Char, and Anthony Silvaggio. 2018. "Reading the Tea Leaves." In *Where There's Smoke: The Environmental Science, Public Policy, and Politics of Marijuana*, edited by Char Miller, 213–22. Lawrence, KS: University of Kansas Press.

Miller, Cheryl. 2018. "The Marijuana Lobby: Who Got the Work." *The Recorder*, February 1. Accessed June 21, 2018. www.law.com/therecorder/sites/therecorder/2018/02/01/the-marijuana-lobby-who-got-the-work/?slreturn=20180620030152.

Mills, Evan. 2012. "The Carbon Footprint of Indoor Cannabis Production." *Energy Policy* 46: 58–67.

Miron, Jeffrey. 2010. "The Budgetary Implications of Drug Prohibition." Report funded by the Criminal Justice Policy Foundation, Harvard University, Boston, MA. Accessed March 12, 2018. www.economics.harvard.edu/faculty/miron/files/budget%202010%20Final.pdf.

Northern California High Intensity Drug Trafficking Area Drug Market Analysis. 2011. "U.S. Department of Justice National Drug Intelligence Center." Retrieved March 21, 2018. https://www.justice.gov/archive/ndic/dmas/Northern_CA_DMA-2011(U).pdf.

O'Hare, Michael, Daniel L. Sanchez, and Peter Alstone. 2013. "Environmental Risks and Opportunities in Cannabis Cultivation." *BOTEC Analysis Corp. I-502 Project #430–5d*, June 28. https://lcb.wa.gov/publications/Marijuana/SEPA/BOTEC_Whitepaper_Final.pdf.

Potter, Gary W., Larry Gaines, and Beth Holbrook. 1990. "Blowing Smoke: An Evaluation of Kentucky's Marijuana Eradication Program." *American Journal of Police* 9 (1): 97–16.

Raphael, Ray. 1985. *Cash Crop. An American Dream*. Mendocino, CA: Ridgetop Press.

Raskin, Josh. 2012. *Marijuanaland*. New York: Trans High Corporation.

Reklaitis, Victor. 2019. "Cannabis Industry's Lobbying on Track to Hit a New Record." *Marketwatch*. Accessed July 27, 2019. www.marketwatch.com/story/cannabis-industrys-lobbying-on-track-to-hit-a-new-record-2019-07-25.

Reuter, Peter. 1983. *Disorganized Crime: The Economics of the Visible Hand*. Cambridge, MA: MIT Press.

Riding, Alan. 1978. "Mexico Won't Halt Marijuana Spraying." *Sarasota Herald Tribune*, Tues May 23, Pg. 8A. Accessed June 21, 2018. https://news.google.com/newspapers?nid=1755&dat=19780523&id=akk0AAAAIBAJ&sjid=c2cEAAAAIBAJ&pg=6770,3068056&hl=en.

Ruskin, Zach. 2019. "Weed's Waste Problem: The Perils of Plastic May Haunt the Cannabis Industry." *Merry Jane*, May 1. Accessed June 12, 2019. https://merryjane.com/culture/weeds-waste-problem-the-perils-of-plastic-may-haunt-the-cannabis-industry.

Shepard, Edward M., and Paul R. Blackley. 2007. "The Impact of Marijuana Law Enforcement in an Economic Model of Crime." *Journal of Drug Issues* 37 (2): 403–24.

Silvaggio, Anthony. 2012. "Google Earth: Environmental Damage of Industrial Cannabis Agriculture." Accessed March 10, 2013. www.youtube.com/watch?time_continue=2&v=Ewv5xeI4uug.

———. 2018. "Cannabis Agriculture in California: The Environmental Consequences of Prohibition." In *Where There's Smoke: The Environmental Science, Public Policy, and Politics of Marijuana*, edited by Char Miller, 13–28. Lawrence, KS: University of Kansas Press.

Sims, Hank. 2015. "Arcata Sez: Grow House Electricity Tax Has Driven Out Hundreds of Weed Operations." *Lost Coast Outpost*, June 16. Accessed May 13, 2018. https://lostcoastoutpost.com/2015/jun/16/arcata-sez-grow-house-electric-tax-has-driven-.

Staggs, Brooke. 2018. "So Far, California Has 6,000 Licensed Cannabis Businesses. Here's What That Looks Like." *Orange County Register*, April 27. Accessed June 21, 2018. www.ocregister.com/2018/04/27/so-far-california-has-6000-licensed-cannabis-businesses-heres-what-that-looks-like/.

Ward, Spencer. 2018. "Marijuana Packaging Waste Is the New Water Bottle." *Rooster*, July 11. Accessed July 21, 2018. https://therooster.com/blog/wasteful-nature-marijuana-packaging-new-water-bottle.

21

Energy Use by the Indoor Cannabis Industry

Inconvenient Truths for Producers, Consumers, and Policy Makers

Evan Mills and Scott Zeramby

Cannabis Legalization Is Necessary but Not Sufficient for Addressing Energy Waste

Decades spent in the shadows of the black market created few opportunities to understand the patterns of energy use associated with indoor cannabis cultivation, let alone compel the industry to manage consumption and thus keep its environmental consequences in check.[1] Cannabis production, distribution, and sale involve a myriad of energy uses, some of which are direct and others indirect (Figure 21.1). Drivers of energy demand and the associated greenhouse-gas emissions include creating the inputs and energy used during production, processing, managing waste, downstream retail activities, and transportation. Key decision makers and stakeholders include policy makers, planners, producers, investors, industry analysts, and consumers.

Although the impacts of outdoor cultivation on ecosystems have received considerable attention (and do not primarily involve energy), those associated with far more energy-intensive indoor cultivation have only rarely been evaluated and integrated into policymaking, even in the post-prohibition era. Indeed, cannabis cultivators continue to be passed over by almost every energy policy instrument developed since the first modern energy crisis of half a century ago. Moreover, many instances of post-prohibition cannabis policies are inadvertently driving energy use upwards, while the "financial incentives" for energy efficiency being offered to indoor cultivators by electric utility companies represent a counter-productive subsidy and legitimization of a polluting activity that could be done much more sustainably outdoors, which could meet all U.S. demand with only 0.01% of current farmland.[2]

The anti-competitive repercussions of ill-conceived policy and scant evaluation of policy adequacy demonstrate that legalization is necessary—but not sufficient—to address the associated environmental issues. These considerations intersect with more prominent cannabis policy issues such as taxation, public health and safety, interstate commerce, testing and product labeling, broader agricultural policy, water resources, and solid waste management. Particularly vexing is that even the most basic analyses are impeded by lack of rigor and lingering uncertainties about the structure and drivers of energy use and how far energy efficiency and renewable energy can realistically go towards mitigating the associated undesirable impacts. For example, stemming from fundamental data gaps,

DOI: 10.4324/9780429320491-21

Direct and indirect drivers of energy use and greenhouse-gas emissions from the cannabis industry

Inputs	• Energy (embodied) • Industrial CO2* • Water production and supply • Soil, amendments, fertilizers • Artificial growing media • Pesticides, herbicides, fungicides, rodenticides • Plastics (bagging, mulch, greenhouse sheeting, containers, irrigation, etc.)	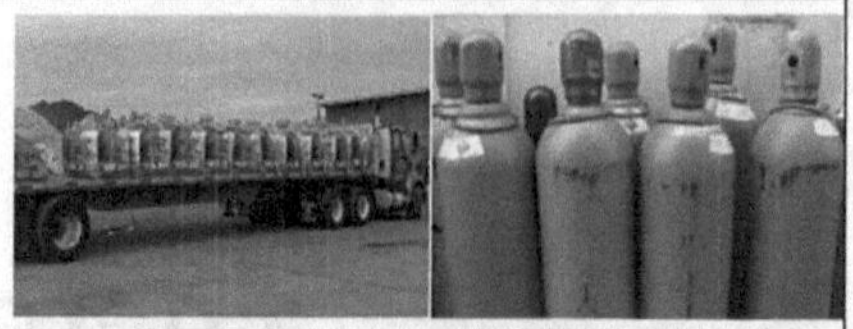
Production	• Outdoor • Small structure (windowless)* • Large structure (windowless) • Greenhouse • Energy: lighting, cooling, heating, ventilation, odor control, CO2 generator, dehumidification, water heat, pumping, IT, plug loads*	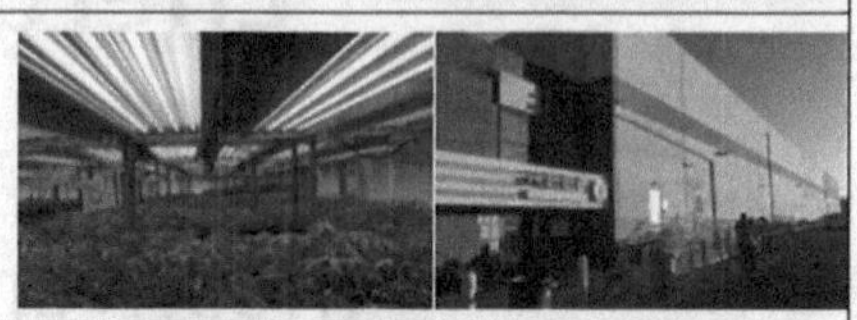
Processing	• Flower drying* / freezing • Energy for producing extracts; solvents (butane, propane, ethanol, isopropyl alcohol) • Cooking/baking • Packaging • Testing labs	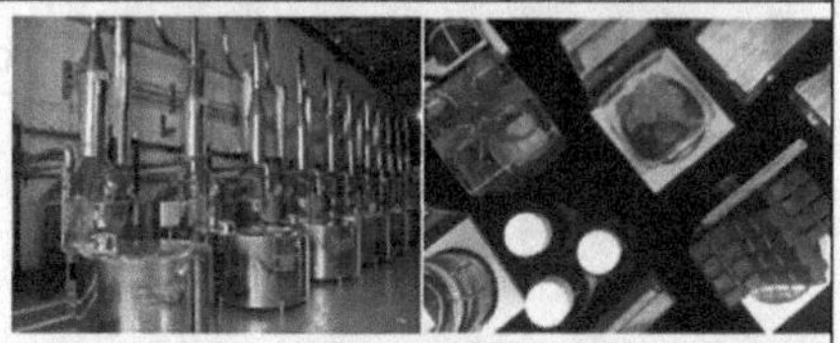
Waste	• Failed/interdicted crops • Material not passing inspection • Single-use soil or artificial growing media • Plastics • Hydroponic water effluent to waste-treatment plant • Biomass residu	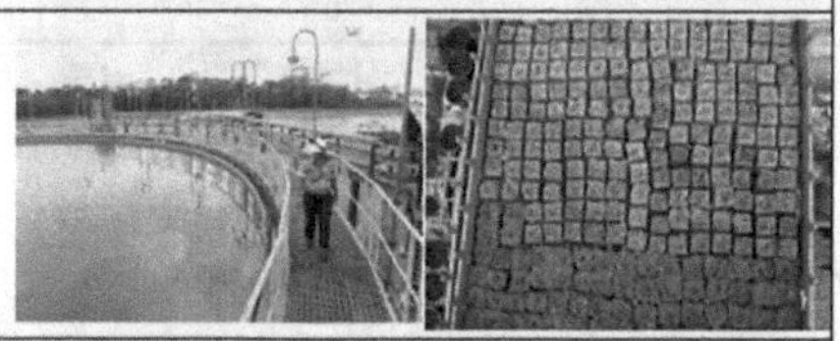
Retail	• Facility construction • Lighting • Heating • Cooling • Ventilation • Refrigeration	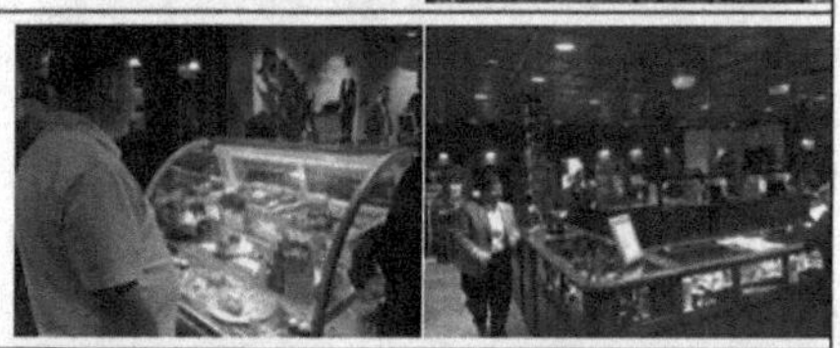
Transport	• Materials to jobsite • Workers to jobsite* • Product to intermediaries • Product to retail* • Consumer to retail* • Delivery services • Waste disposal	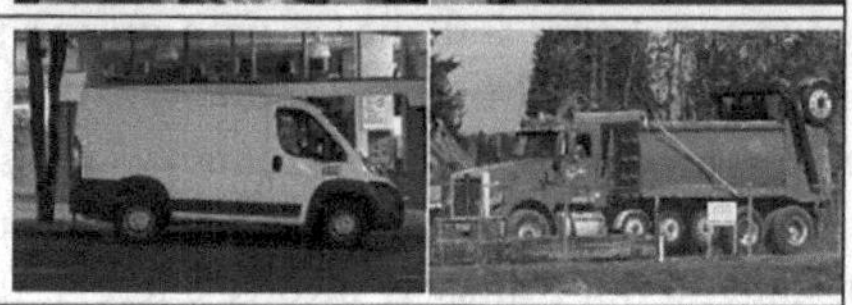

** Items accounted for in energy-use estimates by Mills (2012).*

Figure 21.1 Modes of energy use associated with cannabis production, distribution, and sale

Sources: Photos (from top to bottom, left to right): (a) "Big bags of soil is the new dumptruck" by Roberrific is licensed under CC BY-NC 2.0. (b) "CO_2 Tanks" by jercraigs is licensed with CC BY-NC 2.0. (c) "Distillation" by nathangibbs is licensed under CC BY-NC-SA 2.0. (d) "Water treatment—Hydro Alunorte" by Norsk Hydro ASA is licensed under CC BY-NC-SA 2.0. (e) "Rockwool" by wormjava is licensed with CC BY-NC-ND 2.0. (f) "White Van" by Curtis Gregory Perry is licensed under CC BY-NC-SA 2.0. (g) "Peterbilt Dump Truck" by born 1945 is licensed under CC BY 2.0. Others by authors.

even baseline studies often omit key considerations and unwittingly suffer from unquantified biases due to problems with data collection and verification.

This chapter pinpoints blind spots in regulation, outlines research and analysis needs, argues for consumer information and protections against greenwashing and industry capture of regulatory and green-certification processes, and offers recommendations for incorporating energy considerations into the broader tapestry of cannabis policy. The balance of evidence suggests that even at ostensibly high energy efficiencies and intensive use of renewable energy, indoor cultivation "optimizes the suboptimal" and cannibalizes renewable resources previously developed for other purposes, which is untenable in a carbon-constrained world. Outdoor cultivation—which has sufficed for millennia—is the most technologically elegant, sustainable, ethical, and economically viable approach for minimizing the rising energy and environmental burden of cannabis production.

The Cannabis Conundrum: Drug Policy Is Decoupled From Environmental Policy

Few public policy issues are as multifaceted as that of cannabis production and consumption. Quantifying the energy use and carbon footprint associated with producing cannabis and its derivative products is one of the primary and least explored policy-relevant questions. When confined to the black market, this sector could not readily access relevant expertise and information-sharing networks. However, little progress has been made in the wake of legalization efforts. To our knowledge, no state has initiated a comprehensive approach to the problem, and federal engagement is nonexistent.

Windowless cannabis factory farms constantly battle local weather conditions to maintain stable round-the-clock temperatures and pump out acres of electric light brighter than the summer sun, day or night. Such industrialized cannabis cultivation facilities—whether in Fairbanks or Phoenix—must simulate and maintain artificially cloudless tropical environments while suppressing disease-causing humidity year round. Industrially manufactured carbon dioxide (an added energy-intensive input and greenhouse gas in its own right, increasing carbon footprint on the order of 5%—more if and as energy efficiency improves) is often injected to artificially boost plant growth. Operating the equipment[3] needed to create and maintain these artificial environments can require as much energy as a similarly sized data center. Indoor cultivators cite debatable reasons for this practice: security, a more predictable product, buffering from weather and other crop hazards, maximized cash flow due to year-round production, the need for fewer employees, legislative restrictions, and the ability to achieve multiple harvests per year.[4]

As with most other environmental issues, those associated with cannabis are "shaded out" by other seemingly more pressing concerns faced by policy makers (in this case taxation, zoning, child safety, etc.). Together with the highly technical and complicated nature of how energy is used in the industry and how to quantify energy efficiency, few policy makers are even equipped to engage effectively. As a case in point, the IRS has been thwarted in pursuing tax-fraud cases since it cannot readily correlate reported sales volumes with utility bills.

The Environmental Footprint of Cannabis Production: Demonization or Double Standard?

Energy-intensive indoor cultivation has been conducted within the black market for decades. The original shift to the practice was, in part, a product of prohibition enforcement efforts that pushed growers indoors to avoid detection (Silvaggio 2021, Chapter 20, this volume). As will be outlined later, legalization does not intrinsically address the energy issues and can even compound them by encouraging the rapid scale-up of indoor facilities and otherwise altering patterns of energy use in unexpected ways.

Some industry advocates have complained that cannabis is singled out for scrutiny, while other sectors are left to their devices or otherwise pollute more. This argument is spurious (Mills 2016), as cannabis is in actuality one of the vanishingly few segments of the economy that has been largely overlooked in energy and environmental policy. Moreover, as is well established in the climate change mitigation field, there is no "silver-bullet" solution, and a multitude of energy uses must be simultaneously addressed in order to meet society's important emissions-reduction targets. It is a false choice to argue that one energy use should be addressed in lieu of another. There is no single cause of climate change, and thus no single solution. Meanwhile, the cannabis sector is arguably decades behind the rest of the economy when it comes to energy efficiency. In any case, adequate technical fixes are unlikely to be available if the demand for extraordinary levels of artificial illumination persists.

A key starting point for establishing a context for good decision-making is quantifying the level of energy use and associated greenhouse-gas emissions, and how that compares to other activities. Until less than a decade ago, no peer-reviewed public-domain assessment of cannabis energy use had been published. Early work on this question included a national scoping estimate of the issue based on the largely pre-recreational-legalization policy environment, where virtually all large-scale cultivation was conducted outdoors and indoor cultivation was predominantly windowless (Mills 2012). That said, small indoor operations were (and still are) numerous and generally not designed with energy efficiency considerations in mind.

Based on best-available information at the time, a "bottom-up" model was created based on interviews with practitioners, equipment retailers, and published guidelines for growers (e.g., Rosenthal 2010) (Mills 2012). The boundary conditions (inputs and activities resulting in energy use and greenhouse-gas emissions) represented only a subset of those depicted in Figure 21.1. The per-facility results compared favorably to measured data available for indoor growing operations, and the aggregate energy demand estimates compared well with those subsequently made by others, including the long-range planning authorities for the Northwest power system (Northwest Power and Conservation Council 2016).

From a national vantage point, Mills (2012) found that indoor cannabis consumed 20 billion kilowatt-hours of electricity annually, with additional amounts from direct fuel use, together corresponding to 15 million metric tonnes of CO_2 released into the atmosphere each year.[5] This in turn corresponded to an expenditure of $6 billion per year on energy, nationally, which amounted to 9% of California household electricity use, 3% of total statewide electricity use (all sectors), and 1% of electricity use nationally. Other independent estimates have found similar economy-level results. For example, indoor cultivation is estimated to require 0.6% of statewide electricity use (all sectors) in Colorado and 4% in the city of Denver (Hood 2018).[6] Washington State also reports that indoor cultivation is responsible for 1% of the state's overall electricity consumption (Jourabchi 2014), a number that has probably risen in the intervening years. As early as 2004, it was reported that indoor cannabis cultivation was responsible for 1% of electricity use in British Columbia (Easton 2004), which was long before the recreational legalization decision in Canada. Others have estimated cannabis energy use constitutes 3% of electricity demand in parts of Washington and 0.5% to 1% in Colorado (Remillard and Collins 2017).

For context, the aforementioned national estimate was equivalent to the emissions of 1.7 million average U.S. homes or three million cars and was more than four times the aggregate U.S. pharmaceutical industry energy expenditure.[7] While part of this difference arises from the lower energy prices paid by industrial users compared to residentially based cannabis producers of the time, it is noteworthy that the average primary energy intensity of pharmaceutical facilities (approximately 3,600 kBTU/sf-y) (Capparella 2013) is well below that of indoor cannabis cultivation facilities at around 5,500 kBTU/sf-y.[8]

An additional key finding was that the "energy intensity" (energy use per unit of floor area) in indoor cultivation facilities was vastly higher than that of other common building types (Figure 21.2).

From a regional vantage point, energy use can also be put in context by estimating how it contributes to per-person carbon emissions in economies where cannabis production is significant. While cannabis has been referred to as the largest cash crop in the U.S. in dollars (Gettman 2006), it is particularly significant in California. The implied per-person carbon footprint for the small populations in many of the cannabis-producing areas is far above the averages in a state otherwise

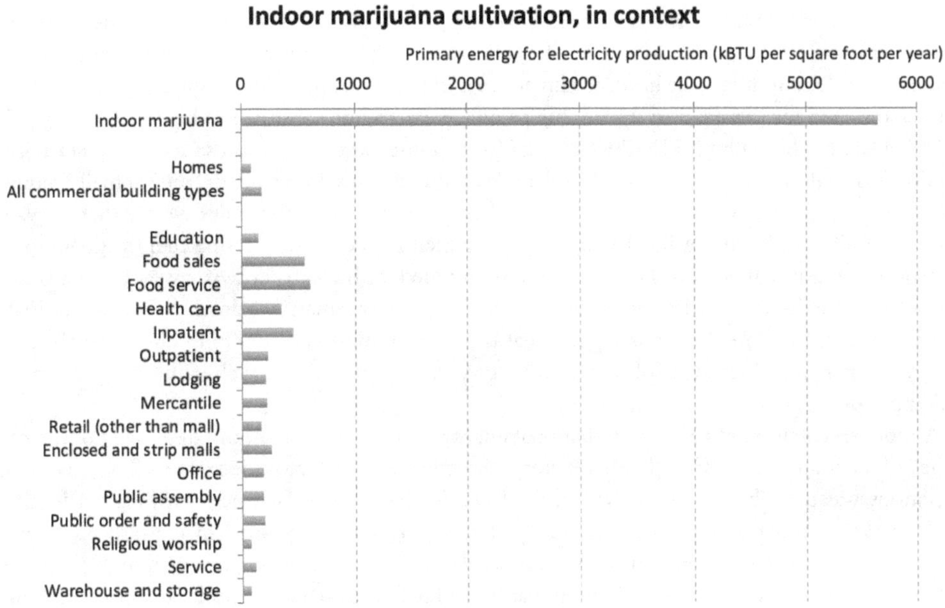

Figure 21.2 Cannabis energy intensity from Mills (2012)

Source: Reference data from U.S. Energy Information Administration. Homes (www.eia.gov/consumption/residential/). Commercial Buildings (www.eia.gov/consumption/commercial/)

known for its energy efficiency—closer to that of the most carbon-intensive "coal" states, despite California's being known as one of the least carbon-intensive states.

From a consumer vantage point, the energy use for growing one 1-gram "joint" creates 10 pounds of carbon dioxide pollution, equivalent to running ten 10-watt LED light bulbs (or one 100-watt incandescent bulb) for 76 hours (Mills 2012). That's as much as driving 22 miles in a 44-mpg Prius. Embedded in each average indoor-grown plant is the energy equivalent of 70 gallons of oil. A small "grow house" with ten grow lights consumes approximately as much electricity as ten average U.S. homes.

All told, the CO_2 emissions of the *average* cannabis user ranges from 16% of their total household carbon footprint in Rhode Island (the state with the nation's lowest consumption rate), where cannabis availability is highly limited, to 59% in Colorado (the nation's highest consumption rate) where it is pervasive. Put differently, the per capita emissions are equivalent to that from powering two high-efficiency refrigerators in Rhode Island and nine in Colorado.[9]

From a producer's vantage point, the cost of energy use varies widely depending on energy prices, efficiency, growing techniques, and strain choice (Arnold 2011), while the business significance of the cost depends on the prevailing wholesale price of the finished product. Circa 2012, the average energy expenditure for indoor cultivation equated to approximately one-quarter to one-half of the wholesale price. As energy prices rise and wholesale prices drop (post-legalization), this ratio will become increasingly unfavorable and could even become a factor in the solvency of some producers. Indoor producers have a far more energy-sensitive business model than outdoor producers or those in other industries and may find themselves in a boom-and-bust scenario given the magnitude of energy expenses.

Widespread cultivation in large-scale greenhouses is a relatively recent development. An analysis of industrial-scale greenhouses found that they, too, are highly energy intensive (Mills 2018), especially if poorly designed and operated. While these "hyper greenhouses" use less energy than do windowless facilities per unit floor area, they still require prodigious amounts of lighting, cooling, heating, and dehumidification in most climates. As evidence of the issue, cannabis greenhouses are one reason cited for the need to update high-voltage electricity transmission lines in Canada (CBC 2019a). Data published by NFD (2018) found greenhouses in the U.S. to use half the electricity of windowless facilities on a per-square-foot basis, yet, due to their lower yields, they actually required only 25% less energy per unit weight of the finished product.[10] An important caveat is that the values reported in that study do not include natural gas, which is a common heating fuel for greenhouses, whereas heating in windowless facilities is often provided with electricity. An assessment in Canada found that greenhouses used only about one-third less energy than windowless facilities did (Posterity Group 2019). The data thus suggest that these greenhouses are anything but "green," as their energy use per unit floor area still tends to be greater than that of virtually any other commercial building type.

A more recent attempt to estimate national energy consumption demonstrated many of the challenges of such analysis (NFD 2018). Of note, the energy used for outdoor as well as greenhouse operations was usefully contrasted with that of windowless indoor facilities, with that of legal and black-market production estimated separately. The report admirably brought forward more measured data on specific facilities than previously available in the public domain, although the sample was small (only two dozen sites with energy and yield data), self-selected, and self-reported. Almost one-third of the sites used LED lights for energy savings, likely far higher than the proportion of sites adopting this technology in the overall marketplace. The analytical scope had narrower boundary conditions (excluding energy sources other than electricity within the facility as well as transportation energy, and cultivation in perhaps more energy-intensive nonindustrial settings such as homes and other informal "small-scale" facilities), did not include off-grid operations often reliant on diesel generators, and was based on a non-randomized sample weighted towards milder climates in the United States. The energy intensity of black-market operations was presumably equated with that of legal operations, embodying an assumption of equivalent efficiencies not verified with actual data. Meaningful direct comparisons to the Mills (2012) study are thus not possible given the narrower boundary conditions and non-representativeness of the sample. The study indicated that some energy-intensity metrics may be improving with the passage of time, as would be expected, although more definitive surveys are sorely needed. Of particular note, the NFD study found roughly a factor of ten variation in key energy intensity metrics (electricity per square foot and per unit of flower yield), indicating enormous non-standardization of existing practices and a correspondingly large potential for energy savings irrespective of historical trends. It is not yet known whether the energy intensity of today's legal production facilities is lower or higher than that of earlier operations, but the recent work of Summers, Sproul, and Quinn (2021) suggests not.

★ ★ ★

There is increasing recognition of the need to manage energy use in cannabis cultivation. While it is encouraging to observe a variety of organizations developing environmental product labeling for cannabis, the methodologies often lack transparency, and there is little or no direct recognition of excellence or penalties for underachievement. Organizational factors create real or perceived conflicts of interest (financial dependence on the industry and users of the product being evaluated, lack of an independent watchdog, and a chronic tension between profit or market share and rigor among certifiers, which can result in the dilution of standards). It has been reported that growers will "shop" for certifications that put their product in the best light (Bennett 2019).

Despite nascent certification and labeling systems, consumers are largely unaware of the energy and environmental impacts of indoor cultivation. It is notable that the "ethical purchasing" movement (consumers seeking to vote with their dollar, e.g., to promote sustainable products) has barely appeared in the cannabis marketplace and, perhaps fearing stigmatization, environmental organizations have conspicuously sidestepped the issue (Bennett 2019). Moreover, cannabis dispensaries have been found to be unreliable sources of information on environmental issues associated with the products they sell, and existing sustainability certifications for cannabis are underdeveloped, vulnerable, and lack credibility (Bennett 2017, 2020, Chapter 17, this volume). Consumers thus operate in an information environment that impedes good purchase decisions.

Many Externalities Compound the Social and Environmental Costs of Indoor Cultivation

In addition to the policy community's need to better understand facility-scale energy use, cannabis operations have various externalities (side effects not reflected in the prices of goods sold) that are not often considered or quantified.

These include moisture damage to buildings, nighttime light pollution, power plant emissions and other environmental impacts, power theft, and power outages and other constraints on the broader grid caused by unchecked electrical load growth. As an example of this latter issue, the city of Portland, Oregon, associated seven power outages over a period of five months with indoor cannabis operations (Pacific Power 2015), and Portland General Electric traced 85% of its residential transformer problems to indoor cannabis growing (Borrud 2015).

In 2010, British Columbia reported that power theft by two-thirds of cannabis producers was costing the utility $100 million per year (BC Hydro 2016). At that time, cannabis was legal only for medical purposes, and most offending facilities were serving the black market.

Unpermitted or uninspected electrical wiring has been the source of a disproportionate number of fires in some localities, and the building stock has been damaged by mold and other consequences of raising humidity in buildings not intended for agricultural operations (Fire Chiefs Association of British Columbia 2008; Mills 2012). Massive fires have occurred even in legal facilities (Reuters 2015).

Cultivating cannabis in areas based on hydropower is often touted as an environmentally benign alternative to carbon-based power. However, attention has recently been given to the likely linkages between hydroelectric power production, reduced salmon populations, and starvation issues facing salmon-eating killer whales (orcas) in the Pacific Northwest (Mapes 2018; University of Massachusetts 2017). Hydroelectric power also results in substantially more water evaporation than do other forms of electricity production.

Adverse Public Health Considerations and Waste Generation Merit More Analysis

Another form of externality—public health impacts related to energy-intensive cultivation practices—also merits close analysis. Cannabis has been widely demonstrated to offer medical benefits under the appropriate circumstances. However, the countervailing health-related dimensions of indoor cultivation—for workers and the general public—have not received much attention, although it is treated elsewhere (Schenker and Langer 2021, Chapter 12, this volume).

Indoor environmental conditions can be an issue for workers and consumers. For example, while mold is a common risk to product viability for indoor and outdoor cultivators alike, indoor environments can be particularly prone to mold growth that can destroy an entire crop. The risk is especially high during power outages or equipment failures when ventilation and dehumidification processes are interrupted. Researchers have noted the potential health risks to workers of the high levels of VOCs (terpenes) emitted from cannabis plants (Plautz 2019). In another example, the doubling or quadrupling of current background carbon dioxide levels (up to 1,500 ppm, to force growth) was once believed to be safe for humans but has subsequently been found to result in CO_2 levels found to significantly reduce nine distinct measures of cognitive and decision-making functioning (Fisk et al. 2013; Allen et al. 2015). Combustion products, such as carbon monoxide, from unvented on-site CO_2 production can also pose health hazards.

Concerns have been raised about the effect of large concentrations of plants in urban areas adversely impacting air quality through their emissions of volatile organic compounds (VOCs), which catalyze other air pollutants. A recent investigation focused on the potential that 600 cultivation facilities within the city of Denver, Colorado, could double the prevailing levels of VOCs, while air pollution in that city already periodically violates federal limits (Wang et al. 2019).

More broadly, energy production itself has well-known health consequences, and of course is the primary source of human-generated greenhouse gases, which bring their own health impacts. Mills (2012) estimated national greenhouse-gas emissions of 15 metric tons of CO_2 each year from indoor cannabis cultivation across the United States. Outdoor practices can also result in greenhouse-gas emissions from land-use change and chemical fertilizers.

Hazardous wastes associated with indoor cultivation are also understudied. The "high-intensity discharge" lamps used for most cultivation contain significant amounts of mercury (~40 mg/lamp). The extent of recycling/recovery of this mercury is unknown, and broken lamps introduce mercury into the growing facility in an uncontrolled fashion. More costly LED lights do not contain mercury. However, recycling programs for LED fixtures are not yet in place.

Indoor practices involving hydroponics (or even traditional irrigation) yield contaminated wastewater that may be introduced into or circumvent wastewater systems. Moreover, non-degrading growing media, such as mineral wool that is saturated with nutrient-laden water, is typically sent to landfill after each harvest. We estimate that an operation with 100,000 square feet of canopy requires 14,000 to 34,000 cubic feet of mineral wool per cycle, which would result in the generation of approximately to 85,000 to 200,000 cubic feet of solid waste to landfill over a year with six growing cycles. For perspective, this results in waste generation of five to 11 times the weight of the processed flowers.[11] Recycling of agricultural mineral wool is not currently available in the U.S. Indoor operations also tend not to reuse soils after each growth cycle, which is yet another large source of solid waste.

Energy Efficiency and Renewable Energy Are Not Enough to Mitigate the Problem

A key challenge intrinsic to the indoor cultivation process, and compounded by seemingly unrelated local ordinances or needs, is that these facilities tend to embody a number of counterproductive design and operational features that make energy use even higher than need be. For example, CO_2 injection requires facilities to be sealed and all air recirculated, which, in turn, boosts energy use significantly. Another example is the sometimes-mandated use of tall opaque walls in front of greenhouses in the name of security, which can also block useful sunlight and thus require added electric lighting energy input. Location of these facilities in or near population centers requires high-resistance air filtration to control odor, which in turn requires increased ventilation energy to counteract the backpressure caused by the dense filter media. Heat is often run at the same time as air conditioning in an effort to control humidity that can otherwise lead to mold growth. Local light-pollution ordinances may require that light-deprivation covers be drawn over greenhouses at night (light may be on during that time, e.g., when the days are short or to capitalize on cheaper power rates), which can trap heat and thus require additional cooling energy. Last are a host of energy-using technologies to remove mold with UV, treat polluted water, recapture and purify waste water, and so on that are ironically used to improve the "sustainability" of indoor cultivation.

Despite these challenges, the industry has begun to look for efficiencies, likely driven more by the squeeze between falling wholesale prices and rising energy costs than by environmental concerns (Pols 2017). Aside from efficiencies (e.g., energy used per given weight of finished product), it is critical to maintain focus on trends in *aggregate* demand, especially for a growing industry. For example, Colorado reports a startling year-over-year increase of 23% in overall production (Hood 2018) and an annual 36% increase in electricity use between 2012 and 2016 (Denver Public Health and Environment 2018). Energy efficiencies cannot improve rapidly enough to offset such growth, and the preceding numbers suggest that energy intensity has actually been increasing. The energy forecasting authority in the Pacific Northwest projects an 82% increase in energy demand despite improving energy efficiency (Jourabchi 2014). A large-scale energy savings study for the province of Ontario, Canada, found a *maximum technical* potential of only 16% energy savings for indoor facilities and 21% for greenhouses (*without* accounting for limited uptake rates or cost effectiveness) (Posterity Group 2019).

Sleek images of energy-saving LED lights and greenhouses look "green" on the surface, but the devil is in the details. These lighting systems are still quite energy intensive.[12] One experiment found that 780 watts of LED were needed to replace 1,000–1,100 watts of traditional lighting (Massoud 2014) in order to maintain yields. Peer-reviewed research dating from the time these alternative lighting sources first started being manufactured suggested that cannabis grown under LEDs may actually take longer to mature and have lower yield and/or potency (Pocock 2015), thus saving little if any energy on a per-weight basis (Nelson and Bugbee 2014). LED performance in these applications appears to be improving, although even more recent studies obtained mixed results (Leichliter, Bisbee, and McGregor 2018). However, product attributes (flower appearance) may be adversely affected by LEDs, which is a palpable market risk for producers. The up-front cost of LED lighting is also vastly higher than conventional lighting, the recovery of which requires a long time horizon for the facility developer. Although the vast majority of indoor cultivation facility space has been constructed since LED fixtures have been available in the market, adoption rates are probably in the low single-digit percentage range. The aforementioned in-depth analysis for Canada found that the technical potential energy savings for LED lighting (without regard for cost-effectiveness or limited adoption rates) was only 7% of entire facility-level energy use (Posterity Group 2019).

These barriers notwithstanding, it is certainly possible to construct cultivation facilities with far higher energy efficiencies than is done at present. Indications of these opportunities as applied to the facility envelope and daylighting are provided a decade ago by Kinney et al. (2012).

That said, there is a degree of naïve optimism and hubris that cultivators need only "go solar" to solve the problem of any remaining energy requirements after efficiencies have been captured. The feasibility of this has not been demonstrated at scale, probably because the required solar array would need to be many times larger than the roof of the facility, and of course could not be on the roof at all if a traditional greenhouse design is used. Even in areas with excellent solar availability, only about 5% of a facility's electricity needs could be generated on the roof (Mills 2018). One noted large-scale facility aiming to be as sustainable as possible achieved a solar contribution of about 30% (Daniels 2019), which presumably required using a very large area of land beyond the building footprint. A state-of-the-art facility in Canada is projecting to offset only 8% to 10% of its electricity use by covering its entire roof (CBC 2019b), emitting approximately 9,000 tons of CO_2 per year instead of 10,000 tons without the solar. One of the nation's largest proposed facilities, with 2.4 million square feet of enclosed "cannabis industrial park," would only provide 4% of the needed electricity from its rooftops, despite being in an optimal solar resource area on the California-Arizona border. Meeting the full electricity demand would require approximately 1,400 acres of photovoltaic panel area.[13] An 80-megawatt dedicated natural gas power plant is instead proposed to provide energy (Kidder Mathews 2019). Such a generator would need to produce 1.23 TWh-y, enough to power 90,000 average U.S. all-electric homes.

While it can be argued that the cannabis industry as a whole can, in principle, be powered with centralized renewable energy, the amounts required are prodigious and for practical purposes (e.g., land-use constraints) rarely achievable. Although California's Coachella Valley is one of the largest wind-energy production areas in that state, cannabis production there (assuming business-as-usual energy efficiencies) will soon eclipse the entire output of all 40 wind power projects located in the area (Figure 21.3). Our "bottom-up" estimate is that projects already in operation consume 13% as much as wind energy in the area produces, although other estimates (Daniels 2019) suggest cannabis facilities in the "west side" of Coachella Valley consume 235 megawatts, which is fully 35% the rated capacity of all wind projects in the area, and far more on an energy basis. Full build-out of existing cannabis facility entitlements would consume far more: 11 times as much electricity as can be produced by all existing wind systems in the area, and more than all the wind power generated across California. It has taken decades and the dedication of vast land areas to build up this level of wind-generation capacity. From a broader public policy vantage point, there is an acute shortage of investment in renewable energy infrastructure to offset even existing carbon emissions, let alone emissions growth from new energy-intensive development. This comparison serves as a poignant illustration of the broader problematic tension between advances in renewable energy supply and unbridled growth in energy demand.

Myths and Market Distortions Bolster Environmentally Detrimental Production Practices

Among the fundamental preconditions for "perfect functioning" of markets is a vibrant information environment for all actors. Unfortunately, energy-relevant information in the cannabis industry is incomplete and often incorrect. One long-standing "myth" is that indoor-cultivated cannabis is superior to its outdoor counterpart. This is a commonly held view in the popular culture, and dispensaries are notorious for "bottom-shelfing" outdoor-grown products as inferior and otherwise favoring and steering customers towards indoor-grown products. Industry experts have argued to the contrary (*San Francisco Bay Guardian* 2011) and medical cannabis produced by the U.S. government is cultivated almost exclusively outdoors.[15]

Economic signals can also distort markets. Energy utilities earn billions of dollars per year from cannabis cultivators. While utilities play a key role in improving energy efficiency in the economy at large (assuming that policy makers ensure that investing in new energy supply is not more profitable than investing in efficient use), utilities benefit far less from outdoor cannabis cultivation and have not been observed to encourage it.

In some areas, indoor cultivators receive the historically low, subsidized electricity prices enjoyed by traditional outdoor farmers (PG&E 2017). Many agricultural customers also receive industrial rates,[16] which are lower than those paid by occupants of other types of buildings (warehouses, data centers, offices, etc.). Subsidies of this sort to indoor growers make them more competitive against outdoor growers while artificially suppressing the profitability of making energy efficiency improvements or investment in renewable energy supply.

Conversely, in order to discourage indoor cultivation, some well-intended policy makers have sought to impose extreme electricity surcharges (*The Arcata Eye* 2012). In practice, however, the expected effect could be to merely trigger relocation. This may "solve" the locality's problem but does not address global energy concerns and can even push cultivators off-grid and onto even more polluting diesel generators for power.

In other contexts, good public policy has often included financial incentives for energy efficiency (rebates, tax credits, etc.). However, in this context, far greater energy savings can be obtained by shifting to outdoor cultivation. A perspective must be maintained that even super-efficient indoor facilities are highly energy intensive when compared to other building types (imagine the values in Figure 21.2

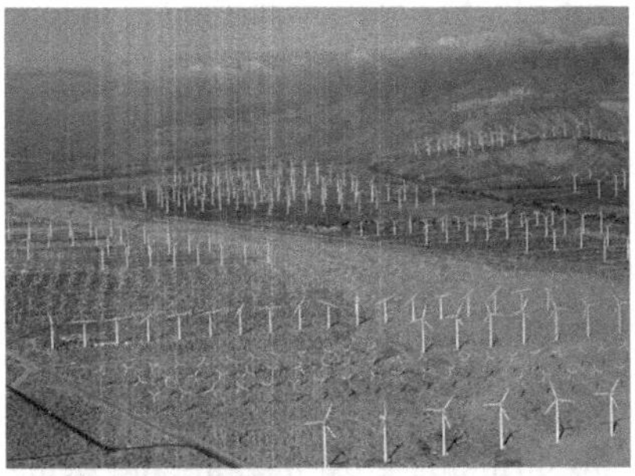

a. 2,229 wind turbines in Coachella Valley, CA

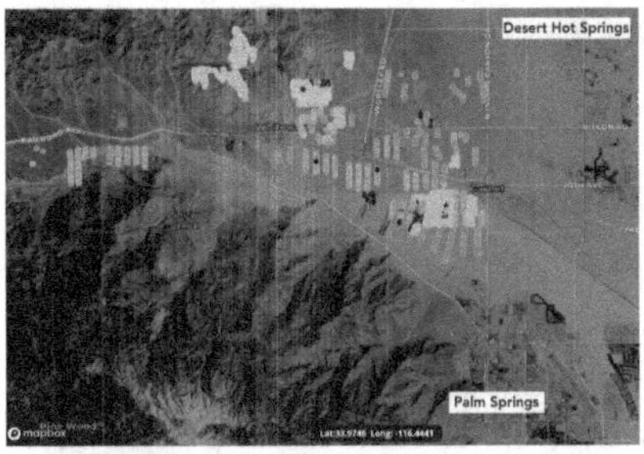

b. 663 megawatts of wind power across 40 projects

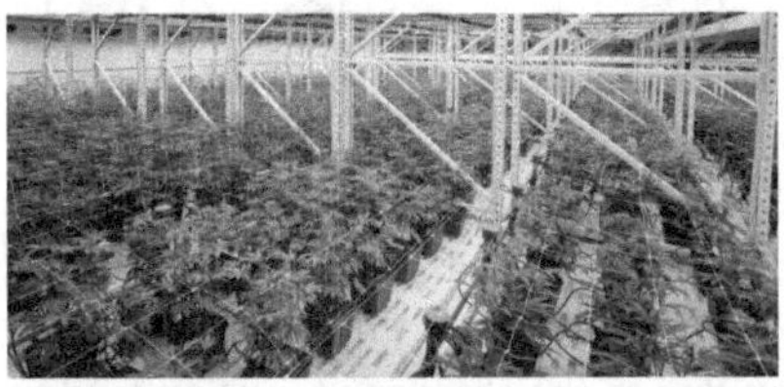

c. Large-scale indoor cannabis cultivation

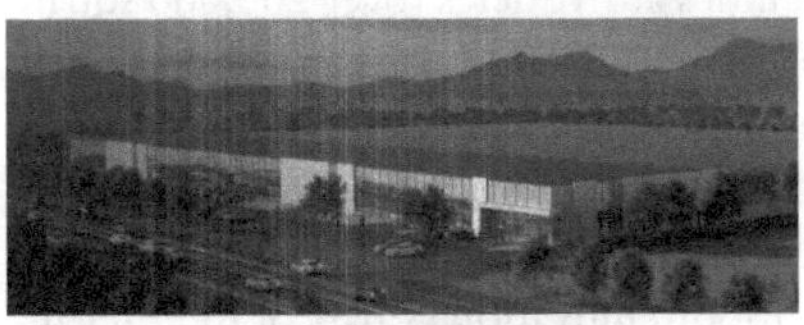

d. Indoor cannabis facility, Cathedral City, CA

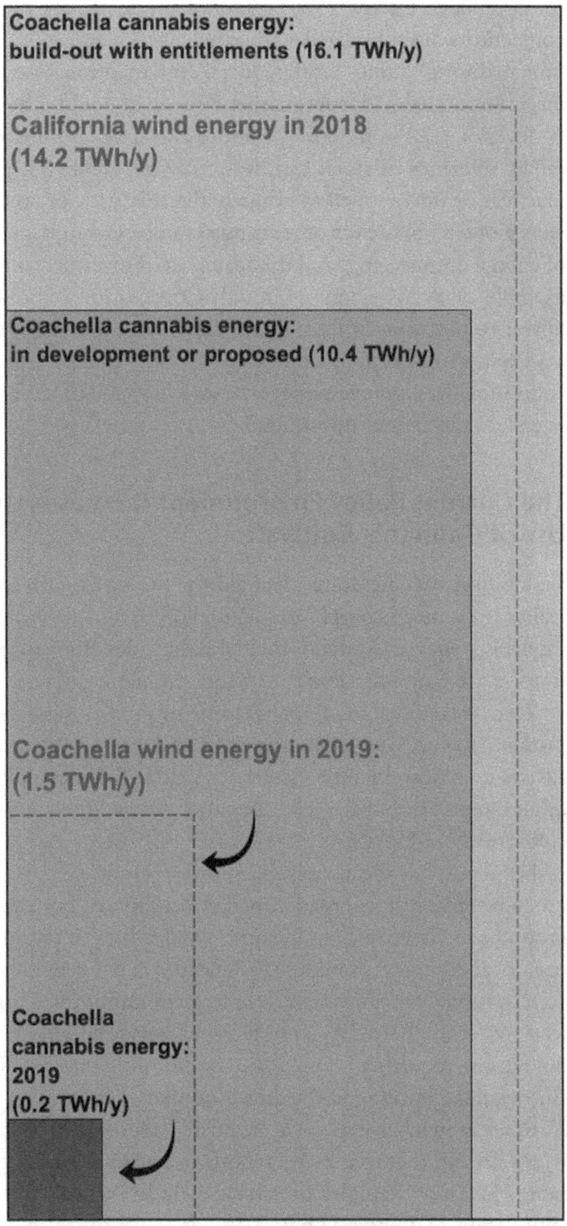

e. Relative Scale of electricity supply and demand

Figure 21.3 California's Coachella Valley is the site of 10% of the state's wind energy production. Cannabis cultivation facilities already in operation in five cities within the Coachella Valley require the equivalent of 13% of the entire electricity production of the 40 wind energy projects (2,229 turbines) located throughout the valley. This will grow to more than 70% of the area's total wind energy output upon completion of cannabis-facility projects proposed or under development. Full build-out per existing entitlements will consume 11 times as much power, significantly exceeding the 14 TWh/year generated by wind power in all of California

Photos: (a) wind turbines from ecoflight.com, with permission; (b) satellite view from Hoen et al. (2018), public domain; (c) interior of cultivation facility photo by the authors; (d) rendering of Venlo-type glasshouse by Sunniva (under construction), with permission; (e) chart shows energy demand for various levels of cannabis development in the Coachella Valley in comparison with wind power generation in that area and statewide.[14]

being reduced by, say, 75%). Outdoor producers are disadvantaged when their well-funded indoor competitors are subsidized with efficiency incentives such as rebates that are, in turn, paid by consumers through utility tariff "adders" (the traditional way of financing utility rebate programs). Such incentives arguably disrupt market forces that could otherwise lead to optimally reduced energy use.

Investor roles in indoor operations also have an impact. Enormous cash infusions following initial public offerings of stock can disincentivize efficiency, particularly if investors are unaware of best practices or unequipped to evaluate the adequacy of cultivation practices. Losses arising from inefficiency of energy use (or other inputs) can be camouflaged by lack of transparency, investor ignorance of energy engineering, and the readiness of investors to infuse more capital if there are shortfalls. An example of this is Canopy Growth Corporation, who, despite shrinking gross margins and being unable to post a profit from their primarily indoor-cultivation-based business, was still able to attract a $4 billion investment from Constellation Brands (Alpert 2019). Compounding these problems, cultivation-facility investors tend not to have the time horizons needed to amortize energy efficiency or renewable energy investments.

The Current Policy Environment Increases the Energy Use of Cannabis Cultivation

Prohibition was previously blamed for the environmental impacts of cannabis cultivation, but the reality is far more complicated (Vitiello 2016). Indeed, owing to the lack of coordination between cannabis policy and environmental policy, decisions inadvertently being made in the post-prohibition era are compounding the energy problem.

That said, there are ample reasons to pursue regulation. For example, historically, some black-market growers have been rumored to leverage the fact of their undocumented income to take advantage of low-income electricity tariffs. This not only created an unintended cross-subsidy from other ratepayers, but the low rates also reduced their incentive to invest in energy efficiency or shift cultivation outdoors.

Local control of cannabis market regulation (e.g., at the city or county level) can lead to perverse outcomes that distort broader market conditions. For example, as noted earlier, the Coachella Valley in southern California has become a major hub of production due to the absence of caps on facility size, local efforts to promote the industry, and a generally permissive regulatory environment. Conversely, local ordinances set a very large minimum size for facilities at five acres (over 200,000 square feet) (Maschke 2018). As a result, very large-scale indoor cultivation is taking place in this extremely hot region, requiring far more air conditioning than in climates more naturally suited for cultivation. An engineer working in the area is quoted as estimating that cannabis cultivation facilities use about 25 times as much energy as a "standard industrial" development (Daniels 2019).

Perversely, there are many reports of localities banning outdoor cultivation as part of their legalization process, examples of which include Nevada County, California (Riquelmy 2016) and the entire state of Illinois (Thill 2019). Regulations also require all production to occur indoors in Canada (CBC 2019b). These measures are presumably taken with security in mind. Yet, if giant internationally sanctioned opium poppy plantations for pain-management drugs can be secured outdoors (Bradsher 2014), surely cannabis farms can do so as well. License fees are typically assessed on a per-square-foot basis, and some localities stipulate equal limits to the allowable cultivation area for indoor and outdoor cultivation, thus strongly biasing choices towards high-density, energy-intensive indoor operations where more crops can be produced each year.

Local officials and others have cited the odors arising from outdoor cultivation as a significant problem and suggest the activity be restricted to indoor facilities (Johnson 2019). This of course also entails the implementation of high-resistance air filters for odor control, which, as noted earlier, increase ventilation energy needs. This concern may be unfounded, as massive VOCs measured in the Denver regional air basin have been traced to indoor grow operations (Wang et al. 2019).

Providing an example of the aggregate effect of these market distortions, an estimated 80% of licensed cannabis production in California is conducted indoors (McVey and Cowee 2018). Once indoor cultivation is endorsed (or mandated), it becomes incumbent on policy makers to ensure that the resultant energy use is not excessive. Virtually all building types and the equipment in them are subject to energy codes and standards in the United States, yet comprehensive ones appropriate for cannabis cultivation facilities have not been promulgated, and the supporting research essential for standards analysis has not been conducted. Massachusetts is among the early states to grapple with this. The state has determined that a single (massive) indoor cultivation facility could result in an increase in lighting demand equal to the energy saved over many years by the state's effort to convert over 130,000 streetlights from conventional high-intensity lamps to LEDs.[17] However, the state's efforts at setting energy standards have been clumsy, for example seeking to specify wattage limits on individual light fixtures, which could easily result in operators installing more fixtures than would otherwise be the case (Davis 2019a).

In another example of unintended energy consequences, mandatory product testing—which is certainly a potentially appropriate policy intervention—can uncover long-standing practices that yield unacceptable contamination levels in the final product. Tainted cannabis products must be destroyed, thus entailing all associated energy to be reallocated to materials that pass testing. The safety thresholds stipulated by the regulations are not necessarily based on scientific study, nor are they consistent with standards for other consumer products. For example, there are no standards or testing for heavy metals in tobacco, despite it being known to contain them, yet testing is done at the parts-per-billion level for cannabis. Researchers have described the lack of studies on the health risks of heavy metals in tobacco (Caruso et al. 2014).

Some previously black-market cultivators have found the new permitting processes under legalization to be onerous and so time-consuming that they cannot transition their businesses to the regulated market. This already appears to be having the effect of driving some legal producers back to the black market, and thus away from access to policy inducements for environmentally improved practices. As of April 16, 2019, roughly 3,000 temporary cultivation permits had expired and the California Department of Food and Agriculture (CDFA) had issued only 62 annual licenses and 564 provisional permits. Reports indicated that less cannabis was sold (legally) in the year after recreational laws went into effect than before. As an indicator of the size of the black market, the most recent official estimates of California's cannabis production, a report published in 2018 by the California Department of Food and Agriculture, showed the state producing as much as 15.5 million pounds of cannabis and consuming just 2.5 million pounds (ERA Economics 2017). The balance is presumably illegal export to areas where prevailing retail prices are higher.

Even where states legalize cannabis cultivation, localities that thwart implementation further reinforce black-market activity. For example, there are many counties in California where a public majority voted to legalize cannabis yet local government has banned most if not all cannabis-related business activities. According to Schroyer and McVey (2019), only 161 of California's 482 municipalities and 24 of the 58 counties allow commercial cannabis businesses. Illinois—the most carbon-intensive cannabis producer in the U.S. (Summers, Sproul, and Quinn 2021)—has banned outdoor cultivation statewide.

A key example of the consequences of a resurgent black market are that off-grid cultivation using diesel generators results in an even higher "carbon footprint" (carbon per unit of electricity produced and consumed) than the electric grids in many areas—for example 2.5 times higher in the case of California (Mills 2012).

Relevant to indoor and outdoor cultivation alike, cannabis regulatory practices also counterproductively influence transportation energy use. In the California regime, for example, the product is typically transported at least four times between the point of cultivation and the point of consumption. Regulations require farmers to transport their product to processors, who then transport to distributors, who then transport to dispensaries. Retail consumers then transport the final product from the dispensary. Shipments of only 25 to 40 pounds between farmer and processor are not atypical. The amounts transported become progressively smaller along the supply chain, which multiplies the amount of embodied transport energy per unit weight.

Transport energy notwithstanding, one fundamental policy barrier to reducing energy use is restrictions on interstate commerce. A comparison of electricity use per unit yield in seven states found a variation of 3.4-fold and that for greenhouse-gas emissions of 26-fold, and this did not include the full range of climate severity or power plant emissions factors seen across the whole country (NFD 2018). Were the nation's supply of cannabis grown in climatically benign locations, energy use would be vastly reduced, as would pressures to grow indoors.

The Case of California: A Cannabis-Climate Train Wreck Driven by Ill-Informed Policymaking

California is a beacon of progressive environmental thought and has long been an engine for innovative environmental technologies and policies. State legislators have passed some of the most far-reaching climate change policies and targets in the world, notably the California Global Warming Solutions Act of 2006 (SB-32), designed to reduce statewide greenhouse-gas emissions to a level 40% below 1990 levels by the year 2030.[18]

Yet, the regulatory structure established for the cannabis industry now works at cross-purposes to these overriding goals (Mills 2019). Seemingly prior to any rigorous analysis of energy impacts, the state inexplicably dictated that indoor cultivation was integral to the broader goal of legalization, creating a preordained legal "purpose" that seemingly cannot be questioned by subsequent environmental considerations. This binding purpose led to the explicit rejection of "environmentally superior" outdoor cultivation alternatives identified in the official Environmental Impact Report (EIR), despite a recognized lack of data that precluded more than cursory quantitative environmental impact analysis (California Department of Food and Agriculture 2017) and conclusions in other official reports that environmental impacts would be "negligible" (Bureau of Cannabis Control 2017).

The EIR takes several leaps of faith to conclude that the legalization program will be "beneficial" towards attaining the state's greenhouse-gas emission reduction goals. They achieve this feat by assuming, remarkably, that overall cannabis production levels would not rise materially following legalization, while the legal fraction of production will increase from approximately 5% to 10% of statewide totals (the rest remaining in the black market) and that this increment will automagically conform with the state's SB-32 emissions-reduction target, thus rendering aggregate emissions slightly lower than without legalization.

The net effect of these analytical contortions—juxtaposed with the market and policy failures outlined earlier in this chapter, particularly the forcing of indoor cultivation in many local jurisdictions—is that California has thus far failed to grasp a rapidly closing window of opportunity to manage energy use and greenhouse-gas emissions from the cannabis industry. Few localities have made efforts to manage energy use and emissions (California Department of Food and Agriculture 2017). A highly limited building energy standards-setting process is slowly being explored, but the earliest date for possible implementation will be 2022—a full 25 years after the state's initial legalization of cannabis for medical use (California Energy Commission 2019b).

A Large Research Vacuum Remains

Although it has been many years since the energy issues of cannabis cultivation were first identified (Mills 2012), very little subsequent research has been conducted, and thus policymaking proceeds in an information vacuum. Contributing to this problem, the cannabis industry and energy suppliers are not always forthcoming with information about current practices and are selective about what they do release. Early work pointed out the need for open-source energy benchmarking using measured data (Mills 2012). Some studies have come forward with information of this sort, often with small samples limited to a certain region or type of cultivation (e.g., County of Boulder 2018), while other efforts are pooling and standardizing the information, although based on self-selected participants and limited public access to the proprietary data.[19] Also needed are improved estimates of market-scale drivers (numbers and types of cultivation facilities, consumption trends, etc.). Much more data (and modeling) are needed to get a strong handle on trends in national energy use associated with indoor cannabis production and to understand the potential for improved energy efficiency and greenhouse-gas reductions. More broadly, measured data alone does not help improve efficiency unless it compels the adoption of improved practices and technologies.

Among the critical policy-relevant questions remaining unanswered:

Are newer large industrial-scale facilities more or less energy efficient than traditionally smaller indoor cultivation practices?

No definitive data have been presented in answer to this question. On the one hand, more efficient heating and cooling systems can be expected, but on the other hand higher ceilings and wider lanes for vehicles and equipment result in far greater volumes of air being space-conditioned. Pressure for maximum yields, which includes six or more crops per year, may also entail greater aggregate energy inputs but less per final unit weight.

How much energy is used in manufacturing extracts and other derivative products?

These processes can be energy intensive, involving equipment that creates high pressures and temperatures, post-processing, etc. In some cases, raw materials are frozen and stored prior to extraction, using added energy. Post-harvest freezing becomes more likely when there is oversupply or inertia in bringing fresh product to market due to overproduction or policy obstacles.

What is the added water burden of indoor cultivation with respect to electricity production and wastewater treatment?

Conventional wisdom is that less direct irrigation water is needed for indoor cultivation, thanks to reduced evaporation, and irrigation efficiencies may be improving with industrialized processes. However—and of particular relevance to the many drought-stricken parts of the country—the massive amounts of water steadily evaporated from dams and cooling towers while producing the electricity destined for indoor cultivation facilities vastly exceeds the direct irrigation water needed to grow outdoors. Based on a rule of thumb of one gallon of water per plant per day and the water intensity of average U.S. electricity production at the electricity intensities of Mills (2012) and seven liters of cooling water per kilowatt-hour (per Torcellini, Long, and Judkoff 2003), indoor cultivation indirectly consumes about 18 times as much water (~1,300 gallons per plant) as the amount used for direct irrigation. Amounts will vary locally depending on practices and electric generation mix in the grid. Ironically, the most water-intensive mode of electricity production is otherwise environmentally lower-impact hydroelectric power. Meanwhile, the greenhouse-gas emissions associated with the electricity used to power indoor grows are fueling future droughts. The demands on wastewater treatment plants (and their energy use) must also be considered.

How much energy and emissions are embodied in inputs, equipment, and facilities used for cultivation?

The energy use in making soils (or single-use growing media), soil amendments, and pesticides for cannabis production has not been quantified, nor has it for constructing facilities and the mechanical equipment that goes into them. Soils or other growing media are typically discarded after each indoor growing cycle, making this an ongoing stream of solid waste and embodied energy. As an illustration, we estimate that the mineral wool often used as a growing media in hydroponic indoor cannabis-cultivation operations increases the overall carbon footprint of the final cannabis product by approximately 5% to 11%, depending on cultivation practices (and likely more given that it is manufactured in areas with substantially higher electricity-related greenhouse-gas emissions than those assumed here).[20] In another example, peat that is mined as a soil amendment destroys an important stable carbon sink in the environment. Meanwhile, agricultural activities of all kinds consume about a billion pounds of plastic, a petrochemical product, annually in the United States alone (Grossman 2015).

How much energy is embodied in producing cannabis products that never reach market?

The cannabis industry has been engaging in overproduction. Recent reports from Canada indicate extraordinary levels of overproduction, with only 4% of cannabis produced there reaching the market (McBride 2019). Technical problems during cultivation cycles (temperature excursions and mold outbreaks) can result in total crop losses, and, for black-market actors, interdiction also results in product not reaching the market. Product failing quality testing must be destroyed. The additional energy consumption associated with these factors has yet to be estimated but could be very significant.

How much transportation energy is involved, and how can that be minimized?

The smaller the quantity of cannabis transported, the greater are the per-unit transportation emissions. In the original 2012 study (Mills 2012), transportation energy amounted to about 15% of the total carbon footprint. Vertically integrated operations (with co-located production, processing, and retail) may well reduce transportation energy requirements.

What is the ongoing role of black-market cultivation, which escapes measurement?

There is a tendency to assume that with legalization "all" production shifts to a new footing. In practice, black-market cultivation has remained dominant and may well have a distinctly different energy and carbon profile than industrialized operations. Misdirected policy measures appear to be *enlarging* the black-market share of total production, which escapes regulation altogether. In California, for example, permitting has resulted in large amounts of paperwork and long periods of suspended operations. Fees in that state for a "medium" indoor facility (10,001–22,000 square feet) can be $80,000 per year, which can discourage participation in the regulated market (Bodwitch et al. 2019). NFD (2018) estimates that black-market operations are still responsible for three-quarters of the energy used to produce cannabis nationally. Non-uniform policy among the states is a significant driver of the black market, and also fosters illegal transportation to states without legalization.

Policy Solutions

Previously, policy makers' focus on the environmental impact of cannabis has been centered on outdoor cultivation, and even those efforts have been deemed highly inadequate by some observers (Carah et al. 2015). The past California lieutenant governor's 2015 report on the topic doesn't once mention energy considerations (Blue Ribbon Commission on Marijuana Policy 2015).

Solutions to the problems of indoor cultivation must begin with earnest policy maker engagement. Sadly, as leading promulgators of energy R&D and policy at the national level, the U.S. Department of Energy and the U.S. Environmental Protection Agency, federal entities with decades of jurisdiction and impactful work on energy efficiency through all segments of the economy, remain silent on the topic. Due to the absence of legalization at the federal level, these agencies even back away from research on issues that could have significant public health and welfare implications (Plautz 2019). Moreover, vanishingly few policy makers at the state level, even in states with varying degrees of legalization, have embraced the issue. Notable exceptions are Massachusetts and Illinois, which have taken initial steps, although the quality of the outcomes is uncertain.

Following are some key needs and opportunities in the policy sphere.

Gather and publish more representative and useful energy data. A start has been made on collecting measured data for actual facilities, but it is far from being representative of the market or having the resolution necessary to evaluate specific regions, cultivation practices, or facility types. It is essential to have third-party quality control and to ensure that these data are unbiased. An acute challenge here is that energy data in this industry—as for any energy-intensive industry—is regarded as highly proprietary. Producers as well as utilities are reluctant to disclose information. Lessons may be taken from the IT sector, in which there is now ample transparency of energy use in data centers and other high-tech facilities, despite prior concerns about the sensitivity of this information. In any case, raw data on energy use doesn't in and of itself identify rates of adoption of efficient technologies, best practices, or help facilities know how to improve. Action-oriented benchmarking can achieve these latter objectives (Mills 2015).

Improve transparency and require energy-use disclosure. Mandatory public disclosure of total energy use as well as efficiency metrics for many types of non-residential buildings is becoming widespread nationally,[21] but the cannabis industry has thus far been passed over by these initiatives. Disclosure of this information could fill information voids that currently impede sound decision-making on the part of investors, energy companies, local authorities, cultivators, and consumers. More transparency regarding the role of energy expenses in business cost structures can help identify inefficiencies that create energy waste, as well as help to develop best practices. Permitted cultivators are typically required to report plant counts, the number of cropping cycles, and the total amount harvested from each crop. Requiring cultivators to report the facility type and equipment deployed during each cropping cycle along with the aggregate energy used as well as energy per unit crop finished weight could provide additional valuable data for policy analysts.

Create an improved consumer information environment, including product labeling. Policy attention should be focused on consumer education and credible product labeling to enable more informed consumer choice and guard against the greenwashing that is today prevalent. Prior to distribution, producers are generally required to submit their products for testing and to make some of that information available to consumers through product labels. It would be a benefit to consumers to also have information regarding the methods used to produce the products and the associated carbon footprint. Dispensaries have a key role to play in this process and can help encourage energy efficiency by educating customers and promoting products that are produced using the most environmentally benign methods.

Eliminate anti-competitive market distortions favoring indoor cultivation. Subsidies to indoor cultivators (grants, tax credits, energy rebates, etc.) mask price signals that would otherwise help markets function correctly. Awarding preferential electricity tariffs or cash incentives for new equipment disadvantages outdoor growers who have a vastly lower carbon footprint. Subsidies of all forms should be eliminated when they result in added energy use. Alternatively, it has been proposed that instead of utilities providing financial incentives to "efficient" indoor growers, they should incentivize outdoor cultivators, which achieves the greatest energy savings (Davis 2019b).

Allocate a portion of licensing fees to help address externalities. Licensing fees for indoor operations are often higher than are those for outdoor operations. This "signal" could be further improved by incorporating some fee proportionality to energy intensity, with an appropriate portion of resulting fees reinvested in improving energy efficiency. Note that there is a tremendous loophole in the current California license fee structure: Greenhouses, regardless of how many supplemental lights they incorporate, are virtually exempt from indoor cultivation fees, yet, as noted earlier, their energy use is substantial.

Develop science-based product-testing standards to avoid unnecessary crop destruction. To minimize unnecessary destruction of energy-intensive finished products, more effort is needed to ensure that required residue levels are realistic and in line with other consumer products such as tobacco and alcohol. Rather than requiring immediate destruction of products, quarantined products should be remediated where possible. Methods such as advanced distillation and microfiltration have been used to remove pesticides, heavy metals, mold, and other contaminants.

Conduct market-relevant publicly funded R&D. Public-sector R&D has a long and successful track record of compensating for market failures where private industry does not independently pursue technological pathways that are in the broader public interest (Mills 1995). Where there is lack of political will to mandate that all production be conducted outdoors, R&D can inform strenuous interventions to address the damage of any compromise position. These include better engineering and design tools for designers, labeling of energy using componentry, and mandatory efficiency standards. Other promising avenues include plant genetics to minimize energy (and water) requirements, development of large-scale energy benchmarking and disclosure initiatives, impartial technology assessments, and peer-reviewed best-practice guidelines.

Where policy makers insist on subsidizing indoor growers—to the anticompetitive disadvantage of outdoor growers—the thresholds for eligibility should be uncompromising. Arguably, only "net zero" facilities, that is, those that generate all their energy on-site with zero-carbon methods (typically solar photovoltaic cells), should be allowed. Hundreds of net zero non-residential buildings have been constructed around the country (NBI 2018), but there is no evidence that this has yet been accomplished for cannabis production.

Conclusions

Cannabis policy and environmental policy must be harmonized. Until then, some of the nation's hardest-earned progress towards climate change solutions is at risk as regulators continue to ignore this industry's mushrooming carbon footprint. Thanks to this inattention, producers have enjoyed a climate-change double standard (and lack of support) while being passed over by a host of policies and programs successfully improving energy efficiency and deploying renewable energy into virtually every other segment of the economy.

Those citing climate pollution as a reason not to legalize cannabis are missing the point: legalization is necessary—but not sufficient—for addressing the problem. Yet, if done poorly, legalization can make the problem far worse. Indeed, history may judge today's cannabis policy makers as betraying the public trust by enabling an industry with such a large carbon footprint.

Many are eager to see an industry more forthcoming about its carbon footprint and one that signals more hands-on interest in managing it and raising consumer awareness. A key factor in this process are individual consumer choice and expectations, which send signals back to the market that ultimately help shape production choices and processes.

The continuation of indoor cultivation does not appear to be defensible on energy and environmental grounds. It may be argued that energy use can be reduced with large investments in energy efficiency or offset with renewable energy generation. However, this is an optimization of a sub-optimal activity. These resources could be used more productively in other arenas where essentially zero-energy methods (i.e., outdoor cultivation, which has met humankind's needs for five millennia) are not available. Meanwhile, zero-net-energy indoor cannabis production facilities have not been demonstrated, presumably because of the enormous area (and cost) of the required solar arrays. Even with zero-net-energy indoor practices, other issues such as mercury in lighting, embodied energy in buildings and equipment, water use, and solid waste production would remain concerns.

Proficiency in accomplishing the unnecessary will not yield true sustainability. Myopic optimization of an activity that does not have to be conducted in the first place is not a legitimate response to the very real risks society faces from climate change. The ethical integrity of indoor cultivation—even at the greatest imaginable "stretch" levels of energy efficiency and renewable propulsion—is in question. This is a pressing issue for producers, policy makers, and consumers alike.

Notes

1 This chapter expands on a presentation entitled "Policymakers' Primer on Addressing the Carbon Footprint of Cannabis Production," delivered by E. Mills to the Council of State Governments annual meeting in December 2017 (Mills 2017).

2 Based on NFD's estimate of 34.4 million pounds/year consumption, 1300 pounds/acre-year yield, and agricultural land area in the US of 312 million acres.

3 The primary energy users are heating and cooling, dehumidification, and lighting. With conventional lighting, most of the input energy results in heat generation, which needs to be immediately removed by air conditioning. Other miscellaneous energy loads can include irrigation pumps, water pre-heaters or coolers, air disinfection systems, motors to operate light-deprivation curtains, and crop dryers. Transportation (during and after production) and post-cultivation product manufacturing further contribute to energy use and carbon footprint.

4 This latter argument is not material, as outdoor growers using light-deprivation methods also achieve multiple harvests per year. Moreover, reducing labor intensity is contrary to the job-creation objectives of most policy makers.

5 This analysis represented the typical small- to mid-scale indoor cultivation practices of the time and associated energy tariffs.

6 The City of Denver reports that 45% of its total growth in electricity demand stems from cannabis (Walton 2015).

7 Note that the original study (Mills 2012) put this at six times, but the value noted here is adjusted for approximately 25% of pharmaceuticals being consumed by Americans that are produced offshore (Altstedter 2017).

8 This cautiously assumes that the source of pharmaceutical industry energy is reporting in "site" energy units, that is, not including the losses due to the inefficiencies of electricity production in power plants. The source's estimate of 1,210 kBTU/sf-year translates to approximately 3,600 kBTU/sf-year when adjusting for this conversion factor.

9 Per capita cannabis consumption from *MJ Business Daily* (https://mjbizdaily.com/chart-of-the-week-average-annual-mmj-purchases-by-state-vary-widely/). State-specific household emissions from U.S. Department of Energy, Energy Information Administration. Assuming cultivation carbon footprint per Mills (2012).

10 Average reported values were 0.79 grams of dried flower yield per kWh for indoor facilities and 1.07 grams/kWh for greenhouses. Values elsewhere in the NFD report suggest the greenhouses were even less favorable.

11 See assumptions later in the discussion of mineral wool embodied energy.

12 One advantage of less-efficient high-intensity discharge lamps is that the heat-producing ballasts can be remoted outside the conditioned space, thereby reducing air conditioning needs. LED ballasts are integral to the fixture and cannot be remotely located.

13 Array area range represents the annual electricity intensity estimated by Mills (2012) also similar to that measured in a site in nearby Nevada (NFD 2018). Solar output per unit area estimated by Sage Energy using Helioscope simulation software.

14 Calculation notes: Estimated cultivated area development status in five Coachella Valley cities based on Simmons (2019), with 350,000 square feet of "canopy" as of April 2019, 19.4 million square feet proposed or under development, and 30 million square feet entitled. Energy intensity is that calculated by Mills (2012). Note that while NFD (2018) cites lower average electricity intensity for some states, their value for the adjacent desert state (Nevada) in their sample is virtually identical to that used here for a California desert location. Wind energy generating capacity values are from Hoen et al. (2018) and associated energy production from California Energy Commission (2019a): average wind energy production rates for 26 projects (475 MW) in the area (2.23 GWh/MW) are applied to the total installed 663 MW for the area to estimate total electricity production.

15 See https://pharmacy.olemiss.edu/marijuana/

16 See www.eia.gov/todayinenergy/detail.php?id=16231

17 Cannabis Energy Overview and Recommendations, MA Department of Energy Resources Energy and Environmental Affairs, 2/23/18, slide 6.

18 https://leginfo.legislature.ca.gov/faces/billNavClient.xhtml?bill_id=201520160SB32

19 See https://powerscore.resourceinnovation.org

20 Per Mills (2012), the grid-based electricity related emissions of CO_2 are 8.1 kg CO_2 per square foot for each indoor cannabis growth cycle. Per Bribian, Capilla, and Aranda Uson (2010), the lifecycle emissions of mineral wool are 1.511 kg CO_2 per kilogram for average European conditions. This emissions factor depends heavily on electricity generation mix. A value of 2.736 was determined by Aivazidou (2013) for conditions in Greece (where the electric system is heavily dependent on lignite coal). Much U.S. manufacturing occurs in Mississippi and West Virginia, where electricity-related CO_2 emissions are much higher than U.S. averages, which, in turn, are substantially higher than European-average emissions upon which Bribian et al.'s analysis is based. Mineral wool usage calculations are based on specific weight of 1.8 kg per cubic foot of mineral wool (per Grodan manufacturer's specs) and a range of material use in cultivation of 0.14 to 0.34 cubic feet (0.26 to 0.61 kg) per square foot of growing area per growing cycle. This yields 0.38 to 0.92 kg CO_2/sf-cycle, or 5% to 11% of the energy-related emissions. This analysis generously assumes that yields are two pounds per light per cycle in industrial grow operations.

21 See https://database.aceee.org/state/building-energy-disclosure

References

Aivazidou, Eirini. 2013. "Development of a Methodological Framework for Carbon Footprint Management in the Supply Chain: The Case of FIBRAN S.A." Diploma Dissertation (in Greek), Aristotle University of Thessaloniki, Greece.

Allen, Joseph G., Piers MacNaughton, Usha Satish, Suresh Santanam, Jose Vallarino, and John D. Spengler. 2015. "Associations of Cognitive Function Scores with Carbon Dioxide, Ventilation, and Volatile Organic Compound Exposures in Office Workers: A Controlled Exposure Study of Green and Conventional Office Environments." *Environmental Health Perspectives* 124 (6): 805–12.

Alpert, Bill. 2019. "Constellation Brands Was Tired of Losing Money on Canopy Growth. Now the Marijuana Company's CEO Is Out." *Barrons.*

Altstedter, Ari. 2017. "Where the U.S. Actually Gets its Drug Supply." *Bloomberg.*

The Arcata Eye. 2012. "Measure I, The Grow House Electricity Tax: City Council Resolution, Municipal Code Section, City Attorney Analysis and Ballot Argument in Favor—August 3, 2012."

Arnold, Jessica. 2011. "Investigation of Relationship between Cannabis Plant Strain and Mass Yield of Flower Buds." *Humboldt State University Proposal.*

BC Hydro. 2016. "Letter from Greg Reimer, Executive Vice President, Transmission, Distribution & Customer Service, BC Hydro." *Company News Release.*

Bennett, Elizabeth A. 2017. "Extending Ethical Consumerism Theory to Semi-legal Sectors: Insights From Recreational Cannabis." *Agriculture and Human Values* 35: 295–317.

———. 2019. "Passing on Pot: When Environmental Organizations Disengage from Political Consumerism in Highly Stigmatized Sectors." *Environmental Politics* 28 pp.

———. 2021. "Consumer Activism, Sustainable Supply Chains, and the Cannabis Market." In *The Routledge Handbook of Post-prohibition Cannabis Research*, edited by Dominic Corva, and Joshua Meisel. New York: Routledge.

Blue Ribbon Commission on Marijuana Policy. 2015. *Policy Options for Regulating Marijuana in California*, 93 pp. Blue Ribbon Commission on Marijuana Policy. Sacramento, CA: State of California and the American Civil Liberties Union.

Bodwitch, Heikia, Jennifer Carah, Kent M. Daane, Christy Getz, Theodore E. Grantham, Gordon M. Hickey, and Houston Wilson. 2019. "Growers Say Cannabis Legalization Excludes Small Growers, Supports Illicit Markets, Undermines Local Economies." *California Agriculture* 73 (3–4): 177–84.

Borrud, Hillary. 2015. "Power Needs of Pot." *The Astorian*.

Bradsher, Keith. 2014. "Shake Up on Opium Island." *New York Times*, July 19.

Bribian, Ignacio Zabalza, Antonio Valero Capilla, and Alfonso Aranda Uson. 2010. "Life Cycle Assessment of Building Materials: Comparative Analysis of Energy and Environmental Impacts and Evaluation of the Eco-efficiency Improvement Potential." *Building and Environment* 46: 1133–40.

Bureau of Cannabis Control. 2017. *Commercial Cannabis Business Licensing Program Regulations: Initial Study/Negative Declaration*, 491 pp. Sacramento, CA: Bureau of Cannabis Control.

California Department of Food and Agriculture. 2017. *CalCannabis Cultivation Licensing: Final Program Environmental Impact Report*, 534 pp. Sacramento, CA: California Department of Food and Agriculture.

California Energy Commission. 2019a. *Electricity from Wind Energy: Statistics and Data*. Sacramento, CA: California Energy Commission.

———. 2019b. *First Utility-Sponsored Stakeholder Meeting: Covered Processes (Controlled Environmental Horticulture): 2022 TITLE 24 CODE CYCLE, PART 6: Statewide CASE Team: September 19, 2019*. Sacramento, CA: California Energy Commission.

Capparella, Josh. 2013. "Energy Benchmarking in the Pharmaceutical Industry." *Pharmaceutical Engineering* 33 (5): 1–6.

Carah, Jennifer K., Jeanette K. Howard, Sally E. Thompson, Anne G. Short Gianotti, Scott D. Bauer, Stephanie M. Carlson, David N. Dralle, Mourad W. Gabriel, Lisa L. Hulette, Brian J. Johnson, Curtis A. Knight, Sarah J. Kupferberg, Stefanie L. Martin, Rosamond L. Naylor, and Mary E. Power. 2015. "High Time for Conservation: Adding the Environment to the Debate on Marijuana Liberalization." *BioScience* 65 (8): 822–29.

Caruso, Rosalie. V., Richard J. O'Connor, W. Edryd Stephens, K. Michael Cummings, and Geoffrey T. Fong. 2014. "Toxic Metal Concentrations in Cigarettes Obtained from U.S. Smokers in 2009: Results from the International Tobacco Control (ITC) United States Survey Cohort." *International Journal of Environmental Research and Public Health* 11 (1): 202–17.

CBC. 2019a. "Windsor-Essex Greenhouses Will Need More Power Than Currently Available. Canadian Broadcasting Corporation." *CBC News*, January 5.

———. 2019b. "Solar Pot: Alberta Cannabis Producer Unveils Rooftop Solar System. Canadian Broadcasting Corporation." *CBC News*, November 12.

County of Boulder. 2018. "Boulder County Energy Impact Offset Fund (BCEIOF) Demand Side Management Study." City of Boulder, Colorado, 41 pp.

Daniels, Melissa. 2019. "A Model of Sustainable Commerce: Carbon Footprint, Grid Concerns Push SoCal Weed Industry to Be More Green." *Desert Sun*, October 10.

Davis, Fred. 2019a. Letter to CannabisCommission@State.MA.US on draft Massachusetts energy standards for indoor cannabis cultivation. August 15.

———. 2019b. "Energy & Environment Working Group." Letter to Commissioner Kay Doyle, Massachusetts Cannabis Control Commission, and Alex Pollard, Massachusetts Department of Energy Resources. January 24.

Denver Public Health & Environment. 2018. *Cannabis Environmental Best Management Practices*, 66 pp. Denver Public Health & Environment.

Easton, Stephen T. 2004. *Marijuana Growth in British Columbia*, 78 pp. Vancouver, British Columbia: Simon Fraser University.

ERA Economics. 2017. *Economic Impact Analysis of CalCannabis Cultivation Licensing Program Regulation*, 113 pp. Davis, CA: ERA Economics, LLC.

Fire Chiefs Association of British Columbia. 2008. *Eliminating Residential Hazards Associated with Marijuana Grow Operations and The Regulation of Hydroponics Equipment, British Columbia's Public Safety Electrical Fire and Safety Initiative*, 108 pp. Quesnel, British Columbia: Fire Chiefs Association of British Columbia.

Fisk, William J., Usha Satish, Mark J. Mendell, Toshifumi Hotchi, and Douglas Sullivan. 2013. *Is CO_2 an Indoor Pollutant? Higher Levels of CO_2 May Diminish Decision Making Performance*. Berkeley, CA: Lawrence Berkeley National Laboratory Report No. 6148E.

Gettman, John. 2006. *Marijuana Production in the United States*, 29 pp. Lovettsville, VA: Bulletin of Cannabis Reform.

Grossman, Elizabeth. 2015. "How Can Agriculture Solve its $5.87 Billion Plastic Problem?" *GreenBiz*, April 6.

Hoen, Ben D., J. E. Diffendorfer, J. T. Rand, L. A. Kramer, C. P. Garrity, and H. E. Hunt. 2018. "United States Wind Turbine Database (ver. 3.2, October 14, 2020)." U.S. Geological Survey, American Wind Energy Association, and Lawrence Berkeley National Laboratory data release. https://doi.org/10.5066/F7TX3DN0. Aerial view of Coachella Valley from https://eerscmap.usgs.gov/uswtdb/.

Hood, Grace. 2018. "Nearly 4 Percent of Denver's Electricity Is Now Devoted to Marijuana." *Colorado Public Radio*.

Johnson, Julie. 2019. "Sonoma County Begins to Process Backlog of Applications for Outdoor Cannabis Farms." *Press Democrat*, June 21.

Jourabchi, Massoud. 2014. *Electrical Load Impacts of Indoor Commercial Cannabis Production*. 11 pp. Portland, OR: Northwest Power and Conservation Council Memorandum.

Kidder Mathews. 2019. *Prospectus for Palo Verde Center Cannabis Industrial Park, Blythe, California*, 15 pp. Seattle, WA: Kidder Matthews.

Kinney, Larry, John Huston, Michael Stiles, and Gardner Clute. 2012. "Energy-Efficient Greenhouse Breakthrough." In *Proceedings of the 2012 ACEEE Summer Study on Energy Efficiency in Buildings*, 13–176 to 13–188. Washington, DC: American Council for an Energy-Efficient Economy.

Leichliter, Katie, Dave Bisbee, and Matt McGregor. 2018. *Amplified Farms 2017 Indoor Horticulture Lighting Study*. 36 pp. Sacramento, CA: Sacramento Municipal Utility District.

Mapes, Lynda V. 2018. "Changes to Dams on Columbia, Snake Rivers to Benefit Salmon, Hydropower and Orcas." *Seattle Times*, December 18.

Maschke, Alena. 2018. "Lawsuit Could Protect Valley Weed Investors." *The Desert Sun*, January 26.

McBride, Stephen. 2019. "Aurora Cannabis Is Dumping Its Pot, Which May Be A Sign It's All Over." *Forbes*, October 21.

McVey, Eli, and Maggie Cowee. 2018. "Where Does California's Recreational Marijuana Supply Come From?" *Marijuana Business Daily*, December 3.

Mills, Evan. 1995. "From the Lab to the Marketplace: Government's Role in R&D and Market Transformation for Energy Efficiency in Buildings." Proceedings of the ECEEE Summer Study on Energy Efficiency in Buildings, Mandilieu, France. European Council for an Energy-Efficient Economy, Stockholm.

———. 2012. "The Carbon Footprint of Indoor Marijuana Production." *Energy Policy* 46: 58–67.

———. 2015. "Action-oriented Benchmarking for Non-residential Buildings." *Proceedings of the IEEE* 104 (4): 697–712.

———. 2016. "A Low Point for High Times." *Letter to the Editor, High Times*, April 4.

———. 2017. "Policymakers' Primer on Addressing the Carbon Footprint of Marijuana Production." *Council of State Governments, Las Vegas*, December 14.

———. 2018. "Not-so-Green Greenhouses for Marijuana Hyper-Cultivation." *Energy Associates*, 5 pp.

———. 2019. "California: A Cannabis-climate Train Wreck in Progress." *LinkedIn Post*. www.linkedin.com/pulse/california-cannabis-climate-train-wreck-progress-evan-mills/.

NBI. 2018. *Getting to Zero Status Update and List of Zero Energy Projects*, 33 pp. New Buildings Institute.

Nelson, Jacob A., and Bruce Bugbee. 2014. "Economic Analysis of Greenhouse Lighting: Light Diodes vs. High Intensity Discharge Fixtures." *PLos One* 9 (6).

NFD. 2018. "The 2018 Cannabis Energy Report." *New Frontier Data*, 63 pp. Washington, DC.

Northwest Power and Conservation Council. 2016. "Seventh Power Plan." Portland, OR.

Pacific Power. 2015. "Marijuana Growing Legal in Oregon and Washington, but Safety, Electric Capacity Issues Remain." Website.

PG&E. 2017. "Agricultural Cannabis Growers Now Eligible for PG&E Ag Rate and Programs." *Pacific Gas and Electric Company, News Release*, March 1.

Plautz, Jason. 2019. "The Growth of Legal Pot Farms Drives Smog Worries." *Science* 363 (6425): 329.

Pocock, Tessa. 2015. *Tuning the Spectrum for Plant Growth. Presentation*. Troy, NY: Rensselear Polytechnic Institute.

Pols, Mary. 2017. "Did You Know Marijuana is America's Most Energy-intensive Crop?" *Press Herald.*

Posterity Group. 2019. *Greenhouse Energy Profile Study*, 170 pp. Ottawa, ON: Independent Electricity System Operator and Posterity Group.

Remillard, J., and N. Collins. 2017. "Trends and Observations of Energy Use in the Cannabis Industry." 2017 ACEEE Summer Study on Energy Efficiency in Buildings, American Council for an Energy Efficient Economy.

Reuters. 2015. "Fire Guts Seattle's First Legal Marijuana Growing Operation." April 8.

Riquelmy, Alan. 2016. "Nevada County Marijuana: Supes Pass Outdoor Grow Ban in 4-to-1 Vote." *The Union*, January 15.

Rosenthal, ed. 2010. *Marijuana Grower's Handbook: Your Complete Guide for Medical and Personal Marijuana Cultivation*. San Francisco, CA: Quick American Archives.

San Francisco Bay Guardian. 2011. "Green Buds: Environmental Cost of Growing Indoors Is Luring the Marijuana Industry Back into The Sunshine." 14–18. August 11.

Schenker, Marc, and Chelsea Eastman Langer. 2021. "Health and Safety of Cannabis Workers." In *The Routledge Handbook of Post-Prohibition Cannabis Research*, edited by Dominic Corva, and Joshua Meisel. New York: Routledge.

Schroyer, John, and Eli McVey. 2019. "Chart: Most California Municipalities Ban Commercial Cannabis Activity." *Marijuana Business Daily*, February 18.

Silvaggio, T. 2021. "The Environmental Impact of Cannabis Liberalization: Lessons From California." In *The Routledge Handbook of Post-Prohibition Cannabis Research*, edited by Dominic Corva and Joshua Meisel. New York: Routledge.

Simmons, Heidi. 2019. "Cannabis Commerce in the Coachella Valley." *Coachella Valley Weekly*, April 17.

Summers, Hailey M., Evan Sproul, and Jason C. Quinn. 2021. "The Greenhouse Gas Emissions of Indoor Cannabis Production in the United States." *Nature Communications*. https://doi.org/10.1038/s41893-021-00691-w.

Thill, David. 2019. "Illinois Marijuana Growers Will Face Energy Efficiency and Reporting Rules." *Energy News Network*, September 16.

Torcellini, Paul, Nicholas Long, and Ronald Judkoff. 2003. "Consumptive Water Use for U.S. Power Production." National Renewable Energy Lab, U.S. Department of Energy, 18 pp.

University of Massachusetts. 2017. "Replace Hydropower Dams to Save the Southern Resident Orca Whale Population!" *Debating Science.*

Vitiello, Michael. 2016. "Legalizing Marijuana and Abating Environmental Harm: An Overblown Promise?" *U.C. Davis Law Review* 50: 773–812.

Walton, Robert. 2015. "Marijuana Grow Houses May Cause 3% Demand Spike for Seattle Utility." *Utility Drive.*

Wang, Chi-Tsan, Christine Wiedinmyer, Kirsti Ashworth, Peter C. Harley, John Ortega, Quazi Z. Rasool, and William Vizuete. 2019. "Potential Regional Air Quality Impacts of Cannabis Cultivation Facilities in Denver, Colorado." *Atmospheric Chemistry and Physics* 19: 13973–87.

22

Two Rural Industries Intersecting Over Time

Cannabis Production and Ecological Restoration in the Mattole Valley, California, USA

Erin Clover Kelly and Marisa Lia Formosa

Keywords: Cannabis production, rural economic development, restoration economy, shadow economy, back-to-the-landers

Introduction

In this chapter, we explore the intersections and impacts of two economic sectors, cannabis production and ecological restoration, in a rural place. This chapter emerged from a research project focused on the economic contributions of ecological restoration (the "restoration sector") in the Mattole Watershed of Northern California (Mattole), where we conducted interviews. Though we explicitly decided not to focus on cannabis production, through interviews we consistently found inextricable links between the restoration and cannabis sectors. In other words, it became clear to us that in order to understand the economic context of restoration, we also needed to understand cannabis production. The interactions between the cannabis and restoration sectors in the Mattole illustrate how legal and illegal sectors can complement and compete with each other economically, including in terms of employment and human capital. We trace the complicated history of the two sectors, and in the process, we raise more questions than answers as we seek to understand how the two sectors work in this rural place and how the cannabis sector has had both positive and negative impacts on the restoration sector and the Mattole community more broadly.

The restoration sector has generated substantial research interest, in part because of its capacity to contribute to rural economic development, including in communities historically dependent on extractive industries (Baker and Quinn-Davidson 2011; BenDor et al. 2015; Dabson 2012; Davis, Sundstrom, and Moseley 2011; Egan, Hjerpe, and Abrams 2011; Nielsen-Pincus and Moseley 2013), of which the Mattole is a representative case. BenDor et al. (2015) found that there were more workers directly employed in restoration in the U.S. than in coal mining, logging, and steel production, and that restoration projects tended to create localized, relatively well-paying jobs. The sector can

DOI: 10.4324/9780429320491-22

be divided into at least three types: mitigation restoration, which is required by law to mitigate for development or resource extraction (e.g., Aronson et al. 2010; BenDor et al. 2015; Kimball et al. 2015); public lands restoration, which includes restoration activities on public lands conducted primarily through government agencies like the U.S. Forest Service (Daniels et al. 2018; Tidwell and Brown 2011); and community-based restoration, in which restoration is primarily funded through competitive grants awarded by state or federal agencies to nonprofit community groups, tribes, local government entities, or individual landowners (Baker 2005; Davis, Sundstrom, and Moseley 2011; Lurie and Hibbard 2008; Nielsen-Pincus and Moseley 2013).

For this chapter, we include all three as part of the restoration sector, though our study mostly focused on the community-based model, the most common type in the Mattole. The jobs created in the restoration sector are often seasonal and short term, and while there is evidence that some of the restoration economy has professionalized in order to better capture competitive grants (e.g., Baker and Quinn-Davidson 2011), at a household level, many still complement restoration jobs with other employment. In the case of the Mattole, the restoration sector has long operated within the context of cannabis production.

Cannabis production, in contrast to restoration, has received little academic attention from researchers interested in rural economic development. Cannabis production is historically part of the broader shadow economy (also called the alternative, undocumented, or informal economy). Though these terms vary slightly, they all describe economic activity "tak[ing] place outside formal state institutions" (Nordstrom 2000, 36). Gibson-Graham (2008) identified the importance of what they termed "alternative economic activities," including legal activities such as gleaning and illegal activities such as theft and poaching. However, cannabis production was not listed as an alternative economic activity. Most researchers focused on rural economic development and land use have ignored cannabis production entirely or dismissed its economic significance. In discussing the undocumented economy in Saskatchewan, Swanson and Bruni-Bossio (2018) lump together all "drug trade" as harmful. Somerville, Smith, and McElwee (2015) characterize "illicit forms of entrepreneurship" as a threat to rural communities and at odds with notions of rurality. Paoli, Decorte, and Kersten (2015) focus on the harms of cannabis production, including violence, theft, and corruption. Others have noted cannabis production among "hippies" in some locations but largely dismissed it as a central economic driver (e.g., Holmes and Argent 2016). One notable exception to this is a paper by Corva (2014), which illustrates the role of cannabis in helping residents form social networks and maintain solidarity in the face of federal surveillance and shared risk. Another exception is from research in Morocco, in which cannabis production was found to have positive impacts on rural landowners who could invest in infrastructure and stay in place (Afsahi 2011). In this chapter, we highlight the importance of cannabis production for rural economies and its influence on other sectors.

Methods

Case Study

The Mattole is located in Humboldt County, part of the "Emerald Triangle," which has relied on cannabis production as its dominant economic sector for decades. In 1990, cannabis production was estimated to have an annual value of $1 billion in the county, dwarfing its other natural resource-based industries of ranching, milk production, and timber (Leeper 1990). Cannabis production has flourished here through a combination of cultural acceptance, clustering of human and physical capital utilized for its production, and remoteness, which has minimized surveillance and enforcement from authorities. For purposes of this chapter, the cannabis sector consists of the cultivation and sale of cannabis into both legal and illegal markets (recognizing that, in the eyes of the federal government, all cannabis production is illegal).

The Mattole is isolated, with rugged, mountainous terrain and poor roads. It has no incorporated municipalities, professional police or fire department, or hospitals. Because of seasonal migrant labor for cannabis production, its population is difficult to estimate but was estimated at approximately 2,000 people in 2009 (Mattole River and Range Partnership 2009). The restoration sector in the Mattole has been led since the 1980s by three nonprofit community-based watershed restoration groups (watershed groups): the Mattole Salmon Group (established 1980), the Mattole Restoration Council (established 1983), and Sanctuary Forest (established 1987). Both authors have connections to the Mattole and its restoration sector. The first author is a former board member of the Mattole Restoration Council and, since 2015, has taught an annual graduate-level field course on rural socioeconomic change in the Mattole. The second author is a fifth-generation Mattole resident and worked for the watershed group Sanctuary Forest from 2007 to 2016, where she worked closely with the community to elicit ideas, knowledge, concerns, and support for restoration projects.

Interviews

We conducted a series of 20 semi-structured interviews with key stakeholders (Table 22.1) involved in Mattole watershed restoration ("restorationists"), based on the authors' knowledge of the sector and subsequent snowball sampling. Our sample, therefore, is composed of people who identify with the restoration sector, though we note that most interviewees, at one time or another, have also participated in cannabis production. In our sample, eight people identified as part of the back-to-the-land movement, which was the influx of young, idealistic people in the 1960s and 70s, often from urban areas. Back-to-the-landers started restoration in the Mattole and established the three watershed groups.

Interviews were semi-structured and followed an interview template with questions focused on the restoration sector (e.g., how did you get involved with restoration work and how has the restoration economy changed?). Though questions about cannabis production were not part of the interviews, all 20 interviewees without prompting spoke about cannabis extensively.

Interviews lasted between 1.5 and 3 hours and took place in interviewees' homes and places of work, in restaurants, and at restoration sites. Interviews were transcribed and analyzed for key themes, in which we identified three eras in the sectors' evolving relationship since about the 1960s: from (1) mutual support to (2) competition and antagonism to (3) potential for re-partnering. Within each era, we found evidence for linkages between the sectors in terms of their economies (labor and resources), which we focus on here.

We refer to cannabis farms as "grows" and farmers as "growers," in keeping with the local lexicon. Cannabis production in the Mattole is generally outdoor in greenhouses set on "pads" (flattened areas, often dug into hillsides). It often involves intensive cultivation, including use of soil amendments, supplemental lights and light manipulation, and irrigation.

Table 22.1 Interviewees and their primary role within the restoration sector

Interviewee Role	*Number of Interviewees*
Past employee or board member	8
Current employee or board member	9
Past consultant	1
Community elder	1
Agency staff	1
TOTAL:	20

Results

Complementary Sectors Creating the "Radical Rural"

The cannabis and restoration sectors were established almost in tandem, and both were initially small scale and operated largely at the margins of society, with little state oversight or taxation. Both sectors, which largely arose from the efforts of idealistic, anti-capitalist, and anti-establishment back-to-the-landers who settled in the Mattole beginning in the 1960s, fit with the notion of the "radical rural" as described by Halfacree (2007). Interviewees described the back-to-the-landers as predominantly white, middle-class people who moved to rural areas to live simpler lives in a "conscious effort to start a new model" that rejected mainstream economic models and built new ones based on idealized visions of rural living. While interviewees indicated that they came to "reinhabit a landscape" and "relearn how to be good stewards," what they encountered was a region that had undergone ecological degradation in the wake of a boom in industrial timber harvesting (House 1999) and economic decline with the loss of timber jobs. In the words of one back-to-the-lander:

> The economy was always an issue for the back-to-the-landers, because there wasn't any. There were a few provisional jobs. There was a stud [timber] mill, the last mill operating in the Mattole valley . . . so there was a significant need for a source of employment, also sources of employment that were consummate with our values. Because environmental values were strong with the back-to-the-land movement.

Thus, while restoration was described as "a passion," it provided little revenue or stable employment and was mostly volunteer based. Cannabis production became the primary revenue source, a financial tool in the words of one interviewee, who said because "they were growing weed, they had the money to do these [restoration] projects." Cannabis production "allowed undeniably a lot of people to settle in and build homes and to raise their children." From the restorationists' perspective, cannabis was supportive of the restoration agenda of the back-to-the-landers, at least from the 1960s through about the 1990s. Generally small-scale, illegal cultivation provided the financial capital needed to allow residents to found community nonprofit organizations, including the three watershed groups, which required a great deal of volunteer labor:

> Everybody just put in the time that they could . . . I think we enjoyed that out here for many years because we had, as a valley, an income source that didn't take a ton of our time that we could make a reasonable living doing, and then volunteer the rest of our time . . . that all kind of correlated with the start of the restoration movement.

This lifestyle was changing in the minds of interviewees. As one younger restorationist said, "some of the old timers are getting nostalgic of how it used to be, what they say is like, yeah, I would grow a few plants and use that to fund my theater project, or fund my community betterment project." Interviewees indicated that both sectors began to change in the 1990s, becoming more integrated with formal economies and abandoning their radical roots.

The restoration sector changed from a largely volunteer workforce wherein workers had seasonal, "multiple, informal jobs" and "growing some weed on the side" to a grant-dependent model, with a small number of full-time, living-wage jobs for professional staff who implemented complex projects and navigated state-mandated permitting processes. Restoration therefore became increasingly tied to the state and state funding. The cannabis sector, meanwhile, pivoted to a more large-scale, "industrial" model—what interviewees called "the green rush," in which cannabis production linked to capitalist markets and many producers embraced consumer culture, visible in new trucks, large houses, and the ability to migrate, living part-time in the Mattole and part-time elsewhere. In the words of one back-to-the-lander, "industrialism has come in. It was bound to happen though."

Divergent Sectors Under the Green Rush

While the term "the green rush" was in use in the 1980s (Raphael 1985), most interviewees in our research used this term to describe the booming economic profile of cannabis in the region after the 1996 California Compassionate Use Act, which legalized cannabis production at the state level for medical purposes and eventually led to less aggressive enforcement of cannabis production laws. Interviewees described an "explosion" of cultivation, with increasing numbers of producers, area of land cultivated, and overall economic value of the industry.

Restorationists continued to arrive in the Mattole after the green rush, drawn by the vibrant restoration economy and the reputation and success of the three watershed groups. They arrived in tandem with large numbers of green rush growers, who came to the area to pursue profit through cannabis production. The green rush therefore was linked to "outsiders" who came to the region solely for the purpose of growing: "people from outside of the area, from Texas to Bulgaria, to God knows where . . . the growth has been so exponential." Many restorationists acknowledged as well that local growers, or the "grandsons of mom and pop," were also tending toward high-impact cultivation practices, consumerism, and the pursuit of maximized profit: "just like balls-to-the walls, big truck, just hit it with diesel and greenhouses and all that stuff."

Within the context of this labor market, the restoration sector struggled to find employees. Restoration was described by one interviewee as "a low-income career path, [with] seasonal work most of the time," while cannabis production offered "more money than most of them would ever have made had they gone off to college." One restorationist said, "finding a solid crew these days is almost impossible. Everyone is growing and I don't blame them," while another lamented that "with cannabis, for a while you had to be limited [in size], and so people had more time. But now, where we're at, everybody is putting everything into it, one hundred percent, and we don't have any time for managing our landscapes."

Interviewees indicated that cannabis production pulled both labor and resources away from restoration, leaving the restoration sector struggling. While green rush growers continued to contribute financially to the restoration sector, "throw[ing] a little bit of cash at the restoration organizations so we can tread water," they were seen by many as not committed to the Mattole or to restoring the Mattole. Several interviewees described the green rush as just the latest in a series of land use and natural resource "booms" that needed to be addressed through ecological restoration. The environmental consequences of increasing cannabis production have been well documented, including the delivery of sediment, petroleum products, and pesticides into streams; water diversions, contributing to dewatered streams; and loss of habitat due to forest clearing (Bauer et al. 2015; Butsic and Brenner 2016). The gravity and extent of these consequences continue to be debated within the Emerald Triangle but were not doubted by our interviewees, who consistently described "a race to the bottom," with cannabis cultivation at odds with the work of the restoration sector.

Interviewees indicated that while the back-to-the-landers had introduced the cannabis economy to the Mattole, they also had lost control of it. Though most of our interviewees participated in both the cannabis and restoration sectors, they said that cannabis production had come to compete with, and ultimately harm, the efforts of restorationists.

Uncertainty and Re-Partnering With Legalization

With legalization of cannabis for recreational purposes approved by California voters in 2016, many interviewees indicated that the cannabis sector could reduce in scale, allowing people to "return" to restoration. One young restorationist said, "My vision for the future (of the Mattole) includes much less emphasis on the cannabis economy. Either because it's non-effective, like can't make money, or just because there are priorities in other places." Another said,

> Maybe the hope and dream for the future is finding the balance where cannabis is a valuable source of income but it doesn't crowd out everything else. The old hippies talk about it, how there was a time when it was that way. There should be a scenario where cannabis can be the main local industry, it can provide people a good livelihood, but it's not the only thing that drives everything else.

In the meantime, however, interviewees saw a need for more restoration, because "we're going to be left with all these parcelized working lands with tons and tons of environmental cleanup." This was seen by many as an opportunity for the restoration sector; interviewees indicated that the watershed groups were in a unique position to help landowners "form road associations, form tributary collectives, work together to secure grant funding, to fix some of the problems [from cannabis production]."

Many interviewees expressed a hope for renewed restoration–cannabis partnerships as cannabis growers came into regulatory compliance under legalization. The restoration sector could thus shift (at least partially) from grant funding to funding from landowners seeking compliance, with both (nonprofit) watershed groups and for-profit contractors and engineering firms helping landowners to get permits. One engineer said this was already happening as landowners paid their company to "come in and help them get into compliance . . . [Doing] road upgrades, getting up to industry standards. Properly sized culverts to pass 100-year flows. Pretty standard stuff." This engineer indicated that the work they had done once under state funding was now coming from private sources, as "the people, cannabis growers, are being forced into paying for restoration. So, it's a different economic funding source for restoration."

Though many restorationists expressed optimism in the wake of legalization, the changing economic landscape was also characterized by uncertainty. Some interviewees said that small-scale, more environmentally benign growers would be left out of the new compliance market. Some predicted that large-scale timberland ownerships might reconsolidate; others envisioned just a reduced economy overall, with "fewer people living here, fewer cars on the road."

Conclusions

We expected this group of interviewees, all of whom were involved with the restoration sector, to speak about restoration when asked about restoration. For our research, we had excluded the cannabis sector to focus on the impacts of the restoration sector. But our interviewees made clear that the two sectors were so intertwined that they could not be understood separately. The cannabis and restoration sectors grew together to allow the back-to-the-landers to "live in the hills" and to realize their vision of an anti-establishment, anti-capitalist utopia. But rather than escaping capitalist logic, cannabis producers under the green rush came to embody it, transforming the economic lives of Mattole residents and redirecting labor from a patchwork of seasonal and part-time jobs, with time for both volunteer and paid work in the restoration sector, to full-time immersion in intensive cannabis production. With legalization, many restorationists saw hope for the re-partnering of the two sectors, largely because of requirements to achieve compliance.

The most important insight of this research is perhaps simplistic, but nonetheless worth stating: the cannabis sector is important for rural livelihoods and economies. Though the economics and community impacts of cannabis production have been inherently difficult to study, and researchers may still view the topic as taboo, its relative invisibility in scholarly work means that we do not understand the economies of many rural places. We therefore end with questions about the cannabis sector for future researchers, though many more questions exist.

Developing the Rural

As "traditional" rural economies such as ranching and forestry have declined across the U.S., there have been many who have called for reinvestment in the rural (e.g., Stauber 2001). We wonder about the implications of cannabis production for rural economic development; how has it contributed to rural economies, but also how will it continue to contribute?

- How do the permitting and regulatory frameworks developed by county, state, and (eventually) federal agencies encourage or inhibit local, small-scale cannabis production? How can policies be structured to maintain cannabis production in cannabis-dependent communities under legalization, when cannabis producers may have economic motivations to move out of remote locations?
- How does cannabis production interact with the multiple forms of capital that are required for rural economic development—not only financial but social, cultural, political, built, and human capital?
- How and under what circumstances has cannabis production counteracted the rural brain drain (the migration of young people to urban places for economic opportunity, see Carr and Kefalas 2010)?
- Who is working in and benefiting from the cannabis sector, and how will this change with legalization? How is cannabis production gendered and racialized—that is, how do people of different genders and races negotiate their roles in the economy?

Considering the Impacts of Cannabis Production on Other Sectors

Cannabis production and restoration are not the only sectors that have intersected over time. It is important for researchers to recognize how the cannabis sector has complemented and competed with other sectors.

- How do market signals encourage or discourage the replacement of some crops (e.g., avocados, timber) with cannabis? How does this impact land use and land values? How does this impact the agricultural sector and, ultimately, farmers' livelihoods?
- What are the multipliers (the indirect and induced benefits) of cannabis production? For example, what proportion of the revenue from cannabis production is spent in local restaurants, hardware stores, and gas stations, and what proportion leaks out of the local economy?
- What are the impacts of the cannabis sector on rural entrepreneurialism? What other businesses have been started or supplemented through cannabis revenues?

The rural economies of the Emerald Triangle are undergoing transformation within the context of legalization, but one thing is certain: the economy and people's livelihoods in places like the Mattole will continue to center on cannabis production, at least for the foreseeable future. Researchers should be examining how cannabis impacts rural places in order to contribute to policy discussions about how to create a fair and reasonable cannabis regulatory framework. There is a growing need to recognize and maintain the economic and community benefits of cannabis, while also grappling with the real challenges of bringing the sector out of the shadows.

References

Afsahi, Kenza. 2011. "Cannabis Cultivation Practices in the Moroccan Rif." In *World Wide Weed: Global Trends in Cannabis Cultivation and its Control*, edited by Gary Potter, Martin Bouchard, and Tom Decorte, 39–53. New York: Routledge.

Aronson, James, James N. Blignaut, Suzanne J. Milton, David L. Maitre, Karen J. Esler, Amandine Limouzin, Christelle Fontaine, Martin P. De Wit, Worship Mugido, Philip Prinsloo, Leandri Van Der Elst, and Ned Lederer. 2010. "Are Socioeconomic Benefits of Restoration Adequately Quantified? A Meta-analysis of Recent Papers (2000–2008) in *Restoration Ecology* and 12 Other Scientific Journals." *Restoration Ecology* 18 (2): 143–54.

Baker, Mark. 2005. "Socio-economic Characteristics and Contributions of the Natural Resources Restoration System in Humboldt County, California." *Ecological Restoration* 23 (1): 5–14.

Baker, Mark, and Lenya N. Quinn-Davidson. 2011. "Jobs and Community in Humboldt County, California." In *Human Dimensions of Ecological Restoration*, edited by Dave Egan, Evan E. Hjerpe, and Jesse Abrams, 221–37. Washington, DC: Island Press.

Bauer, Scott, Jennifer Olson, Adam Cockrill, Michael van Hattem, Linda Miller, Margeret Tauzer, and Gordon Leppig. 2015. "Impacts of Surface Water Diversions for Marijuana Cultivation on Aquatic Habitat in Four Northwestern California Watersheds." *PLoS One* 10 (3): e0120016. doi:10.1371/journal.

BenDor, Todd T., William Lester, Avery Livengood, Adam Davis, and Logan Yonavjak. 2015. "Estimating the Size and Impact of the Ecological Restoration Economy." *PloS One* 10 (6): 1–15.

Butsic, Van, and Jacob C. Brenner. 2016. "Cannabis (*Cannabis sativa* or *C. indica*) Agriculture and the Environment: A Systematic, Spatially-explicit Survey and Potential Impacts." *Environmental Research Letters* 11: 044023.

Carr, Patrick J., and Maria J. Kefalas. 2010. *Hollowing Out the Middle: The Rural Brain Drain and What it Means for America*. Boston, MA: Beacon Press.

Corva, Dominic. 2014. "Requiem for a CAMP: The Life and Death of a Domestic U.S. Drug War Institution." *International Journal of Drug Policy* 25: 71–80.

Dabson, Brian. 2012. *Transitioning to a Restoration Economy: A Case Study of Oregon's Forestry Sector*. Columbia, MO: Rural Futures Lab.

Daniels, Jean M., Max Nielsen-Pincus, Michael Paruszkiewicz, and Nathan Poage. 2018. "The Economic Contribution of Stewardship Contracting: Two Case Studies from the Mt. Hood National Forest." *Journal of Forestry* 116 (3): 245–56.

Davis, Emily J., Shiloh Sundstrom, and Cassandra Moseley. 2011. *The Economic Impacts of Oregon's South Coast Restoration Industry*. Working Paper Number 34. Ecosystem Workforce Program and Institute for a Sustainable Environment, University of Oregon.

Egan, Dave, Evan E. Hjerpe, and Jesse Abrams. 2011. "Why People Matter in Ecological Restoration." In *Human Dimensions of Ecological Restoration*, edited by Dave Egan, Evan E. Hjerpe, and Jesse Abrams, 1–19. Washington, DC: Island Press.

Gibson-Graham, J. K. 2008. "Diverse Economies: Performative Practices for 'Other Worlds'." *Progress in Human Geography* 32 (5): 613–22.

Halfacree, Keith. 2007. "Trial by Space for a 'Radical Rural': Introducing Alternative Localities, Representations and Lives." *Journal of Rural Studies* 23: 125–41.

Holmes, John, and Neil Argent. 2016. "Rural Transitions in the Nambucca Valley: Socio-demographic Change in a Disadvantaged Rural Locale." *Journal of Rural Studies* 48: 129–42.

House, Freeman. 1999. *Totem Salmon: Life Lessons from Another Species*. Boston: Beacon Press.

Kimball, Sarah, Megan Lulow, Quinn Sorenson, Kathleen Balazs, Yi-Chin Fany, Steven J. Davis, Michael O'Connell, and Travis E. Huxman. 2015. "Cost-effective Ecological Restoration." *Restoration Ecology* 23 (6): 800–10.

Leeper, Joseph. 1990. "Humboldt County: Its Role in the Emerald Triangle." *California Geographical Society* 30: 93–109.

Lurie, Sarah, and Michael Hibbard. 2008. "Community-Based Natural Resource Management: Ideals and Realities for Oregon Watershed Councils." *Society and Natural Resources* 21 (5): 430–40.

Mattole River and Range Partnership. 2009. *Mattole Integrated Coastal Watershed Management Plan: Foresight 2020*. Accessed November 3, 2018. www.mattole.org/wp-content/uploads/2014/08/WatershedPlan_Final_w_Cover.pdf.

Nielsen-Pincus, Max, and Cassandra Moseley. 2013. "The Economic and Employment Impacts of Forest and Watershed Restoration." *Restoration Ecology* 21 (2): 207–14.

Nordstrom, Carolyn. 2000. "Shadows and Sovereigns." *Theory, Culture & Society* 17: 35–54.

Paoli, Letizia, Tom Decorte, and Loes Kersten. 2015. "Assessing the Harms of Cannabis Cultivation in Belgium." *International Journal of Drug Policy* 26 (3): 277–89.

Raphael, Ray. 1985. *Cash Crop: An American Dream*. Caspar, CA: Ridge Times Press.

Somerville, Peter, Robert Smith, and Gerard McElwee. 2015. "The Dark Side of the Rural Idyll: Stories of Illegal/Illicit Economic Activity in the UK Countryside." *Journal of Rural Studies* 39: 219–28.

Stauber, Karl N. 2001. "Why Invest in Rural America and How? A Critical Public Policy Question for the 21st Century." *Economic Review* 86 (2): 33–63.

Swanson, Lee A., and Vincent Bruni-Bossio. 2018. "A Righteous Undocumented Economy." *Journal of Business Ethics* 160: 225–37. https://doi.org/10.1007/s10551-108-3878-2.

Tidwell, Tom, and Hutch Brown. 2011. "Moving Towards a Restoration Economy." *Journal of Forestry* 109 (7): 386–90.

23

Cannabis Seed in the Rif Region of Morocco

The Commodification of Nature and the Construction of a Contested International Market[1]

Kenza Afsahi

Keywords: Cannabis seed, hybrids, contested markets, environmental justice, Morocco

Introduction

In Morocco, various players, including intermediaries and cannabis users, have participated in the introduction and circulation of new cannabis seed varieties. More recently, seeds have been imported from Europe or the USA on a more frequent basis by transnational players or seed professionals, known as "breeders" (Afsahi 2017a). The commodification of seeds by players in industrialized countries has benefited from a context in which cannabis production was increasingly local in industrialized countries, with close access to consumer markets. Hence, some players specialized in commodifying a new product, with the export of cannabis seed. How do players define acceptable and unacceptable standards for the cannabis seed market? Seeds are contested commodities, in the sense that they have a strong symbolic value, with their production and marketing raising ethical and rhetorical controversies (Duval and Garcia-Parpet 2012). Among the controversies raised by the issue of seed, let us cite the conflict between those who want to have rights as inventors in order to benefit from their work and those who consider it to be a sacrilege to patent living things (Berlan 1983), as well as the debates concerning the environmental consequences and impacts on human health triggered by the development of the seed industry—in particular GMO seeds—and the intensive use of plant health products generally associated with so-called variety improvement.

In the past twenty years, economic sociologists have looked at a variety of markets raising ethical issues and at how some products find themselves on the market or how some players demand that certain products be commodified in the name of morality. A number of studies concerning contested markets have thus emerged (Zelizer 1992; Radin 1996; Callon 2009; Healy 2004; Muniesa, Millo, and Callon 2007; Steiner 2010; Steiner and Trespeuch 2013, 2015; Karpik 2013; Rao 2009), relating to subjects such as organs, children, the deceased, life insurance and gambling. But there are still very

DOI: 10.4324/9780429320491-23

few studies available concerning cannabis markets, particularly when these concern issues specific to Southerncountries. In countries that have recently legalized cannabis for medical use or otherwise, the new legislation, which has emerged in different national contexts (Uruguay, USA, Canada, EU, etc.), has led to new forms of cannabis commodification, for which states attempt to create regulated markets at every stage, from growing to consumption. The objectives are simultaneously to reduce illegal trade, add economic value to the product via taxation, protect human health, impose barriers on players at the outset (price increases) and determine which commodities may circulate and be used. These experiences imply a redefinition of standards, narratives, trade and commodities, and so on and raise questions relating to the construction of the market. While some studies have emerged concerning the positive (economic contribution of new markets, weakening of the black market) or negative (increased consumption) effects of the decriminalization and legalization of cannabis, some researchers are just starting to look at cannabis markets as a contested market (Dioun 2018; Cadigan and Harris 2018; Bergeron and Nouguez 2015). Several of these studies demonstrate the continued existence of illegal markets in parallel with the new legal ones.

These different market systems that have emerged are not harmonized and coexist with illegal markets, which have their own regulations. Based on the case of Morocco, this chapter focuses on the emergence of the cannabis seed trade and supplements studies in the economics of conventions and economic sociology concerning contested markets. Defining the contested subjects triggers disputes between producers, intermediaries, the state and all the players involved in the process of idea and knowledge production and the valuation of goods (Bessy and Chateauraynaud 2010).

Transformations in the cannabis cultivation environment (technical, relationships, legislation, etc.) are observed over the long term, even if the changes are rapid in terms of the dynamics of illegal drug market players. That is why it is impossible to measure the effects of new seed varieties over a period of just a few years. Furthermore, the seed issue is difficult to grasp on the scale of just one social group. Its analysis needs to be carried out on several levels (geographic, historic, etc.) and to take into account the diversified players (local farmers in Southern countries; intermediaries, mediators and "breeders" or seed selectors or producers from Northern countries). These different levels also need to be linked together in order to observe the exchanges between very localized players, with little mobility, such as cannabis growers in Southern countries, and transnational players, some of whom have a very high level of technical knowledge and demonstrate strong mobility, such as breeders, operating in very diverse areas and regulatory contexts (legalization, decriminalization, illegality). These various levels make it possible to reflect on the construction of contested markets that create marked economic, social and legal inequalities between players.

This chapter is part of ongoing research on the development of the cannabis seed market. Starting in 2013, we observed the introduction of seeds of hybrid cannabis varieties into the Rif region (Chouvy and Afsahi 2014). I subsequently became interested in technical changes, production and exchanges of knowledge surrounding these new varieties (Afsahi 2017a).

The chapter is based on observations and informal, semi-structured interviews conducted with the various stakeholders (growers, intermediaries, associations, breeders, etc.). Besides the cannabis growers in the Rif region, those involved in the seed supply considered here are all men and have had a link with Morocco at some point in their past. They all have experience in breeding and/or growing cannabis, but only the breeders have become professional and are recognized in the field (Afsahi 2017a). The so-called transnational actors come from diverse backgrounds, often with experience in militancy and very good knowledge of the world of cannabis. Those players, including breeders, have a capacity to evolve in diversified spaces and regulatory frameworks, particularly with respect to legalization, decriminalization and illegality. This capacity to evolve in different spheres gives them a high level of mobility and numerous connections, including in the legal market or with institutions. Several of these players have strong links with Dutch coffee shops, for example (Afsahi 2017a).

This seems to be of benefit to farmers in the Rif region, who recognize these players as distributors of seeds and growing methods but also as the people who buy their products and make them known outside their borders.

From some twenty interviews, we have chosen the five most representative in relation to the issue of the article, conducted over the last two years. In order to gather in-depth perspectives, some people were interviewed several times, at different moments and about different aspects of their story: their learning process, knowledge and more technical aspects of cannabis seeds and cultivation, the perception of their work, and the way in which they justify their practices morally to perceive this as a legitimate market. The interview excerpts are anonymous without any indication of age or nationality. The data have been supplemented by very recent observations in the Rif region of Morocco, on the websites of seed banks and breeders and on growers' discussion forums. In the first section, I consider the arguments put forward by the transnational players operating in the seed markets, which are still under construction, concerning the value of hybrids and their commitment to cannabis growers in Morocco. This legitimization has benefited greatly from the cannabis prohibition context. In the second part, I explore how local players have created, in their recent history, a context favorable to the introduction of hybrid seed varieties and the conditions to increase the ethics of their activities. I also examine how, at the same time as becoming vulnerable populations, they are currently constructing a narrative hinged around environmental issues, highlighting the advantages of traditional *kif* (called *Beldiya*).

Part I: Transnational Seed Players and Raising the Ethical Standards of Practices

The Production of Information and Hybrid Varieties

Today's cannabis market is characterized by a lack of scientific knowledge when it comes to the issue of cannabis varieties, created by the prohibition context. Very few botanists or plant biologists, ethnologists, economists or agronomic specialists have worked on the question of the varietal diversity of cannabis.

For psychotropic varieties, knowledge concerning these varieties and seeds has been gathered and developed in informal laboratories for decades without any institutional control, by players who have operated in "gray areas" in terms of the regulations after collecting original varieties in the South. Using these new seeds, transnational players have created seed banks[2] and a hybrid seed market.

In a previous paper (Afsahi 2017a), we focused on breeders and their professionalization. Breeders are recognized players in the environment, as professionals or experts. The cannabis seed market reveals the capacity of these players to create their own research and development system. The development of new seed varieties is not simply a matter of competition or changing consumer tastes. It is also related to the development of genetic selection and cultivation methods associated with cannabis in industrialized countries where indoor production techniques make it possible to optimize cannabis growing conditions and hybridize cannabis varieties from traditional growing countries. The hybrid varieties now created include regular, feminized and autoflowering varieties, which all require a particular work organization and specific growing methods. After becoming popular in industrialized countries, fully feminized varieties are now also popular in Southern production regions. This player offers the following explanation:

> Even amateur cannabis growers are now almost all switching to feminized varieties. It's hard work to keep mother plants for cuttings. The mother plants are kept under constant light for

> 18 hours to stop them from flowering so that regular cuttings can be taken under lamps, in controlled cultivation conditions. The best phenotype is chosen and it is then multiplied an infinite number of times . . . You need to have "elite" plants to produce cuttings that you then treat so that male glands develop and give you feminized seeds. . . . It's a technical process. Ordinary growers don't know how to do it. They have to buy each time. It's the same for autoflowering plants. It's not so simple to do.
>
> *(interview with a transnational player, 2017)*

Breeders also enable us to consider how knowledge is kept in the hands of a very small network of illegal drug market players. They translate knowledge, but in a partial and selective manner, and also form a global network, while relying on the help of local players (Afsahi 2017a).

As suggested by certain studies concerning the circulation of seed (corn and sorghum) within specific local farming communities, the seed needs to be acquired from donors fully trusted by the growers and with whom there is the greatest cultural proximity in order to have viable, high-quality information (Garine, Barnaud, and Raimond 2014). The seed transfer networks for local varieties lost with the arrival of hybrid varieties are important since they influence the mechanisms underpinning the genetic diversity of plants (Idem 2014). Yet we can see that it is difficult to retrace the history of hybrid varieties in the Rif region. Their real nature is only known by international seed producers, who hold the information at the other end of the chain or via certain intermediaries who pass on the seed to the local farmers, along with the information required to grow the plants (Afsahi 2017a). As recounted by these two breeders, it is difficult to assess the number of hybrid varieties currently grown:

> For the hybrids or polyhybrids you find in the Rif region, you can talk about all varieties in general: they buy without even knowing the real origin, but the most common ones are there: Critical, Critical Bilbo, Critical Mass, Amnesia and Og Kush, but the list is very long for the other, less common seeds.
>
> *(breeder interview, 2017)*

> Currently in the Rif region, a huge amount, and too many different hybrids are grown, and unfortunately, there are more and more new ones every year. I could tell you that more than 10 varieties are being grown.
>
> *(breeder interview, 2019)*

So local farmers are getting hold of hybrid seeds for which they do not have all the information and constructing their own personal knowledge based on their experience. They are also changing their names: for example, *Critical* has become known as *Trikita* to Moroccan peasant farmers. This name has even become the name of a Moroccan hashish (cannabis resin) sold in Europe. We questioned several breeders about the origins of Critical or its current place in cannabis cultivation:

> Critical is an old European variety that was bred by the famous Shantibaba, more than 15 years ago. Very popular in Spain, the flowers soon became a commercial product produced in large quantities and, following the Spanish, the Moroccans were given the chance to try it. It has come a long way. I would say that since 2010 Critical seeds have been planted on a large scale in the Rif region.
>
> *(breeder interview, 2019)*

> Nowadays, Critical is no longer the most widespread variety at all and has been quickly replaced by other varieties, such as Nicole, Bubblegum, Kosher Tangie or Tangie, etc.
>
> *(breeder interview, 2019)*

While several hybrid varieties are currently grown in the Rif region, some of them, before Critical (Trikita for local farmers), became very popular and were grown for several years in succession: *Pakistana* and *Khardala* in particular (Afsahi 2017b). They are abandoned, however, once yields become too poor—the harvest from the hybrids is less in subsequent years. It is nonetheless worth noting an evolution from Khardala to Critical, which, according to this transnational player, is due to the switch from regular varieties (with male plants) to feminized varieties: "Khardala is the last conventional hybrid to be grown on a large scale. Production is now 100% feminized or on female cuttings" (transnational player interview, 2017).

The Technical Arguments in Favor of the Expansion of Hybrids in the Rif Region

The interest in the research and development of hybrid seeds has mainly been driven by breeders, who are keen to demonstrate the benefits of hybrids to local farmers in the Rif region. The introduction of these seeds over a number of years did not immediately result in their commodification. It took varying amounts of time to convince farmers and to test the seeds and the techniques associated with these seeds.

A first series of arguments in favor of the introduction of hybrids concerns the rapid increase in yields and the THC content of the cannabis (Chouvy and Afsahi 2014) compared to local varieties. This increased productivity (as regards THC) to make Moroccan hashish more competitive and meet European demand.

Another series of arguments concerns the need for Rif farmers to change their growing methods, not suitable for hybrids, and, consequently, the introduction of methods better suited to "more potent" cannabis (Chouvy and Afsahi 2014). New practices have also emerged concerning the use of underground water and the digging of wells to irrigate hybrid varieties, or the adoption of new irrigation systems, such as drip systems and the expansion of water reservoirs in the Rif landscapes (Afsahi 2017a; Chouvy and Macfarlane 2018). The changes have also affected the use of fertilizers and plant health products, now more intensively used since these new seeds are more vulnerable than the Beldiya variety. Some changes have also affected sowing methods, as this transnational player tells us:

> Millions of feminized seeds went off from Spannabis[3] for Morocco. They are grown on vines, with a hole every 50 cm. This creates big hills, covered with weed.
>
> *(transnational player, 2017)*

It has thus become crucial for local farmers to master new methods imported from industrialized countries. This is, in any case, another of the arguments put forward by transnational players, who demonstrate their capacity to develop a system for on-site technical assistance and crop supervision in the Rif region.

Hence, some breeders produce their seeds in the Rif region and supervise the growing of these seed varieties:

> I have several varieties growing at present, including some new ones that I am trying out and that I hope to adapt to best suit your climate [in Morocco]. Yes, depending on my varieties, there are four that adapt very well, but I'm still working to do the best possible.
>
> *(breeder interview, 2019)*

Attentive to both quality and the environment, some justify their presence on-site by the fact that local farmers are finding it difficult to cope with the introduction of feminized seeds and the speed with which new methods have been introduced:

> Feminized seeds have changed a lot of things: water and fertilizer requirements, the purchase cost but higher yields at the end for some varieties. But they are much more sensitive to the climate and plant care, drying and storage conditions. Above all, for more than half of the varieties used, feminized seeds have not been tested and are very sensitive to mold and fungal diseases related to the climate. The result is irrevocable and the final product is full of mold, which the Moroccans cannot identify and is very bad and dangerous for consumers. So knowing what we should and can grow on this land is essential for the future of cannabis growing in the Rif region . . . To start with, the new methods involve huge water stores, demand much more complete and expensive fertilizers, require ground watering systems using irrigation instead of spraying in the air, involve terracing of land to level it, etc.
>
> *(breeder interview, 2019)*

Growing and extraction methods are also being introduced by numerous transnational players moving to the Rif region to farm, attracted both by the climate and growing expertise, as well as very cheap local labor. Farms have therefore been moved to the Rif region:

> My biggest fear is that the traffickers import qualified labor. Both as a crop manager and to transform. . . . In some cases this is the case, in others they do it all and pay a rent. . . . Sometimes they lose everything too . . . But when the Colombians or Italians set up a large-scale operation, they see it through. . . . Yes, they really do it all without Moroccans, except as low-end assistants. There are also freelancers, who mainly provide training so they can have a better final product to buy and traffic. It's the same thing in Jamaica.
>
> *(breeder interview, 2017)*

> I've given loads of advice to growers and their families and I am trying to improve their conditions, as well as yields and efficiency. Whether it concerns their soil to be protected, water, fertilizer, watering times and methods, the tests to be carried out and the various problems they encounter depending on the regions and genetic varieties they grow. Unfortunately, the exchange is a poor one since their knowledge is limited. Fortunately, today, with the help of the internet, many progress quickly and, in fact, recently our exchanges have become more interesting and we can learn and grow together.
>
> *(breeder interview, 2019)*

The preliminary results of our research suggest that transnational seed market players employ a variety of measures in an attempt to justify the development of seed as being ethically acceptable and beneficial for the plant and the environment, or using "noble" arguments related to sharing (Ducos, Joly, and Moreaux 1985) and exchange. It is not impossible either that they recognize the adverse effects on the environment and local populations. In addition, breeders indicate that getting into the new more technical cultivation methods associated with hybrids requires more expertise than growers in Southern countries currently have. Therefore, they need advice and technical support. They consequently set themselves the mission of providing Rif farmers with the logistics that isolated Moroccan growers—incapable of measuring the scientific and technical scope of new cannabis varieties—do not have access to.

Part II: The Vulnerable Populations of the Rif region and the Genetic Resources of Beldiya

The Adoption of New Seed Varieties and New Techniques for the Production of Hashish

In the historic cannabis-growing region in the Rif Mountains, as well as in other small-scale cannabis growing areas in Morocco, for generations growers used local cannabis seed, producing, depending on the regions, traditional varieties of *kif*, such as *Ktamiya*, grown by the people of Ketama. The peasant farmers did not buy the seed; they kept seeds from their previous harvest to reseed their fields or got it from their families or neighbors. The seeds were sown using the broadcast method (by scattering). The way the seeds were selected, stored and scattered on land of variable quality, along with the associated cultivation methods, preserved the genetic diversity of Moroccan *kif*.

It was during harvest that the farmers built up their seed stores. According to the elders, who remember the period prior to the production of hashish, before the 1960s, the entire farming period, from sowing to harvesting, was subject to rituals and contributed to a moment of solidarity. The seed-harvesting period was a time of celebration, with lots of birds of various species coming to feed on the seeds too. Everyone involved in collecting the seeds could take seed for themselves, since they had free access to it. Mouliéras (1895) recounts that the families of Ketama who had the biggest fields had to use the *touiza* method (collective farm labor) to sow and harvest.

As objects that circulate, seed carries the imprints of those having worked it, helping to create a tight-knit network of humans and plants. Selecting the seed on the farm creates a sense of belonging to a peasant world far removed from the modern farmer (Demeulenaere and Bonneuil 2011). In addition, the old varieties are associated with specific seed storage methods and farming processes (Idem 2011).

The end of the 1960s—and especially the 1980s—marked the beginning of the end for the preservation of local varieties. It was then that growers of the Rif region appear to have begun adopting new varieties from Lebanon for the production of hashish intended for the European market, as recounted by this player:

> But we [Europeans] made lots of oil, which was good at the time, because the quality of the weed was too variable. Except the market wanted weed. Hash oil is awkward to transport. . . . So they were left with stock on their hands. . . . So the importers suggested that the peasant farmers should send one son per family to the Bekaa Valley. To learn how to cultivate, sieve and bring back bags of seeds. A huge success in the early years, before the invention of the international soap bar,[4] this poisonous crap that invaded the market in the early 1990s.
>
> *(transnational player interview, 2017)*

Until the 1980s, the Ketama growers are said to have been some of the first to adopt these new Lebanese seeds and the methods of cultivation and transformation of the *kif* into hashish, before they were adopted on a larger scale in various provinces in the north of the kingdom. During the same period, Westerners are also said to have introduced modern seeds into Morocco and to have crossed them with the traditional *kif* of the Rif region to increase profitability. In the space of ten years, the characteristics of Western "improved" varieties were observed in almost all Rif populations (Clarke and Merlin 2016).

The dried flower sieving/threshing phase has become the key phase in the collection of seeds. Cannabis plants are usually dioecious and produce flowers that may be male (pollen) or female (seeds) (Idem 2016). They are also anemophilous, or wind-pollinated, depending on the wind to spread the pollen from male plants to female plants.

Growers thus abandoned *kif* cultivation, switching to *sinsemilla* (seedless) cultivation, a practice dating from the early 1970s that was to become widespread towards the end of the decade. This practice consisted of eliminating the male plants from the fields when growing cannabis, to only leave unfertilized female plants. Instead of producing seeds, the females produce only trichomes and therefore active ingredients, including THC (Idem 2016). Despite the adoption of this method, most growers kept male plants in their fields, reporting better fertilization of female plants. It would appear that for decades growers thus created and used a new cannabis seed, which is a mixture of Moroccan and Lebanese varieties. *Kif* was associated with a cultivation method, producing seeds.

The Multiplication of Hybrids

For the past ten or so years, growers have been adopting various hybrid varieties of cannabis, the seeds of which have been imported in large quantities from Europe, and, more recently, North America. It was following the introduction of the hybrids, new usages and methods, that the name Beldiya emerged to refer to the local variety, commonly known as *kif*.

At the time of their introduction, hybrids met with only limited success among the farmers, who did not yet master the growing methods and the new growing calendar (Afsahi 2017a). Thereafter, the speed with which the new seeds were adopted was stupefying, although not all farmers immediately introduced them, either because they did not have access to or master the methods or because they were resistant to introducing a new product into the heart of the traditional growing region. For the past few years, all fields have been sown with new hybrid forms, in the majority of cases feminized (*hejala-veuve*), no longer involving the thinning out phase. According to one breeder:

> On the plantations as a whole, there are now 70% to 80% feminized seeds, marketed by the seed banks, with the rest being traditional Moroccan plants. In 2012, there were only 10% feminized seeds.
>
> *(breeder interview, 2019)*

In Morocco, the hybrid varieties were regular ones and, more recently, feminized ones, but on our most recent observations in the Rif region in 2019, growers were trying autoflowering varieties. These varieties have been developed by seed producers to start flowering once the plants reach an early plant growth stage rather than wait for daylight to reduce to trigger flowering (Clarke and Merlin 2016). They are ready to be harvested just ten weeks after germination. According to some of the people I spoke to, they are reputed to be the varieties aimed at amateur growers wishing to grow a few plants, those just starting out in the growing process, those who do not have the time or patience to get involved in a long, costly venture, or those who are not very experienced. The quest for profitability could encourage the growing of these varieties in the Rif region, since they could allow three harvests per year (early May, early August and early October):

> A. is testing autoflowering varieties grown in a small field next to a larger parcel of land, sown with the "second-generation" Critical variety. One of the grower's contacts abroad had brought him seed from a French seed bank. The grower appeared to take the trial very seriously: in particular, he had indicated the name of each of the varieties planted in the ground. Two of the plants grown were not successful.
>
> *(field diary 2019)*

Concerning the methods for transforming dried cannabis into hashish (cannabis resin), growers have gradually become interested in new methods:

> B., a Ketama grower, showed me what he had carefully hidden in his bedroom: several packets of seeds, sold 2 to 5 seeds at a time, as is the case for domestic growing in industrialized countries. These seeds came from a French seed bank and a Californian seed bank, the Humboldt Emerald Triangle. He also had a box with a Secret Smoke brand iced water extraction machine (Ice-O-Lator), a vaporizer and various samples of weed or hashish of different varieties placed in a plastic box. He was pretty proud to show me that he had access to different Western use, growing, and processing methods.
>
> *(field diary 2019)*

However, for some transnational players, the changes in hashish production methods remain very limited:

> All the producers still use sieving and threshing to harvest the material. However, they are increasingly trying new methods, such as cold methods and more elaborate drying techniques, extraction machines, etc.
>
> *(breeder interview, 2019)*

Rif growers have shown an interest in and curiosity for new methods and seeds that they have themselves brought back from trips or that have been introduced by relatives or customers living abroad, particularly in the Netherlands or Spain, two countries very involved in domestic cannabis growing and the production of new seed (Chouvy and Afsahi 2014). They can have a dual discourse with respect to hybrids: one that excludes exogenous plants (because they affect the local environment) and another that includes them and makes them competitive players. The social media, and internet in general, have also contributed to greater access to what was happening in industrialized countries. This results in a do-it-yourself (DIY) approach when selecting seeds or implementing the associated methods, without a rational protocol. There are so many new hybrids introduced each year, sometimes by players speaking a different language from the local people. Yet these hybrids, which require adaptation to the environment and new methods, sometimes find themselves in the hands of growers without any information or instructions. This grower expresses a common view: "Today, everything is all mixed up. It's insane."

The Protests of Local Farmers and the Return of Beldiya

The protests following the introduction of hybrids relate to the various costs that did not exist previously and the ecological crisis generated by the hybrids, more specifically concerning the increasing rarity of the local variety, Beldiya.

Sowing new seeds each year is too expensive. So the farmers reduce these costs by replanting the hybrids. This practice is called *maaouda* (repeated) and explains why feminized varieties have a lower yield the following years and why the fields contain male plants, since the feminized plants are pollinated by the male plants from nearby fields. The female plants are fully fertilized by the male plants growing nearby, and the "best" improved seed is sown the following year (Clarke and Merlin 2016). In this way, local varieties are quickly submerged by invading genes and are therefore replaced by a nonselected cross-mixture of Western varieties that are poorly suited to the local environmental conditions and treatment methods. According to Clarke and Merlin (2016), Mexico, Jamaica and Thailand have also lost a large number of their local cannabis varieties.

The growing methods for *kif* (now called Beldiya) made it possible to keep the seeds regular and preserve local variety resources. New methods, such as sowing in pots, clash with growing methods different from those used by local farmers, such as broadcast sowing. "You also need to buy the pots (full of plastic). If you want to keep regular ones, you need to scatter the seeds, even if this is not an optimized method."

According to the people we spoke to, the commodification of hybrid seed also creates an intense dependence and a loss of autonomy of growers to the benefit of players who previously bought the harvest from growers but who today establish "tacit contracts" with them. The seeds are sold with, in return, a guarantee that they will buy back the crop. These players may also sell compost from Germany to growers, along with fertilizers and chemical plant health products. They offer cultivation advice and technical support and, in a large number of cases, impose their growing methods, often characterized by an intensive farming system. Consequently, local farmers become reliant on seed players and tend to lose their empirical knowledge of seed, along with the associated selection and technical practices.

In this new context, some local farmers are beginning to object, based on environmental arguments and a desire to defend local varieties. They try to attach new value to the local variety, to defend the associated knowledge and growing and use methods, the therapeutic benefits (uncut, it would be a product that is good for health) and also environmental benefits. Beldiya has become an omnipresent subject of conversation, feeding narratives based on a nostalgia for how the environment was before the arrival of the hybrids, especially in the historic growing area.

Through the stories gathered about Beldiya, I tried to understand why it was still present in the narrative of growers, despite the fact that they participated in the introduction and spread of hybrids in the Rif region. The conditions in which it is grown close to hybrids that pollinate the fields mean that it is not possible to preserve it correctly. Some narratives even defy the laws of botanics: "I only grow Beldiya." This statement comes from a grower whose brother grows Critical in the fields neighboring his own, thereby encouraging pollination between the varieties. Other narratives reflect the resistance of growers who apparently protect the seeds that they know to be important: "My Beldiya [by that he means their seeds]: I keep it, I hide it," while here too certain botanists are talking about a drop in the germination rate depending on the storage conditions and, over time, for seeds that are not sown each year. There therefore seems to be a widespread sense of mistrust towards new seeds, sustained by an increase in the value of Beldiya, sold at 15,000 dirhams per kg of hashish.

For some players in the historic growing area, it is not only a matter of protecting vulnerable populations but also the environment and the native plant, which they deem to be endangered. In their collective work: *Marchés contestés* ("Contested Markets"), Philippe Steiner and Marie Trespeuch (2015) highlight how, in the process of calling into question the existence or absence of a market, "causal entrepreneurs" appeal to fragile populations, that need to be protected by creating a market or preventing it, for example with children that are protected from the dangers of drugs, pornography or gambling, who would be threatened by a dangerous and unscrupulous population.

These new practices have led to an ecological crisis related to the depletion of soil and water, as well as an economic and social crisis as a result of the debt generated by new production costs and a lack of control of the methods used to grow these new seeds. A number of other issues are also being raised, such as health problems linked to the use of fertilizers and pesticides, sometimes bought illegally, water contamination or the disappearance of traditional crops that were a staple food for local people and the disappearance of the botanical diversity of Moroccan cannabis. The process of well-digging has resulted in numerous conflicts between farmers due to the privatization of underground water: for the first time, according to several of the people we talked to, there were a number of homicides in the area of Issaguen linked to water-related conflicts. Many local players also mention unsold stocks of Critical and what that implies in terms of visibility and an increased risk with the authorities.

Through Beldiya, the local farmers are realizing that the hybrids have not only generated a loss of market and a deterioration in the environment, but also that they have had an adverse effect on social cohesion and ancient agricultural knowledge.

Today, Beldiya is loaded with symbolic meaning, reactivated by the narratives, and a banner for opposition against a new farming system imposed by hybrid crops, characterized by stock losses, seed fraud and increased poverty among growers, potentially leading to suicide or the mortgaging of their land (*rahn*), along with new violence related to water access.

Therefore, forms of resistance have emerged on the part of those who are determined to preserve the native plant:

> The problem with the arrival of new seeds is that it creates a natural imbalance. Everybody is trying to make money from it. In other areas (new growing areas), the forests of Ouazzane and Chaouen have been decimated. A desert is being created. Humankind is destroying itself, committing suicide.
>
> *(grower interview, 2019)*

A player from an association mentions actions to promote the development of the region and the preservation of the original *kif* plant, as well his project to restore the homes in his original village using hemp bricks:

> I want it to be a model for people using the native plant, because it has always existed; to preserve our traditions, smoke with a sebti pipe, and save our architecture of the past. The ancients used *kif* stems, straw. Hemp has been found in old houses. They knew how to use it, they made rope with it and it was a cycle of nature. They respected the water source, they constructed small reservoirs, in Charij [water source], in the mountains, with winter water. In the past, the water was slowed down by plants in the mountains, but now, these plants are no longer there and the water runs straight onto the road. . . . When we talk about the native plant, we're talking about the parent plant, which was born there, which has been there for centuries and is extraordinarily adaptable since it is in its own environment . . . What we are seeking is to preserve natural heritage.
>
> *(player from an association interview, 2019)*

According to him, this resistance appears to be winning over several growers in the historic growing area:

> With the arrival of winter and snow, people have understood that they need the forest. How will they keep warm otherwise? The indigenous people still preserve their natural and physical environment. For example, there are plants they use in the winter, such as the dwarf oak. They cut off branches to feed their cows and goats in the winter, when it snows. The leftover wood is dried for food preparation purposes. They have known about permaculture for centuries. . . . But if you take a native plant out of its environment, it is no longer the same. There is a danger to survival. The native plants that used to exist need to be replanted because otherwise there will be landslides, and an impact on the sea too, with the mud that comes down.
>
> *(player from an association interview, 2019)*

Depending on the cannabis growing regions, the local peasants have developed a narrative hinged around the benefits and detrimental effects of hybrid seeds. The narrative may concern the seeds themselves, the growing methods or the economic and environmental consequences. As highlighted by Steiner and Trespeuch (2015), here the ethical protest is based on the designation of fragile populations, who could be endangered by the emergence of contested markets:

> There is hardship now. The Europeans are cultivating their raw material on our land. And here, they are selling their poison (the new seeds). For small growers, their economic situation is getting worse and worse. Their natural environment is being destroyed; people are becoming poorer. There is a crisis in the Ouezzane area and other regions; they can't get rid of their stock . . . What's more, there are Europeans renting land here, who are in the process of making reservoirs.
>
> *(player from an association interview, 2019)*

Only a few local or transnational players are resisting, aware of these inequalities and of the ecological consequences of the seed market, as recounted by this local farmer and association member, who is seeing a growing awareness among several farmers, sometimes encouraged by a demand for the traditional product:

> All smokers and connoisseurs are coming back to Beldiya today. Now there's not a gram of Beldiya on the market; others have produced other varieties. Beldiya sells like gold. . . . The fashion has come and gone, especially in areas like Bab Berred, which was one of the first to plant, then spreading to Ouazzane.

A breeder involved in the dissemination of new hybrid varieties is no less aware of the need to preserve the heritage of the original seeds, while taking onboard new knowledge in terms of farming methods:

> Unfortunately, Beldiya and Tibizla seeds are increasingly difficult to find and I hope that some families are preserving them carefully. For my part, I believe that it is one of the most important parts of your heritage. It's still possible to find a little of the original genetic Beldiya from the olden days, but younger generations are all turning towards feminized seeds. . . . For those who preserve these seeds, their motivation is one of heritage and, above all, the low water and fertilizer requirements and the ease with which they withstand your harsh, dry climate; their capacity to grow in these conditions after years make them real champions. I would be really sorry to see them disappear and it would be a catastrophe. The medicinal capacities of Beldiya and Tibizla, as well as Pakistana and Mexicana, are immense and are perfectly suited to the environment, both to preserve it and for the survival of the Rif people. It would be far better to grow Beldiya using new methods and organic fertilizers than all the new varieties that have been grown in recent years.

Then he explains:

> The characteristics of Beldiya are its resistance to the climate, its requirement for little water and the small amount of ramification and branching. . . . It has small flowers and narrow leaves, good resin production and a host of other qualities. Tibizla is another variety similar to Beldiya but slightly better quality. It is also very robust and very suited to your climate.

He does not deny, however, that new hybrid varieties similar to Beldiya are also suitable for the Moroccan climate:

> There is also Hardala (Khardala), a mixture of Beldiya and Pakistana, which over the years and as habits have changed, has ended up being called Hardala. There are also other names, like King Hassan or Caramelo, which are also a guarantee of quality and are typical varieties of the Rif region. They are mixes: ancestral growing methods allowed a few male plants to pollinate

the flowers in order to have seeds to replant for the next season, something that is now being lost because feminized seeds must not be pollinated in order to be able to produce more and a better-quality product.

The introduction of new hybrid varieties is causing a loss of local farming identity (Mendras 1992 [1967]). Henri Mendras observed the changes triggered by hybrid corn varieties in France, in particular the loss of know-how and social cohesion associated with the reproduction of seed on the farm. The new seeds result in a new, more individual and market-oriented working organization. For farmers, it generates a new reference frame for legitimization (agronomic science instead of tradition) and new knowledge (from knowledge about nature to mechanical and management knowledge) (ibid. 1992 [1967]).

By changing their farming practices, cannabis growers are giving up local knowledge built up over centuries, knowledge that has helped forge their identity. Since the new growing methods are not adapted to local conditions, the local variety is losing its attributes.

In contrast with the controversy related to the plant varieties system Thomas (2006),[5] in the case of the cannabis seed market, no questions concerning biological patents have been raised, either by local farmers or governments. The players who could contest the seed trade are peasants from Southern countries; vulnerable, invisible people, often threatened with arrest for growing cannabis, which is illegal in their country. Since the activity of the peasant farmers is illegal, the states are stigmatized for their production and cannot protect populations against the appropriation and use of their local resources by players themselves outside any form of control (breeders) or the major cannabis firms that are developing in industrialized countries.

Conclusion

As in the wheat example studied by Bertrand (2018, 31), the peasant ontology of cannabis "suggests that local farming knowledge is an exercise mobilizing a very broad range of knowledge to forge a singular science of places and times." The knowledge of the Rif farmers is rendered invisible by that of transnational players, and there is risk that it could become even more so with the technical agronomic knowledge employed for the purpose of economic profitability. Hence, the commodification of seed and the introduction of hybrids oppose two different types of knowledge.

The development of hybrid seed does not correspond to the local realities of Moroccan farmers. And yet, today, this market represents the main seed source for local farmers. Farmers are now confronted with a seed market in its own right, sometimes independent and parallel to the hashish market, with transnational players specializing in seeds. This type of market did not exist previously. Local farmers are now reliant on these players and the knowledge they bring relating to the seeds.

In contrast with Bergeron and Nouguez (2015), who show how a cannabis market is still confined to certain places and certain people, as in the Netherlands, we have seen in this chapter that the cannabis market in the Rif region has been built as a mirror image to a highly complex international network. It is not defined by its containment but by its involvement in a global, supranational, evolving context, which is constantly being redefined and in which various supply and demand players interact, along with transnational players who contribute to the production and circulation of knowledge relating to the use, cultivation and distribution of seed.

In this chapter, the consideration of different levels of scale also allows us to observe markets with different regulations, within a context of globalization. It also enables us to question the changes that the world cannabis market has been undergoing in the past few years in terms of the growth in cannabis cultivation in industrialized countries, changes in cannabis legislation in certain countries and their consequences for the cultivation of cannabis, particularly in Southern countries. These players reflect the global reality of the cannabis market currently, in terms of both changes in cannabis cultivation itself and the legislative changes relating to its use.

In the seed market, our observations also reveal the mechanisms of stratification between illegal and legal players (including in the field of research) in industrialized countries and between Southern players and industrialized country players. These findings are consistent with other research (Cadigan and Harris 2018) that documents links between the criminal justice system and economic institutions in legal US cannabis markets, where the regulations and moralizing practices on the market create categories of people with variable levels of legitimacy to access a new market. Hence, some citizens could more legitimately have access to lucrative opportunities (those whose activities were not related to the cannabis market), whereas players who were previously involved in illegal markets would be excluded and seen as criminals. This has consequences, in particular, for people of color seeking to enter the legal market and who were disproportionately affected by the criminalization of cannabis.

Until now, the commodification of seed has occurred outside the framework of new legislation. But new cannabis regulations will help to create a contested seed market, which could come under state control and legal private interests, as has been the case for the seeds of other plants (Quin 2013). This is already resulting in numerous North/South inequalities in terms of environmental justice and loss of biodiversity. Thus, the components underpinning the seed market have been put in place. The construction of this seed market demonstrates strong economic, social, legal (patents, intellectual property) and environmental inequalities between Northern and Southern players. With the legalization of cannabis in several industrialized countries and the arrival on the market of multinational and pharmaceutical companies, Southern farmers are no better protected. The new seeds being developed today in informal laboratories will benefit from the new regulations in industrialized countries that thousands of seed banks will be able to take advantage of.

The new regulatory context of cannabis markets has an impact on the preservation of plant diversity and the work of small growers, as recounted by this transnational association player campaigning for the legalization of cannabis:

> Our main fear is that the cannabis industry meets the same fate as the American corn or soy industry, where we have seen the disappearance of small-scale growers, replaced by monopolies set up by large corporations who manage to gain control over plant genetics.
>
> *(interview, 2017)*

It is now urgently necessary to rethink the issue of environmental justice and the loss of biodiversity in the case of cannabis seed and in an international context of evolving regulations. Today, the changes in the cannabis market are such that they offer industrialized countries the chance to patent varieties if they manage to prove that the variety is new, stable and uniform. Numerous patents have been filed, even in a context in which cannabis is banned, in a variety of fields, including medicine (medicinal products containing cannabinoids, such as Sativex), agriculture (lighting or ventilation systems), food (such as honey or coffee containing cannabis), cosmetics and e-liquids, among many other areas.

There is a risk that Southern farmers could become the main victims since they lose the usage of original cannabis seeds, one of the foundations of their cultural heritage. For the majority of farmers, a seed "is not merely the source of future plants and food; it is a vehicle through which culture and history can be preserved" (Shiva 2001, 69). The anthropology of nature and archaeological research related to the defense of local seeds are enabling farmers' voices to be better heard today (Bertrand 2018).

Moroccan farmers are beginning to realize the detrimental effects of hybrid varieties on their environment and their culture, but their room for maneuver is small since their legislative systems do not yet enable them to cope with this market. Growers have genetic resources and unique knowledge that need to be protected from the introduction and expansion of hybrid varieties and new growing methods. Traditional varieties have been contaminated by the hybrids introduced, particularly due to cross-pollination. Pure original varieties have become rare in all traditional cannabis-producing countries (for example, Jamaica, Mexico, Morocco and Thailand). This situation makes the collection of traditional seed varieties more and more difficult, whereas their preservation and reproduction are issues that have become more important than ever to protect genetic diversity (Clarke and Merlin 2016).

Finally, some studies show correlations between biological and cultural spheres and conclude, "culturally diversified humanity is more capable of producing biological diversity than standardized humanity," particularly using advanced technologies. According to Thomas (2011, 131) "this issue . . . is clearly related to the issue of production systems, consumption patterns and cultural domination."

Notes

1 I thank all the anonymous actors who have agreed to exchange with me. I would also like to thank Julien L. and Abdellatif Adebib for their availability and our exchanges.

2 From the 1980s onwards, numerous seed banks were created in the Netherlands, where cannabis growing for the production of seed and the sale of this seed were tolerated. In fact, the Convention on Narcotics Drugs (1962), which had acted as a legislative framework on a global scale, stipulates that cannabis is an illegal substance but does not explicitly mention cannabis seeds. Cannabis seeds, which do not contain any narcotic substances, are "technically" legal in all EU member states according to international law. However, cannabinoid substances that are banned by international conventions develop during the cannabis cultivation process. Furthermore, as long as it is not proved that they are intended for private or commercial growing purposes or as long as there has been no germination, various players consider that it is legal to market the seeds. While this approach applies in Europe, once a product enters a specific country, it is subject to the laws of the country in question. It is therefore possible to buy seeds that are banned in one country but legal in another.

3 Spannabis is considered a major event in the cannabis scene in Europe. It takes place every year over three days in Barcelona.

4 Several kinds of hashish packaging exist, more or less famous in the market. Here the interlocutor designates by soap bar a packaging of hashish in the form of soap.

5 It was not until 1992 that local knowledge concerning the genetic resources of plant varieties was formally recognized in international conventions (Convention on Biological Diversity, CBD) and 1995 for the agreement on trade-related aspects of intellectual property rights (TRIPS). Several countries are in the process of changing their laws relating to access to genetic resources and this knowledge, so that the property rights of indigenous communities over the resources that they have preserved from one generation to the next can be recognized. However, according to Thomas (2006), the biodiversity preservation mechanisms of the 1990s were set up for biotechnologies, in order to guarantee access to biodiversity and impose on the world the recognition of the biological patent system of the USA and Europe (which hold 95% of patents). The mechanisms for sharing the profits with local populations do not always work.

References

Afsahi, Kenza. 2017a. "Ketama et Amsterdam: passeurs et développeurs de savoirs dans la production de haschich." *Autrepart* 2 (82) (Dossier "Circulation des savoirs et espaces d'apprentissage au Sud"): 161–77.

———. 2017b. "Quand la Khardala et les hybrides bouleversent le Rif." *Revue Santé, réduction des risques et usages de drogues (Swaps)* 87 (2-numéro spécial "Géopolitique et drogues, hommage à Alain Labrousse"): 21–25.

Bergeron, Henri, and Etienne Nouguez. 2015. "Les frontières de l'interdit: le commerce de cannabis." In *Marchés contestés. Quand le marché rencontre la morale*, edited by Marie Philippe Steiner, 121–50. Toulouse: Presses universitaires du Mirail, Département De Sciences Sociales Trespeuch.

Berlan, Jean-Pierre. 1983. "L'industrie des semences, économie et politique." *Économie rurale* 158: 18–28.

Bertrand, Aliénor. 2018. "Le blé des physiocrates. Contribution à une histoire politique de l'ontologie végétale." *Cahiers philosophiques* 1 (152): 9–36.

Bessy, Christian and Francis Chateauraynaud. 2010. "Le savoir-prendre. Enquête sur l'estimation des objets." *Techniques & Culture* 54–55 (1): 689–711.

Cadigan, Michele, and Alexes Harris. 2018. "Deserving Cannabis Entrepreneurs: How the State and Workers Define Who Gets to Be Legal." Conférence Contested Markets: Lessons from Cannabis Legalization, HEC, Paris, June 2018.

Callon, Michel. 2009. "Civilizing Markets: Carbon Trading between *in Vitro* and *in Vivo* Experiments." *Accounting, Organizations and Society* 34 (3): 535–48.

Chouvy, Pierre-Arnaud, and Kenza Afsahi. 2014. "Hashish Revival in Morocco." *International Journal of Drug Policy* 25 (3): 416–23.

Chouvy, Pierre-Arnaud, and Jennifer Macfarlane. 2018. "Agricultural Innovation in Morocco's Cannabis Industry." *International Journal of Drug Policy* 58: 85–91.

Clarke, Robert C., and Mark Merlin. 2016. "Cannabis Domestication, Breeding History, Present-day Genetic Diversity, and Future Prospects." *Critical Reviews in Plant Sciences* 35 (5–6): 293–327.

Demeulenaere, Elise, and Christophe Bonneuil. 2011. "Des semences en partage: Construction sociale et identitaire d'un collectif "paysan" autour de pratiques semencières alternatives." *Techniques & Culture Éditions de la Maison des sciences de l'homme* 57 (2) (2011–2012): 202–21.

Dioun, Cyrus. 2018. "Negotiating Moral Boundaries: Social Movements and the Strategic (Re) Definition of the Medical in Cannabis Markets." *Research in the Sociology of Organizations* 55 (1): 55–84.

Ducos, Chantal, Pierre-Benoît Joly, and Michel Moreaux. 1985. "Hybrides et lignées pures: le marché et l'entreprise privée sont-ils intrinsèquement pervers?" *Économie rurale* 165: 46–50.

Duval, Julien, and Marie-France Garcia-Parpet. 2012. "Les enjeux symboliques des échanges économiques." *Revue Française de Socio-Économie* 2 (10): 13–28.

Garine, Eric, Adeline Barnaud, and Christine Raimond. 2014. "Quel pourrait être le territoire des semences des sorghos que cultivent les Duupa du Massif de Poli (Nord du Cameroun)?" *Les Cahiers d'Outre-Mer* 265: 67–92.

Healy, Kieran. 2004. "Sacred Markets and Secular Ritual in the Organ Transplant Industry." In *The Sociology of the Economy*, edited by F. Dobbin, 308–31. New York: Russell Sage Foundation.

Karpik, Lucien. 2013. "Réalité marchande et réputation." *Communications* 1 (93): 121–29.

Mendras, Henri. 1992 (1967). *La Fin des paysans*. Arles: Actes Sud.

Mouliéras, Auguste. 1895. *Le Maroc inconnu. Première partie: Exploration du Rif.* Oran: Imprimerie Fouque.

Muniesa, Fabrice, Yuval Millo, and Michel Callon. 2007. "An Introduction to Market Devices." *The Sociological Review* 55 (2): 1–12.

Quin, Annabel. 2013. "la grande transformation des semences." In *Penser une démocratie alimentaire*, edited by Sunder the Supervision of François Collart Dutilleul and Thomas Bréger, Volume I. Inida, Costa Rica: Instituto de Investigacion en Derecho Aliment.

Radin, Margaret Jane. 1996. *Contested Commodities*. Cambridge: Harvard University Press.

Rao, Hayagreeva. 2009. *Market Rebels: How Activists Make or Break Radical Innovations*. Princeton, NJ: Princeton University Press.

Shiva, Vandana. 2001. *Protect or Plunder? Understanding Intellectual Property Rights*. London and New York: Zed Books.

Steiner, Philippe. 2010. *La Transplantation d'organes: un commerce nouveau entre les êtres humains*. Paris: Gallimard, coll. "Bibliothèque des sciences humaines."

Steiner, Philippe, and Marie Trespeuch. 2013. "Maîtriser les passions, construire l'intérêt. Les jeux d'argent en ligne et les organes humains à l'épreuve du marché." *Revue française de sociologie* 1 (54): 155–80.

——— (dir.). 2015. *Marchés contestés. Quand le marché rencontre la morale*. Toulouse: Presses universitaires du Midi.

Thomas, Frédéric. 2006. "Biodiversité, biotechnologies et savoirs traditionnels. Du patrimoine commun de l'humanité aux ABS (access to genetic resources and benefit sharing)." *Revue Tiers Monde* 4 (188): 825–42.

———. 2011. "Cosmologies, diversité bioculturelle et préservation de l'environnement." *Natures Sciences Sociétés* 2 (19): 129–32.

Zelizer, Viviana. 1992. "Repenser le marché. La construction sociale du 'marché aux enfants' aux États-Unis." *Actes de la recherche en sciences sociales* 4 (94): 3–26.

Section 5
Culture and Social Change

In each of our previous sections, we have emphasized research agendas that center two dynamics opened up by the emergence of cannabis legalization with, not after, prohibition: the persistence of prohibition as a problem and problems created by efforts to incorporate legal cannabis into normal cultural contexts, rather than change what it means to be normal. We are especially interested in research questions about cannabis legalization that explore, rather than assume, how the meaning of cannabis changes and/or is changed by processes of legalization. Legalization carves out particular spaces where the plant, as a commodity, is tolerated in society, but it does not necessarily bring people who value the plant in different, historically "deviant" ways, along with it.

When it comes to the relationship between prohibition and legalization, this section offers researchers opportunities to consider how the meaning of cannabis, in this particular moment, recombines with prohibition culture, which has stigmatized the meaning of cannabis as an exceptional danger to society. Legal cannabis, in the context of ongoing prohibition, carves out institutional exceptions to different kinds of cannabis stigmatization but does not remove it. When it comes to broader social problems, the post-prohibition cultural landscape presents at least two points of entry for researchers that pivot around the concept and practice of cultural normalization. Social movements to legalize cannabis can be more reformist when they focus on convincing others that cannabis is meaningful for "normal" people exercising individual liberty to achieve therapeutic outcomes or recreational pleasure. And they can be more radical when they focus on interrogating cannabis practices to critique what—or who—is normal.

Given the centrality of medical stigma to the legitimation of Prohibition 2.0, we begin with a chapter of original research on how the stigma of cannabis use interrupts the meaning of cannabis as a medical subject. In "Flipping the Script on Cannabis Stigma: Legitimacy Strategies of Medical Cannabis Patients," sociologist Michelle Newhart and medical cannabis activist William Dolphin draw on extensive interview research to investigate how stigmatization shapes patient experiences with medical cannabis. Their patient-focused research highlights how stigma associated with "legitimate" versus "problematic" cannabis use may influence health outcomes. They also critically examine what the ongoing stigmatization of cannabis as a therapeutic in public health institutions may mean for helping people heal. To the extent that medical cannabis is becoming socially legitimate, Newhart and Dolphin explore the implications of that change for recreational or non-catastrophic therapeutic use. Their interviews also examine the reconstruction of patient stigma as an unintended consequence of medical cannabis commercialization, for which claims about therapeutic efficacy may be cartoonishly exaggerated in the pursuit of profit.

Cultural studies scholar Ingrid Walker, in "Pleasure and the New Normal of Recreational Cannabis in the United States," examines issues of cannabis stigmatization by critically unpacking the limits of cultural "normalization" as a counter-strategy in discussions of recreational adult use. At the heart of the matter, she argues, are underdeveloped analyses of pleasure and deviance in drug policy discourses of health and safety. The "dangerous" political subject of drug use for pleasure is normalized by carving out and identifying legal use as "recreational," a safely acceptable, simplified form of pleasure. At the same time, the integration of regulated cannabis markets into normal, formal, circuits of capitalism funnels the politics of cannabis use into practices of neoliberal consumerism. Walker's work points researchers to examine cultural assumptions about the politics of normalization under conditions of continuing, generalized drug prohibition.

In "Changing the Face of the Stoner: Images of Race and Gender in Cannabis Legalization Campaigns in the United States," sociologist Katie Kaufman Rogers also focuses on how the politics of normalization may repurpose tropes of normality and stigmatized identities in ways that rework, rather than necessarily reduce, subjects of prohibition stigma. She utilizes discourse analysis to examine popular representations deployed in cannabis industry media for the purpose of normalization. Those images explicitly draw on stigmatic representations of "stoners" to associate legal cannabis use and business with white, upper-class identities. The mobilization of privileged identities explicitly reproduces the exclusion of deviant subjects and racial minorities from discourses of legal cannabis legitimacy.

Aguiar and colleagues investigate how Uruguayan attitudes towards cannabis legalization shifted from minority to majority support over the course of its first five years. Like Canada, Uruguayan legalization was organized at the national level but absent initial public support for this top-down governance reform initiated by President Mujica, a former left-wing guerilla. Public support for cannabis legalization was cultivated not before but during the implementation of legal cannabis. The authors ask how this happened and apply quantitative analysis of media frames to generate data for analysis. Their chapter is an excellent primer on legalization in Uruguay and is also valuable as an international case study for researchers doing comparative research on the relationship between legal policy implementation and public support.

Social work scholar and Flow Cannabis director of development Amanda Reiman's chapter, "The Intersection of Cannabis Reform and Other Progressive Movements: Opportunities for Interdisciplinary Researchers," provides researchers with an overview of potential opportunities for solidarity between regulated cannabis industries and broadly institutionalized ongoing social movements descended from the 1960s. While not formally auto-ethnographic, Reiman's introduction draws on her remarkable professional and personal journey through key sites and organizations associated with cannabis policy reform. Reiman's hybrid experience as a researcher, scholar, high-level reform professional, and corporate development officer puts her in a unique position to highlight and advocate for corporate social responsibility in the service of broader social policy reform.

Naturopathic doctor and clinical researcher Michelle Sexton uses auto-ethnography to parse out the meaning of cannabis "citizen science" as a reaction to public health stigma about cannabis as medicine but co-opted by the commercialization of therapeutic claims about cannabis in the absence of professional research engagement. Citizen science drew upon pre-prohibition healing practices that incorporated cannabis as botanical medicine, as part of a wider trend towards institutional acceptance of integrative medicine. Sexton's deep personal experience navigating medical cannabis advocacy through rapidly commercializing environments in Washington and California reveals once again the value of activist research to outline the emergence of an anti-prohibitionist critique of medical cannabis commercialization. In this case study, she identifies the "second track" route to the marketization of medical cannabis in the explosion of CBD products shaped by institutionalized nonregulation of nutritional supplement supply chains and brand claims.

The chapters in this section each map out ways of researching the relationship between cannabis legalization and social change beyond "good or evil" representations mobilized by advocates of continued prohibition or cannabis legalization. They ask us to consider how negative stereotypes developed under conditions of prohibition are transformed and reworked under conditions of legalization. They call for critical public health research that can address marketing claims about therapeutic efficacy without a fixation on toxicity. And they ask us to consider the cultural politics of "what is normal" in society, rather than insisting on normalization as a necessarily progressive process. Cannabis legalization reflects shifting social norms, but those shifts can be useful for varieties of legalization that differ in their acceptance of cultural differences in society.

24

Flipping the Script on Cannabis Stigma

Legitimacy Strategies of Medical Cannabis Patients

Michelle Newhart and William Dolphin

Keywords: Stigma, medical cannabis, medicalization, normalization, legitimacy

Introduction

Medical cannabis patients in the U.S. navigate a complex set of stigmas, from interpersonal social judgments based on stereotypes about marijuana users to structural discrimination that derives from the drug's legacy as an illicit substance. Drawing on in-depth, semi-structured interviews with 40 patients aged 30 to 68 who were enrolled in Colorado's medical marijuana program, this chapter explores strategies that midlife medical cannabis patients use to navigate the uncertainties in attitudes and laws, flip the script on stigma, and create legitimacy for the therapeutic use of medical cannabis.[1]

Stigma is a foundational concept across social science disciplines. At its most basic, it retains Goffman's (1986 [1963]) characterization from more than a half century ago: stigma is a discrediting attribute that invokes the "interrelated components of labeling, stereotyping, setting apart, status loss, and discrimination in the context of differences in social power" (Link 2017, 660). Generally, stigmatization is theorized as interactional. One person ascribes a discrediting attribute to another person, creating a rationale for discrimination in formal and informal ways (Jones et al. 1984; Link and Phelan 2001, 365). Contemporary theories have expanded the concept to acknowledge that stigma exists "outside of a model in which one person does something bad to another" (Link 2001, 382). This structural or institutionalized stigma includes broader, macro-social applications of labeling and judgment that can produce "negative outcomes outside the context of interpersonal interactions," as well as within them (Hatzenbuehler 2016, 743; Lynne-Landsman, Livingston, and Wagenaar 2013). When public or private institutions adopt practices that restrict opportunities and espouse ideologies that rationalize these restrictions (Corrigan 2004, 481; Hatzenbuehler 2016), stigma becomes embedded in the structure of society, enforcing and legitimizing the stigmatization of specific identities.

DOI: 10.4324/9780429320491-24

Throughout the 20th century, cannabis users have confronted both structural and interpersonal stigma. The rules around cannabis have been shaped by the policy and posturing of the federal government, which has characterized cannabis as a dangerous drug of abuse with no medical value. This has justified the curtailment of civil liberties and trivialized even medicinal use of cannabis as a sign of "abuse" or "addiction." Until recently, most medical practitioners and their professional associations have aligned with the government's position about medical cannabis use, emphasizing the paucity of evidence for its use as a medicine and its potential dangers. Agreement among legal and medical sectors of authority has helped reinforce and perpetuate the stigmatization of cannabis users. The stability of structural stigma around cannabis has allowed official characterizations of users to establish norms and influence what information is considered factual.

Despite institutional rhetoric, many see cannabis as relatively harmless. Its use has been widespread for 50 years, and claims about its dangers from prior eras are widely acknowledged as exaggerated (Hathaway, Comeau, and Erickson 2011; Asbridge et al. 2016). Starting in the mid-1990s, some researchers have asserted that cannabis use is accommodated with increasing cultural acceptance and no longer signifies membership in a "distinct deviant sub-group" (Hammersley, Jenkins, and Reid 2001; Parker 2005; Dahl and Heggen 2014; Hathaway, Comeau, and Erickson 2011). While nonconforming subcultures may still engage in cannabis use as a signal of mainstream subversion and "cool" rebellion, many cannabis users are in the mainstream, and cannabis use may be their only act of nonconformance (Hammersley, Jenkins, and Reid 2001, 132; Athey 2018). Nonetheless, cultural stereotypes about users persist and may include "hippie" associations and concerns with factors that affect competence, such as intelligence, motivation, and judgment.

State medical cannabis programs have been created in the context of increased normalization of cannabis use (Parker 2005; Hammersley 2005; Hathaway, Comeau, and Erickson 2011; Mostaghim and Hathaway 2013). When something that was previously considered nonmedical is incorporated into the medical domain, it is referred to as *medicalization* (Conrad 2007). Normalization and medicalization are both pathways that mitigate stigma, but with different implications. Normalization indicates greater acceptability and willingness to reduce formal restrictions, even as it shifts some responsibility to individuals, who must establish that doing so does not introduce or exacerbate social problems. Medicalization reorganizes management of the issue under a separate domain of social control (Conrad 2007). Historically, medicalization has been a part of normalization, destigmatizing other previously prohibited substances (Hathaway, Comeau, and Erickson 2011).

Overcoming Internalized Cannabis Stigma to Adopt Medical Use

The medical cannabis patient identity introduces new meanings and challenges to associations between cannabis use and identity at both the structural and the interpersonal level. Historically, cannabis use has been associated with youth, yet the fastest growing group of medical cannabis users is among middle age and older patients with chronic health problems (Bobitt et al. 2019; Lloyd and Striley 2018).

Many of the midlife patients in our study described having prior beliefs that reflected common stereotypes and stigma about cannabis and its users, only to have these ideas dispelled by experience. Others already believed official narratives about cannabis to be false, but even those with extensive prior experience with cannabis expressed skepticism of medical benefit prior to exploring it as a medical option. In order to adopt therapeutic use and claim a medical cannabis patient identity, they first had to overcome their own internalized stigma about cannabis. Wes, a diabetic for over 30 years, says:

> I grew up a very non-believer [in cannabis]. I believe in my government and things like that, that [cannabis] was all bad, bad, bad. So, I did more research and found out that it was actually

> beneficial to diabetics and neuropathy and all that. . . . I was seeing that [my wife] benefited from it, and I had already experienced some benefits from it, but . . . I was 42 or 43 years old, and so I had had 40 years of the government brainwashing me on how bad it is. So, I was still kind of, yeah, it probably helps, but there may be some bad stuff to it or whatever. A little apprehensive about it.

When patients revised their beliefs about the therapeutic potential of cannabis, many felt betrayed by what they had been told by various institutional actors who are often expected to serve as sources of authoritative information. A good example is Mark, a tech writer in his early 40s who developed severe neuropathy that resisted treatment. Mark shares:

> There's a certain stereotype that I grew up with. . . . [Cannabis is] the gateway drug or the source of all evil. You're going to be a worthless loser sitting on a sofa all day if you partake of it. It's going to introduce you to heroin and opium. The list goes on. . . . I'm just now getting mostly over the anger I felt for being fucking lied to my whole life about something that could be so [beneficial].

Mark achieved more than pain control with cannabis. A self-identified "problem drinker" who had been on antidepressants for over a decade, Mark reported that once he initiated medical cannabis use, he reduced his drinking "by 80 or 90%" and stopped using antidepressants. Mark's experience departed dramatically from his expectations, triggering a "conversion" in which his prior cultural belief was abruptly abandoned (Bicchieri 2017, 137). Experiencing relief directly or witnessing improvement by a close friend, spouse, or relative typically led to a rapid revision in viewpoint.

Legitimacy Strategies of Medical Cannabis Patients

Once patients adopted medical cannabis use, they faced potential stigma. Strategies for managing stigma varied. Patients often engaged in medical behaviors, adopting dosage, timing, and situational strategies consistent with the use of other medicines. Because medical cannabis use is a concealable behavior, some patients chose to conceal use to avoid being stigmatized. Others chose to disclose their use and claim the patient identity (Newhart and Dolphin 2019). These patients employed various coping strategies to manage stigma, which included resisting cannabis stigma or deflecting it when it was invoked. Individuals often utilized one primary strategy, but many combined multiple strategies based on the contingencies of the situation, as has been found in other studies of stigmatizing identities (Thoits 2011).

Deciding to Conceal or Disclose Medical Cannabis Use

Concealment is an identified coping strategy for those with stigmatized identities (Turan et al. 2019, 4). Revealing cannabis use includes risks, so patients weighed carefully their choice about disclosure (Jones et al. 1984; Lau et al. 2015). Identifying as a medical cannabis patient is not an either/or proposition: most individuals disclosed cannabis use selectively and chose not to disclose their use in at least some situations. A few patients in our study reported not identifying publicly out of a fear of specific reprisals. Gary, a resident in public housing, worried that public advocacy could lead to eviction, so he was discreet, only disclosing medicinal cannabis use anonymously online. Other patients reported similar concerns with risks related to child custody, employment, or federal benefits that prevented open identification.

Most patients not only disclose within close networks of family and friends, but they also relied on others when deciding whether to try medical cannabis, as they did with other healthcare matters.

Patients frequently recounted that trying cannabis was a "family decision" that included parents, adult children, significant others, or spouses. Of those who were married, only a few patients had spouses who were medical or recreational cannabis users. Patients overwhelmingly said they would not have decided to use cannabis had their spouse objected.

Many patients preferred being open about their medical cannabis status, but even those who identified openly still recounted instances that called for discretion, such as around children. Frank is a good example. A retired college professor who had openly used cannabis in his younger years, Frank had few reasons for hiding its part in his treatment regimen for stage-four colon cancer. Yet when asked if there were any situation in which he would hide his use, Frank says:

> I've got this decision to make here in about a week from Thursday because all of my kids are bringing in their kids, . . . and the kids are going to stay here. So, I've got four [grandkids]. I mean, the oldest is fifteen, and the youngest is one. . . . I don't think that they have enough information to make a logical decision. Is grandpa just crazy or what?

Others limited disclosure out of concern that family members would experience "courtesy stigma," the spillover of prejudice and discrimination as a result of association (Goffman 1986 [1963]). For instance, Jason, an upper-middle-class married dad with young kids, uses cannabis to treat gastroesophageal reflux disease (GERD). He has disclosed use to close friends and family but preferred to be discreet and avoided discussing it directly.

INT: In what situation would you feel uncomfortable if somebody outed you as a medical marijuana user?

Jason: At my kid's school. Or in front of my in-laws. But they all know. All of them know anyway, but it's not something that I feel comfortable talking to them about.

INT: Do you think it would change their impression of you in some way?

Jason: No, because they've known me since I was 16, or since I was in the fourth grade. So, they know me anyway. But my kid's friends' parents don't. And I don't want them to think, "Oh gee, I can't let my kid go over to their house because their dad is a stoner."

Because cannabis use is concealable, episodic, and usually done in private, revealing it provides an opportunity to frame one's use as medical but may also cue "stoner" stereotypes. The reception of one's claim to medical use is often uncertain and may remain so even after discussing it. Opting to not discuss it can be a way to limit opportunities for stigmatization.

Deciding to conceal or reveal medical cannabis use is also tied to the disclosure of a medical condition, another characteristic that can result in stigmatization. Medical conditions range widely in their cultural meaning. Some may not be seen as serious enough to support a claim to medicinal use of cannabis. Others may be serious enough to raise questions about the person's ongoing capability to perform various roles competently, a concern that may be compounded by similar stereotypes about compromised function from cannabis use. Patients may not wish to reveal intimate information about health conditions to others when it may result in embarrassment or change how they are treated.

The ability to defy stereotypes about medical cannabis use is influenced by other identity characteristics that determine their fit with stereotypes of "stoners." Those who diverge from the stereotype of a "typical" cannabis user and those with serious or visible medical conditions are less vulnerable to cannabis stigmatization and more likely to be seen as legitimate medical users. By contrast, legitimacy is more difficult to establish for those with medical conditions that are not visible or not considered "serious" enough to warrant an unconventional treatment. These include, for example, those with conditions that signal "deviant" lifestyle choices, those in poverty or from racial and ethnic groups historically stereotyped as associated with cannabis use, and those with a history of drug problems. These groups are caught in intersections of potentially discrediting attributes that may compound how stigma is experienced, influencing their willingness to disclose use.

Deflecting Stigma

Disclosing medical cannabis use may result in stigma, but as Thoits (2011) points out in her research on mental health stigma, many "labeled individuals resist stigma and stereotyping rather than accept or adapt to it" (6). One way that patients resist stigma is through deflection. This strategy has been reported across a range of stigmatizing identities (Thoits 2011; Hathaway 2011). Instead of confronting stigmatizing views, patients may sidestep them, using self-presentation, behaviors, and other identities to assert that the characterization does not fit them personally (Thoits 2011). Individuals may mitigate stigma by downplaying the identity to "differentiate themselves from the more conspicuous stigma bearing persons" (Thoits 2011). For example, Jason, a financial advisor, had used cannabis recreationally prior to becoming a medical user. Culturally, he distanced himself from other cannabis users, expressing annoyance at hippies and social-cause protestors. When asked directly about how his cannabis use shaped his outlook, he de-emphasized it as a marker of identity:

> I have never really considered marijuana to be that influential in anything really in my life, except for making me happy. Or not stressed. It's really more of a stress reliever than anything for me. I don't have an upset stomach when I use it; I don't have heartburn; I don't get pains in my side.

In summarizing what his status as a qualified patient means, Jason says, "The only thing it's really done is made me a little more comfortable and not feel like I'm just hiding anything. I just feel more comfortable now, that it's more accepted."

Other patients used speech, behavior, and social identifiers such as age, jobs, military service, and community affiliations to indicate their lack of fit with stereotypes. Some aspects of the cannabis identity may be embraced while attributes deemed discrediting are downplayed or rejected. Another illustration is Julie, a schoolteacher who uses cannabis for muscle spasm and chronic pain. She discusses her enjoyment of cannabis culture, which in part comes from defying expectations:

> I look very much forward to going to the 420 Rally, and I go to the Cannabis Cup every year, Kush-Con, any type of event—I am there. For one, I don't fit the typical profile of the stoner chick, so I enjoy attending those events. I've been up to the state house many times testifying up there, and I've heard people say it's real refreshing to know we have somebody highly educated that stands up for what she's doing.

Julie knows that the expectations for teachers include morally upright behavior and assumptions about intelligence but may also suggest being less culturally "cool." Julie mixes these two identities with different moral valences and attempts to claim the positive aspects of each, even as she reinforces stigmatizing judgments that she distances herself from. When non-stereotypical individuals identify as medical cannabis users, they reveal what has been hidden by structural stigma: cannabis users are threaded invisibly through everyone's family, workplace, and social networks. This revelation, and the communication about cannabis it elicits within one's network, can work powerfully to reduce stigma.

Resisting Stigma

Similar to other stigmatized groups, medical cannabis patients are acutely aware of the stereotypes they may face. Anticipating or experiencing a stigmatizing encounter can lead patients to learn more about the issue and connect with others who share the identity, discovering a diversity of patients who provide counterexamples to stereotypes. In an atmosphere of structural stigma, medical cannabis education travels laterally among networks of family, friends, and acquaintances, animated by compelling personal testimonials. We have argued elsewhere that this engenders the emergence of a "thought community" among patients where counternarratives form and are repeated (Newhart and Dolphin 2019). This loose affiliative transfer of knowledge provides an alternative source of authority and legitimacy for stigma revision and public action.

Patients often actively resist stigma by claiming superior knowledge. In interactions, they will dispute the accuracy of information that is used to justify stereotypes and stigmatization. Instead of experiencing stigma as discrediting or shameful, they reinterpret such interactions as ignorance on the part of the individual, a product of biased and outdated information passed down from institutional sources. Because many patients remember their own views prior to adopting medical cannabis use, which may have included similar assumptions, they often see such encounters as an opportunity to educate others, or at least dispute misrepresentations about cannabis and its users. Brett illustrates this:

Brett: "Stoner" is. . . . It can be a fun term, but it oftentimes is a more negative term meaning a person that doesn't get a lot done, not very bright, long hair, lot of smoking pot, instead of cannabis. And I completely refute that. I have friends of mine that are partners in law firms that medicate daily. I have a friend of mine that's a plastic surgeon. He's a world-renowned physician. He medicates on a daily basis, so. . . .

INT: I mean, what do you do when you're confronted? Do you feel you are ever directly confronted with those stereotypes?

Brett: Oh yeah, and I welcome it. I welcome it.

INT: How do you handle those situations?

Brett: You know, I try very much to gauge where the people are at. If they're completely not ready for the information and the wall is up, you know, I'm not going to frustrate them or myself. . . . The one thing I won't allow anybody to do is to put any kind of judgment on me or to try to give me information that's not accurate. . . . I have to correct the inaccuracy. But if they don't have the information and they don't want it . . . God bless you. That's "so be it."

Patients also resist structural stigma by invoking alternative markers of legitimacy, such as the state medical cannabis program or their doctor's advice. Jason provided a useful example when he reported that receiving his medical card not only left him feeling less guilty about his cannabis use, but also increased his perception of legitimacy around his condition (GERD):

> I felt like, after meeting the doctor, that it was legit, that I had a legitimate disorder. I do have a legitimate disorder that is covered under [Colorado's medical cannabis law], and I felt, I didn't feel like I was fooling anybody or trying to get around the system or anything like that because I have one of the [qualifying conditions].

Not all medical cannabis patients experience the same degree of stigmatization, so the differential effects of cultural and subcultural identities and affiliations are worthy of further investigation (Satterlund, Lee, and Moore 2015). For those whose social positioning otherwise insulates them from stigma, a stigmatizing interaction with an authority figure may be mobilizing in ways that increase their willingness to claim identity and group identification, yet even patients with multiple marginalized identities used similar strategies, referencing common counternarrative talking points about cannabis and representing them as superior knowledge.

Flipping the Script Through Attribution

To challenge structural stigma, patients may try to establish that associated stereotypes are not free-standing facts about the world but are claims with authors and promulgators. Assigning authorship to specific claims allows those who are vulnerable to stigma to contest an accepted cultural belief and assert that it is motivated and prejudicial. This can be successful to the degree that others accept the counterclaim as accurate.

Medical cannabis patients identify multiple institutional actors responsible for creating and maintaining structural stigma around cannabis use. Patients tend to focus on pharmaceutical companies, politicians, and law enforcement, although other industries that might face competition from legal cannabis, such as alcohol, paper, petroleum, and cotton, may also be included. These industries are typically described as motivated by profits. As Carl says:

> If they can't replicate it, they can't control the market. They can't have a patent on it. And that comes right down to money and money only. For pharmaceutical companies. I think pharmaceutical companies put more money into campaigns and more money in to fight it [cannabis legalization] just for the reason of money.

Many midlife patients come to medical cannabis as a last resort, after ample experience with pharmaceuticals that were ineffective or increasingly problematic. In retrospect, patients report these experiences as traumatic and detrimental to their health, functioning, and families. As Ron says:

> We don't have medicine to help people. We've got medicines to addict people on multiple medicines that continually get one more to take care of the last symptom that the last med gave you, and then you need one more, and one more.

Patients routinely reported reducing or eliminating prescription drugs once they added medical cannabis to their treatment regimen (Lucas and Walsh 2017; Reiman, Welty, and Solomon 2017; Piper et al. 2017), and this robust substitution effect is perceived as Big Pharma's motive to either oppose cannabis access or attempt to control and pharmaceuticalize it. As Brett says:

> You know, the pharmaceutical industry is set up so that there's a different pill for every ailment. That's profitable. One pill for nausea, another pill for inflammation, another pill for pain, another pill to handle the side effects of the other pills. Cannabis handles . . . a wide variety of them—nausea, inflammation, pain, migraines. . . . They don't want a multipurpose medicine.

Other organizational actors are often seen as complicit with pharmaceutical companies in the suppression of information about cannabis, either through ignorance or shared greed. As Ron says, "The doctors don't know, and pharmaceutical companies don't care, because it's just ka-ching, ka-ching, ka-ching, ka-ching. It's all about money." Similar to Ron, many patients saw their doctors as victims of structural stigma who are uneducated about medical cannabis, despite their substantial medical educations. Government officials and agencies, on the other hand, were portrayed as willing institutional partners in protecting pharmaceutical profits and their own positions. As Tina says:

> The government knows what is in these pills. They also know the good that medical marijuana, that marijuana does. They know it's medicine. They've known for years. . . . It infuriates

> me. . . . What's going on, really? To me, the whole reason I see behind it, I can't think of any other humane reason—and you can't put money on a human life—but that's what it is. It's about money.

Carl makes equally explicit connections between profits and policy maker motives:

> [Money is] getting all the politicians to fight it. That should be banned. All these contributions should be banned, totally, from unions, from pharmacies, because it's. . . . What do they call it when you can't try a case because you're involved with it or whatever? Conflict of interest. It's a total conflict of interest, everything they're doing, every law they're making, because they're either drawing their paycheck by doing this, or they want to draw their paycheck.

Whether the government, corporations, or specific stakeholders are identified as the author(s) or proponent(s), assigning them responsibility for circulating stigmatizing associations of cannabis use helps show that it is not a universal truth but instead a campaign of influence by "moral entrepreneurs" who possess the power to make labels stick and who benefit economically or in terms of social power when they are successful (Becker 1953). Systems are ascribed different motives than individuals, with making profit, reducing competition, and maintaining control being the most common. When system actors value institutional goals despite significant costs to people's health, freedom, and civil liberties, the motives can be framed as immoral and prejudicial, thereby calling into question the legitimacy of their authority.

Conclusion: Flipping the Script on Cannabis

Medical cannabis patients employ multiple strategies to manage stigmatizing interactions and structural stigma. Some conceal use, especially when disclosure could risk the loss of resources they need, such as subsidized housing or employment. Others disclose their medical cannabis use selectively, compartmentalizing the identity and adopting medicalized behaviors for cannabis consumption in ways that reinforce the moral evaluation of their use as appropriate. Patients also resist stigma and stereotypes through deflection or challenge. The broadest challenge may go beyond interpersonal management to redefining stigma as embedded into the fabric of institutions whose motives are illegitimate. When patients resist stigma and attest to the medical utility of cannabis, they contribute to the redefinition of cannabis as having benefits, not just harms. These claims counter structural stigma, but for social change to occur, others must agree. Public opinion polling indicates that agreement is building. Since state medical cannabis programs began, support for the legalization of all adult use has risen sharply from 31% to more than 60% (Hartig and Geiger 2018; McCarthy 2018; NORC 2018; Quinnipac 2019).

Many participants in our study extoll the potential of education to undermine prejudice and misinformation and transform norms and policy, and other studies find a similar emphasis on education among stigmatized groups (Lau et al. 2015; Newhart and Dolphin 2019; Bobitt et al. 2019). In an environment where the usual arbiters of legitimacy—government and medical institutions—are considered inaccurate, education resonates as a solution. However, other stigma researchers warn that education—in the sense of introducing more factual information—is often overrated and rarely reverses stigma (Corrigan 2018). This is because the moral evaluations on which stigma is based are usually unaffected by the introduction of facts (Corrigan 2018). Education that recategorizes the moral dimensions of a problem may be more effective. For many types of stigma, personal interactions are a meaningful part of reducing interpersonal stigma. As more people identify themselves as medical cannabis users and engage in interactions about it, they help to redefine the meanings and symbolism associated with use and revise ideas about who uses it, in what context, and for what purpose.

Medicalization coexists with recreational use as it undergoes greater normalization, influenced in part by the new calculus of risk and reward that medical use has introduced. The shifting identities around both medical and recreational cannabis use are made more complicated by the intermixing of formal identity, conferred by the state, and the reasons for use, which may or may not align. State medical cannabis programs qualify patients under specific criteria, which in most states include a defined list of symptoms or diagnoses. The patients in our study were all registered with a qualifying diagnosis, but many reported also using cannabis medicinally for additional conditions that were not formally recognized as qualifying.

Classifications of cannabis use as "medical" or "recreational" cannot be reduced to whether an individual has registered as a patient with a state program. The patients in our study saw the decision to try using cannabis therapeutically and registering with the state as distinct and separable. A 2016 survey asked over 1,000 users without a medical card who accessed two Colorado adult-use retail stores about their use, and found that 65% were using it for pain and 74% for sleep, with 88% reporting they were substituting cannabis for pharmaceutical medications (Bachhuber, Arnsten, and Wurm 2019). Others have also found that the line between recreational and medical use of cannabis blurs in practice (Bostwick 2012; Athey 2018). Patients in our study reported the distinction between therapeutic and putatively recreational use to be arbitrary at times, with several saying they timed cannabis dosing to enhance activities such as going to a movie or watching a sitcom. Institutional logics rely on bright-line distinctions that can be applied systematically, but in the lived experience of patients there may not be a clear way of demarcating differences between minimizing symptoms and side effects and enjoyment.

Some have suggested that adult-use access obviates the need for identifying medical use, but reducing all policies to general legalization overlooks the importance of cultural meaning and its effect in influencing behavioral models for use. Retaining medical use as a category affects individual decisions, allowing more stigma-sensitive patients a point of entry. Medical classification also has important institutional consequences, supporting the further research and development of innovative treatments.

Attitudes about cannabis and its uses are evolving, but changes in social norms do not necessarily change structures of power. Institutions possess powers that individuals do not. They can suppress contradictory positions, set rules that enforce a stigmatizing story, and ignore, delay, or disrupt attempts to present credible alternative narratives. Medicalization weakens that structural stigma. State laws that allow medical cannabis use create contradictions with federal law and scheduling classifications. Other cases of social change indicate that disrupted categories create confusion and contradictions that "provide opportunities to push for change" (Armstrong and Bernstein 2008). As norms change, those who defend structural stigma may come to appear to be acting illegitimately, eroding trust in those institutions.

In this chapter, we have discussed cannabis stigma as both interpersonal and structural. Medical cannabis stigma is always layered and modified by other identity characteristics, which include one's fit with stereotypical cannabis identities, one's vulnerability to marginalization due to other stigmatizing identities, and the characteristics of one's medical condition, which may or may not support claims to medical cannabis identity. Future research could contribute a clearer understanding of how these different sources of stigma affect individual coping strategies. Sensitivity to cannabis stigmatization is another area to explore, as is the role of communities in buffering stigma. In practical terms, it is worth considering how stigma affects choices to disclose in consequential settings, such as in medical treatment, where failing to disclose may affect health outcomes.

Cannabis is being reintegrated in society in a multilayered way, making the study of cannabis stigma both complex and rich for insights well beyond the medical realm. Additional study might explore the unintended consequences of the medicalization and normalization processes, such as how commodification and cultural diffusion pose threats to those who have claimed cannabis as a meaningful marker of identity, community, and subcultural opposition to mainstream values. Future research can build on existing studies to better understand how policy choices and attendant rhetorical framing modify, extend, or dismantle the historical narrative of harm and the stigma around cannabis.

Note

1 To recruit the widest range of patients across gender, medical condition, past cannabis use, and location, study recruitment took place at dispensaries and events throughout Colorado and through advertising in Colorado medical cannabis publications. This sample was 70% male and 30% female, mirroring gender representation among Colorado's program at the time. The sample was overwhelmingly white, with only 10% of participants identifying as multiracial/multiethnic. Interviews lasted one to three hours and were recorded, transcribed, and analyzed using NVivo 10 software. More details on methods, sample, and findings, can be found in *The Medicalization of Marijuana: Legitimacy, Stigma, and the Patient Experience* (Newhart and Dolphin 2019).

References

Armstrong, Elizabeth A., and Mary Bernstein. 2008. "Culture, Power, and Institutions: A Multi-Institutional Politics Approach to Social Movements." *Sociological Theory* 26 (1): 74–99. www.jstor.org/stable/20453096.

Asbridge, Mark, Jenna Valleriani, Judith Kwok, and Patricia G. Erickson. 2016. "Normalization and Denormalization in Different Legal Contexts: Comparing Cannabis and Tobacco." *Drugs: Education, Prevention & Policy* 23 (3): 212–23.

Athey, Nicholas. 2018. "A Profile of Medical Cannabis Users Residing in Canada and the United Kingdom: Accounting for Policy and Experience." PhD dissertation, School of Criminology, Simon Fraser University, Burnaby, British Columbia, Canada.

Bachhuber, Marcus, Julia H. Arnsten, and Gwen Wurm. 2019. "Use of Cannabis to Relieve Pain and Promote Sleep by Customers at an Adult Use Dispensary." *Journal of Psychoactive Drugs*. doi:10.1080/02791072.2019.1626953.

Becker, Howard S. 1953. "Becoming a Marihuana User." *American Journal of Sociology* 59 (3): 235–42.

Bicchieri, Cristina. 2017. *Norms in the Wild*. New York, NY: Oxford University Press.

Bobitt, J., S. H. Qualls, M. Schuchman, R. Wickersham, H. D. Lum, K. Arora, G. Milavetz, and B. Kaskie. 2019. "Qualitative Analysis of Cannabis Use among Older Adults in Colorado." *Drugs & Aging*. doi:10.1007/s40266-019-00665-w.

Bostwick, J. Michael. 2012. "Blurred Boundaries: The Therapeutics and Politics of Medical Marijuana." *Mayo Clinical Proceedings* 87 (2): 172–86. doi:10.1016/j.mayocp.2011.10.003.

Conrad, Peter. 2007. *The Medicalization of Society*. Baltimore, MD: The Johns Hopkins University Press.

Corrigan, P. W. 2018. *The Stigma Effect: Unintended Consequences of Mental Health Campaigns*. New York: Columbia University Press.

Corrigan, Patrick W., Fred E. Markowitz, and Amy C. Watson. 2004. "Structural Levels of Mental Illness Stigma and Discrimination." *Schizophrenia Bulletin* 30 (3): 481–91.

Dahl, Silje Louise, and Kåre Heggen. 2014. "Negotiating Identities." *Young* 22 (4): 381–98. doi:10.1177/1103308814548106.

Goffman, Erving. 1986 [1963]. *Stigma: Notes on the Management of Spoiled Identity*. First Touchstone Edition, 1986 ed. New York: Simon and Schuster, Inc.

Hammersley, Richard. 2005. "Theorizing Normal Drug Use." *Addiction Research & Theory* 13 (3): 201–3. doi:10.1080/16066350500053471.

Hammersley, Richard, Richard Jenkins, and Marie Reid. 2001. "Cannabis Use and Social Identity." *Addiction Research & Theory* 9 (2): 133–50.

Hartig, Hannah, and A. W. Geiger. 2018. "About Six-in-Ten Americans Support Marijuana Legalization." *Pew Research Center FactTank*. www.pewresearch.org/fact-tank/2018/10/08/americans-support-marijuana-legalization/.

Hathaway, Andrew D., Natalie C. Comeau, and Patricia G. Erickson. 2011. "Cannabis Normalization and Stigma: Contemporary Practices of Moral Regulation." *Criminology and Criminal Justice* 11 (5): 451–69. doi:10.1177/1748895811415345.

Hatzenbuehler, Mark L. 2016. "Structural Stigma: Research Evidence and Implications for Psychological Science." *American Psychologist* 71 (8).

Jones, Edward E., Amerigo Farina, Albert H. Hastorf, Hazel Rose Markus, Dale T. Miller, and Robert A. Scott. 1984. *Social Stigma: The Psychology of Marked Relationships*. Hillsdale, NJ: Lawrence Erlbaum Associates.

Lau, Nicholas, Paloma Sales, Sheigla Averill, Fiona Murphy, Sye-Ok Sato, and Sheigla Murphy. 2015. "Responsible and Controlled Use: Older Cannabis Users and Harm Reduction." *International Journal of Drug Policy* 26 (8): 709–18. doi:10.1016/j.drugpo.2015.03.008.

Link, Bruce G. 2017. "Commentary On: Sexual and Gender Minority Health Disparities as a Social Issue: How Stigma and Intergroup Relations Can Explain and Reduce Health Disparities." *Journal of Social Issues* 73 (3): 658–66. doi:10.1111/josi.12236.

Link, Bruce G., and Jo C. Phelan. 2001. "Conceptualizing Stigma." *Annual Review of Sociology* 27 (1): 363–85. doi:10.1146/annurev.soc.27.1.363.

Lloyd, Shawnta L., and Catherine W. Striley. 2018. "Marijuana Use among Adults 50 Years or Older in the 21st Century." *Gerontology & Geriatric Medicine* 4. doi:10.1177/2333721418781668.

Lucas, Philippe, and Zach Walsh. 2017. "Medical Cannabis Access, Use, and Substitution for Prescription Opioids and Other Substances: A Survey of Authorized Medical Cannabis Patients." *International Journal of Drug Policy* 42: 30–35. doi:10.1016/j.drugpo.2017.01.011.

Lynne-Landsman, Sarah D., Melvin D. Livingston, and Alexander C. Wagenaar. 2013. "Effects of State Medical Marijuana Laws on Adolescent Marijuana Use." *American Journal of Public Health* 103 (8): 1500–6. https://doi.org/10.2105/AJPH.2012.301117. http://dx.doi.org/10.2105/AJPH.2012.301117.

McCarthy, Justin. 2018. "Two in Three Americans Now Support Legalizing Marijuana." *Gallup Poll Social Series*.

Mostaghim, A., and A. D. Hathaway. 2013. "Identity Formation, Marijuana and 'the Self': A Study of Cannabis Normalization among University Students." *Frontiers in Psychiatry* 4: 160. doi:10.3389/fpsyt.2013.00160.

Newhart, Michelle, and William Dolphin. 2019. *The Medicalization of Marijuana: Legitimacy, Stigma, and the Patient Experience*. New York, NY; Abingdon, OX: Routledge.

NORC. 2018. "Support for Marijuana Legalization Continues to Rise." *General Social Survey (GSS)*.

Parker, Howard. 2005. "Normalization as a Barometer: Recreational Drug Use and the Consumption of Leisure by Younger Britons." *Addiction Research & Theory* 13 (3): 205–15. doi:10.1080/16066350500053703.

Piper, Brian J., Rebecca M. DeKeuster, Monica L. Beals, Catherine M. Cobb, Corey A. Burchman, Leah Perkinson, Shayne T. Lynn, Stephanie D. Nichols, and Alexander T. Abess. 2017. "Substitution of Medical Cannabis for Pharmaceutical Agents for Pain, Anxiety, and Sleep." *Journal of Psychopharmacology* 31 (5): 569–75. doi:10.1177/0269881117699616.

Quinnipac University. 2019. "U.S. Voters Oppose Trump Emergency Powers on Wall 2–1 Quinnipiac University National Poll Finds; 86% Back Democrats' Bill on Gun Background Checks." https://poll.qu.edu/national/release-detail?ReleaseID=2604.

Reiman, A., M. Welty, and P. Solomon. 2017. "Cannabis as a Substitute for Opioid-Based Pain Medication: Patient Self-Report." *Cannabis Cannabinoid Res* 2 (1): 160–66. doi:10.1089/can.2017.0012.

Satterlund, Travis D., Juliet P. Lee, and Roland S. Moore. 2015. "Stigma among California's Medical Marijuana Patients." *Journal of Psychoactive Drugs* 47 (1): 10–17. doi:10.1080/02791072.2014.991858.

Thoits, Peggy A. 2011. "Resisting the Stigma of Mental Illness." *Social Psychology Quarterly* 74 (1): 6–28. doi:10.1177/0190272511398019.

Turan, Janet M., Melissa A. Elafros, Carmen H. Logie, Swagata Banik, Bulent Turan, Kaylee B. Crockett, Bernice Pescosolido, and Sarah M. Murray. 2019. "Challenges and Opportunities in Examining and Addressing Intersectional Stigma and Health." *BMC Medicine* 17 (1): 7. doi:10.1186/s12916-018-1246-9.

25

Pleasure and the New Normal of Recreational Cannabis in the United States

Ingrid Walker

Keywords: Drugs and pleasure, cannabis legalization, cannabis normalization, cannabis use and pleasure, non-problematic cannabis use

Introduction

Cultural silence about drug pleasures in the United States, an important consequence of both drug prohibition and medicalization, tacitly complies with the dominant social narrative that "drugs are harmful." While the majority of people who use drugs do not use them problematically or with negative consequences, the misconception that drug use is fundamentally harmful influences health care and policy, as well as how users themselves disclose even legal drug use (Walker 2017). Critical drug studies, an interdisciplinary field that examines the social factors and systems that influence drugs and their users, has increasingly focused on pleasure as intrinsic to drug use.[1] Many scholars in this field argue that intoxication and other drug pleasures are a benefit and end point in themselves to be recognized without being problematized.[2] Research that explores the varied pleasures and negative consequences of normalized cannabis use made possible in legalized contexts holds out the potential for different understanding of and discourses about drug use, particularly non-problematic drug use. This chapter poses questions about the implications of the normalization of regulated recreational cannabis use for critical drug research. Specifically, how has the issue of pleasure—a driving force in cannabis use—been subsumed into a cultural process of normalization of cannabis? And, as a result, how might critical drug studies need to reframe and theorize drug pleasures?

Regulated Cannabis

At least five years into the reality of recreational cannabis in Washington and Colorado in the United States, there is still a distinct disorientation to the experience of engaging in a legal commercial activity that previously took place in criminalized subcultures. For those of us in the United States able to purchase recreational cannabis legally as part of other routine errands, it can be surreal. The dazzling array of products and the sheer volume of business resonate as the abundant choice of U.S.

DOI: 10.4324/9780429320491-25

capitalism, from the scores of smokable "flowers," vape cartridges, or dabs to edible or topical cannabis in drinks, candy, baked goods, salves, oils, and tinctures. The convergence of cannabis commodification and the freedom to pursue one's high in a regulated context has brought those of us who benefit from a legal recreational market into a strange but welcome new world. In this sense, the integration of regulated cannabis into everyday life can be a uniquely normalizing drug experience.

To be clear, this cultural "normalization" is partial at best. The politics of legalized recreational cannabis sustain many of the social inequities and injustices prioritized and amplified by prohibition—issues that continue to need to be addressed even in states that have reformed cannabis policies (Alexander 2012). While arrest rates for cannabis possession among both black and white adults decreased significantly post-legalization in Washington, the relative racial disparities in arrest rates doubled (from 2.5 times to 5 times higher for black Americans than whites) (Firth et al. 2019). States that have legalized marijuana have been slow to legislate and implement expungement and vacation policies for hundreds of thousands of misdemeanor convictions for marijuana possession. Even as the drug war continues to be waged disproportionately on people of color and poor people, the landscape of the legal weed industry is predominantly white and middle to upper class (McVey 2017). Critics of the new legal recreational market have pushed for policy reform to directly address the racialized legal and socioeconomic fallout of the drug war, calling out early states' failure to bring communities most harmed by criminalization into the privileged environment of legalized cannabis (Wang and Mays 2019; Rouse 2019). Thus, even as an emergent legal cannabis market has become integrated and legitimized for some Americans, the broader culture has yet to cross that barrier.

In this environment of sociopolitical disparity, the rapid assimilation of legal cannabis into U.S. capitalist culture represents familiar dynamics that both reflect and respond to drug war politics. On the one hand, recreational cannabis legalization signifies a distinct desire for normalized, regulated drugged pleasures. On the other, it reflects some of the worst injustices and restrictions of a neoliberal marketplace that casts citizens as consumers (Gershon et al. 2011; Foucault 1975). Legalization's focus on rationality and self-discipline align tightly with an ideology of choice and social freedom. Yet, despite the intoxicating pleasures of cannabis use, the freedom to consume cannabis has become—in the legal, recreational environment—an act of self-governance (Reith 2004). The creative act of cannabis consumption is contained by the self-regulating consumer. In this sense, the pleasures of legal cannabis are more implicit than explicit, even in a market that produces endless products for precisely this purpose. Policy, then, is just one factor in untangling the consequences of U.S. drug prohibition. As cannabis legalization evolves, it is important for drug research to consider what cannabis "normalization" means in U.S. culture, particularly its implications for drug users. U.S. policy reform and research have elided a focus on a full spectrum of drug use, especially the legitimacy of drugged intoxications.[3] As cannabis becomes normalized, drug research has a role in establishing alternative ways of thinking about drug use, better understanding the complex motivating factors and outcomes of cannabis use—from self-regulating use practices to the experiential, embodied aspects of drugged pleasures.

Cannabis Normalization

Borrowing the concept from disability studies, drug scholars have employed "normalization" to examine how users and nonusers progress from perceptions of drug use as an abnormal, outsider activity to its acceptance as normative behavior (Parker 2005; Parker, Williams, and Aldridge 2002; Duff 2005; Measham, Aldridge, and Parker 2001; South 1998; Shiner and Newburn 1997). More broadly, normalization describes a process by which the cultural meaning of recreational drug use transitions from deviant to commonplace as part of the cultural landscape. Measures of normalization include drug access and availability, rates of drug experimentation and use, attitudes about self-regulating use, and the degree of accommodation of illegal drug use by nonusers (Measham, Aldridge, and Parker 2001; Parker, Williams, and Aldridge 2002). While early studies focused more on youth practices and perceptions of drug use, self-regulated drug use, and cultural change, the normalization thesis extends to adult drug use practices (South 1998). In the case of legalized cannabis, normalization describes the social perception of cannabis use as unremarkable for adults over the age of 21. Further, normalization includes a recognition that, in a continuum of drug use, most people have a healthy, that is, non-problematic, relationship with illegal drugs—whether used as a medical therapy and/or as a recreational pleasure (Walker 2017).

Even as normalization displaces pejorative cultural associations of cannabis use, it overlays experiences of pleasure and intoxication with expectations of self-discipline. David Moore argues that, in this process, the discourse of normalization poses a threat to our categorical understanding of drug use (Moore 2008). Recreational cannabis regulation has sidestepped the expansiveness and aim of its intoxicating pleasures by framing drug use as a process of *self*-regulation. Normalization depathologizes a now-legal drug practice: cannabis use shifts from a deviant activity to one associated with a rational consumer. Expectations of the "rational" subject are framed by risk management and self-restraint. These discourses of freedom, scholars argue, are employed to contain discourses of pleasure, producing self-regulating, governable citizens (Duff 2015; Bancroft 2013; Moore 2008; Rose, O'Malley, and Valverde 2006; O'Malley and Valverde 2004; Reith 2004). In fact, users of illegal drugs sometimes deliberately employ the terms of neoliberal discourse to convey controlled and functional consumption, to avoid stigmatization by signaling the possibility of a use practice that is distinct from addiction (Askew and Salinas 2018). Normalization's disciplinary effects are also expressed in the way that state control requires industry to enact strict regulations that cover cannabis from production to in-store merchandise, advertising restrictions, packaging and labeling rules, quality assurance, and even budtender training (Jensen and Roussell 2016). Discourses of control extend beyond industry and user self-regulation to new voices, such as an etiquette book by the great-great-granddaughter of Emily Post that advises readers on dispensary behavior and appropriate conversation topics with a cannabis delivery person (Post 2019).

The framework of drug normalization is complicated by the multitude of ways in which people access and use cannabis. In practice, the conceptual and regulatory domains of the "recreational" and "medicinal" uses for cannabis have been far more complex than our attempt to separate them suggests (Kiepek and Beagan 2018). Determining the factors that motivate cannabis use is challenging, especially as each state has policies that may or may not discern the rationales for cannabis use (Roffman 2016; Schnuer et al. 2014). For example, in a detailed study comparing recreational and medicinal use, the RAND Western States Survey of Colorado, Washington, Oregon, and New Mexico contrasted states with legal recreational cannabis with their neighbors, finding that 76% of medicinal users who have doctor's recommendations for medical use also used recreationally (Pacula, Jacobson, and Maksabedian 2016). In other words, people who use cannabis consume it for a variety of reasons—motives that may change day to day or even hour to hour. Categories like "recreational/medicinal" or "pain/pleasure" have more to do with ideological distinctions and policy efforts than the use-value of cannabis (Walker 2017; Parker, Aldridge, and Measham 1998; Hammersley, Jenkins, and Reid 2001). Drug use practices are embedded in other life practices and require a more nuanced approach as part of broader, complex lived experiences (Hammersley 2005). The normalization of a formerly criminalized and medicalized psychoactive substance has the potential effect of homogenizing what might be better understood as distinctive aspects and even a complex spectrum in the vast practices of cannabis use. With little research on non-problematic drug use, the legalization and subsequent normalization of cannabis provide an opportunity for drug research to explore a continuum of drug use practices and to better understand the diversity and complexity of embodied drug experiences within the context of other experiences and life contexts (Askew 2016; Schnuer 2013).

Pleasure in Critical Drug Research

Critical drug research has widely shown how prohibition and public health practices have tried to constrain "the messiness of pleasurable human embodiment" (Coveney and Bunton 2003, 3). Some scholars argue that drug use should be studied as a practice that can evoke both pleasures and pain, benefits and harms, with positive and negative outcomes (Taylor 2016; Hammersley 2011; Race 2009). Others challenge the ontology of public health's rational actor in understanding intoxicating pleasures (Duncan et al. 2017; Duff 2004, 2008; Keane 2008; Moore 2008; O'Malley and Valverde 2004; Schnuer 2013). Explorations of the antithetical relationship between addiction and pleasure find that people with substance use disorder articulate intricate pleasures about their drug use (Maclean 2005; Duncan et al. 2017; Dennis and Farrugia 2017). A growing body of scholarship focuses on what Duncan et al. have identified as "the embodied, performative, situated, and affective dimension of drug use and the positive relations that pleasure produces" (Duncan et al. 2017, 3). Scholarship on drug pleasures has come to conceive of pleasure as emergent, contingent on a range of contextual elements, and performative practices that assemble in a particular drug experience (Dilkes-Frayne and Duff 2017; Race 2009). Critical drug studies continues to develop a multivalent set of concepts for thinking about drugs, users, and drug pleasures (Thompson and Coveney 2018). Drug consumption can be understood as a creative, symbolic force that plays a key role in shaping identity as a fluid construct (Reith 2004).

In the last decade, two special issues of the *International Journal of Drug Policy* (*IDJP*) focused explicitly on drug pleasures, opening wide a conversation about pleasure and theorizing social and material coproduction of drug experiences (Holt and Treloar 2008; Dennis and Farrugia 2017a). In the 2017 issue, Race proposed that the indeterminacy of pleasure may function as a radical intervention in research knowledge-making if we consider drug use as experiments taken with an end in mind, with the deployment of particular sources of information, and with particular effects. An instance of drug use is exploratory (much like research) in that its end is unfixed; a user is making choices based on previous experiences and information and often engages others in the sharing/experience of outcomes. Malins described the dynamics and complex set of factors engaged in any instance of drug use, taking issue with "pleasure" as a finite category for drugged experiences:

> Humans (and other animals) take a range of drugs for a range of different reasons . . . to experiment with what the body can do, or to make the body function better or differently. They are used to slow down or speed up time, or to engage with new modes of thinking and perceiving. They are used to connect differently with one's environment, to find new ways of relating to friends or lovers, to get in the right zone to write poetry or music, or to feel the body become one with the music, lights and a dancing crowd. They are used to generate novel forms of sociality, to dismantle the limits of autonomy, identity, and the individual self, to find a liminal zone where the self and its boundaries dissolve. They are used to pose a challenge to fascism and its control over our bodies, our thoughts, and our modes of desiring. These are things that unsettle us, that provoke or transform us, may indeed bring pleasure, but to confine their affect to an emotion of pleasure—or similarly to an experience of pain-relief—would be to limit them, and our understanding of them.[4]

This catalog of the potential diversity and dynamism of drug desires suggests that the kind of user "experiments" Kane sees people engaging in are far more complex than drug research has thus far expressed. I cite Malins's description in full because rarely in academic work do researchers attempt to capture the complex phenomenology of drug use as what Cameron Duff has called a "practice of the self" (Duff 2008, 386–87). This frontier of drug research is far more accessible to researchers with the legalization of recreational cannabis, if we take care not to default to reductionism in the pursuit of understanding how and why people use cannabis.

Studying Regulated Cannabis Pleasures

What do we want to understand about drug pleasures, particularly cannabis pleasures, and how might the normalization of cannabis use facilitate the exploration of those questions? Conversely, how does the factor of cannabis normalization reframe drug use, and what might be obscured or lost in this new framing? What can we learn from people who use drugs about the many uses they make of cannabis? What would an ethics of "making pleasure matter" in drug research look like (see Dennis and Farrugia 2017)? While these questions are less typical of U.S. drug research, cannabis normalization may help scholars turn to the project of explicitly researching drug pleasures in this emergent context.

Centering research design on the participatory influence of people with lived experience will raise epistemological questions about what we think we know and what we might learn about drug use (Walker and Netherland 2019; Lancaster, Ritter, and Diprose 2018). As people who use drugs co-create research design, Helen Keane writes, the role of empirical description will hang in tension with theoretical methods (Keane 2017). Beyond interviews and other informative social science methods, narratives and the artistic exploration of user experience by users themselves offer a critical aperture to ontologies of desire and/or pleasure. For example, ethnographic work and first-person narratives of poly-drug use, including regulated cannabis, will likely reframe drug pleasures in revealing ways. While the participant-observer role is a difficult one, such subjective knowledge or familiarity is at least implicit in studies of other kinds of embodied experiences. The issue of having firsthand experience of drug pleasures and a closeness to one's research may present challenges (Race and Brown 2016). It could also open up new ways of discussing drug pleasures: using one's experience with cannabis as a position from which to make critical claims could lead to different expressions of drug pleasure and knowledge translation.

Cannabis normalization raises questions about the study of drugged pleasures that are less normalized. For example, how might it either sustain or destabilize differential normalization: where functional drug use is accepted, but excessive or dysfunctional drug use is rejected (Shildrick 2002)? In a protracted overdose crisis in which injection drug use has become even more stigmatized, the normalization of cannabis demonstrates differentiated values regarding kinds of use, drugs used, and those using them. The scholarship of drug pleasures has spoken to that divide and may bridge rather than reinforce a distinction between what are seen to be different user populations (Duncan et al. 2017; MacLean 2005). While normalized cannabis use may lead to a scholarly focus on pleasure with the most accessible users, there is a likelihood of missing poly-drug use as a part of a larger continuum of experiences. Or, the implications of normalization for "recreational" cannabis users may reinforce the sorting of users into groups and the stigmatization of other drug use. Among the many outcomes of prohibition's enforced silencing of people who use drugs is that they are interpellated in a variety of ways, including as being unified in identity and experience. Dennis and Farrugia speak to this ethos of care in scholarship, specifically "how to make drug consumers matter" (Dennis and Farrugia 2017, 87). Recognizing many kinds of drugged pleasures, because of and despite cannabis normalization, will be important to the study of poly-drug use pleasures.

Further, the normalization and commodification of cannabis may render it a different kind of pleasure altogether—especially for new users as well as all who benefit from a legalized market. In this context, the meaning of pleasure and drug use shifts to emphasize something closer to "well-being" rather than pathology or criminal behavior. The normalization of cannabis use may eventually codify it in our cultural understanding as simply another available intoxicant, as alcohol has been codified. In such contexts, the drug practices of the self that are engaged in and inextricably bound up with related practices (music, sex, spirituality, exercise, experiencing the natural world) become less reduced to a "drug experience" and more one feature of a broader life. Further, in the aftermath of legalization, we may be unwittingly giving a "pass" to critical issues of how commodified markets themselves frame cannabis use. If consumers are not entirely passive actors in a market, how they engage in co-production of meaning in their choices and cannabis use practices is relevant (Race 2009). For example, cannabis legalization potentially evokes the ideological concerns of its users and its subcultures, from racial and socioeconomic equity to the impact of cultivation on workers and the environment.

While reductionist discourses of self-control can be a type of cultural constraint, people who use drugs—especially cannabis—do manage their experiences. The Global Drug Survey published a "Net Pleasure Index" in 2014 in which people who use drugs answered questions that demonstrated the net of the cost/benefit analysis they perform in making choices to use particular drugs. After discounting the downsides, cannabis had almost a 50% net pleasure rating (Winstock 2014). In other words, people who use cannabis found it to offer the most pleasure for the least cost (lower than only MDMA and LSD, and nearly consistent with mushrooms). It is likely that this factor in cannabis use and experience, the least costs combined with more pleasures, will shift thinking in the U.S. about drug harms and pleasures. In this sense, the normalization of cannabis will inform not just health research but also understanding motivations for a wider spectrum of cannabis (and other drug) pleasures.

One counterintuitive function of cannabis normalization is that it may facilitate its erasure as a noteworthy practice, either obscuring cannabis use altogether or rendering it less perceptible than when it was criminalized. As socially situated, co-constructed embodied experiences, drug pleasures find a range of expression. The role of critical drug studies in the study of normalized cannabis use may be to push beyond binary discourses of medical therapeutics, self-regulation, or dangerous intoxication. The new accessibility to cannabis users opens exploration of many topics that remain relatively unstudied in the U.S., especially drug pleasures (Walker and Netherland 2019). How do the majority of cannabis users experience non-problematic drug use? What is the role of cannabis in contexts of polysubstance pleasures? How will the incorporation of expertise from people who use cannabis in research design, data collection, and analysis help scholars differently understand pleasures in their multiplicity? And what is it we want to learn, ultimately, about drug pleasures?

Notes

1 Critical drug studies, an interdisciplinary field that examines drugs and the people who use them, includes perspectives from cultural studies, sociology, anthropology, philosophy, criminal justice, critical race studies, women's studies, psychology, public health, and addiction studies.

2 For critical drug scholarship on drugs and pleasure, see Moore 2008, as well as Duncan et al. 2017; Thompson and Coveney 2018; Walker 2017; Askew 2016; Bunton and Coveney 2011; Holt and Treloar 2008; Moore 2008; O'Malley and Valverde 2004; Coveney and Bunton 2003.

3 See, for example, the research in note 1.

4 Malins 2017, 130. Malins pointedly argues that in describing the dynamics of drug use, the concept of Deleuzian "desire" is a more comprehensive dynamic to reference than pleasure.

References

Alexander, Michelle. 2012. *The New Jim Crow: Mass Incarceration in the Age of Colorblindness*. New York: New Press.

Askew, Rebecca. 2016. "Functional Fun: Legitimising Adult Recreational Drug Use." *International Journal of Drug Policy* 36: 112–19.

Askew, R., and M. Salinas. 2018. "Status, Stigma and Stereotype: How Drug Takers and Drug Suppliers Avoid Negative Labelling by Virtue of Their 'Conventional' and 'Law-Abiding' Lives." *Criminology & Criminal Justice* 19 (3): 311–327.

Bancroft, Angus. 2013. *Nudge Policy, Embodiment and Intoxication Problems*. Basingstoke: Palgrave Macmillan.

Bunton, Robin, and John Coveney. 2011. "Drugs' Pleasures." *Critical Public Health* 21 (1): 9–23.

Coveney, J., and R. Bunton. 2003. "In Pursuit of the Study of Pleasure: Implications for Health Research and Practice." *Health* 7 (2): 161–79.

Dennis, Fay, and Adrian Farrugia, eds. 2017a. "Drugged Pleasures." Special issue, *International Journal of Drug Policy*, 49.

Dennis, Fay, and Adrian Farrugia. 2017b. "Materialising Drugged Pleasures: Practice, Politics, Care." *International Journal of Drug Policy* 49: 86–91.

Dilkes-Frayne, Ella, and Cameron Duff. 2017. "Tendencies and Trajectories: The Production of Subjectivity in an Event of Drug Consumption." *Environment and Planning D: Society and Space* 35 (5): 951–67.

Duff, C. 2004. "Drug Use as a 'Practice of the Self'": Is There Any Place for an 'Ethics of Moderation'in Contemporary Drug Policy?" *International Journal of Drug Policy* 15 (5–6): 385–93.

———. 2005. "Party Drugs and Party People: Examining the 'Normalization' of Recreational Drug Use in Melbourne, Australia." *International Journal of Drug Policy* 16 (3): 161–70.

———. 2008. "The Pleasure in Context." *International Journal of Drug Policy* 19 (5): 384–92.

———. 2015. "Governing Drug Use Otherwise: For an Ethics of Care." *Journal of Sociology* 51 (1): 81–96.

Duncan, Tristan, Cameron Duff, Bernadette Sebar, and Jessica Lee. 2017. " 'Enjoying the Kick': Locating Pleasure within the Drug Consumption Room." *International Journal of Drug Policy* 49: 92–101.

Firth, C., J. Maher, J. Dilley, A. Darnell, and N. Lovrich. 2019. "Did Marijuana Legalization in Washington State Reduce Racial Disparities in Adult Marijuana Arrests?" *Substance Use & Misuse*: 1–6.

Foucault, M. 1975. *Discipline and Punish*. A. Sheridan, Tr., Paris, France: Gallimard.

Gershon, I., A. J. Cohen, K. Ho, T. Sanders, K. Sykes, S. Wright, and I. Gershon. 2011. "Neoliberal Agency." *Current Anthropology* 52 (4): 537–55.

Hammersley, R. 2005. "Theorizing Normal Drug Use." *Addiction Research & Theory* 13 (3): 201–3.

———. 2011. "Developing a Sociology of Normal Substance Use." *International Journal of Drug Policy* 22 (6): 413–14.

Hammersley, R., R. Jenkins, and M. Reid. 2001. "Cannabis Use and Social Identity." *Addiction Research & Theory* 9 (2): 133–50.

Holt, Martin, and Carla Treloar, eds. 2008. "Pleasure and Drugs." Special Issue,. *International Journal of Drug Policy* 5 (19): 349–52.

Jensen, E., and A. Roussell. 2016. "Field Observations of the Developing Legal Recreational Cannabis Economy in Washington State." *International Journal of Drug Policy* 33: 96–101.

Keane, Helen. 2008. "Pleasure and Discipline in the Uses of Ritalin." *International Journal of Drug Policy* 19 (5): 401–9.

Keane, Helen. 2017. "Female Vulnerability and Susceptible Brains: Gendered Discourses of Addiction." *The Social History of Alcohol and Drugs* 31 (1): 126–39.

Kiepek, N., and B. Beagan. 2018. "Substance Use and Professional Identity." *Contemporary Drug Problems* 45 (1): 47–66.

Lancaster, K., A. Ritter, and R. Diprose. 2018. "Recasting Participation in Drug Policy." *Contemporary Drug Problems* 45 (4): 351–65.

MacLean, S. 2005. " 'It Might Be a Scummy-Arsed Drug But it's a Sick Buzz': Chroming and Pleasure." *Contemporary Drug Problems* 32 (2): 295–318.

Malins, Peta. 2017. "Desiring Assemblages: A Case for Desire Over Pleasure in Critical Drug Studies." *International Journal of Drug Policy* 49: 126–32.

McVey, E. 2017. "Percentage of Cannabis Business Owners and Founders By Race." *Marijuana Business Daily*, September 11. https://mjbizdaily.com/chart-19-cannabis-businesses-owned-founded-racial-minorities/.

Measham, F. C., J. Aldridge, and H. Parker. (2001). *Dancing on Drugs: Risk, Health and Hedonism in the British Club Scene*. London: Free Association Books.

Moore, David. 2008. "Erasing Pleasure from Public Discourse on Illicit Drugs: On the Creation and Reproduction of an Absence." *International Journal of Drug Policy* 19 (5): 353–58.

O'Malley, Pat, and Mariana Valverde. 2004. "Pleasure, Freedom and Drugs: The Uses of 'Pleasure' in Liberal Governance of Drug and Alcohol Consumption." *Sociology* 38 (1): 25–42.

Pacula, R. Liccardo, M. Jacobson, and E. Maksabedian. 2016. "In the Weeds: A Baseline View of Cannabis Use Among Legalizing States and Their Neighbours." *Addiction* 111 (6): 973–80.

Parker, Howard. 2005. "Normalization as a Barometer: Recreational Drug Use and the Consumption of Leisure by Younger Britons." *Addiction Research & Theory* 13 (3): 205–15.

Parker, H., J. Aldridge, and F. Measham. 1998. *Illegal Leisure: The Normalization of Adolescent Recreational Drug Use*. London: Psychology Press.

Parker, H., L. Williams, and J. Aldridge. 2002. "The Normalization of 'Sensible' Recreational Drug Use: Further Evidence from the North West England Longitudinal Study." *Sociology* 36 (4): 941–64.

Post, L. 2019. *Higher Etiquette: A Guide to the World of Cannabis, From Dispensaries to Dinner Parties*. Berkeley, CA: Ten Speed Press.

Race, Kane. 2009. *Pleasure Consuming Medicine: The Queer Politics of Drugs*. Durham, NC: Duke University Press.

Race, Kane, and Rebecca Brown. 2016. "Cultural Studies Perspectives [on Drugs and Alcohol]." *The Sage Handbook of Drug and Alcohol Studies* 1.

Race, Kane. 2017. "Thinking with Pleasure: Experimenting with Drugs and Drug Research." *International Journal of Drug Policy* 49: 144–49.

Reith, Gerda. 2004. "Consumption and its Discontents: Addiction, Identity and the Problems of Freedom." *The British Journal of Sociology* 55 (2): 283–300.

Roffman, Roger. 2016. "Legalization of Cannabis in Washington State: How is it Going?" *Addiction* 111 (7): 1139–40.

Rose, Nikolas, Pat O'Malley, and Mariana Valverde. 2006. "Governmentality." *Annual Review of Law and Social Science* 2: 83–104.

Rouse, K. 2019. "Racial Justice Drives Fight for, and Against, Legal Pot in New Jersey." *New York Times*, March 11. www.nytimes.com/2018/03/11/nyregion/nj-legal-marijuana-racial-justice.html?module=inline.

Schnuer, G. 2013. "Pleasure and Excess: Using Georges Bataille to Locate an Absent Pleasure of Consumption." *Addiction Research & Theory* 21 (3): 258–268.

Schnuer, Gillian L., Brian A. King, Rebecca E. Bunnell, Gabbi Promoff, and Timothy A. McAfee. 2016. "Toking, Vaping, and Eating for Health or Fun: Marijuana Use Patterns in Adults, US, 2014." *American Journal of Preventive Medicine* 50 (1): 1–8.

Shildrick, Tracy. 2002. "Young People, Illicit Drug Use and the Question of Normalization." *Journal of Youth Studies* 5 (1): 35–48.

Shiner, Michael, and Tim Newburn. 1997. "Definitely, Maybe Not? The Normalisation of Recreational Drug Use Amongst Young People." *Sociology* 31 (3): 511–29.

South, N., ed. 1998. *Drugs: Cultures, Controls and Everyday Life*. Newbury Park, CA: Sage.

Taylor, Stuart. 2016. "Moving beyond the Other: A Critique of the Reductionist Drugs Discourse." *Cultuur and Criminaliteit* 6 (1): 100–18.

Thompson, Lee, and John Coveney. 2018. "Human Vulnerabilities, Transgression and Pleasure." *Critical Public Health* 28 (1): 118–28.

Walker, I. 2017. *High: Drugs, Desire, and a Nation of Users*. Seattle, WA: University of Washington Press.

Walker, I., and J. Netherland. 2019. "Developing a Transformative Drug Policy Research Agenda in the United States." *Contemporary Drug Problems* 46 (1): 3–21.

Wang, V., and J. Mays. 2019. "Black Lawmakers to Block Legalized Marijuana in N.Y. If Their Communities Don't Benefit." *New York Times*, March 11. www.nytimes.com/2019/03/11/nyregion/marijuana-legalization-african-americans.html.

Winstock, A. 2014. "The Global Drug Survey 2014. Findings." *Global Drug Survey*. Accessed September 5, 2019. www.globaldrugsurvey.com/past-findings/the-global-drug-survey-2014-findings/.

26

Changing the Face of the Stoner

Images of Race and Gender in Cannabis Legalization Campaigns in the United States

Katie Kaufman Rogers

Keywords: Race, gender, cannabis legalization, discourse analysis

Introduction

Cannabis legalization was an unpopular idea in the United States for most of the last century. Over the last two decades, support for legalization skyrocketed, favored by a majority for the first time in 2013 and by two-thirds of those polled in 2018 (Jones 2019). At the time of this chapter's publication, 91 percent of U.S. adults say cannabis should be legal in some form (Van Green 2021), and congressional Democrats are considering legislation that would nationally decriminalize the plant. Rising public favorability toward cannabis, alongside a wave of state legalizations, fuels the popular narrative that weed[1] is being destigmatized, allowing consumers to "come out of the closet" (e.g., Margolin 2018; Rittenhouse 2018; Weiss 2015).

Movements to affect drug policy aim to reconfigure prevailing ideas about drugs and drug users, which are racialized and gendered (Alexander 2010; Campbell 2000; Lassiter 2015; Roberts 1997, 2016). Cannabis is no exception. Since the early 1900s, U.S. news, media, political discourse, and popular culture have drawn on racist, sexist imagery to construct cannabis use as a socially stigmatized practice (Alexander 2010; Chasin 2016; Chapkis and Webb 2008; Dufton 2017; Himmelstein 1983). Images of dealers and users of color, particularly black and Latino men (Alexander 2010), were used to justify prohibition and criminalization by portraying cannabis as a threat to white women, white children, and the white patriarchal order (ibid. 2010; Chasin 2016). Discourse on "stoners," a stigmatic identity marker ascribed to cannabis users (see also "potheads" [Chapkis and Webb 2008, 86; Himmselstein 1983]), constructs them as drains on society, defined by joblessness and amotivation (ibid. 2008, 1983), a "schlubby" physical appearance (Clark-Flory 2010), and a white masculinized immaturity (e.g., the Seth Rogen "man-child" [*Rolling Stone* 2014; White 2019]). Stigmatic constructions of cannabis users vary over time (Himmelstein 1983) and continue to evolve (e.g., Newhart and Dolphin Chapter 24, this volume). Recent shifts in attitudes and policy on cannabis raise a new question: How are race and gender deployed in cannabis legalization campaigns?

In this chapter, I investigate how race and gender are depicted in campaigns to legalize cannabis, through a qualitative content analysis of the Yes on 19 and Yes on 64 campaigns for adult-use

DOI: 10.4324/9780429320491-26

cannabis legalization in California. Drawing on a systematic analysis of campaign materials, articles, and news reports, I use discourse analysis to uncover racialized and gendered subtexts of these legalization campaigns. My analysis focuses on how these campaigns highlighted stories, images, and voices that *change the face of "the stoner"* by framing white women and children as sympathetic beneficiaries, rather than victims, of cannabis use. I argue that depictions of class-privileged white women enjoying cannabis for its recreational and medicinal properties served to launder and legitimize the image of the industry by severing connections to the stoner as a stigmatic identity. These findings raise questions about the perils and possibilities of pursuing "normalization" as a means to shape opinions and policy on cannabis, particularly when grounded in capitalist ideologies that are themselves racist, sexist, and heteronormative. This study underscores the importance of foregrounding an analysis of race and gender in mapping the changing political economy of cannabis, post-prohibition and beyond.

Race, Gender, and Cannabis Policy Debates in the United States

Race and gender shape prevailing ideas about which groups deserve sympathy and protection from the state. Who is labeled a victim and who is labeled a perpetrator are patterned to construct hegemonic archetypes of "ideal criminals," assumed to be guilty, and "ideal victims," assumed to be innocent (Carlson 2014; Dirks, Heldman, and Zack 2015; Eastman 2015; Heitzeg 2015; Hollander 2001; Madriz 1997; Snedker 2012). Such has been the case in the context of cannabis, where activists have lobbied to change laws by constructing sympathetic figures as victims of the current policy regime (Chapkis and Webb 2008; Chasin 2016; Dufton 2017; Herzberg 2020; Lassiter 2015). Campaigns for decriminalization, legalization, and prohibition sought to persuade the public that policy change was needed to protect these groups (ibid. 2008, 2015, 2016, 2020). Nationwide drug scares (Reinarman and Levin 1989; Reinarman 2015), drug problems (Jensen and Gerber 1998), and drug debates (Dingelstad et al. 1996; Rosino and Hughey 2017) vilify consumers and distributors through racialized and gendered controlling images (Collins 2005, 2009) such as the image of "the thug" (Dow 2016), "the felon" (Alexander 2010), and "the crack mom" (Roberts 1997 [2016]). These images are used to justify harsher punishments and increased surveillance for communities of color, particularly black and Latinx communities (Alexander 2010; Serrano 2013; Steinmetz, Schaefer, and Henderson 2016).

Meanwhile, white women and children are frequently characterized as "victims" of drug policy (Daniels, Netherland. and Lyons 2018; Lassiter 2015; Netherland and Hansen 2016, 2017). Propaganda such as the film *Reefer Madness* (Gasnier 1936) and cultural touchstones like TV's *Weeds* (2005–2012) represented cannabis spaces as violent, hyper-masculine, and sexually dangerous for white women, specifically (Chasin 2016; Serrano 2013). These campaigns played on colonial anxieties that see men of color as threatening the "innocent" and "pure" sexualities of white women, who are viewed as white men's property (Chasin 2016; Davis 1981; McClintock 1995). Likewise, white children were rendered as victims of cannabis policy. Anti-cannabis "parent movements" of the late 1970s and early 1980s opposed cannabis on the grounds that it endangered (white) children, laying groundwork for the punitive backlash of the Reagan era (Dufton 2017). These movements were spearheaded by white, middle-class women, many of them liberal Democrats, who argued that decriminalizing pot was reckless and harmful to their kids (ibid. 2017).

As such, interlocutors in cannabis policy debates have deployed images of race and gender to further their agendas. However, we know less about how the "face" of cannabis consumption is constructed in the present context of *post-prohibition*, a sociopolitical landscape in which individual state legalizations emerge against the backdrop of federal prohibition (as well as state prohibitions). As I will show, considering how these images are racialized and gendered is vital to understanding the trajectory of cannabis policy in the United States.

Methods

This chapter presents findings from a qualitative content analysis of race and gender in cannabis news reports, op-eds, and legalization campaign materials. I focused on materials circulating in the years surrounding two campaigns for legalization in California: Proposition 19, which failed to legalize in 2010, and Proposition 64, which legalized cannabis for adult use in 2016. At the time of both campaigns, Californians were already enjoying medicinal-use cannabis, legalized by Proposition 215 in 1996. This chapter's analysis is not meant to compare the efficacy of these campaigns or identify a "tipping point" for the passage of adult-use legalization. Rather, my goal is to uncover racialized and gendered subtexts of discourses proffered by both campaigns, forming a piece of a broader picture of cannabis legalization in the United States.

Data come from two sources. First, I conducted a systematic analysis of online campaign content published by the National Organization for the Reform of Marijuana Laws (NORML), including both national NORML and the NORML Women's Alliance (NWA). I focus on NORML because it is the largest and most well-resourced cannabis lobbying group in the country (Dufton 2017). I accessed campaign materials no longer online (e.g., earlier iterations of the NORML homepage, the website for the Yes on 64 campaign, etc.) via The Wayback Machine (https://archive.org/web/), a digital archive of information on the internet that saves web pages over time. I accessed pages archived between January 2008 and December 2016 (beginning with the year immediately preceding Prop. 19 and ending with 2016, when Prop 64 was passed). Second, I assembled a sample of news reports on cannabis using Google Alerts, a tool that monitors the internet for mentions of a given topic (or set of topics), then alerts the user via email. I configured Google Alerts to notify me via email whenever it identified a news report about cannabis. Over the course of roughly three and a half years (February 2016–September 2019), I reviewed 643 emails as they were received, containing a total of 4,501 links (most emails contained multiple links). For the years preceding the 2016–2019 range, I purposively sampled news reports, op-eds, and features by entering codes manually via Google search.

I focus my analysis on pro-legalization discourses across two domains: (a) *the family* and (b) *the market*. I chose these domains because they are commonly invoked in anti-drug campaigns, which claim drug use prevents women and people of color from fulfilling their socially prescribed roles in these realms (Campbell 2000; Chapkis 2013; McCorkel 2013). Such campaigns mobilize racist, sexist controlling images (Collins 2005, 2009) associated with each of these domains to marshal support for their agendas. These images—including the neglectful "bad mother," the hypersexual "crack whore," and the jobless "welfare queen"—are used to manage, shame, and punish drug-using women, particularly black women, by painting them as unfit to mother their children and as relying on welfare and sex work to fund their drug use (Collins 2005, 2009; McCorkel 2013; Roberts 1997, 2016). Regulation of drug-using women thus reflects broader racialized norms of womanhood, reproducing a system in which women's access to rights and resources hinges on "fulfill[ing] their responsibilities as contingent workers, consumers, and caretakers" (Campbell 2000, 4).

Domains of the family and the market are not mutually exclusive but inextricably intertwined, overlapping, intersecting, and co-constitutive (Nakano Glenn 1992). However, by analyzing them as discrete categories, I investigate how, within each of these domains, cannabis legalization campaigns *change the face of the stoner* by discursively distancing cannabis from stigmatized characteristics and stereotypes associated with cannabis users.

Marijuana Moms: Normalizing Cannabis vis-à-vis the Family

Mothers featured prominently in California legalization campaigns, as cannabis consumers and advocates for children. These mothers were overwhelmingly white, middle class, and married to men. I find two patterns in these representations of motherhood. First, mothers delivered the argument that *prohibition*, not legalization, endangers children and threatens the institution of the family. Second, mothers who use cannabis themselves insisted that it does not hinder their performance in the domestic sphere, and in some cases, enhances it.

Cannabis legalization campaigns mobilized mothers to deliver the message that legalization protects and benefits children. In the months preceding the vote on Prop. 19, the newly formed NORML Women's Alliance called on mothers to take up the activist mantle. It was one of the first acts of the NWA, a self-described "nonpartisan coalition of prominent, educated, successful, and geographically diverse[2] professional women" who oppose prohibition. According to an NWA statement, mothers understand that prohibition is "child-endangering" policy that "undermines the American family" and fuels a trend of "children selling marijuana en mass [sic]." Mothers also backed legalization on behalf of kids with chronic illnesses like epilepsy and fibromyalgia, who rely on medicinal cannabis for treatment. Over the course of 2009–10, NORML national and the NWA featured a number of mothers advocating legalization on these grounds. These included Jessica Corry, a married, pro-life Republican who spoke at NORML's San Francisco conference "wearing an American flag lapel pin, a triple strand of pearls and a gold marijuana leaf pin" (Parker 2009). Such tactics promoted legalization by drawing on conservative gender ideologies defining women's role as primary caretakers.

Mothers who use cannabis themselves were also featured in legalization campaigns. Through quotes, first-person narratives, and op-eds, these women defended their ability to function as domestic caretakers while high. The NWA built on these, claiming cannabis makes mothers *better* parents to their children, encouraging qualities like "patience, empathy, understanding, and playfulness." One mother, writing anonymously in *Jezebel* (2012), said cannabis enabled her to giggle her way through the "totally vacant, rule-less games" she plays with her baby. "Anybody who thinks that weed makes parents ignore their children has clearly never been high around one," she wrote. "I've never had a glass of wine and been captivated by children's books like I have after smoking a bowl." Mothers also argued that weed is harmless relative to drugs like alcohol, which many parents vocally and legally enjoy. "Being judged for doing something nontoxic and totally organic, enjoying a god-given plant, by moms who suck back two bottles of Chardonnay like sports drinks feels like shit," complained one pot-smoking mom to a reporter for *The Today Show* (Binns 2012).

Mothers also argued that weed helps them enjoy the tedious duties of domestic life and mitigates familial conflict. In a blog post, the NWA christened cannabis "mother's new little helper," borrowing a moniker popularized by the Rolling Stones' song "Mother's Little Helper" (Jagger and Richards 1966), about the rise in anti-anxiety drugs prescribed to housewives. ("Mother's Helper" is also the name of a popular cannabis strain, now sold legally in dispensaries.) "[Smoking weed] can make folding a pile of laundry fun," one mother told *Today* (2012). Others say cannabis takes the edge off their "bitchiness" and frustration in the household. "That is *exactly* the kind of shit that would've irrationally pissed me off if I hadn't smoked," said another, describing a potential conflict with her husband. "Instead, I just laughed." Another mother puts it simply to *Marie Claire* (Kohen 2009): "I got kind of uptight [during my weed hiatus], and my husband was like, 'Actually, I liked you better when you smoked.'"

The "marijuana moms" in these stories were overwhelmingly depicted as white, middle class, cisgender, normatively feminine, and married to men. Non-white, poor, single, and/or queer, trans, and gender-expansive parents who proudly use cannabis were rarely represented, and when they were, they were almost never celebrated. One exception is a *Blavity* profile of Shonitria Anthony, a journalist and black mother of two. "I decided to start Googling 'stoner moms' [and] 'moms who smoke weed' just to see what it would bring up," Anthony told *Blavity*. "But all the women I found were white, so I was just very confused." Now, Anthony hosts a podcast called *Blunt Blowin' Momma*, which combats controlling images associated with cannabis and black motherhood. "The narrative is always black women having too many abortions, or black women having too many kids," she explained. "When you see these white moms [in the media] who are consuming cannabis—I don't see anyone attacking them."

These representations of mothers demonstrated that cannabis does not necessarily jeopardize (and can even improve) women's ability to fulfil their role as caretakers and housekeepers in the white heteropatriarchal family. By showing how cannabis can help women be more nurturing parents, they distanced pot-using mothers from the racialized stereotype of the neglectful "bad mom" who uses drugs. However, it remains an open question whether discourses that normalize cannabis consumption for rich, married, straight white mothers can help change the stigma faced by mothers who do not check these boxes. Further, in suggesting that cannabis can *increase* women's capacity for reproductive labor, these images constructed legalization as compatible with the racial gendered division of labor that structures the U.S. economy at large.

Stiletto Stoners: Normalizing Cannabis vis-à-vis the Market

Traditional stoner stereotypes construe cannabis users as shiftless slacker dudes who contribute little to society (Chapkis and Webb 2008; Himmelstein 1983). Legalization campaigns, by contrast, highlighted cannabis-using women and depicted them as productive agents in the U.S. economy, both as high-functioning professionals and consumers of commodities. Through their relation to the market, these women stoners were represented as embodying dominant norms of white, class-privileged femininity, such as maintaining a thin body, wearing designer clothing, and incorporating products into a daily beauty regimen.

Legalization campaigns depicted women cannabis users as productive members of society by highlighting their participation in the paid-labor market. One year before Californians voted on Prop. 19, *Marie Claire* published an article called "Stiletto Stoners" (Kohen 2009). It profiled "smart, successful" women with "killer careers and enviable social lives" who smoke weed to decompress after work. According to the article, these women are "career animals" (e.g., corporate lawyers, publicists, TV producers, and insurance agents) who unwind with joints instead of Chardonnay or prescription drugs. The piece also described stiletto stoners as "slim and athletic," looking "nothing like the blotto hippie teens of *Dazed and Confused* or the unemployed, out-of-shape schlubsters who are a staple of the Judd Apatow canon."

The story caught fire. Stiletto stoners were featured in *The New York Times*, *The Huffington Post*, *Salon*, *Elle*, *The NY Daily News*, *Jezebel*, and more. Matt Lauer described stiletto stoners on *The Today Show* as "educated, career-minded women who regularly smoke marijuana," and *Marie Claire*'s editor-in-chief appeared to reassure Lauer, "We're talking about highly functioning women. These are not people who are lying on park benches." The message was clear: Cannabis legalization is compatible with capitalism *and* hegemonic norms of femininity.

This coverage caught the attention of national NORML and the NWA, which began promoting stiletto stoner articles on their websites and incorporating the imagery into their own messaging. In 2010, the NWA issued a press release announcing a partnership with *Pot Couture* ("the first online magazine for sophisticated lady stoners"). Together, they launched an "aesthetic" campaign to support California's Prop. 19. The goal was to "give Mary Jane a makeover"—to "reframe the perception of the marijuana legalization movement, and the stereotype of those involved" by spotlighting "professional" women who use cannabis. Central to this campaign was a "high-style" photoshoot featuring seven light-skinned, femme-presenting women posing in stilettos and elegant dresses—all of them "activists and professionals who support Proposition 19."

These legalization campaigns also portrayed women cannabis users as productive consumers. While NORML's "High Society" campaign did not immediately succeed in achieving legalization (Prop. 19 failed in 2010), the revelation that middle-class white women smoke weed left its mark on the industry. By the time Prop. 64 appeared on the 2016 ballot, such women were appearing everywhere. Abbi and Ilana stashed pot in their vaginas on TV's *Broad City* ("nature's pocket!"), and high-end dispensaries stocked an array of cannabis-infused products marketed to women—skincare, cosmetics, menstrual-pain-relief oils, bubble baths, lubricants, aphrodisiac teas, low-dose edibles, tinctures, and beyond. This commercial landscape does not attach a negative connotation to cannabis use. Instead, these firms work to redefine cannabis as the basis for wellness, beauty, and productivity. In these narratives, smoking pot is not only "normal," it is a new way to express upper-class white femininity through the consumption of commodities. Products containing cannabidiol (CBD)—said to alleviate chronic pain, anxiety, insomnia, and inflammation—were rapidly incorporated into the beauty and wellness industries. In this consumer-capitalist context, the activist commitment to "self-care" (Lorde 1988; Nelson 2013) is co-opted to sell CBD products, marketing them as rejuvenating to workers laboring under capitalism. These marketing tactics also help portray cannabis businesses as legitimate, upscale operations that sell high-end products to white-collar consumers.

These narratives also work to make cannabis compatible with an embodiment of white femininity that can be expressed through consumption of commodities. This commodified version of white femininity encourages women to make purchasing decisions that bring their bodies closer into alignment with racist, sexist standards of beauty. Kohen's (2009) "Stiletto Stoners" article, for instance, revels in physical descriptions that detail its subjects' slim physiques, designer office wear, and lavish symbols of heterosexuality (e.g., a "3-carat cushion-cut engagement ring"). By framing weed as a commodity whose use expresses a high-class femininity, these discourses frame wealthy, thin, heterosexual white women as a sympathetic face of cannabis consumption. They construct women as "deserving" (Chapkis and Webb 2008) cannabis consumers on the condition that they participate in the market economy and appear desirable by white heteronormative standards.

Images of stiletto stoners demonstrate that legalization aligns with existing norms of the regulated economy. These images reject the stereotype of the state-dependent "pothead" (Chapkis and Webb 2008; Himmelstein 1983) by redefining women cannabis users as upper-class professionals who maintain independence in the formal labor market. Additionally, by framing pot as something that can harness the buying power of wealthy white women, the stiletto stoner narrative constructs weed as a commodity that can be incorporated into existing markets targeting these consumers.

Conclusion

Public support for U.S. cannabis legalization has trended steeply upward since 2000, with 91 percent of U.S. adults now favoring medical and/or recreational legalization (Van Green 2021). This trend, alongside a spate of state legalizations, feeds the popular claim that cannabis use is being normalized, enabling stoners of all identities to "come out of the closet." However, by identifying racial and gendered subtexts of legalization campaigns, my findings raise questions about the limitations and potentialities of "normalization" as a mechanism of achieving a just, egalitarian cannabis policy.

Pro-legalization campaigns and news reports utilize race and gender to "normalize," "de-stigmatize," and "mainstream" cannabis consumption by *changing the face of the stoner*. These discourses work to center white women and children as sympathetic beneficiaries, rather than victims, of the cannabis legalization movement. By defining white, class-privileged mothers and women professionals as the new face of cannabis use, these images and narratives affirm that legalization will not threaten the white patriarchal institutions of the family or the market economy, enabling women to continue fulfilling their socially prescribed roles in these domains. They construe cannabis consumption as a practice that is not only acceptable for class-privileged white women but can also improve their performance as mothers, wives, workers, and consumers.

The tone and point of view relayed in these stories encourage readers to view white mothers who smoke weed not as criminals or social deviants but as relatable, responsible individuals whose drug use has negligible or even positive effects on their domestic relationships. These representations solicit sympathetic feelings towards these mothers, who say their cannabis use is harmless, yet unfairly exposes them to reputational and legal risks that other drug-using mothers (e.g., wine drinkers) do not face. However, this framing elides the protections afforded to white "marijuana moms" by virtue of their racial categorization, class status, and rootedness in the hetero-patriarchal family. Mothers who are queer, of color, or poor or working class are dramatically more likely to be targeted by the state for their parenting practices. For black mothers, especially, accusations of neglectful parenting tied to drug use result in lifelong, structural consequences, including criminal charges, forced or coerced sterilization, and loss of their children to child protective services (Roberts 1997, 2016).

Further, the message that rich, white, straight-sized, married, and/or normatively feminine women deserve to smoke pot because they fulfil societal demands of women upholds a regime that shames and punishes women who do not adhere to these dictums. Because these weed normalization discourses are grounded in capitalist ideologies, they do less to dismantle racist, sexist stereotypes associated with cannabis use than they do to enable a small, elite group to reconfigure their own cannabis use as "normal," through a process of reifying and distancing themselves from traditional pot stereotypes. Broadly, these discourses demonstrate legalization's value-add to white patriarchal institutions like the family and the formal economy. In this way, bourgeois white femininity works as a mechanism for laundering the image of the cannabis industry, promoting legalization as a boon to the labor market and consumer capitalism.

These findings highlight the need for analyses on cannabis' changing culture, social landscape, and political economy that foreground the intersection of race and gender. Future research should address at least two areas of inquiry: First, studies must investigate the experiences of cannabis consumers across race, class, gender, and sexuality, in various states and regulatory contexts. How do cannabis consumers experience stigma in a post-prohibition era, where cannabis remains criminalized at the federal level and racial disparities persist in cannabis-related arrests (ACLU 2013, 2020)? To what extent can discourses that normalize cannabis use for wealthy, white, straight, married, and so on consumers benefit consumers who are *not* structurally privileged along these lines? Second, future research must address the implications of these cannabis normalization discourses for workers, professionals, and entrepreneurs in the U.S. cannabis industry, particularly as it moves into state-regulated economies. Regulated weed markets in the United States are predominantly, visibly white (McVey 2017, 2019), and men occupy the lion's share of leadership positions in the space (ibid. 2017, 2019). Research is needed that not only identifies barriers to entry for people of color (especially women of color) seeking to participate in cannabis business but that also documents their experiences as workers, entrepreneurs, and executives in a white-male-dominated industry.

Notes

1 Language used to discuss cannabis is politicized and contested. Some activists, journalists, and licensed cannabis businesses are moving away from terms like "weed" and "pot" as a way of distancing the plant from stereotypes and controlling images (Collins 2005, 2009) used to justify prohibition and criminalization (e.g., Bethea 2019; Holson 2019; Lissner 2018; Schmich 2019). In this chapter, I use the terms *weed* and *pot* interchangeably with *cannabis*, because they still enjoy wide usage among consumers, in popular discourse, and in the content analyzed for this study. Further, as this chapter seeks to explore, these discursive shifts may themselves constitute a form of whitewashing, obscuring the drug war's racial injustices as a white- and male-dominated cannabis industry flourishes in the regulated economy.

2 There is no publicly available information on the racial makeup of the NWA. As of 2015, the NWA's website (https://normlwomensalliance.org/) indicated its board of directors included three women of color and a white man.

References

ACLU (American Civil Liberties Union). 2013. *The War on Marijuana in Black and White*. New York: ACLU.

———. 2020. *A Tale of Two Countries: Racially Targeted Arrests in the Era of Marijuana Reform*. New York: ACLU.

Alexander, Michelle. 2010. *The New Jim Crow: Mass Incarceration in the Age of Colorblindness*. New York: The New Press.

Anonymous. 2012. "I'm a Mom and I'm Stoned Right Now." *Jezebel*, June 26.

Bethea, Charles. 2019. "Don't Call it 'Weed,' and Other Tips from the Cannabis Media Summit." *The New Yorker*, January 14.

Binns, Corey. 2012. "Pot-Smoking Moms Are Tired of Being Judged by Wine Drinkers." *Today*, July 16.

Campbell, Nancy. 2000. *Using Women: Gender, Drug Policy, and Social Justice*. New York: Routledge.

Carlson, Jennifer. 2014. "The Equalizer? Crime, Vulnerability, and Gender in Pro-Gun Discourse." *Feminist Criminology* 9 (1): 59–83.

Chapkis, Wendy. 2013. "The Trouble with Mary Jane's Gender." *Humboldt Journal of Social Relations* 35: 71–88.

Chapkis, Wendy, and Richard J. Webb. 2008. *Dying to Get High: Marijuana as Medicine*. New York: New York University Press.

Chasin, Alexandra. 2016. *Assassin of Youth: A Kaleidoscopic History of Harry J. Anslinger's War on Drugs*. Chicago, IL: University of Chicago Press.

Clark-Flory, Tracy. 2010. "Meet the 'Stiletto Stoners,'." *Salon*, October 21.

Collins, Patricia Hill. 2005. *Black Sexual Politics: African Americans, Gender, and the New Racism*. New York: Routledge.

———. 2009. *Black Feminist Thought: Knowledge, Consciousness, and the Politics of Empowerment*. 2nd ed. New York: Routledge.

Daniels, Jessie, Julie C. Netherland, and Alyssa Patricia Lyons. 2018. "White Women, U.S. Popular Culture, and Narratives of Addiction." *Contemporary Drug Problems* 45 (3): 329–46.

Davis, Angela Y. 1981. *Women, Race, and Class*. New York: Random House.

Dingelstad, David, Richard Gosden, Brian Martin, and Nickolas Vakas. 1996. "The Social Construction of Drug Debates." *Social Science Medicine* 43 (12): 1829–38.

Dirks, Danielle, Caroline Heldman, and Emma Zack. 2015. "'She's White and She's Hot, So She Can't Be Guilty': Female Criminality, Penal Spectatorship, and White Protectionism." *Contemporary Justice Review* 18 (2): 160–77.

Dow, Dawn Marie. 2016. "The Deadline Challenges of Raising African American Boys: Navigating the Controlling Image of the 'Thug'." *Gender & Society* 30 (2): 161–88.

Dufton, Emily. 2017. *Grass Roots: The Rise and Fall and Rise of Marijuana in America*. New York: Basic Books.

Eastman, Jason T. 2015. "The Wild (White) Ones: Comparing Frames of White and Black Deviance." *Contemporary Justice Review* 18 (2): 231–47.

Gasnier, Louis J. (Director). 1936. *Reefer Madness* [Film]. G&H Productions.

Heitzeg, Nancy A. 2015. "'Whiteness,' Criminality, and the Double Standards of Deviance/Social Control." *Contemporary Justice Review* 18 (2): 197–214.

Herzberg, David. 2020. *White Market Drugs: Big Pharma and the Hidden History of Addiction in America*. Chicago, IL: The University of Chicago Press.

Himmelstein, Jerome L. 1983. "From Killer Weed to Drop-Out Drug: The Changing Ideology of Marihuana." *Contemporary Crises* 7: 13–38.

Hollander, Joceyln A. 2001. "Vulnerability and Dangerousness: The Construction of Gender through Conversation about Violence." *Gender & Society* 15 (1): 83–109.

Holson, Laura M. 2019. "Common Name for Cannabis is Making an Industry Wince." *The New York Times*, July 8, B4.

Jagger, Mick, and Keith Richards. 1966. "Mother's Little Helper." [Song]. On *Aftermath* [Album]. Decca Records.

Jensen, Eric L., and Jurg Gerber. 1998. "Social Construction of Drug Problems: An Historical Overview." In *New War on Drugs: Symbolic Politics & Criminal Justice Policy*, edited by E. L. Jensen, and J. Gerber, 1–23. Highland Heights, KY: Academy of Criminal Justice Sciences.

Jones, Jeffrey M. 2019. "U.S. Support for Legal Marijuana Steady in Past Year." *Gallup*, October 23.

Kohen, Yael. 2009. "Stiletto Stoners." *Marie Claire*, October 1.

Lassiter, Matthew D. 2015. "Impossible Criminals: The Suburban Imperatives of America's War on Drugs." *The Journal of American History* 102 (1): 126–40.

Lissner, Caren. 2018. "As Marijuana Goes Mainstream, Reporters Wrestle with Terminology." *Columbia Journalism Review*, September 26.

Lorde, Audre. 1988. *A Burst of Light: And Other Essays*. Ithaca, NY: Firebrand Books.

Madriz, Esther I. 1997. "Images of Criminals and Victims: A Study on Women's Fear and Social Control." *Gender & Society* 11 (3): 342–56.

Margolin, Madison. 2018. "The Future of Cannabis is Female, and These Groups Aim to Ease the Way." *LA Weekly*, February 26.

McClintock, Anne. 1995. *Imperial Leather: Race, Gender and Sexuality*. New York: Routledge.

McCorkel, Jill A. 2013. *Breaking Women: Gender, Race, and the New Politics of Imprisonment*. New York: New York University Press.

McVey, Eli. 2017. "Chart: Percentage of Cannabis Business Owners and Founders by Race." *Marijuana Business Daily*, September 11.

———. 2019. "Women & Minorities in the Cannabis Industry." *Marijuana Business Daily*.

Nakano Glenn, Evelyn. 1992. "From Servitude to Service Work: Historical Continuities in the Racial Division of Paid Reproductive Labor." *Signs* 18 (1): 1–43.

Nelson, Alondra. 2013. *Body and Soul: The Black Panther Party and the Fight Against Medial Discrimination*. Minneapolis, MN: University of Minnesota Press.

Netherland, Julie, and Helena B. Hansen. 2016. "The War on Drugs That Wasn't: Wasted Whiteness, 'Dirty Doctors,' and Race in Media Coverage of Prescription Opioid Misuse." *Culture, Medicine and Psychiatry* 40 (4): 664–86.

———. 2017. "White Opioids: Pharmaceutical Race and the War on Drugs That Wasn't." *Biosocieties* 12 (2): 217–38.

Parker, Kathleen. 2009. "Today's Marijuana Lobby is More Hockey Mom Than Hippie." *Washington Post*, October 21.

Reinarman, Craig. 2015. "The Social Construction of Drug Scares." In *Constructions of Deviance: Social Power, Context, and Interaction*, edited by Patricia A. Adler and Peter Adler. 8th ed., 155–65. Boston, MA: Cengage Learning.

Reinarman, Craig, and Harry Gene Levin. 1989. "Crack in Context: Politics and Media in the Making of a Drug Scare." *Contemporary Drug Problems* 16: 535–77.

Rittenhouse, Lindsay. 2018. "Marketers Are Putting a New Face on Weed as They Navigate Regulations and Battle Stoner Stigma." *Adweek*, September 30.

Roberts, Dorothy. 1997 (2016). *Killing the Black Body: Race, Reproduction, and the Meaning of Liberty*. New York: Vintage Books.

Rolling Stone. 2014. "Seth Rogen's Stoner Empire: Inside *Rolling Stone's* New Issue." *Rolling Stone*, December 3.

Rosino, Michael L., and Matthew W. Hughey. 2017. "Speaking through Silence: Racial Discourse and Identity Construction in Mass-Mediated Debates on the 'War on Drugs'." *Social Currents* 4 (3): 246–64.

Schmich, Mary. 2019. "Marijuana? Cannabis? Weed? Pot? Dope? What Do You Call That Stuff?" *Winona Daily News*, July 11.

Serrano, Alfonso. 2013. "Weed All About It: The Origins of the Word 'Marijuana'." *Al Jazeera America*, December 14.

Snedker, Karen A. 2012. "Explaining the Gender Gap in Fear of Crime: Assessments of Risk and Vulnerability Among New York City Residents." *Feminist Criminology* 7 (2): 75–111.

Steinmetz, Kevin F., Brian P. Schaefer, and Howard Henderson. 2016. "Wicked Overseers: American Policing and Colonialism." *Sociology of Race and Ethnicity* 3 (1): 68–81.

Van Green, Ted. 2021. "Americans Overwhelmingly Say Marijuana Should Be Legal for Rereational or Medical Use." *Pew Research Center*, April 16.

Weiss, Jeff. 2015. "The Making of the Modern Stoner." *Vulture*, June 29.

White, Adam. 2019. "How Seth Rogen Went from Schlubby Slacker to the Saviour of Mainstream Comedy." *The Independent*, August 20.

27

Marijuana in the Media During the Regulation Era in Uruguay, 2013–2017

Sebastián Aguiar, Mauricio Coitiño, Florencia Lemos, and Clara Musto

Keywords: cannabis regulation, Uruguay, framing analysis, public opinion, media analysis

Introduction

On December 10, 2013, Uruguay became the first country in the world to comprehensively regulate the marijuana market. The debate and parliamentary approval of Law 19172 had a huge media impact, as shown by the numerous covers and headlines that international media dedicated during 2013 to Uruguay, to its then President José Mujica, and to this unique experiment.

The legal reform had been promoted for more than a decade by social movements and finally catapulted into Parliament in 2012. However, public opinion did not support the project at all. Its approval did not reach 25% in any of the surveys until 2016. Prior research (Cruz, Boidi, and Queirolo 2017) noted this surprising stability in public opinion and studied the determinants of opposition. However, between 2016 and 2017, four years after the approval, public opinion seems to have changed abruptly (Figure 27.1). Three independent surveys indicate that support for regulation rose almost 20 percentage points, in a relatively short period of time since 2016. The question then is obvious: what happened during this period?

There is broad consensus that the media play a key role in the debate of public issues. By selecting and highlighting certain issues, the press has an agenda-setting function towards political actors and policy makers. As well, the media is a key element in public opinion formation around the issues in the public agenda. Given the importance of media coverage for opinion formation, several studies have explored the specific relationship between media and drug policy, specifically media definitions of drug use as a major problem in the United States in the 1970s (see Elliott and Chapman 2000; Stryker 2003; Roberts, Henriksen, and Christenson 1999; Slater, Long, and Ford 2006; Taylor 2008; Hawdon 2010).

In relation to the analysis of cannabis media coverage, various studies have taken this approach. Shepherd (1981) has analyzed the selection of scientific sources used in journalistic coverage. Haines-Saah et al. (2014) described the privileged normalization of the use of cannabis in the Canadian press from 1997

DOI: 10.4324/9780429320491-27

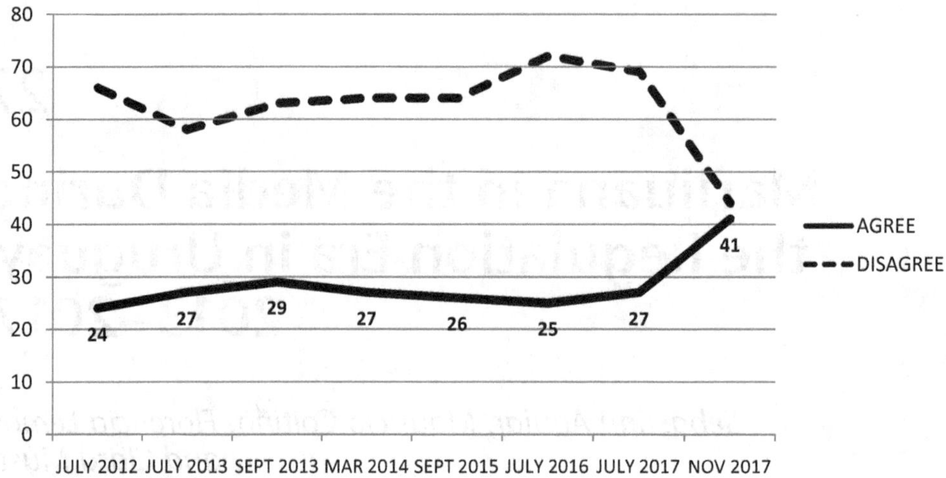

Figure 27.1 Evolution of public opinion about cannabis regulation in Uruguay

Source: Based on survey data by CIFRA (2012, 2014, 2015, 2016, 2017), Equipos Mori (2013), Factum (2013), and First National Survey on Cannabis Regulation (Monitor Cannabis 2018a)

to 2007. Acevedo (2007), on the other hand, analyzed the change in the definition of the problem of cannabis during the public debate on the reclassification of the substance in Great Britain in 2004–2005. Sznitman and Lewis (2015) found that in the case of cannabis for medicinal use in Israel, the ratio of news pieces that showed a frame of cannabis as medicine and those that showed a frame of cannabis as an illegal drug evolved in a manner consistent with public opinion on the matter at a given time but without any significant relationship to the number of medical cannabis licenses granted by the government.

We also draw on studies on public opinion and media coverage on cannabis and cannabis regulation in Uruguay. Filardo et al. (2012) identified a series of recurring topics on news pieces related to cannabis published on Uruguayan media in 2011. Cruz, Boidi, and Queirolo (2016) studied the determinants of public support to cannabis regulation in Uruguay. Finally, Coitiño, Queirolo, and Triñanes (2017) carried out a comparative content analysis of the coverage of cannabis and alcohol regulation in Uruguayan media from 2013 to 2015, finding a set of recurring framing elements in at least 5% of their corpus.

This chapter analyzes media coverage during the 2013–2017 period to identify the main elements and turning points in the public discussion of cannabis regulation in Uruguay and how the framing of cannabis and cannabis regulation evolved in the content of media coverage. We ask to what extent changes in the framing of the debate contributed to the recent shift in public opinion about this policy.

For Entman (1993), frames perform one or more of four functions: defining problems in terms of the actions of a causal agent that have costs and benefits; identifying the forces that create the problem; making moral judgments about the causal agents of the problem and its effects; and proposing and justifying treatments for the problem and predicting their effects. We could then say that frames are sets of elements of evaluation of certain issues used by actors and which appear publicly at specific moments.

Methods

The corpus comprises 11,445 news pieces (articles, short news, editorials, columns, etc.) compiled from 86 Uruguayan national and local media containing the word "cannabis" and/or "marijuana," published between December 10, 2013, and December 10, 2017. Most of the pieces come from national print media (54.4%), followed by national digital media, local print media, and local digital media. The proportion between print and digital pieces evolved from mostly print pieces in 2014 to mostly digital pieces in 2017.

For the content analysis, we considered only the subset of pieces published either in the print or digital versions of the main national print media: *El País*, *El Observador*, *La Diaria*, and *La República* (Open Society Foundations 2013). The subset of pieces of these media (n = 4,005) represents 35% of the corpus and 82.5% of national print media pieces. Within the selected subset, we identified the main sources, mentioned actors through correspondence analysis, and grouped them through multi-dimensional scaling using Wordstat™. The topics discussed were identified through topic extraction with Wordstat™ and dictionaries run with QDAMiner™.

Analysis

Media Milestones

What were the milestones in cannabis media coverage in the 2013–2017 period? Do these milestones reflect the steps taken by the Uruguayan government to implement the Cannabis Regulation Law? Figure 27.2 shows the distribution of the news pieces in the corpus based on their date of publication, with an overlay of the main policy milestones. The biggest media milestone during the entire period corresponds to the start of cannabis dispensation at pharmacies on July 20, 2017: 188 pieces on the event were published on that day and the following.

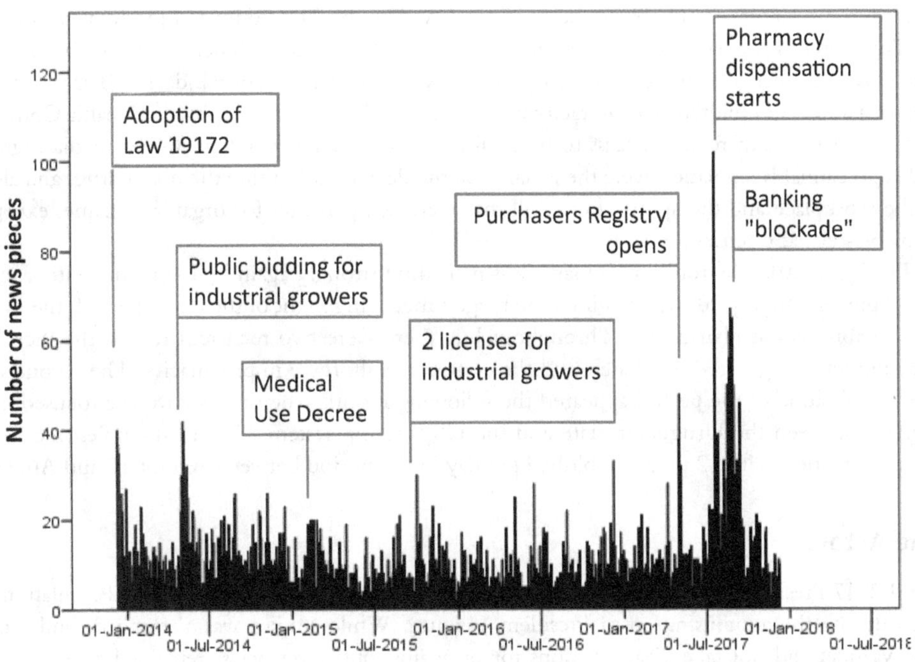

Figure 27.2 Distribution in time of pieces in the corpus, 2013–2017
Source: Prepared by the authors based on the full database (11,445 items)

The second major media milestone of the period can also be identified in 2017: the "banking blockade" of implementation by which local banks reported that they would close the accounts of pharmacies that dispensed cannabis, so as not to risk their relations with the US banking system. This milestone began on August 3, 2017, and its media presence increased, reaching a total coverage of 67 pieces on August 24.

From December 2013 to December 2014, while most pieces focused on the debate of political representatives among themselves and with international actors about Law 19172, the three major media milestones identified—where coverage peaked—focused on implementation. The first, in February 2014, corresponds to the call for interested parties to apply for five-year licenses for the production of psychoactive cannabis for sale in pharmacies. In this same month, a second media milestone corresponds to the appointment of the Scientific Advisory Committee created in charge of monitoring the functioning of the new legal framework. The third media milestone of 2014 appeared in March, when regulatory decree No. 120/014 was introduced, establishing the regulations for accessing recreational cannabis through domestic cultivation, cannabis clubs, and purchase at pharmacies.

During 2015 and 2016, the first two years of the second administration of President Vázquez, the implementation of cannabis virtually fell into media silence. The most covered development of this period was in March 2015, when President Vázquez decided to postpone the start of cannabis sales at pharmacies indefinitely (Vázquez quiere que venta de marihuana en farmacias sea "prolija" 2015). The President had already declared that it seemed "unbelievable" for him to sell cannabis at pharmacies, but he accepted that because it was a law and "it will have to be done eventually" (Es increíble que se venda 2014). In 2015, two key news stories were the issuance of the regulatory decree for medical cannabis in February and the granting of two licenses for the production of psychoactive cannabis for sale in pharmacies in October. The corpus shows a significant increase in police news about seizures, prosecutions, and closure of drug houses, where cannabis is mentioned. Indeed, the amount of cannabis seized by the police grew by 71% compared to the previous year.

This trend in media coverage of police news continued in 2016. There were 46 days in which cannabis was a recurring topic. In July, a major story was the hearing of Fundación Batar, an association of parents of children with refractory epilepsy and West syndrome, by the Health Committee of the Parliament to request access to medical cannabis for their children. Other media highlights linked to cannabis regulation were the issuance of the decree prohibiting the use of drugs and alcohol at the workplace and the approval of a bill that increased penalties for organized crime, except for cannabis-related offenses.

Finally, in 2017 the topic of cannabis was picked up strongly again by the media with a total of 3,710 pieces. On July 20, we identified the biggest media highlight of the entire period: the first day of cannabis sales at pharmacies. Throughout July there were two recurrent topics: the increase in the number of registered purchasers and the continuous shortage in pharmacies. The second major media milestone of the period appeared the following month when news coverage focused on the conflict between the Uruguayan state and the US banking system. This media milestone had the longest duration with 12 pieces published per day in the period between August 17 and August 31.

The Actors

Until 2017 President José Mujica was the most cited actor regarding the Cannabis Regulation Law, even during the administration of President Vázquez. While Mujica was a strong defender of the law, Vázquez did not take clear positions for or against but nevertheless remained a relevant actor mentioned with reference to the implementation process. The National Drug Board (JND), under the Presidency Office, was the most mentioned institution, both through its chair, Juan Andrés Roballo, and the three secretaries general who succeeded each other during the period: Julio Calzada (2010–2015), Milton Romani (2015–2016), and Diego Olivera (2016 to present).

At a second level, Jorge Basso and Cristina Lustemberg, respectively minister and undersecretary of public health, together with Minister of the Interior Eduardo Bonomi, were the other government figures most mentioned. This may derive from the historical preeminence of drugs as a matter of health and safety, handled by doctors, lawyers, and the police, rather than as a problem of education orsocial or economic development.

A third set of authorities participated in the debate from civil society and academia, all of them positioned in favor of the new law: Julia Galzerano and Raquel Peyraube, medical doctors specialized in medical cannabis and founders of the Uruguayan Society of Endocannabinology; Martín Collazo (activist of Proderechos and researcher with Monitor Cannabis Uruguay), Bruno Calleros (activist of the Movement for the Liberalization of Cannabis), Laura Blanco (activist of the Association of Cannabis Studies, AECU), and Eduardo Blasina (cannabis entrepreneur and founder of the Museum of Cannabis of Montevideo).

Just as in the period prior to the enactment of the law, the authorities who opposed the legal reform were not civil society actors but political actors linked to a specific sector of evangelical legislators of Partido Nacional (Musto 2018). On the opposite side, along with ruling party representative Sebastián Sabini, pro-government Luis Gallo emerged as an advocate within the Frente Amplio party, following up on the implementation, in particular regarding the medical uses of cannabis, from Parliament.

An institutional analysis shows that the government remained the main reference throughout the period. The Institute of Regulation and Control of Cannabis (IRCCA), the regulatory agency created by Law 19172, progressively increased its presence, and in 2017 became the most mentioned government agency. IRCCA even surpassed the presidency in mentions, which in turn was steadily present throughout the period (in 2014 and 2016 it was the most mentioned government institution).

At a second level of occurrence, the presence of partisan political institutions was identified. Other institutions mentioned in the period were the Pharmacies' Chamber (Centro de Farmacias), with an almost marginal appearance in 2014 but identified as a relevant actor in 2017; and intergovernmental organizations, in particular the UN, the UN International Narcotics Control Board (INCB; mainly in 2014), and the Organization of American States (OAS). Finally, civil society organizations had a marginal presence compared to government institutions and political parties, appearing mainly in the first two years of implementation.

The presence of nine clusters of actors was identified by means of a dendrogram of the institutions and authorities (Figure 27.3). This technique visually groups text elements (institution and authority names) based on their tendency to co-occur within the corpus. The two conglomerates at the top correspond to civil society actors: the first is composed of actors and organizations devoted to cannabis activism for home growing and cannabis clubs. The second includes the organizations and political actors advocating for a comprehensive regulation. There is a third conglomerate of civil society at the bottom composed of medical and industrial cannabis experts. A fourth conglomerate reflects the government institutions and authorities in charge of public health, while the fifth conglomerate is composed of the University of the Republic and National Drugs Observatory actors, both data production and analysis institutions.

Government institutions and authorities make up two distinct conglomerates: conglomerate six brings together high-ranking authorities and institutions and political parties (presidency, Ministry of the Interior, political parties, Parliament, etc.), while in conglomerate seven direct managers of implementation (National Drug Board, IRCCA) are identified together with other actors involved in the process of cannabis sale at pharmacies, as the Pharmacies' Chamber. Finally, the eighth conglomerate corresponds to the appearance of international organizations (INCB, UN, and OAS), and the ninth conglomerate is made up of the institutions and actors in charge of controlling and supervising the use of cannabis in drivers (UNASEV[Road Safety Unit], Gerardo Barrios).

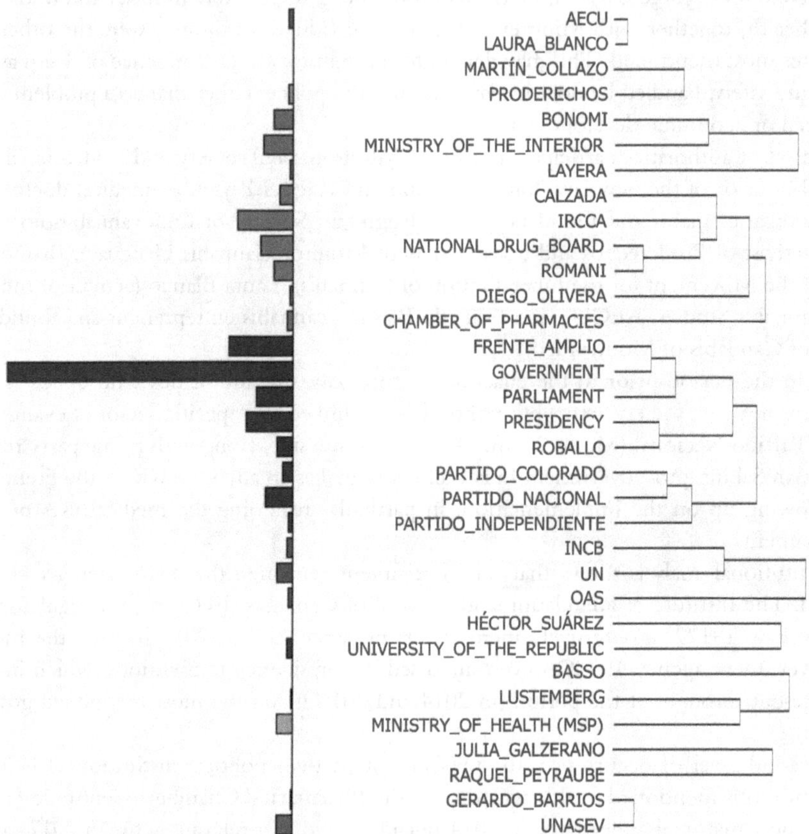

Figure 27.3 Dendrogram of authorities and institutions

Source: Prepared by the authors based on the full database (11,445 items)

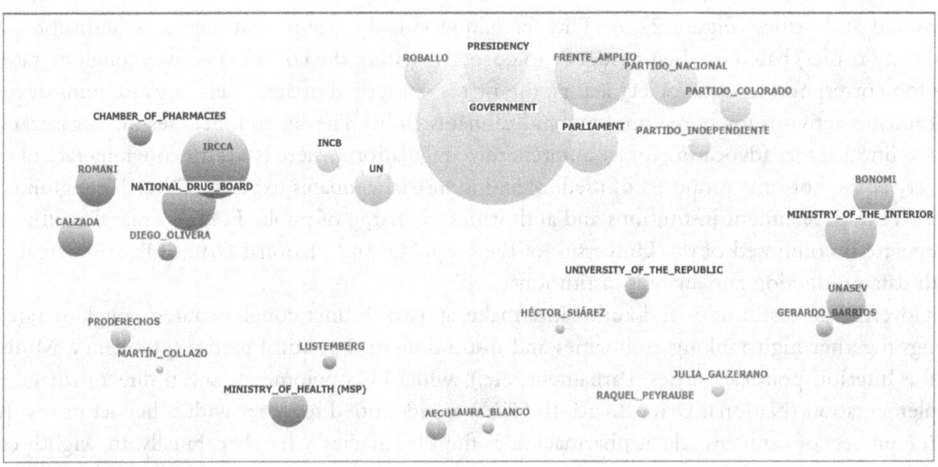

Figure 27.4 Multidimensional scaling of actors

Source: Prepared by the authors based on the full database (11,445 items)

In order to validate the conglomerates described previously, we used multidimensional scaling to visualize the actor's and actor group's closeness by plotting them in a Cartesian space. Multidimensional scaling calculates the relative distances between elements (actor names) based on their joint appearance in the pieces of the corpus. As Figure 27.4 shows, political parties (Partido Nacional, Partido Colorado, Frente Amplio) are positioned close to the government, which in turn is close to the bodies of drug policy implementation (National Drug Board, IRCCA). Relatively far from these appear the actors linked to security (Ministry of the Interior and Minister Bonomi), road safety (UNASEV), and health (Ministry of Public Health and Minister Lustemberg). Some of the latter, particularly those focused on medical cannabis (Julia Galzerano, Raquel Peyraube), are located close to activist organizations (AECU, Proderechos), which in turn are far from the parties and the government at the top of the graph.

The Topics

To inductively identify the main topics covered in the subset of pieces from the four main print media, we ran a topic extraction analysis. This is done through software by constructing a correlation matrix of all words in the corpus, then measuring their actual association in the data and their relative distances to other words, which produces a series of "word packages" or thematic clusters. We identified 14 relevant thematic clusters, whose strength of association can be represented by their eigenvalue: the greater the eigenvalue, the more intense is the relationship between the words of each "word package" in the matrix.

In decreasing order by their eigenvalue, Cluster 1 refers to the implementation of the sale in pharmacies. Cluster 2 groups the debates and positions of parliamentarians and party authorities, both from the ruling party and the opposition. Cluster 3 corresponds to the coverage of aspects of the repressive drug trafficking policy and criminal incidents that involved marijuana in some way. Cluster 4 reflects the coverage of the implementation of cannabis clubs and domestic cultivation. Cluster 5 corresponds to the topic of access to medical cannabis. Cluster 6 summarizes the international repercussions of Uruguayan regulation at the level of multilateral organizations: basically the UN INCB and the OAS. Cluster 7 refers to the implementation of cannabis consumption controls on drivers by UNASEV. Cluster 8 gathers the positions of the actors of the social movement that supported the approval of Law 19172.

Cluster 9 reflects the approach of scientific studies on cannabis and the opinion of scholars and experts. Cluster 10 corresponds to the government-party defense of the reform at Parliament and to government announcements on the implementation of the three ways of access. Cluster 11 reflects the National Drug Board's approach to regulation, mainly through the voice of its secretaries. Cluster 12 reflects the aspects related to the implementation of the registries of the three ways of access, and the monitoring of the sale in pharmacies. Cluster 13 refers to the public health aspects of the policy, and the main voices are the highest-ranking health authorities. Cluster 14 covers administrative aspects of implementation, mainly developed by the regulatory agency (IRCCA).

In order to have thematic categories that are more comprehensive of the media milestones throughout the period and to avoid categories that only represent a circumstantial topic, we merged some of the initial clusters based on their thematic closeness to produce nine simplified clusters. For instance, the simplified cluster of government implementation includes the word packages of user registration, preparation for sale at pharmacies, and problems of the sale at pharmacies (initial clusters 1, 12, and 14). This operation is described in Table 27.1, along with the eigenvalues and number of appearances of each cluster. Simplified clusters are sorted by their number of appearances in the corpus, and initial clusters are sorted according to their simplified cluster.

Table 27.1 Simplification of thematic clusters

Initial Clusters	*Eigenvalue*	*Appearances**	*Simplified Cluster*	*Appearances**
1. Problems of the sale at pharmacies	5.04	1,548	Government implementation	3,374
12. User registration	1.28	1,383		
14. Preparation for sale at pharmacies	1.18	443		
10. Government's law	1.42	2,727	Law	2,727
13. Public health issues	1.27	1,057	Health	2,453
5. Medical cannabis	1.88	1,396		
3. Security and drug trafficking	2.13	1,636	Security	1,636
9. Scientific approaches	1.48	1,164	Evidence	1,164
2. Political discussion of the reform	2.69	1,090	Political debate	1,090
6. International repercussions	1.69	817	International	817
11. National Drug Board statements	1.31	487	Presidency	577
7. Road safety	1.64	90		
4. Cannabis clubs	1.99	435	Civil society	531
8. Reformist civil society	1.52	94		

Source: Prepared by the authors based on the subset from the main print media (4,005 items)

* Number of appearances of two or more key tokens

Discussion: The Framing of Cannabis

To describe the evolution of frames of communication on the regulation of cannabis, we integrated the three dimensions surveyed in the previous sections: the media milestones, the actors, and the main topics of the public conversation.

Frames belong to the actors and correspond to their definitions of problems, their moral judgments about the agents that cause them, and their preferences for treatment of the problem (Entman 1993). But these frames appear in the media content as a result of the treatment of certain topics that make it possible for the discourse of those actors containing those frames to be reflected in the media. Each media milestone is, from this perspective, an opportunity for the media positioning of the communication frames of certain actors, depending on the topics associated with that milestone.

In order to approximate the evolution of communication frames, we grouped the actors based on their shared evaluation within each simplified thematic cluster. Where actors showed conflicting evaluations, they were split into two groups ("positive" and "negative"). Figure 27.5 shows the evolution of the occurrence of thematically grouped actors in this subset of the corpus. The X-axis has been labeled with a series of chronologically ordered topics associated with the main media milestones. The Y-axis indicates the percentage of occurrences within the total of the whole period.

Figure 27.5 allows us to summarize the evolution of actors' frames. As is further developed later, at the end of the period there was a decrease in the occurrence of negative evaluation frames and an increase in the occurrence of informative and positive frames, which could be associated with the shift in public opinion detected at the end of 2017.

Those actors that debated the validity of the approved law (political and international, both positive and negative) and projected competitive elements of framing (regulation as a bold solution vs. regulation as an intensifier of the consumer problem/breach of international law) gradually lost weight, especially at the end of the period. The group of actors associated with the issue of security linked to drug trafficking gained considerable weight in 2015 and especially in 2016, in the midst of media milestones that put the Ministry of the Interior and, to a lesser extent, the political opposition, in the limelight.

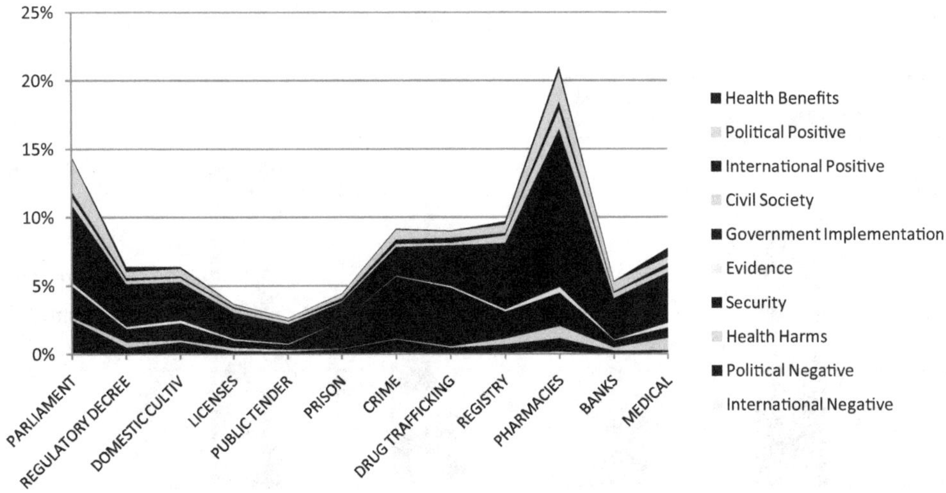

Figure 27.5 Evolution of the occurrence of grouped actors by topic evaluation (frames)

Source: Prepared by the authors based on the subset of pieces from the main print media (4,005 items)

Both actor groupings of health maintained a discreet weight through the period but grew visibly in 2017 in the context of the discussion about developments in medical cannabis implementation. The media coverage of these developments opened a significant space for clinical experts and patients to project the framing of the health benefits of cannabis. The academics who monitor this aspect of the policy, and share a framing of health benefits, also grow in weight in this same context. In a context of direct responsibility for the implementation developments that structured the media milestones of 2017, the government's discourse regains its predominance. This also implies a greater projection of the framings of the state's extraordinary efforts to implement a reform that can be later evaluated.

As frames imply positions and evaluations of the actors on topics, we can collapse the ten actor groups into "positive" (i.e., supportive of regulation), "negative," and "neutral" or "informative" frames.

As shown in Figure 27.6, the negative frames of health harms, negative international repercussions, critical political actors, and the association of cannabis with public security problems represented at least a third of the total occurrences each year until 2016, but then decreased to less than a fourth in 2017.

Meanwhile, the positive frames of the political actors that defended the reform, positive international repercussions, and the actors supportive of medical cannabis were proportionally more stable, with highs in 2014 and 2017.

Finally, the informative frames comprised more than half of the occurrences of all frames in 2017, compared to only a third in 2016. Moreover, half of all the occurrences of informative frames in the period were concentrated in this year (1,934 out of 3,871). These are the frames of government and regulation authorities related to the various aspects of implementation, as well as the evidence-based discourses from academic and independent experts (though marginal in their occurrence).

But inasmuch as they support the theory of change behind cannabis regulation, either scientifically or by taking it as a given, these informative framings could be attributed a positive value. In that case, the results of these analyses show that 2017 saw the sharpest contrast in the proportion of

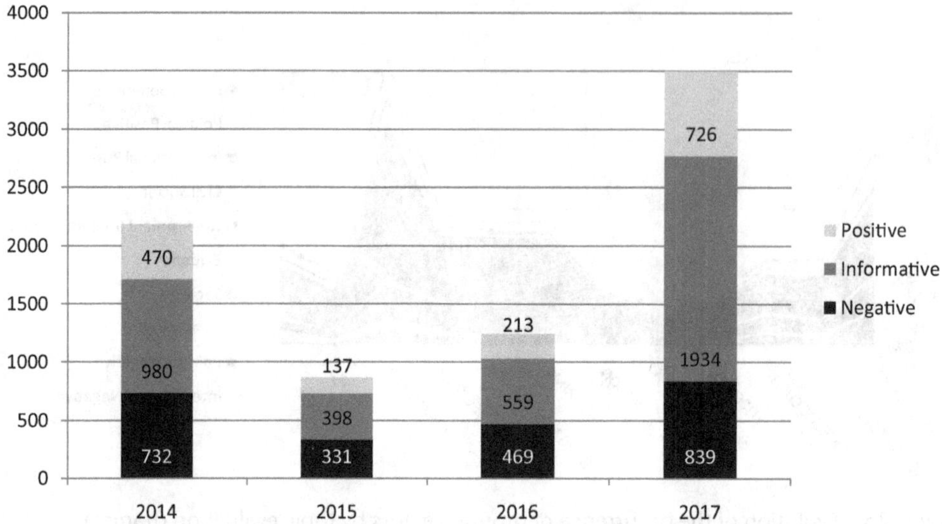

Figure 27.6 Evolution of simplified frames per year (number of occurrences)

Source: Prepared by the authors based on the subset of pieces from the main print media (4,005 items). Data from December 2013 is excluded for clarity.

negative and positive frame occurrences (839 versus 2,660 occurrences) in the period, in line with the shift to a more supportive public opinion.

Conclusions

Our analyses show that the media coverage offers a relevant image of the public discussion of the issue of cannabis regulation. We can also see that media coverage was consistent with key developments in the implementation process, which explains the timing in the shift in public opinion.

The framing elements of the regulators, the positive governmental framing of implementation, and the health benefits of medical cannabis occurred with greater frequency in the corpus towards the end of the study period. All these elements of framing could contribute to positive opinion about the regulation of cannabis and its effects.

On the other hand, the topics of media coverage in 2017 did not favor the media presence of actors whose framing elements were linked to the disapproval of cannabis regulation (Cruz, Boidi, and Queirolo 2016). The explosion of medical cannabis coverage likely reduced the space for actors associated with health harms (Ministry of Public Health, political opposition, the presidency) who were not authorities on the topic of health benefits. Thus, the framings of the harmful effects of consumption ("Marijuana is a substance that is harmful to health"; "Marijuana is a gateway to hard drugs") tended to occur less in 2017.

Additionally, the implementation of pharmacy sales and the subsequent banking blockade opened space in the media coverage to the frames of the actors of government (the presidency and IRCCA) from the perspective of implementation, and in turn reduced the space for the negative political frame of regulation as an intensifier of the "consumer problem" ("Cannabis users are a threat to society").

Finally, the overall occurrence of the security actors dropped sharply in 2017 to its lowest level of the entire period, and we can assume that this was also the trajectory followed by the elements of framing associated both with the Ministry of the Interior and the political opposition, which question the theory of change of the legal reform as a partial solution to the problem of drug trafficking ("The regulation will not be effective to reduce the illegal sale of marijuana"). These developments seem to be consistent with the inflection in public opinion detected in 2017, where approval has risen from an average of 25% during the study period to 41%–44% in 2017.

The major media milestones of 2017 focused on key elements of regulation. First, the beginning of the sale at pharmacies demonstrated the viability of the policy, which until then was uncertain. Second, the blockade from the US banking system framed the defense of cannabis regulation as a matter of national sovereignty. For its part, the increased coverage of access to medical cannabis introduced a topic on which almost 90% of public opinion had a positive view in 2017 (Monitor Cannabis 2018b).

Showing the viability of the regulatory model, presenting the measure as a national enterprise, and prioritizing access to medical cannabis seem to have been pivotal aspects in the turn of public opinion towards greater support. On the other hand, the topics of security and drug trafficking, particularly in a model that was not yet fully operational, seem to have been associated with the stability of negative opinion before 2017.

Overall, the political discussion that characterized the first year after the adoption of the law gave way to a public conversation based on specific aspects, where several of the most relevant negative frames lost space. For example, spokespersons who highlighted the health harms of cannabis switched from talking about cannabis as a diffuse threat to public health to referring to specific issues, such as the risk of normalization and problematic consumption. This turn is particularly marked in 2017 with the beginning of the sale at pharmacies and an in-depth discussion about medical cannabis.

The informative government discourse frames increased the most in the 2016–2017 period and may have contributed to the change in public opinion. This type of discourse seems to promote a better public evaluation of the initiative in a cumulative way: once people learn why it is possible to regulate and how it is actually being done, they may be prone to drift away from negative framing elements. Other governments developing similar initiatives may see an improvement in public opinion of cannabis regulation if their actors manage to take advantage of the media interest in implementation developments to widely project an explanatory and informative discourse through the media.

Finally, this study tests an innovative media analysis procedure that can be replicated for other issues or contexts: frames are operationalized as evaluations of actors projected to media contents as a result of the treatment of certain topics in media coverage. As well, software-based content analysis techniques allow one to process a high number of news pieces and carry out objective comparative studies. In particular, the comparison with other countries could be valuable, for example in terms of the weight of government actors in media coverage or the role of security in the public debate on cannabis regulation.

It would be useful to supplement this analysis with qualitative approaches such as through focus groups, in order to appraise the importance attributed by citizens to the elements described in this study, and to better understand the relationship between the "frames in communication" and the "frames in thought" (Chong and Druckman 2007) of the relevant actors in media coverage.

References

Acevedo, B. 2007. "Creating the Cannabis User: A Post-Structuralist Analysis of the Re-Classification of Cannabis in the United Kingdom (2004–2005)." *International Journal of Drug Policy* 18: 177–86. https://doi.org/10.1016/j.drugpo.2006.11.008.

Chong, D., and J. Druckman. 2007. "Framing Theory." *Annual Review of Political Science* 10: 103–26. https://doi.org/10.1146/annurev. polisci.10.072805.103054.

CIFRA. 2012. "La legalización de la venta de marihuana." http://www.cifra.com.uy/index.php/2015/09/02/marihuana/.

———. 2014. "Los uruguayos y la marihuana." https://web.archive.org/web/20150325171933/http://www.cifra.com.uy/novedades.php?idNoticia=233.

———. 2015. "Survey on Public Opinion About Cannabis Regulation." In *Cannabis legal en Uruguay. Estado de situación perspectivas*, edited by M. F. Boidi, R. Queirolo, and J. M. Cruz, 2016. http://ucu.edu.uy/sites/default/files/facultad/dcsp/presentacion-lamrimontevideo-agosto16.pdf.

———. 2016. "El consumo de la marihuana y su venta en farmacias." http://www.cifra.com.uy/index.php/2016/06/29/el-consumo-de-marihuana-y-su-venta-en-farmacias/.

———. 2017. "El consumo de marihuana y su venta en farmacias." https://www.cifra.com.uy/index.php/2017/08/17/el-consumo-de-marihuana-y-su-venta-en-farmacias-2/.

Coitiño, M., R. Queirolo, and A. Triñanes. 2017. "Dos drogas, diferentes mensajes: los medios y la regulación de la marihuana y el alcohol en Uruguay." *Contratexto* (28): 119–46. https://doi.org/10.26439/contratexto2017.n028.1566.

Cruz, J. M., M. F. Boidi, and R. Queirolo. 2016. "Saying no to Weed: Public Opinion Towards Cannabis Legalisation in Uruguay." *Drugs: Education, Prevention and Policy* 25 (1): 67–76. doi:10.1080/09687637.2016.1237475.

———. 2017. "The Status of Support for Cannabis Regulation in Uruguay 4 Years after Reform: Evidence from Public Opinion Surveys: Support for Cannabis Regulation." *Drug and Alcohol Review* 37 Suppl 1. doi:10.1111/dar.12642.

Elliott, A., and S. Chapman. 2000. " 'Heroin Hell their Own Making': Construction of Heroin Users in the Australian Press 1992–97." *Drug and Alcohol Review* 19: 191–201. doi:10.1080/713659328.

Entman, R. M. 1993. "Framing: Toward Clarification of a Fractured Paradigm." *Journal of Communication* 43: 51–58. doi:10.1111/j.1460-2466.1993.tb01304.x.

Equipos Mori. 2013. "Dos de cada tres uruguayos en contra de la regulación de la marihuana." https://web.archive.org/web/20161223205916/http://equipos.com.uy/noticias_despliegue.php?i=135.

"Es increíble que se venda marihuana en farmacias." 2014. *El Observador*, October 16. https://www.elobservador.com.uy/nota/-es-increible-que-se-venda-marihuana-en-farmacias-2014101614470.

Factum. 2013. "Las dudas y contradicciones de la sociedad sobre la legalización de la marihuana." https://web.archive.org/web/20131202050441/http://www.factum.edu.uy/node/1080.

Filardo, V., S. Aguiar, C. Musto, and D. Pieri. 2012. "La marihuana provoca esquizofrenia. Espacio público y drogas en Uruguay." In *Aporte universitario al debate sobre drogas*, edited by N. A. Paraskevaídis. Montevideo: Comisión Sectorial de Investigación Científica.

Haines-Saah, R. J., J. L. Johnson, R. Repta, A. Ostry, M. L. Young, J. Shoveller, and P. A. Ratner. 2014. "The Privileged Normalization of Marijuana Use—An Analysis of Canadian Newspaper Reporting, 1997–2007." *Critical Public Health* 24 (1): 47–61. http://dx.doi.org/10.1080/09581596.2013.771812.

Hawdon, J. 2010. "The Role of Presidential Rhetoric in the Creation of a Moral Panic: Reagan, Bush, and the War on Drugs." *Deviant Behavior* 419–445.

Monitor Cannabis. 2018a. "Primeros resultados sobre la aprobación de la regulación." https://web.archive.org/web/20200224160205/http://monitorcannabis.uy/cambios-en-la-opinion-publica-sobre-la-regulacion-del-cannabis/.

Monitor Cannabis. 2018b. "Cannabis medicinal: la revolución silenciosa." https://web.archive.org/web/20200304060329/http://monitorcannabis.uy/cannabis-medicinal-la-revolucion-silenciosa/.

Musto, C. 2018. "Regulating Cannabis Markets. The Construction of an Innovative Drug Policy in Uruguay." PhD thesis, Utrecht University – Kent University, Kent, UK.

Open Society Foundations. 2013. *Trazando un mapa de los medios digitales: Uruguay*. London: Author.

Roberts, D. F., L. Henriksen, and P. G. Christenson. 1999. *Substance Use in Popular Movies and Music*. Washington, DC: Office of National Drug Control Policy. http://www.health.org/govstudy/mediastudy/new.htm.

Shepherd, R. G. 1981. "Selectivity of Sources: Reporting the Marijuana Controversy." *Journal of Communication* 31: 129–37. doi:10.1111 / j.1460-2466.1981.tb01236.x.

Slater, M. D., M. Long, and V. L. Ford. 2006. "Alcohol, Illegal Drugs, Violent Crime, and Traffic-Related and Other Unintended Injuries in US Local and National News." *Journal of Studies on Alcohol* 67 (6): 904–10. https://doi.org/10.15288/jsa.2006.67.904.

Stryker, J. E. 2003. "Media and Marijuana: A Longitudinal Analysis of News Media Effects on Adolescents' Marijuana Use and Related Outcomes 1977–1999." *Journal of Health Communication* 8: 305–28. http://dx.doi.org/10.1080/10810730305724.

Sznitman, S. R., and N. Lewis. 2015. "Is Cannabis an Illicit Drug or a Medicine? A Quantitative Framing Analysis of Israeli Newspaper Coverage." *International Journal of Drug Policy* 26 (5): 446–52. https://doi.org/10.1016/j.drugpo.2015.01.010.

Taylor, S. 2008. "Outside the Outsiders: Media Representations of Drug Use." *Probation Journal* 55: 369–87. https://doi.org/10.1177/0264550508096493.

"Vázquez quiere que venta de marihuana en farmacias sea 'prolija'" 2015. Espectador, March 4. http://historico.espectador.com/politica/310690/vazquez-quiere-que-venta-de-marihuana-en-farmacias-sea-prolija.

28

The Intersection of Cannabis Reform and Other Progressive Movements

Opportunities for Interdisciplinary Researchers

Amanda Reiman

Keywords: Cannabis, social change, environmentalism, gender, economic justice, racial equity

Conflict of Interest

Dr. Reiman is currently the director of development for Flow Cannabis, a cannabis company licensed in California.

Introduction

Cannabis policy development intersects with social policy issues such as environmentalism, gender equity, economic justice and racial discrimination. Social and racial justice in particular have become talking points for 2020 U.S. presidential candidates when they speak about legalization (Reiman 2019; Gabriel 2019). And, because of the interest in and focus on cannabis from the media to the legislature, cannabis policy can be developed to amplify the urgency of and interest in policy reform movements. This is an opportunity that was unavailable when I first began studying cannabis in 2002. The narrow view of drug use and drug policy in the 1980s and 90s stymied many conversations about the broader context of drug use and enforcement. I chose to study social welfare because of the emphasis on person in environment. Different from psychology, social work looks at the impact of social and environmental forces in the development of mental health resilience. Drug policy has traditionally gone against this philosophy, focusing instead on drug users as a population with a brain disease and sellers and manufacturers of drugs as criminals without consideration of powerful structural and environmental forces. For me, the movement to legalize cannabis has uncovered many socioeconomic and environmental aspects of drug use, drug markets and policy development. I have studied these in my role as a public health postdoctoral fellow, as the director of research for

DOI: 10.4324/9780429320491-28

one of the oldest dispensaries in the country, and as the manager of marijuana law and policy at the Drug Policy Alliance. And through this work in research, practice and policy in the emerging field of cannabis, I have concluded that cannabis reform will not reach its full potential for change unless we look beyond the plant and into how this social change can matter in a greater context. The investigation of cannabis as a catalyst for change is in the tradition of the social work profession.

Cannabis industry regulation is a unique process compared to the regulation of other agricultural commodities, with rules that diverge from the norm when it comes to the oversight of the cultivation, processing, manufacture and sale of cannabis products. Those writing about the transition to legalization point out inconsistencies in how similar industries are regulated (Paniello 2018). There is an opportunity to capitalize on this divergence and bring new data into the fields of environmental science, sustainable agriculture and social justice work. Opportunities also exist for researchers in these fields to study the industry as it evolves, related to their fields of expertise.

This chapter will first explore how cannabis research and policy intersect with other social policy reform movements. Then, potential research collaborations and opportunities in this context will be presented along with sample research questions. The goals of this chapter are to examine cannabis policy design as a catalyst for empowering and engaging reformers and researchers working in the fields of environmentalism, gender equity and racial and economic justice. Specifically, this chapter will highlight the intersection between cannabis policy reform and social science research by looking at how emerging cannabis markets highlight other reform issues.

Cannabis Policy as a Megaphone for Social Change

Using cannabis policy reform as a catalyst to bring progressive social issues and their camps together can breathe new life into old causes and mobilize new resources brought on behalf of a fledgling formal economy (Jenkins 1983). Advocacy fatigue is real, even among the most passionate, due to resource scarcity, a sense of urgency not always embraced by the public and funding paradigms that support alternate approaches. For reformers and researchers, discovering a new nuance or connection to the cause can help re-energize the work, bring new members into a movement and help those already there see things in a new and different way (McCarthy and Zald 1977; Basas 2014). While the issue of cannabis policy reform is a topic that can be studied with complete focus, it can also serve as a platform or frame that amplifies the efficacy of other policy reform efforts.

Cannabis and . . .

The Schedule I status of cannabis in the United States has, until recently, kept the issue of cannabis policy reform under the purview of the criminal justice system and research institutions only interested in harms. The National Institute of Drug Abuse (NIDA) has a mission to "to advance science on the causes and consequences of drug use and addiction and to apply that knowledge to improve individual and public health" (NIDA 2019). Therefore, funding related to cannabis research has been focused on studying dependence and the negative impact on the lives of consumers. In response, reformers began touting the harms of prohibition as they contribute to other social problems. Jack Herer, one of the leading advocates for the many uses of hemp and a key figure in the reform movement, spoke of the environmental benefits of hemp, and the Drug Policy Alliance drew attention to the racist nature of cannabis laws (Bourque 2019; Drug Policy Alliance n.d.). Part of the challenge was connecting the issues of environmentalism and racial justice to cannabis prohibition and illustrating how legalization and the development of responsible and evidence-informed cannabis policies can advance their causes as well. This can be done with research that uses the experiment of state-level cannabis legalization to test theories, programs and practices developed to address inequity and harm. Research can inform both the development of the cannabis industry and the reform of other industries and institutions. The following sections outline how this approach can be used in the areas of environmentalism, gender equity and racial and economic justice.

Environmentalism

A structural effect of prohibition was indoor cultivation (Mills 2012; Miller 2018). Not wanting to be discovered, cultivators went underground, and indoor cultivation became the norm. Today, this practice is exacerbated by the fact that cannabis cannot be legally shipped across state lines, so states such as Michigan are forced to cultivate in environments with short growing seasons and harsh winters. Because of this, and the fears that still exist around cannabis, those who care about the environment have had little opportunity for influence thus far. Times are changing, but there is still a huge disconnect for people who care about the environment yet do not connect their environmentalism to support sun-grown, sustainable cannabis production (see Mills and Zeramby Chapter 21, this volume).

Private certification programs and energy initiatives exist in the cannabis industry to help environmentally conscious farmers appeal to ecologically ethical consumers. They include Clean Green, Patient Focused Certification, Dragonfly Earth Medicine and others. Recently, the iconic soap brand Dr. Bronner's launched a regenerative cannabis certification program/initiative called Sun and Earth Certified. Farms that receive this certification practice regenerative farming methods such as sun grown, rain catchment, integrated pest management, polyculture and closed loop systems. Closed loop means that the farm uses no outside amendments, soils or energy to maintain it. Another aspect of the certification is fair wages paid to farmers and employees. The farms that meet the standard are sold under the Brother David's line. All of the profits from Brother David's go to help other farms reach the regenerative standard (www.brotherdavids.com).

Under prohibition in the United States, cannabis farmers were lumped into one category. Environmental degradation happening at the hands of large grows on public land was being generalized to all cannabis farmers. Campaign Against Marijuana Planting (CAMP), the federal cannabis cultivation eradication program from the 80s, 90s and even recent years did not always differentiate between small family farms stewarding the earth and large clear-cut grows on public land that used harmful poisons and firearms to protect profit (Flock and Scialla 2019; Miller 2018; Corva 2014). The desire to prevent environmental degradation at the hands of cannabis cultivators did not die with legalization. Prop. 64 in California included tax revenues earmarked to address the environmental harms caused during prohibition (Adult Use of Marijuana Act 2016). While the government claims that those causing environmental harms are the targets, there is concern over how the government will prioritize enforcement (MacBride 2019). In 2018, CAMP was active in California, eradicating over 600,000 plants (Sernoffsky 2019). As the licensing process matures, the opportunity will come to support environmentally friendly cultivation practices. Groups working to reduce carbon emissions and high-intensity energy use should pay attention to research and policy development around indoor cultivation.

For example, private sector organizations like the Resource Innovation Institute (RII) are exploring new technologies to reduce the footprint of cannabis agriculture. These technologies can be implemented outside of cannabis by working with those who are also interested in sustainability. RII's mission is "to advance resource efficiency to create a better cannabis future" (Resource Innovation Institute 2019). The group recently partnered with New Frontier, a big data firm focusing on the cannabis industry, to produce the 2018 Cannabis Energy Report. This comprehensive, 65-page document is the first to provide a scientifically based, wide ranging study of energy use and cannabis cultivation in the regulated industry. And while the report is cannabis-specific, it is easily generalizable to other areas of agriculture and manufacturing and includes the development of RII's PowerScore, an online tool for cannabis facilities to assess their carbon footprint and the impact of their sustainable practices (Resource Innovation Institute 2019).

Research on the environmental impacts of various methods of cannabis cultivation is ammunition for groups seeking to curb our reliance on artificial and carbon-intensive energy methods. According to the Cannabis Energy Report, legal cannabis production in the United States uses as much energy as does the city of Anaheim, CA, an estimated 1.1 million megawatt hours. This use is projected to increase 162% by 2022. The recommendations in the report include the development of more energy-efficient technologies, policies that support sustainable practices and reporting requirements and the serious consideration of allowing sun-grown and low-energy-intensive cultivation such as greenhouse cultivation over more intensive methods (New Frontier 2019, 4).

More than just avoiding harms from cannabis cultivation, regenerative cannabis farming methods can be beneficial in other ways. For the past few decades, environmental scientists have begun to question the utility, humanity and impact of large-scale industrial agriculture (Union of Concerned Scientists n.d.; Horrigan, Walker, and Lawrence 2002; and see Dillis et al. Chapter 19, this volume). Concerns about pesticides, animal mistreatment, methane gas emissions and water use have much of the public moving in the direction of conscious food consumerism. Categories such as "fair trade," "organic," "non-GMO" and "biodynamic" can help consumers choose environmentally ethical consumption (see Bennett Chapter 17, this volume).

Gender Equity

Cannabis used to boast a much higher rate of women executives than did other industries, but one study suggests their representation is shrinking. A 2017 survey of 567 founders and executives found that the proportion of cannabis industry executives in the U.S. who were female fell from 36% in 2015 to 27% in 2017 (Harris 2019; McDonough 2018). While that rate is still above the rate of 23% for all U.S. businesses, women are losing ground in cannabis. Scholars who study gender bias have an opportunity to study this in real time.

In addition to hiring, women are less likely to be approved for business loans in general (Fay and Williams 1993; Beck, Behr, and Madestam 2018). Those who work on the issue of gender equity in the workplace should examine the cannabis industry and how it might preserve these gains compared to the general business landscape and address missteps before it's too late. The shift of cannabis from a movement to an industry can be seen in the makeup of those who run it. In advocacy, women are often center stage, while men dominate the business space (Levitt 2011). As the industry consolidates resources and market control as well as "professionalizes" its practices, we are vulnerable to the same gender inequities seen in other industries such as tech and finance (Hicks 2018).

An opportunity exists here to acknowledge and address the institutional biases before they take root. There are substantial ways to use the current cannabis industry experience to address these inequities, but it will take the partnership with and participation of persons and organizations historically dedicated to reforming gender-biased institutions. The regulated cannabis industry provides a specific opportunity to study gender differences and related biases in the business world. The negative impact of a woman's assertiveness style, decision-making and financial proactivity have been studied in the context of gender equity in business, and these phenomena are playing out as the cannabis industry seeks stable footing (Bossuyt and Van Kenhove 2018; Koch, D'Mello, and Sackett 2015; Ongena and Popov 2016).

Race and Transformative Justice

When considering racial equity in business, research suggests that promoting this value is economically beneficial (Turner 2016). And while cannabis equity programs are a supposedly helpful way to bring this issue into the conversation, they rarely accomplish addressing the system that created the problem in the first place. Proposition 64 in California did not address equity specifically, except to say that those who had been convicted of a cannabis crime could not be denied participation in the new industry (Adult Use of Marijuana Act 2016). After the passage of Prop. 64, the discussion of who would be first in line to participate in the regulated industry began to emerge. Cannabis equity programs were pioneered by the city of Oakland, California. The idea behind them is to allow communities most affected by the War on Drugs to have first shot at licenses under a legal regime. These programs take the form of priority licenses, incubation opportunities and reduced costs for entry (Rustin 2019).

While well intentioned, some question whether they are enough to fully address the underlying socioeconomic issues caused by years of cannabis prohibition. The Hood Incubator was formed in Oakland to help those who qualify for equity licenses become successful business people (www.HoodIncubator.org). However, as programs like the Hood Incubator note, simply handing a license over to someone who has experienced a lifetime of inequality and lack of opportunity does nothing to prepare them for business ownership (Hood Incubator 2019). Various models of cannabis equity are beginning to emerge in the U.S., and their outcomes should be evaluated (Ravani 2019; Enwemeka 2018; Pyke 2019).

Today, conversations about cannabis legalization come with a lot of lip service to giving opportunities to those most impacted by the drug war (Dickinson 2019). Can we use cannabis prohibition, something that has negatively impacted the lives of so many in such a long-lasting way, to start a real conversation about transformation in the context of equity?

A real conversation about transformation vs. equity starts at restorative justice. Restorative justice focuses on holding offenders accountable for the harms they have inflicted on a community. In the context of cannabis prohibition, the harms inflicted on communities were often at the hands of law enforcement, driven by militant policies and procedures (Brooks 2019; Valencia 2017). Efforts to acknowledge these harms and engage in restorative justice have appeared in equity programs. But are they really achieving restorative justice? Equity programs may seek to create an equal playing field in the workforce, but restorative justice policies would seek to remove from an individual the stigma and barriers that prevent successful integration into a productive life along with the tools to overcome the barriers instilled by prohibition. Restorative measures can include financial reparations, the expungement of records, retroactive release from prison and other programs that grant land and other opportunities to those who have been oppressed by institutional racism and biases (Zehr and Mika 2014).

An approach that goes beyond restorative justice and speaks to the opportunity for sustained change as a result of the provisions made for harms caused is transformative justice, in which the impacted person is not just restored but actually transformed (Gready and Robins 2014; Johnstone 2011). An example from the cannabis space would be to not simply hand over a business license in an attempt to restore what was taken under prohibition, but to also offer business and life skills training to give the opportunity for personal transformation. These types of programs have been found to have the longest lasting impacts on self-sufficiency and betterment of personal situations caused by structural racism (Evans 2015). In addition to a socioeconomic context, transformative justice has been studied from an agribusiness perspective, which is relevant for farmers who have been impacted by cannabis prohibition and speaks to redistribution of land (Coolsaet 2015). These movements towards transformative justice practices can and should be inclusive in cannabis policy reform, and the impacts of these programs, which often vary from state to state, can be analyzed to determine which program characteristics encourage or hinder success.

After decades of tough-on-crime politics, criminal justice reform is on the national agenda. Since cannabis legalization has been promoted as a way to address racial disparities in the criminal justice system, the two issues are intertwined. Working with organizations such as the ACLU and Black Lives Matter on the issue of transformative justice for cannabis should be an easy sell, and it should be a part of every cannabis legalization bill or initiative. Legalization frameworks should, at a minimum, include automatic expungement of records, retroactive release, employment and ownership protections for those with drug felonies, and provide equity and business training opportunities for those impacted by the drug war. In 2018, Rep. Barbara Lee from California introduced the RESPECT resolution in the U.S. House of Representatives. The resolution called on states to

> adopt best practices and take bold steps referred to in subsection (b) to address disparities in the cannabis marketplace participation and to address, reverse, and repair the most egregious effects of the war on drugs on communities of color, in particular to those who now hold criminal records for a substance that is now legal and regulated.

The steps suggested included

1. Establishing reasonable licensing and application fees.
2. Allowing localities to comply with the minimum requirements of the state and not instituting license caps.
3. Prioritize licensing for those impacted by the drug war.
4. Regulations that favor smaller cultivators.
5. Allowing those with criminal histories to participate in the industry.
6. Automatic expungement.
7. Resentencing options for those currently incarcerated for cannabis.
8. Eliminating suspicionless drug testing.
9. Allowing those currently under state supervision to participate in the industry.
10. Tax revenue earmarked for community reinvestment.
11. Oversight bodies that reflect the demographics of the community.
12. Requirement around the use of ancillary and support businesses run by those impacted by the drug war.
13. Establishing public consumption areas (Lee 2018, 3–7).

Research on the intersection between cannabis-related transformative justice measures and socio-economic and neighborhood effects would be a fascinating research topic.

Economic Justice

For decades, people have been supporting their families and their communities via the underground cannabis economy. Now that the risk is more in picking the wrong business partners than being arrested, are we going to sit by and watch already well-financed people win this game while those with traditionally less opportunity sit on the sidelines? As financial capitalism becomes more involved, the consolidation of the cannabis industry is happening quickly, and thus the chance to study it in its nascent state is short-lived. In 2018 the Democratic Economic Committee released a report on the national cannabis economy, finding that

> The legalization of cannabis has significant implications for state economies, as well as the national economy. The industry totaled more than $8 billion in sales in 2017, with sales estimated to reach $11 billion this year and $23 billion by 2022. There were more than 9,000 active licenses for cannabis businesses in the U.S. in 2017, with the industry employing more than 120,000 people.
>
> *(Joint Economic Committee 2018, 1)*

Cannabis legalization presents a naturally occurring experiment in market formation, and if we don't shine a light on the issue of economic justice, we are missing an amazing opportunity. Capitalism benefits those with means. The economic barriers to entry are high, and usually only those who can afford the financial risk can reap the rewards. And while this issue intersects with racial and gender equity, it also falls heavily on whether it is possible to create an economically equitable space in a society dominated by financial capitalism.

The cost to enter the cannabis space is prohibitive to smaller players (Kovacevich 2019). The initial lack of access to banking, including small business loans and services, makes starting up difficult without private capital to pay the initial licensing fees and operational costs. The high costs of licensure and maintaining compliance poses a financial challenge. Some states such as Florida have instituted caps on licensure (Smith 2019). Because this is intended to limit both the size of the market and the number of players, those who are more well financed will often be the ones who obtain the licenses. There are organizations that focus on access to business services and success for lower income people, such as locally run economic development corporations (www.edfc.org). However, government agencies like the Federal Small Business Administration are prohibited from working with cannabis businesses. Some policy options are being developed to support easier entry into the marketplace, such as allowing businesses to run from homes or to be run collectively. One example is the S license in CA, which allows licensed manufacturers to share the same premises (Gue 2018). The study of whether these policies have been successful in reducing barriers for small cannabis businesses can help drive future policy priorities.

Research Directions and Opportunities

The Schedule I status of cannabis still stymies research. This occurs not just in access to funding for carrying out research, but also in the bias towards studies that are looking for anything other than harms (National Academy of Sciences 2017). Given the growing legitimacy of not just the use of cannabis but the industry being created around it, avenues for research are opening up that did not previously exist (PBS 2019).

Some U.S. states, such as California, will allocate tax revenue from legalized cannabis to support both medical research and public health outcome research once revenue for these programs is produced via taxes. In response to this, universities in California have begun to institutionalize cannabis research centers. UCSD, UCLA, UC Berkeley and UC Davis have all launched cannabis research arms, while Humboldt State University established the Humboldt Institute for Interdisciplinary Marijuana Research before it was legal in California.

Social science think tanks such as Research Triangle International (RTI) and the Pacific Institute for Research and Evaluation are also proposing social science research around cannabis. In 2017, RTI published a study on cannabis consumer decision-making and budtender experience (Peiper et al. 2017).

In the absence of public research funding, the industry plays a role as well. BDS Analytics and New Frontier have become two of the larger "big data" firms in the cannabis space. BDS focuses on market and industry data while New Frontier does more research on the bigger picture of the cannabis industry as it relates to public health and economic and environmental impact. Leafly, a company that works with cannabis labs to provide information and guidance to consumers, has a consumer database of hundreds of thousands if not millions of cannabis consumers' ratings and descriptions of various cannabis strains. Other cannabis data firms include Headset, Zephyr, The Brightfield Group, Jade Insights, Strainprint, Cannabis Benchmarks and Cannabis Big Data (Cannabis Big Data n.d.). Engaging these entities in academic research partnerships can further the science necessary to change policy and develop industry infrastructure from a public health perspective.

Following with the theme of "cannabis and . . ." are research opportunities beyond the cannabis space. Allied organizations across environmental, racial, gender and economic justice fields have an interest in seeing well-written socially and environmentally minded cannabis policies. And while the need for such inquiry may have been rebuffed in the past as inconsequential, it is hard for any organization to now overlook the opportunity to use the excitement around cannabis to further their own cause.

Regarding research focus, helping the public understand not only cannabis use, its impacts and the impacts of various policies, but also the connection of cannabis to these other progressive areas is key if allied relationships are to work. Helping those who care about gender equity and environmentalism understand the connection, similarities and potential of intersecting with cannabis broadens our world and makes the issues about more than just the plant, which, in the long run, is how you build lasting social change.

Sample Research Questions

One of the hopes in writing this chapter is that it can inspire both cannabis researchers and those in the allied fields of environmental science, gender studies, and racial and economic justice work. The opportunities to study the cannabis industry itself and integrate what we learn with existing social policy concerns can breathe new life into some age-old questions. The following are some sample research questions generated from the discussion in this chapter.

Environmentalism:

1. How can energy consumption data from various types of cannabis cultivation techniques inform the discussion of climate change?
2. How do regenerative cannabis farming methods impact land health and carbon suppression caused by the meat industry?

Gender Equity:

1. What is the impact of "professionalization" on gender equity in the cannabis industry?
2. Do women-run cannabis businesses better understand and meet the needs of female and therapeutic consumers?

Race, Transformative and Economic Justice:

1. How has cannabis policy reform impacted indicators of community health?
2. What elements of local cannabis equity programs are related to success among participants and how do we incorporate these elements into broader social programs?
3. How do policing practices change post legalization around both cannabis and other crimes?
4. What are successful policies for ensuring the inclusion and success of small businesses in the cannabis industry?
5. How can the use of land grants, co-op models and other alternative structures provide cannabis cultivation opportunities for economically vulnerable people in rural areas?

Conclusion

Cannabis prohibition is a blip in the plant's lifespan. Used therapeutically across cultures for thousands of years, the war on cannabis and its designation as a dangerous drug with no medical value lasted for less than 100. And while in the context of thousands of years 100 does not seem like such a long time, it did a great deal to set society back in terms of research, development of societal norms around cannabis use and business practices for a cannabis industry.

So, while the plant has a long history, we are just beginning efforts to maximize the benefits and minimize the harms to individuals and their environments as a result of both cannabis use and prohibition. And while public health and medical research are vital to fulfilling that goal, research on the developing industry is just as important for preventing some of the pitfalls of other industries that exacerbate the structural racism and sexism already in place and maintain a consumer-driven, environmentally taxing system of big businesses and bigger bank accounts. Cannabis will not solve these problems, but putting the process of legalization under the microscope and using it to better understand the deeper systems of oppression and destruction at play in other American industries can further the cause by using cannabis as a catalyst for research, discussion and change.

References

The Adult Use of Marijuana Act. 2016. https://static.cdfa.ca.gov/MCCP/document/Comprehensive%20Adult%20Use%20of%20Marijuana%20Act.pdf.

Basas, Carrie. 2014. "Advocacy Fatigue: Self-Care, Disability Discrimination, and Legal Attrition." https://ssrn.com/abstract=2478900.

Beck, Thorsten, Patrick Behr, and Andreas Madestam. 2018. "Sex and Credit: Is There Gender Bias in Lending?" *Journal of Banking and Finance* 87. https://ssrn.com/abstract=2126489.

Bossuyt, Saar, and Patrick Van Kenhove. 2018. "Assertiveness Bias in Gender Ethics Research: Why Women Deserve the Benefit of the Doubt." *Journal of Business Ethics* 150 (3): 727–39.

Bourque, Andre. 2019. "Perhaps Jack Herer Was Right, the Future of Mankind May Be Hemp." *Forbes*, July 8. www.forbes.com/sites/andrebourque/2019/07/08/perhaps-jack-herer-was-right-the-future-of-mankind-may-be-hemp/#33ffc0705d98.

Brooks, Ryan. 2019. "Cory Booker Said His Fight to Legalize Pot Is About 'Restorative Justice' For Communities Hit by The War On Drugs." *BuzzFeed News*, February 28. www.buzzfeednews.com/article/ryancbrooks/cory-booker-legal-pot-2020-election.

Brother David's. n.d. www.brotherdavids.com/.

Cannabis Big Data. n.d. "Data Companies in the Cannabis Industry." https://cannabisbigdata.co/data-insights/data-companies-in-the-cannabis-industry/.

Coolsaet, Brendan. 2015. "Transformative Participation in Agrobiodiversity Governance: Making the Case for an Environmental Justice Approach." *Journal of Environmental and Agricultural Ethics* 28 (6): 1089–104.

Corva, Dominic. 2014. "Requiem for a CAMP: The Life and Death of a Domestic U.S. Drug War Institution." *International Journal of Drug Policy* 25 (1): 71–80.

Dickinson, Tim. 2019. "Why Cory Booker Cares so Much About Legal Weed." *Rolling Stone*, May 2. www.rollingstone.com/politics/politics-features/2020-cory-booker-legal-weed-pot-cannabis-why-826232/.

Drug Policy Alliance. n.d. "Race and the Drug War." www.drugpolicy.org/issues/race-and-drug-war.

Enwemeka, Zeninjor. 2018. "How Mass Plans to Create Equity in its Marijuana Industry." *WBUR*, June 27. www.wbur.org/bostonomix/2018/06/27/massachusetts-marijuana-equity.

Evans, Matthew. 2015. "Structural Violence, Socioeconomic Rights and Transformative Justice." *Journal of Human Rights* 15 (1): 1–20.

Fay, Michael, and Lesley Williams. 1993. "Gender Bias and the Availability of Business Loans." *Journal of Business Venturing* 8 (4): 363–76.

Flock, Elizabeth, and Mark Scialla. 2019. "Illegal Marijuana Growers Poison Forests-These People Fight Back." *National Geographic*, April 8, 2018. www.nationalgeographic.com/environment/2019/04/illegal-marijuana-growing-threatens-california-national-forests/.

Gabriel, Trip. 2019. "Legalizing Marijuana, with a Focus on Social Justice, Unites 2020 Democrats." *New York Times*, March 17. www.nytimes.com/2019/03/17/us/politics/marijuana-legalize-democrats.html.

Gready, Paul, and Simon Robins. 2014. "From Transitional to Transformative Justice: A New Agenda for Practice." *International Journal of Transitional Justice* 8 (3): 339–61.

Gue, Blair. 2018. "New 'Type S' License Information Released by The California Department of Public Health's Manufactured Cannabis Safety Branch." *Rogoway Law Group*, April 4. www.rogowaylaw.com/new-type-s-license-information-released-california-department-public-healths-manufactured-cannabis-safety-branch/.

Harris, Lissa. 2019. "Women Are Disappearing from the Cannabis Industry, Why?" *Green Entrepreneur*, May 26. www.greenentrepreneur.com/article/333207.

Hicks, Mary. 2018. "Why Tech's Gender Problem is Nothing New." *The Guardian*, October 12. www.theguardian.com/technology/2018/oct/11/tech-gender-problem-amazon-facebook-bias-women.

Hood Incubator. 2019. www.thehoodincubator.org.

Horrigan, Leo, Polly Walker, and Robert Lawrence. 2002. "How Sustainable Agriculture Can Address the Environmental and Human Health Harms of Industrial Agriculture." *Environmental Health Perspectives* 110 (5): 445–56.

Jenkins, J. 1983. "Resource Mobilization Theory and the Study of Social Movements." *Annual Review of Sociology* 9: 527–53.

Johnstone, Jerry. 2011. *Restorative Justice: Ideas, Values, Debates*. London: Routledge.

Joint Economic Committee. 2018. "The National Cannabis Economy." www.jec.senate.gov/public/_cache/files/bf473de9-98bb-4465-a310-de992926409a/national-cannabis-economy-final.pdf.

Koch, Amanda, Susan D'Mello, and Paul Sackett. 2015. "A Meta-Analysis of Gender Stereotypes and Bias in Experimental Simulations of Employment Decision Making." *Journal of Applied Psychology* 100 (1): 128–61.

Kovacevich, Nick. 2019. "The Hidden Costs of the Cannabis Business." *Forbes*, February 1. www.forbes.com/sites/nickkovacevich/2019/02/01/the-hidden-costs-of-the-cannabis-business/#3f341bb37da3.

Lee, Barbara. 2018. RESPECT Resolution. https://lee.house.gov/imo/media/doc/LEE.RESPECT.pdf.

Levitt, Dana. 2011. "Women and Leadership: A Developmental Paradox?" *Adultspan* 9 (2): 66–75.

MacBride, Katie. 2019. "Protecting Pleasure: Inside the Fight for Safe Cannabis for All." *Playboy*, July 2. www.playboy.com/read/protecting-pleasure-inside-the-fight-for-safe-cannabis.

McCarthy, John, and Mayer Zald. 1977. "Resource Mobilization and Social Movements: A Partial Theory." *American Journal of Sociology* 82 (6): 1212–41.

McDonough, Elise. 2018. "9 Female Owned Cannabis Companies Crushing it in California." *Leafly*, October 24. www.leafly.com/news/industry/9-female-owned-cannabis-companies-crushing-it-in-california.

Miller, Char. 2018. *Where There's Smoke: The Environmental Science, Public Policy and Politics of Marijuana*. Lawrence, KS: University Press of Kansas.

Mills, Evan. 2012. "The Carbon Footprint of Indoor Cannabis Production." *Energy Policy* 46: 58–67.

National Academies of Sciences. 2017. *Challenges and Barriers in Conducting Cannabis Research*. Washington, DC: National Academies Press.

National Institute on Drug Abuse. 2019. "NIDA's Mission." www.drugabuse.gov/about-nida/strategic-plan/nidas-mission.

New Frontier Data, Scale Microgrid Solution and the Resource Innovation Institute. 2019. "The 2018 Cannabis Energy Report." https://newfrontierdata.com/product/2018-cannabis-energy-report/.

Ongena, Steven, and Alexander Popov. 2016. "Gender Bias and Credit Access." *Journal of Money, Credit and Banking* 48 (8): 1691–724.

Paniello, Andrew. 2018. "5 Things You Need to Know About the Cannabis Industry." *Yahoo Finance*, October 23. https://finance.yahoo.com/news/5-things-know-cannabis-industry-115706903.html.

PBS. 2019. "Why So Many Americans Now Support Legalizing Marijuana, in 4 Charts." *PBS*, February 5. www.pbs.org/newshour/science/why-so-many-americans-now-support-legalizing-marijuana-in-4-charts.

Peiper, Nick, Camille Gourdet, Angelica Meinhofer, Amanda Reiman, and Nicco Reggente. 2017. "Medical Decision-Making Processes and Online Behaviors Among Cannabis Dispensary Staff." *Substance Abuse: Research and Treatment* 11: 1–9. https://doi.org/10.1177/1178221817725515.

Pyke, Alan. 2019. "Illinois' Cannabis Bill is First to Incorporate Reparations—the Dream of Legalization Movement." *Think Progress*, June 26. https://thinkprogress.org/illinois-cannabis-bill-first-to-incorporate-reparations-c0dff8d5f77b/.

Ravani, Sarah. 2019. "Oakland's Groundbreaking Cannabis Equity Program Showing Modest Results so Far." *San Francisco Chronicle*, May 25. www.sfchronicle.com/bayarea/article/Oakland-s-groundbreaking-cannabis-equity-13895654.php.

Reiman, Amanda. 2019. "The Environmental Impact of Cannabis Legalization." *Cannabis Now*, January 21. https://cannabisnow.com/the-environmental-impact-of-cannabis-cultivation/.

Resource Innovation Institute. 2019. https://resourceinnovation.org/about/.

Rustin, Zack. 2019. "How Cannabis Equity Programs are Shaping the Industry's Future." *Civilized*, January 2. www.civilized.life/articles/how-cannabis-equity-programs-are-shaping-the-industrys-future/.

Sernoffsky, Evan. 2019. "Statewide Pot Raids Target Illegal Grows in 39 Counties-52 Arrested." *San Francisco Chronicle*, March 1. www.sfchronicle.com/crime/article/California-pot-bust-police-raid-illegal-grows-in-13282815.php.

Smith, Jeff. 2019. "Florida Judge: State's Medical Cannabis Dispensary Cap Unconstitutional." *Marijuana Business Daily*, February 4. https://mjbizdaily.com/florida-medical-marijuana-dispensary-cap-unconstitutional-judge-rules/.

Turner, Ani. 2016. "The Business Case for Racial Equity." *National Civic Review* 105 (1): 21–29.

Union of Concerned Scientists. n.d. "Hidden Costs of Industrial Agriculture." www.ucsusa.org/food_and_agriculture/our-failing-food-system/industrial-agriculture/hidden-costs-of-industrial.html.

Valencia, Leslie. 2017. "Equitable Cannabis Policy: Economic Equity for Low Income Communities of Color in California." Accessed November 14, 2020. www.dialogue4health.org/resource-library/detail/leslie-valencia-equitable-cannabis-policy-recommendations.

Zehr, Howard, and Harry Mika. 2014. "Fundamental Concepts of Restorative Justice." In *Restorative Justice: Ideals and Realities*, edited by Theo Gavrielides. London: Routledge. https://doi.org/10.4324/9781351150125.

29

Conflict and Consensus When Worlds Collide

The Intersection of Cannabis Citizen Science and Academia

Michelle Sexton

Keywords: Cannabidiol (CBD); citizen science; evidence base; human protections; medical ethics

Introduction: Deceptive Industry Practice Exposed

I opened the first cannabis analytical (potency) testing facility in Washington State in 2010 as a means of formal investigation into the chemical composition of medical cannabis. There was no clear formal path in academia for researching therapeutic benefits. This chemical analysis allowed a means to understand milligram-based dosing and for guiding patients.

A year later a story broke about a young boy in San Francisco whose intractable seizure was alleviated by a cannabidiol (CBD) product (known as CBD-dominant cannabis) purchased at a dispensary. The story spread like wildfire through the pediatric seizure community.[1] Although multiple drugs are typically prescribed for these patients, they suffer from drug side effects and often do not gain seizure control.

My medical practice was subsequently flooded with families seeking guidance in administering CBD-dominant medical cannabis to their children with epilepsy. My naturopathic medical practice had become specialized in medical cannabis since completing a three-year full-time postdoctoral fellowship at the University of Washington. In the Department of Pharmacology, we studied the role of the endocannabinoid system in a variety of health conditions including seizure, brain tumors, ALS and multiple sclerosis and brain inflammation. This immersion in cannabinoid pharmacology had left me very curious about medical cannabis and identifying the potencies and chemotypes[2] that were effective for patients.

One affected family came to my clinic with their five-year-old daughter Haley (not her real name) who had a diagnosis of Dravet syndrome.[3] Because Haley could experience 100 seizures per hour, she and her entire family suffered, as they would be watchful for her even throughout the night. They attended a cannabis farmers' market where a young man had sold them a tub of "CBD"

DOI: 10.4324/9780429320491-29

butter.[4] They took the procured butter home, administered what they described to be "about a teaspoon" and described witnessing what to them was a miracle: Haley slept all night and had no seizures. Both parents were nurses by training and, together, we searched the medical literature and synthesized a dose escalation schedule which was widely adopted ultimately across the US (Porter and Jacobson 2013; Sexton 2012b).

Subsequent chemical analysis revealed, however, that the butter contained no CBD. The cannabinoid content was instead primarily delta-9 tetrahydrocannabinol (THC). We calculated she had been given approximately a 10 mg dose of THC, also known to have anti-seizure benefit (Wada, Sato, and Corcoran 1973). The good news was that Haley slept all night with no apparent harm done. My perspective was that harm, in the form of misrepresentation of the product to a highly vulnerable family, had occurred. I called the vendor who had sold the butter who told me that the CBD must have "boiled off," which I knew was bogus. CBD has been shown to convert to THC, but this requires a strong acid reaction and does not occur simply with heat (Gaoni and Mechoulam 1966; Quarles, Ellman, and Jones 1973; Baek 1985).

The Genesis of the CBD Revolution and the Rise of Cannabis Citizen Science

Cannabis had been bred for high-THC content, but a renaissance in cannabis biodiversity was occurring. Northern California breeders had been breeding cannabis for CBD-dominant chemotypes.[5] Ultimately, one of the families travelled there to secure clones of a specific chemotype, "ACDC," and brought it to the Seattle area. This plant was a cross of "Cannatonic," a chemotype imported from Spain,[6] with "NYC Diesel." A local Seattle grower established ACDC clones that consistently produced 18% CBD with less than 1% THC and used an ethanol extraction process to make a solid extract.[7] The company gave the product away through a program called "Leaf of Hope." The patients using this experienced a range of improvements in seizure occurrence, sleep, motor skills and quality of life.

Over the next decade, cannabis citizen science (CS) began to grow and flourish, creating challenges for doctors and patients. The political (Schedule 1 status) and economic climate of cannabis in the United States led to non-science-based products that have not filled the research gaps. The primary gap has occurred from the prohibition of the medical community from performing research that normally builds the evidence base for therapies.

Traditionally, botanical medicines are created from "whole plant" extractions. This allows for the synergistic effect of many compounds, effects that are not well suited to research methods designed for isolated molecules (Wang et al. 2005).[8] The rise of anecdotal evidence led to the cannabis industry and its citizen scientists skipping some important research steps (pharmacology) and conducting formal safety and efficacy experiments with their products on humans. Enter the uncontrolled clinical trial.

Clinical trials are intended to demonstrate the efficacy of a new treatment by comparing the people treated with an active medicine to a control group receiving a placebo or a compared medication (Sacca 2010). The randomized controlled clinical trial (RCT) is considered to be the gold standard for human research and the ethical foundation governing clinical practice internationally. Historically, this gold-standard evidence base[9] for cannabis scarcely exists. Along with many other botanical medicines, the historical and anecdotal data on its use (over centuries) has served as the safety data.[10]

The large-scale *uncontrolled* clinical trials (no comparison group or placebo control) being conducted by CS with cannabis is a structural effect of the Schedule 1 status. But despite this status, the personal human relationships cultivated with cannabis medicine led this botanical medicine down a very different path from other medical treatments.

Blurring the Lines Between Marketing and Medicine

What occurred as a direct result of both Schedule 1 *and* the CBD renaissance was a chain of events starting with "Charlotte's Web." This is a product named after Charlotte Figi and catalyzed by her story with Dravet syndrome. Her intractable seizures were reported to be 100% controlled by administering the "oil" (a solid extract diluted into olive oil), allowing her to completely discontinue use of all of her anti-epileptic drugs (Maa and Figi 2014). This child, her miraculous response and the product named after her was instrumental in deconstructing the general public's stigma about medical.[11]

The burgeoning cannabis and hemp industries subsequently seized on this opportunity, with a deluge of patient-branded products flooding the market: "Jayden's Juice," "Haleigh's Hope," "Palmetto's Harmony," "Myriam's Hope" and "Riley's Sunshine" (not all children). This was an entirely new marketing ploy: exploitation of a patient's illness, using the patient's name, bringing very emotional messaging to highly vulnerable patients (or their parents). These vulnerable populations are known to be well suited for a heightened placebo effect (Benedetti 2012). This could be considered as a form of disease mongering insofar as those marketing CBD products were aggressively promoting public awareness of the range of conditions allegedly targeted by their concoction and therefore were exploitative of patients. In essence, the evolving cannabis industry, which emerged from the political frame of "compassionate care,"[12] now seems to be mirroring drug companies' corporate processes by forging informal alliances, comprised of patient groups and industry professionals, to widen the market for sales (Wolinsky 2005).

The modern commodification of cannabis can be likened to the patent medicine phenomenon of the early 1900s associated with the term "miracle-cure mania." A 1905 exposé written about this phenomenon led to the first Food and Drug Act in 1906 (Adams 1907). Patent medicine salesmen boasted that their concoctions would cure almost anything (similar to cannabis claims) with products named after the unscrupulous healers marketing them (e.g. "Dromgools Bitters," "Clark Stanley's Snake Oil Liniment," among many others). Here the key motivation was not healing the patient but sales (Young 1961). This is a conflict of interest, illustrated in present time by the opioid crisis, where pharmaceutical companies market opioids with the goal of financial gain (Robertson 2019). The purveyors of new cannabis patent medicines have not identified *or* disclosed financial conflicts of interest to the patients.

So, while cannabis entrepreneurs and enthusiasts stepped into a research void, the CS movement acting in isolation from academics was necessary, but it is not sufficient for protecting human subjects moving forward.

Is Citizen Science Reflective of a Larger Social Shift?

Taken in the context of societal shifts towards "peer-to-peer" (P2P) societies,[13] where tasks previously in the hands of institutions are shared with individuals/collectives, there is a necessary and valuable role for CS (Wildschut 2017). The tools necessary to conduct basic science research (even basic cannabis analytics) have been prohibited in academia.[14] CS became a perfect venue for acquisition of cannabis knowledge disallowed for formal academic researchers.

However, the blurring of lines between the direct marketing of cannabis and ethical considerations are a result of politics causing doctors to ignore the science (Ziemianski et al. 2015; Carlini, Garrett, and Carter 2017; Philpot, Ebbert, and Hurt 2019). The combination of the public dissatisfaction with cannabis prohibition, the lack of research on potential benefits and the government's insistence that cannabis has no medical benefit (Schedule 1 designation) created a "perfect storm" for CS to step in.

The insufficient evidence base, potential ethical considerations, dubious conclusions, out-of-pocket costs for uncontrolled trials and unreserved claims about the medical utility of cannabis products are of concern to the medical community (Ayers, Caputi, and Leas 2019). In the absence of adequately trained licensed healthcare providers to advise patients, uncredentialed individuals[15] stepped in to fill a gap by serving as healthcare provider proxies, promoting and advocating the use of medical cannabis. This scenario has precipitated several potential concerns.

1. Unlicensed individuals often lack formal medical training and therefore are not capable of identifying when medical risk is present.[16] This is highlighted by a story of a patient who was suffering from neuropathic pain with a history of anxiety treated by Xanax.[17] Her doctor had recently rapidly reduced her Xanax dose, greatly exacerbating her anxiety (a withdrawal symptom). She visited a dispensary where a patient "consultant" who calls herself "Dr. Beth" (she has no medical degree) advised her to inhale off of a vaporizer pen (highly concentrated THC $\cong$ 70%) every ten minutes. The patient followed her instructions, inhaling every ten minutes for two hours. She subsequently presented to the emergency department for uncontrolled anxiety.
2. There is substantial competition for cannabis sales, whether adult-use or medical intent, because the various states' regulatory frameworks have made it difficult for companies to succeed.[18] Reports that companies pay commissions to dispensary employees put the dispensary personnel in the position of acting with an undisclosed conflict of interest. These under-the-table payments by cannabis product companies to dispensary personnel are occurring and are unethical.[19] A "budtender" may recommend a cannabis product to a patient, not based on whether it is the best fit for the patient's medical condition, but because they receive a commission for sales.
3. Finally, the industry and dispensary personnel as well as medical consultants are not oriented toward fundamentals of medical ethics, including informed consent regarding other treatment options (Haug et al. 2016). In most instances they are, effectively, practicing medicine without a license. They may be making recommendations that conflict with guidelines from national organizations, and/or have no evidence base.[20] This may actually harm the patient, as illustrated by the two stories shared here (patient with Dravet syndrome and patient with severe anxiety) (Dickson et al. 2018).

Doing No Harm

The Hippocratic oath taken by doctors includes an axiom and tenet of medicine "*primum non nocere*"—"first, to do no harm" (Smith 2005). This is an axiom unrecognized by the supplement industry in general, and the cannabis industry particularly, by those on pro-cannabis crusades and those profiting from sales. While the Dietary Health and Supplement Act (DSHEA), as an arm of the FDA, is tasked with regulating dietary supplements, the enforcement for unscrupulous players is lacking, and there is a need for better quality control (QC) and policing of the entire industry. The scrutiny of cannabis quality, as evidenced by state regulations requiring QC for licensed cannabis and related products, is a harbinger of what is coming for the supplement industry at large.

The commercial interests of both the cannabis and the pharmaceutical industries are "over-medicalizing" patients (Kaczmarek 2019). This occurs by direct marketing of potentially unnecessary interventions, which can be economically or physiologically harmful to the patient.[21] Patients are bombarded with cannabis advertising and claims as a miracle cure (for everything apparently), while having to pay out-of-pocket for these unsubstantiated claims.

Here I am proposing an alternative hypothesis to the "cannabis as miracle cure" hypothesis: cannabis sold as medicine with unverified claims is a potential harm to patients. Awareness needs to be brought to the potential harms of the cannabis-industrial complex. Harms mentioned earlier in the chapter include (1) physical harm (patient who went to the Emergency Department), (2) ethical harm: being lied to (pediatric epilepsy patient and butter with no CB content) and (3) economic harm: selling products that have no known efficacy for the presenting symptom.[22] There is, of course, a great need to expand the evidence base for cannabis, and here is where academic and CS knowledge need to converge.

Human Subjects Research

Cannabis manufacturers and patient advocates have taken on the role of the clinical trial, offering an "uncontrolled" version, often with no medical expertise or training in research ethics and without supervision from those with this training. This can be viewed as a form of medical cultural misappropriation.[23] Previously, academia invited citizens into the data collection process.[24] Now CS has initiated clinical and other research, sometimes despite a lack of training in the methods and ethics used by academic scientists and without the involvement of academia. Conducting human subject research in an academic setting requires satisfying multiple federal policies, put in place to protect human subjects from exploitation. Exploitation of humans, such as that of rural African American men living in poverty in the 1940s Tuskegee Institute,[25] is an example of such exploitation. The National Research Act of 1974 instituted the Internal Review Board (IRB) system to protect human subjects. It has three basic tenets: respect for persons, beneficence and justice (Office of the Secretary 1979).

Informed consent is another important piece of patient protection: a formal process through which specific disclosure occurs. Study subjects must be provided a clear assessment of benefits versus risks and fully informed of any potential for harm: legal, social, physical, psychological or economic; *and* provided information on alternative treatments. These human protections have been entirely bypassed by some CS research. In uncontrolled research, there is the potential for false generalizations, for example, "if one child with epilepsy was cured, then mine will be too." Combined, these considerations beg the question "what are the ethical limits to or benefits from CS?"

As with all drugs, there are responders and nonresponders to medical cannabis.[26] This becomes obvious when a patient is monitored clinically over time, with laboratory results for biomarker changes or imaging data to track either progress or lack thereof. There are outliers who may see complete remission of disease or symptoms, such as seizure or pain, while the majority only have partial benefit. Other outliers see no benefit or experience adverse effects and discontinue use. Those who discontinue use or are unsuccessful with cannabis may be in the majority and are the ones who get no media attention. So, what is marketed is not always generalizable to the population at large.

Likewise, with all nutritional supplements, there are concerns that consumers may not be receiving what is advertised. Because of the federal restriction, there is a lack of oversight of cannabis products by DSHEA, and reports of contamination and public health harms have emerged, including the recent reports of lipoid pneumonia[27] (Lenton et al. 2018; Russo 2016; Dryburgh et al. 2018; Sun and McGinley 2019). A task force was convened by the FDA in 2019 to look into adverse reactions, such as acute psychiatric distress, driving impairment and aggression, in products labeled as CBD or hemp oil. One was found to contain a potent synthetic cannabinoid (4-cyano CUMYL-BUTINACA), highlighting the hazards patients face and the public health implications (Horth et al. 2018). The American Herbal Products Association (AHPA) has issued guidance policies for the cannabis and hemp industries such as Good Agricultural Practices (GAP) and Good Manufacturing Processes (GMP). However, while required by DSHEA for approval of any supplement for human research purposes, these policies are voluntary for cannabis.

The Way Forward: Citizens, Scientists and Beyond

I have previously labeled cannabis the "Gateway Herb" (Sexton 2012a) insofar as the United States seems to be in a revival of natural approaches to health, and cannabis can play an important role.[28]

The National Center for Complementary and Alternative Medicine estimated in 2008 that 40% of adults in the US were using some form of integrative care and spending $33.9 out of pocket, since it is rarely covered by health insurance plans. Many of the tools and herbs Americans access, such as cannabis, massage, and acupuncture, have been used as traditional medicine for centuries.[29] An emerging theme from patients investigating medical cannabis is the need for doctors who work with them toward optimal health to be open-minded to new paradigms of healthcare. Patients want and need this new paradigm, and in this sense, cannabis can be viewed as a gateway.

Millions of people who are primarily oriented to pharmaceutical medicines are for the first time stepping outside the conventional medicine box to explore cannabis. Sometimes the cannabis CS movement has facilitated this move. Cannabis seems to be opening the door to what some may consider a "Pandora's box," but others simply see as Robert Frost saw—the gate to a road "less traveled by." The commodification of cannabis needs the counterbalance of quality control, an evidence base, and either affordability or reimbursement for cannabis medicine. The end of prohibition via removal of cannabis from Schedule 1 will open the door for citizens to again work together with the scientific and medical communities and to provide a bridge across the divide that has existed since cannabis was prohibited in the US beginning in the 1920s (Bewley-Taylor 1999).

In the context of rising demand for social and cultural change in the delivery of healthcare, the P2P movement and academics will do well to collaborate on mainstreaming the countercultural shift. This shift calls foremost for the de-scheduling of cannabis to allow for formal investigation of medical-grade cannabis products and public-private partnerships. Patients need affordable medicine, which means removing taxation of medical-grade product and moving towards a model that could provide for reimbursement by insurance. For now, those involved in the commodification of cannabis need to continue to advocate for patients to ensure access to medical-grade product, to insure that medical cannabis is affordable and that the products they are sold are effective *and* safe. We all need to be vigilant to the unique needs of those who are sick while providing a framework to ensure they are not exploited by unfounded claims. It will take all of the sciences, medicine, psychology, pharmacology (discovery of medicine) and pharmacy (distribution of medicine), among others, collaborating with CS to usher in this new healthcare paradigm. Not only overturning the prohibition of cannabis, but also ending the commercialization of medicine altogether and integrating relevant (human) cannabis research into the academic setting are challenges the community as a whole face together.

Notes

1 Families with children who suffer from various forms of seizure disorder unresponsive to anti-epileptic drugs (AEDs).
2 Chemotype is the term used to describe the variety of chemical compositions of cannabis varieties. The term is not used in botany as "strain" is reserved for microbiology.
3 This is one of many intractable epilepsy diagnoses, caused by a genetic mutation.
4 Cannabis flower extracted by heat into ordinary table butter.
5 Including Lawrence Ringo at his ranch in Blocksburg, CA.
6 From Resin Seeds: bred from the "Reina Madre" genetics.
7 In botanical medicine, a substance derived from mixing an herb with a solvent (typically water/alcohol) and then removing the solvent (by evaporation).
8 Pharmacology methods are suitable for a single compound/single target models. Plant compounds are known to be "promiscuous" (hitting more than one target), and botanical medicine is many compounds working alongside one another.
9 Evidence-based practice is the integration of the best research evidence with clinical expertise and patient values.
10 Because botanical medicines are herbs and therefore plants, they are often perceived as natural and therefore safe. This refers to their potential for toxicity or side effects.
11 Dr. Sanjay Gupta, medical correspondent for CNN, helped to fuel this deconstruction via the documentary series *Weed* beginning in 2013 with the story of Charlotte Figi.

12 Programs such as "Leaf of Hope" provided free cannabis to people with serious illness.
13 "P2P is a process or dynamic that can be found in many communities and movements self-organizing around the co-creation of culture and knowledge. Well known general examples include the free/open source software movement; free culture; open hardware; and open access in education and science" (from https://p2pfoundation.net).
14 Due to the Schedule 1 restriction on cannabis and cannabinoid compounds, academic laboratories typically cannot handle Schedule 1 compounds without a DEA license. This DEA license then explicitly prohibits the handling of any non-DEA obtained Schedule 1 compounds—such as cannabis flower accessed locally.
15 These may be "lay" people (those with no formal medical training) who fancy themselves as healers, self-proclaimed experts on the topic of medical cannabis, those hired to work in dispensaries, among others. There are websites devoted to training these persons, such as Healer.com and True Farma Advocate Program.
16 As a corollary, many medical professionals lack training in cannabinoid medicine.
17 A drug in the benzodiazepine class used to treat anxiety and panic disorder.
18 The high cost of licenses, permits, land, security, other startup requirements, as well as a lack of access to financing, present significant barriers impacting who can enter the industry.
19 This was revealed to me personally by the owner of a licensed cannabis distribution company in California.
20 For instance, the American College of Obstetricians and Gynecologists recommends "Women who are pregnant or contemplating pregnancy should be encouraged to discontinue marijuana use."
21 Watch commercial television on any given night to be bombarded by a series of advertisements for pharmaceuticals.
22 New claims, in the interest of sales, are emerging for minor cannabinoids such as CBG, THCV and CBC, which have very little preclinical data and no human data yet available.
23 Adoption of elements of the medical culture by those who are not formally trained in or members of this culture. Some contend that there can be safety risks due to the lack of many years of training and experience by those misappropriating medical culture.
24 While this has not been the case with cannabis, CS has been defined as "the involvement of the public in scientific research—whether community-driven research or global investigations. The Citizen Science Association unites expertise from educators, scientists, data managers, and others to power citizen science" (citizenscience.org).
25 An infamous and unethical clinical study conducted between 1932 and 1972 by the US Public Health Service on syphilis in African American men (White, R.M. 2000).
26 Treatment response rates for specific therapeutic regimens are known to vary based on age, gender, disease severity (and heterogeneity of disease itself), ethnicity, concomitant medication use, and environmental, genetic and other factors. As with other drugs, some patients have a beneficial response to cannabis, others gain no relief or suffer only side effects.
27 A rare inflammatory condition that occurs when fat particles enter the lungs.
28 A healing-oriented medicine that takes account of the whole person, including all aspects of lifestyle. It emphasizes the therapeutic relationship between practitioner and patient, is informed by evidence and makes use of all appropriate therapies.
29 The Chinese Emperor Fu Hsi (ca. 2900 BC), whom the Chinese credit with bringing civilization to China, referenced *Ma*, the Chinese word for cannabis (Deitch, R 2003).

References

Adams, Samuel Hopkins. 1907. *The Great American Fraud*. Chicago: American Medical Association.

Ayers, J. W., T. Caputi, and E. C. Leas. 2019. "The Need for Federal Regulation of Marijuana Marketing." *JAMA*. doi:10.1001/jama.2019.4432.

Baek, S. H., M. Srebnik, and R. Mechoulam. 1985. "Boron Triflouride Etherate on Alimina—a Modified Lewis Acid Reagent. An Improved Synthesis of Cannabidiol . . ." *Tetrahedron Letters* 26: 1083–86.

Benedetti, F. 2012. "The Placebo Response: Science Versus Ethics and the Vulnerability of the Patient." *World Psychiatry* 11 (2): 70–72.

Bewley-Taylor, D. R. 1999. *The United States and International Drug Control 1909–1997*. New York: Continuum.

Carlini, B. H., S. B. Garrett, and G. T. Carter. 2017. "Medicinal Cannabis: A Survey Among Health Care Providers in Washington State." *American Journal of Hospice and Palliative Care* 34 (1): 85–91. doi:10.1177/1049909115604669.

Deitch, R. 2003. *Hemp: American Histor Revisited: The Plant with a Divided History*. Algora Publishing.

Dickson, B., C. Mansfield, M. Guiahi, A. A. Allshouse, L. M. Borgelt, J. Sheeder, R. M. Silver, and T. D. Metz. 2018. "Recommendations From Cannabis Dispensaries About First-Trimester Cannabis Use." *Obstetrics and Gynecology* 131 (6): 1031–38. doi:10.1097/AOG.0000000000002619.

Dryburgh, L. M., N. S. Bolan, C. P. L. Grof, P. Galettis, J. Schneider, C. J. Lucas, and J. H. Martin. 2018. "Cannabis Contaminants: Sources, Distribution, Human Toxicity and Pharmacologic Effects." *British Journal of Clinical Pharmacology* 84 (11): 2468–76. doi:10.1111/bcp.13695.

Gaoni, Y., and R. Mechoulam. 1966. "Hashish—VII: The Isomerization of Cannabidiol to Tetrahydrocannabinols." *Tetrahedron* 22 (4): 1481–88.

Haug, N. A., D. Kieschnick, J. E. Sottile, K. A. Babson, R. Vandrey, and M. O. Bonn-Miller. 2016. "Training and Practices of Cannabis Dispensary Staff." *Cannabis and Cannabinoid Research* 1 (1): 244–51. doi:10.1089/can.2016.0024.

Horth, R. Z., B. Crouch, B. Z. Horowitz, A. Prebish, M. Slawson, J. McNair, C. Elsholz, S. Gilley, J. Robertson, I. Risk, M. Hill, L. Fletcher, W. Hou, D. Peterson, K. Adams, D. Vitek, A. Nakashima, and A. Dunn. 2018. "Notes from the Field: Acute Poisonings from a Synthetic Cannabinoid Sold as Cannabidiol—Utah, 2017–2018." *MMWR Morbidity and Mortality Weekly Rep* 67 (20): 587–88. doi:10.15585/mmwr.mm6720a5.

Kaczmarek, E. 2019. "How to Distinguish Medicalization from Over-Medicalization?" *Medicine and Health Care Philosophy* 22 (1): 119–28. doi:10.1007/s11019-018-9850-1.

Lenton, S., V. A. Frank, M. J. Barratt, G. R. Potter, and T. Decorte. 2018. "Growing Practices and the Use of Potentially Harmful Chemical Additives Among a Sample of Small-Scale Cannabis Growers in Three Countries." *Drug and Alcohol Dependence* 192: 250–56. doi:10.1016/j.drugalcdep.2018.07.040.

Maa, E., and P. Figi. 2014. "The Case for Medical Marijuana in Epilepsy." *Epilepsia* 55 (6): 783–86. doi:10.1111/epi.12610.

Office of the Secretary. 1979. "The Belmont Report." In *Ethical Principles and Guidelines for the Protection of Human Subjects of Research*. HHS.gov Office for Human Research Protections: Department of Health, Education and Welfare. Washington, DC: U.S. Government Printing Office, 20402.

Philpot, L. M., J. O. Ebbert, and R. T. Hurt. 2019. "A Survey of the Attitudes, Beliefs and Knowledge About Medical Cannabis Among Primary Care Providers." *BMC Family Practice* 20 (1): 17. doi:10.1186/s12875-019-0906-y.

Porter, B. E., and C. Jacobson. 2013. "Report of a Parent Survey of Cannabidiol-Enriched Cannabis Use in Pediatric Treatment-Resistant Epilepsy." *Epilepsy and Behavior* 29 (3): 574–77. doi:10.1016/j.yebeh.2013.08.037.

Quarles, W., G. Ellman, and R. Jones. 1973. "Toxicology of Marijuana: Conditions for Conversion of Canandiol to THC upone Smoking." *Clinical Toxicology* 6 (1): 211–16. doi:10.3109/15563657308990520.

Robertson, C. 2019. "Doctors Accused of Trading Opioid Prescriptions for Sex and Cash." *New York Times*, April 17. www.nytimes.com/2019/04/17/us/doctor-arrested-prescription-drugs.html.

Russo, E. B. 2016. "Current Therapeutic Cannabis Controversies and Clinical Trial Design Issues." *Frontiers in Pharmacology* 7: 309. doi:10.3389/fphar.2016.00309.

Sacca, L. 2010. "The Uncontrolled Clinical Trial: Scientific, Ethical, and Practical Reasons for Being." *Internal Emergency Medicine* 5 (3): 201–4. doi:10.1007/s11739-010-0355-z.

Sexton, Michelle. 2012a. "Cannabis, the Gateway Herb: A Doctor Responds." Accessed April 29, 2019. Multidisciplinary Association of Psychedelic Studies, September 19, 2012. https://maps.org/news/media/3248-cannabis-the-gateway-herb-a-doctor-responds.

Sexton, Michelle. 2012b. "An Ethnographic Report of Cannabis Use in Pediatric Intractable Epilepsy Patients." International Cannabinoid Research Society, Baveno, Italy.

Smith, C. M. 2005. "Origin and Uses of Primum Non Nocere-Above All, Do no Harm!" *Journal of Clinical Pharmacology* 45 (4): 371–77. doi:10.1177/0091270004273680.

Sun, L. H., and L. McGinley. 2019. "Most Vaping-Related Lung Injuries Linked to Marijuana Products, CDC Says." *The Washington Post*, September 27. www.washingtonpost.com/health/2019/09/27/most-vaping-related-lung-injuries-linked-marijuana-products-cdc-says/.

Wada, J. A., M. Sato, and M. E. Corcoran. 1973. "Antiepileptic Properties of 9-Tetrahydrocannabinol." *Experimental Neurology* 39 (1): 157–65.

Wang, M., R. J. Lamers, H. A. Korthout, J. H. van Nesselrooij, R. F. Witkamp, R. van der Heijden, P. J. Voshol, L. M. Havekes, R. Verpoorte, and J. van der Greef. 2005. "Metabolomics in the Context of Systems

Biology: Bridging Traditional Chinese Medicine and Molecular Pharmacology." *Phytotherapy Research* 19 (3): 173–82. doi:10.1002/ptr.1624.

White, R. M. 2000. "Unraveling the Tuskegee Study of Untreated Syphilis." Archives of Internal Medicine 160 (5): 585–98.

Wildschut, D. 2017. "The Need for Citizen Science in the Transition to a Sustainable Peer-to-Peer-Society." *Futures* 91: 46–52.

Wolinsky, H. 2005. "Disease Mongering and Drug Marketing. Does the Pharmaceutical Industry Manufacture Diseases as Well as Drugs?" *EMBO Report* 6 (7): 612–14. doi:10.1038/sj.embor.7400476.

Young, J. H. 1961. *The Toadstool Millionaires: A Social History of Patent medicines in America before Federal Regulation*. Princeton, NJ: Princeton University Press.

Ziemianski, D., R. Capler, R. Tekanoff, A. Lacasse, F. Luconi, and M. A. Ware. 2015. "Cannabis in Medicine: A National Educational Needs Assessment Among Canadian Physicians." *BMC Medical Education* 15: 52. doi:10.1186/s12909-015-0335-0.

30

Post-Prohibition Cannabis Research Futures

Joshua S. Meisel and Dominic Corva

Keywords: cannabis, legalization, strict control, social movements, neoliberalism

The chapters assembled in this handbook described a body of scholarship and focal areas for cannabis scholars that is fixed in time and place yet also reveals potential cannabis research futures. We asked handbook contributors to identify emergent research directions to enrich our understanding of how cannabis intersects with governance, public health, markets and society, the environment, and culture and social change. Our aim was to provide readers with reference points for future cannabis scholarship informing scientific knowledge, public policy, and social action. The first part of this conclusion outlines three topics of considerable significance to post-prohibition research agendas, as we have developed that concept in the framing essays. The second part of this conclusion breaks down that significance for each of our five interdisciplinary subject areas collected in the volume.

The Times, They Are a-Changin' . . . Again

In the first part of this conclusion, we consider three key relational characteristics of the varieties of legalization at the time of this writing. We consider the relationship between cannabis legalization and other social movements that emerged at the end of one historical conjuncture, Keynesian liberalism, but is completing at a time of crisis for the one that followed, neoliberalism. We then consider "strict control" legalization as an intermediary, rather than final, variety of legalization relative to prohibition. Finally, we develop a preliminary critique of cannabis commercialization that is critical of its relationship with legal cannabis capitalism rather than its wider access as a dangerous drug.

Legalization After Neoliberalism: Social Movement Contexts This Time

Cannabis legalization, as an organized social movement outcome, appears as an anachronism in the contemporary landscape. As discussed in the introduction, it emerged in the 1960s out of a network of domestic and international liberation movements that were both political and cultural: against postcolonial imperialism on the one hand and against hegemonic cultural values governing

 DOI: 10.4324/9780429320491-30

the reproduction of everyday life under industrial capitalism on the other (Anders 1990). These included but were not limited to a constellation of social movements that gave birth to the "new left," after the decline of the labor movement: women's liberation, the civil rights movement, the free speech movement, liberation from sexual norms, and freedom from gender conformity more broadly. Within the "new left," the counterculture was never a comfortable fit, focused as it was on creating new ways of being in the world rather than revolutionizing or reforming formal political institutions (Rossman 1971). The politics of cannabis legalization as a singular social movement subject emerged from the countercultural wing of the new left, for which it was a legible node in a web of meaning symbolizing anti-systemic subjectivity connected to many, often global others, in a time of global systemic crisis (Wallerstein 2011). As that crisis resolved in the 1970s, it became professionalized as a singular subject of institutional reform rather than countercultural revolution: a struggle for the right to consume provided by constitutionally protected free speech, connected with the political wing of the new right most associated with libertarian, rather than moral, conservatism.

These minoritarian, anti-institutional elements of liberal and conservative political formations were descendant and ascendant, respectively, when the economic crises of the 1970s created openings for new ideas about how to best govern capitalist societies. The postwar Keynesian consensus contained class warfare by promoting job security through strong unions; strong regulations for industrial capitalism; social safety nets and welfare programs for the poor; and high corporate tax rates to finance what would later be called "big government." After 1980, the "new right" created a new political consensus that would eventually be called neoliberalism: an ideology of governance associated above all with the promotion of market solutions to social problems and, if that didn't work, police and prisons for the socioeconomically disadvantaged rather than social welfare programs (Gilmore 2007). The failure of the libertarian right to bring cannabis consumption along for the ride into the era of market freedom can only be explained by the usefulness of drug crimes for bipartisan neoliberal politics of crime control, a strange alliance between moral conservatism and technocratic social engineering.

The political landscape for the re-emergence of cannabis legalization as a social movement in the 21st century is quite different than it was in the 1970s, but it is similar in the sense that, once again, systemic crises have created openings for change. This time, the system in crisis is the one that was emergent in the 1970s, neoliberalism. The fact that cannabis legalization first succeeded in the United States in 2012, four years after a global financial crisis caused by neoliberal economic governance, is probably not a coincidence. The new old world is once again rapidly changing. The politics of penal expansion, as the security partner of market governance, have been increasingly contested since the turn of the 21st century. There are at least three tendencies driving this process that seem directly connected to the politics of cannabis legalization. On the neoliberal left, the disproportionate impact of policing on people of color demonstrates clear evidence of systemic racism, galvanizing the emergence of the Black Lives Matter movement since 2014. Punishment in society is not colorblind, to paraphrase Michelle Alexander (2020). On the neoliberal right, the ideological contradiction between promoting market freedom and imprisoning people for drugs they choose to consume has become unsustainable. And for neoliberal governance right and left, the "war on terror" has displaced the war on drugs in security discourses and practices since 2001, particularly in the United States.

The politics of market governance, though, are the senior partner of the neoliberal consensus. These, too, have been in crisis and can be directly correlated with the growth of commercial cannabis markets, leading up to the first successful cannabis legalization initiatives in the United States. The 2008 financial crisis increased unemployment, made real estate precarious, and bled public sector budgets dry. On the West Coast of the United States, cannabis markets provided a safety valve for unemployed people and underutilized real estate. Public sector stakeholders became focused on the potential of cannabis taxes to help deal with declining revenues. Unlike the 1970s, material economic conditions related to cannabis and its market value (rather than simply its consumption) are useful for proponents of legalization. Ironically, the tax revenue basis of Prohibition 1.0 appears as a significant argument for, and element of, cannabis legalization.

The advertised promise of public and private revenue under conditions of neoliberal crisis constitutes an ideological financialization of arguments for cannabis legalization. This seems fairly straightforward, except that in contemporary contexts of historic economic crises, the neoliberal prescription of "more capitalism" is less convincing than it was in the 1970s, when "more government" collapsed as a consensus solution for social problems. This tension is all the more apparent when one considers the reality of actually existing legal cannabis market formation, which promotes both more capitalism and more government at the same time: legalization with, not after, prohibition, is characterized by "strict control." Adult consumers may access cannabis for consumption, but they may not access it outside of supply chains that can only be owned by a few, usually white, male, and well-capitalized, business interests: the opposite of a neoliberal "free market" and against the interests of racial and ethnic minorities that have been most impacted by the drug war at large and cannabis criminalization in particular.

Strict Control as an Intermediary Reform

The usefulness of strict control and what its alternatives might be thus emerge as subjects of significant relevance to researchers and policy makers, even while the usefulness of prohibition remains for a generation of public servants and private interests that has profited handsomely from it. The prohibition of a plant from free societies has become, in some cases literally, molecularized. The plant has been partially decriminalized not just through strictly controlled legal markets, but also through the widespread decriminalization of its non-THC cannabinoids, of which cannabidiol (CBD) is the most dominant (see Silber-Coats Chapter 18). So, too, has the criminalization of cannabis as a whole plant become compartmentalized: Any adult in a legal jurisdiction can possess a limited amount of cannabis at a time and is free to consume some or all of it in the privacy of their own home. But under conditions of strict control, unlicensed cultivation remains almost entirely criminalized.

This is the main difference between the practicality of decriminalizing or legalizing cannabis in the 1970s and doing so today. In the 1960s and 1970s, the supply chain between cannabis cultivation and its most substantial consumption markets was international, from rural peripheries to urban cores. Against the grain of most other commodity chain tendencies under conditions of neoliberalism, cannabis cultivation was significantly domesticated. This is most clear on the West Coast of the United States, where California producers captured the lion's share of national supply in the period following medical cannabis decriminalization (Central Valley HIDTA 2010). While this is clearly true for any kind of cannabis cultivation, the supply chain glut that busted wholesale prices for cannabis flower between 2008 and 2016 seems to have been driven by rural outdoor cultivation at larger and larger scales, combined with widespread, pre-legal reductions in criminal penalties and risk of exposure to enforcement for simple possession.

"Strict control" legal cannabis markets, especially in places with a robust history of medical cannabis decriminalization, are finding it much more difficult than expected to capture consumer share. This is because, absent the costs of complying with strict control and the high taxes that come with that, the cost of cannabis production is about the same as the cost of growing tomatoes. The arbitrage between prohibition prices and the "free market" cost of cannabis flower has, over the last 40 years, stimulated domestic cultivation especially in times of economic crisis. Strict control policies retain this incentive by artificially increasing the cost of getting licensed cannabis to market. This "pulls" people into unlicensed cultivation, manufacturing, and distribution. Under conditions of intensive economic crisis, people are also pushed out of the formal economy into informal sectors, including unlicensed cannabis (and other drug) market participation. This is the dynamic that seems to have driven the commercialization of cannabis production this century, certainly to the point at which closed domestic legal markets came to appear not only viable to regulate but potential sources of revenue for declining public sector budgets.

Commercialization and the Politics of Reform

The dynamics of commercialization driving the usefulness of cannabis legalization are more complex than they appear, however. Unlicensed cannabis market activity is both a decentralized livelihood strategy for people on the socioeconomic margins and a speculative, profit-driven industry for larger scale organized crime. Strict control legalization seems fixated on the latter, seeking to replace both equally prohibited activities with commercial industry stakeholders for which the profit motive and industrial tendencies are not only given but expected. At the same time, however, the commercial aspects of legal cannabis capitalism are increasingly indicted by public health institutions, neo-prohibitionists, and social justice movement stakeholders as problems with, rather than desired outcomes of legalization, for different reasons. In a very short period of time, commercialization has turned from an argument for cannabis legalization into a problem associated with it (Himmelstein 2020).

Cannabis legalization as a singular subject of social movement organizing is once again being connected to other, often very different, political and movement agendas—the reverse of what happened in the 1970s. Although strict control frameworks seem to hold many of these interests together, particularly as a criminal justice reform strategy that changes prohibition rather than replaces it, they are already in crisis for diverse ideological and material reasons. If they are "experiments in democracy," the results so far are mixed and therefore of limited relevance as models for federal, national, or global alternatives to prohibition. If the goal is to remove criminal penalties for adults, then decriminalization works just as well. If the goal is to protect the environment, then licensing industrial agriculture at scale, especially indoors, defeats the purpose. If the goal is to eliminate unlicensed activity, then creating barriers to legal market entry is counterproductive. If the goal is to double down on enforcement against unlicensed actors to protect legal markets and public tax revenue, then we are back to the stimulus of prohibition where higher prices incentivize unlicensed production. If unlicensed prices rise to match licensed prices, then diverted products from licensed systems become more significant as sources of unlicensed product exported out of legal jurisdictions.

"Strict control" is materially unsustainable, given contemporary conditions of widespread experience and expertise with cannabis cultivation on the one hand and the declining rate of profit for industrial cannabis agriculture. If there is money to be made in the long run for capitalist commodity chains, it may be in branding, intellectual property, ancillaries and real estate, and most of the profit made thereof will accrue to financial and cultural elites, just as in the rest of the capitalist system. The last frontier of cannabis legalization as a social movement will be about economic justice for socioeconomically marginalized communities for whom cannabis market participation represents informal sector livelihood strategies and who will remain criminalized under regimes of strict control. The problem of racial disproportionality will continue to be relevant on this frontier but is connected to a broader historical stigmatization of cannabis-positive cultivating, distributing, and using demographics. This includes forms and rates of consumption for people who use cannabis spiritually, therapeutically, and as a form of cultural expression that is not capturable by the term "recreational." This is because their rates of use and amounts of possession generally exceed strict control frameworks and because they often control costs by participating in unlicensed cannabis market activities.

A Call for Research Into the Impacts of Cannabis Policy Change

The emergence of strictly regulated cannabis at a time of crisis for "free-market" capitalism raises fundamental questions about how we understand the sources, processes, and impacts of policy change. As drug policy change occurs within the context of specific economic, political, and social conditions, policy impacts must also be understood within those same broader systems and structures. Cannabis policy change then creates openings for research examining the varied meanings and impacts of commercialization on governance, public health, the environment, markets and the economy, and culture and social change.

As articulated in the introduction to this handbook, we deploy the term post-prohibition to characterize structures that are entangled with the objectives, values, discourse, and operational tools of prohibition-era enforcement activities within the context of regulated cannabis. It will be important for cannabis scholars to consider the ways in which regulated cannabis itself might reproduce harmful regimes of prohibition. There are already troubling examples of this process when demographic groups disproportionately impacted by the drug war continue to be excluded from regulated cannabis (ACLU 2020) and targeted by racialized police violence (Hart 2020); when new policing systems are established to enforce regulations enacted *to support* legalization (for example, Sheeler 2020); when the natural environment continues to be exploited through destructive cultivation processes (Miller 2018); when cannabis itself continues to be perceived as a health-compromising drug rather than a therapeutic (Newhart and Dolphin 2019); and when workers continue to be exposed to exploitative and physically dangerous labor practices (see Schenker and Langer Chapter 12). In this way, future research should examine the ways in which post-prohibition cannabis reforms might reorganize, rather than eliminate, systems and logics of exclusionary social control. This analysis of post-prohibition legalization and regulation can borrow from critiques of prisoner reentry as part of broader reform initiatives in the criminal legal system where prisoner reentry "is a socially constructed site of intervention, which is produced by and simultaneously produces the punishment system" (Byrd 2016, 3).

In the period of time that this handbook was in final preparation, we witnessed concurrent and cascading global crises. These events include the crisis of racial injustice in the United States ignited by the police killing of George Floyd, unequal and insufficient health care responses to the public health catastrophe that is the COVID-19 pandemic, ongoing threats to human existence from global climate change and related ecological collapse, and the failure of neoliberal governance to effectively respond to the economic collapse ushered in by these events. The emergence of crises at the time of this handbook's preparation has practical implications for how cannabis research agendas are developed. For example, how can cannabis cultivation technologies and practices minimize or contribute to global climate change? In what ways can the cannabis industry and state regulatory systems disrupt historical patterns of racialized economic exclusion and criminal injustice rooted in cannabis prohibition enforcement tactics? What is the experience and impact of post-prohibition cannabis control on more vulnerable members of society? Finally, how are taken-for-granted assumptions about governance, security, public health, markets, and social change upended by these convergent crises? In the remainder of this chapter, we highlight potential research directions informed by the contributions to this handbook.

Cannabis Legalization as a Neoliberal Reform

Legalization has emerged in the context of neoliberalism in crisis marked by austerity measures, racial injustice, climate change, and reformulations of global power. As noted by Seddon (2020), cannabis law reform is a neoliberal project insofar as it highlights broader cultural and political tensions between the discourse of personal and consumer freedom and the material consequences of state retreat and free markets. This contradiction of legalization is evident when we consider the emergence of intensive regulatory schemes in jurisdictions that have pursued legalization while neoliberalism simultaneously rejects regulation as a threat to free-market capitalism. This throws into sharp relief the contemporary crises of neoliberalism. If cannabis law reform during the 1960s and early 1970s was symbolic of a broader tension between counterculture demands for greater personal freedom and the desire of critics to uphold prevailing standards of public morality, the current post-prohibition moment is characterized by "the broader problem of how to regulate vibrant, globalized 21st century capitalism. At the heart of the matter is finding the optimal balance between state and business" (Seddon 2020, 15). Future cannabis scholarship will need to explore the forces that influence this balance across diverse social and political contexts.

So what does it mean to move cannabis control to a post-prohibition context in which access is subject to state regulation while continuing to restrict access to other illicit substances targeted by strict prohibition? It may be that regulated cannabis strengthens other drug prohibitions by reinforcing their legitimacy and authority. This is more likely as the "soft drug" and "hard drug" false dichotomy is maintained as tobacco, alcohol, and prescription drugs can resist these stigmatizing labels. How does neoliberalism reconcile opposing normative cultural values of mass consumption and moderation? How can neoliberal logics be maintained where "freedom" to grow, sell, and consume cannabis is a geographically specific luxury for some while an existential threat for others? Moreover, how has the emergence of CBD-dominant cannabis with less than 0.3% THC challenged, if not disrupted, cannabis governance? What is the relationship between regulation and enforcement? What types of access and products should be regulated? How should they be enforced? Should there be limits placed on commercialization? What is the difference between livelihood and commercial market activities? Finally, what is the relationship between access and consumption? Post-prohibition governance is rationalized by ongoing claims that legal access to cannabis will drive up rates of consumption. Should consumption increase, is that necessarily a negative outcome, according to what criteria, and who decides?

Ambivalence in Public Health Research

As described by several of the handbook contributors, cannabis public health policy is tethered to the dominant narrative of the prohibition regime: Cannabis is a dangerous drug that inspires violence and other criminal behavior, corrupts youth, and leads to the use of opioids and cocaine. Public health institutions must navigate this prohibition ideology of cannabis as a dangerous drug while concurrently implementing and regulating systems of cannabis therapeutics. This is the context in which public health–informed harm reduction initiatives operate. This is evident in the United States where the claim of cannabis as medicine by U.S. states is in direct conflict with the U.S. Controlled Substances Act. Though the U.S. government rejects the notion of medicinal cannabis and retains THC-dominant cannabis in the most restricted category as a Schedule I controlled substance, much of the ongoing resistance to incorporating drug war harms into public health interventions is the ongoing belief that cannabis has a "high potential for abuse." This ends up stymying efforts to push public health policy, programs, and research beyond concerns about youth exposure and strict control, for example, to public education and consumer-centered harm reduction. For example, oral cannabis products represent relatively recent additions to the cannabis buffet line, and consumers would benefit from knowing how to avoid as well as manage the effects of unintentional overconsumption (Meisel 2020).

One tenet of the prohibition regime that justifies the belief that cannabis has a "high potential for abuse" has been the frequent claim that cannabis use incites users to begin use of harder substances. This "gateway" theory of drug use initiation in popular discourse did not always distinguish between psychopharmacological causal mechanisms or more social pathways created by exposure to illicit markets due to cannabis prohibition. It was not until 2016 that the DEA finally acknowledged, "research does not support a direct causal relationship between regular marijuana use and other illicit drug use" (2016, 53705). Despite this dramatic reversal from the DEA, former U.S. Attorney General Jeff Sessions continued linking cannabis to opioid use (Lynch 2017).

While integration of cannabis into normative supply chains is wholly legal, some are concerned that commercial cannabis might replicate tobacco and alcohol policy models emphasizing demand creation rather than reduction (Barry and Glantz 2016). As one commentator noted (Moodie 2014, 525), these other drug industries undermine evidence-based public health efforts by "biasing research findings; co-opting policymakers and health professionals; lobbying politicians and public officials to oppose public regulation; influencing voters to oppose public health regulation and blatantly ignoring their own codes of conduct." This is a cautionary note indeed for cannabis scholars to consider as they develop research agendas that assume cannabis commercialization will somehow be different from other regulated industries producing other mind-altering substances. We saw evidence of this blurring of public health and commercial interests in the United States where physicians participated in cigarette advertising for almost a quarter century (Gardner and Brandt 2006). More recently, physicians were tapped to promote the use of opioid pain medications that contributed to the rise of opioid dependency and overdoses in the United States (Madras 2017) but also promote race- and class-stratified systems of opioid dependence treatment (Hansen and Skinner 2012).

There remain substantial obstacles (Meisel, Watson, and Wesley 2019) and limited government funding to support scientific research into the therapeutic benefits of cannabis, as the vast majority of support is earmarked for research that contributes to the narrative of cannabis as a dangerous drug (Hart 2020; Piomelli et al. 2019). In what ways then do public health institutions and funders maintain policy and practice that deny research agendas seeking to move beyond cannabis as a dangerous drug to consider cannabis as a therapeutic or even entheogenic substance (Johnstad 2020)? How does public health reconcile reducing the harms of ongoing cannabis criminalization while simultaneously carrying out research into the public health benefits of legalized cannabis use? Is cannabis use a public health threat or a vector for public wellness? How can wellness be reimagined to include non-physiological indicators of well-being, such as spiritual health? What sort of research designs can be employed and methods developed to provide practitioners and consumers with actionable data in the context of state restrictions on cannabis research? What should be the relationship between medical practitioners and the cannabis industry? What are the public health implications of cannabis agriculture and manufacturing not just for those who labor in such industries, but also the communities in which such industries are located?

Limits of Cannabis Market Liberalization

Beyond considering cannabis as a focus of interest—and tension—within public health, cannabis scholarship must also investigate cannabis itself as a commodity chain that delivers legible, rather than hidden, data on employment, profits, and tax revenue. It is the market benefit promises of legalization that have contributed to shifting public support for cannabis liberalization in many countries since the 1990s. Legalization for market benefits conform to the ideology of neoliberalism that offers market solutions for social problems. Yet regulation, especially strict regulation, contradicts the free-market tendencies of legalization. Regulations are also products of political struggles and, in the context of cannabis markets, are shaped by those with the political and financial capital. As was shared by several handbook contributors, cannabis regulations that should protect workers, the public, and the environment are often absent, insufficient, or not enforced.

Cannabis scholarship must investigate whether the economic promises of legalization have been fulfilled and for whom. To what extent are the interests of investors, employees, and the general public aligned, and if they are not, whose interests are privileged? Future research must also consider what kinds of cannabis markets are being created by legalization, and for whom. As legalization unfolds in the context of prohibition, unregulated markets persist in some locations where it "occupies a legal and cultural grey area" (Meisel 2017, 3). In such contexts, what are the experiences of employees faced with dangerous or exploitative workplace conditions? How has legalization changed the material conditions of cannabis work? What are the implications for workers, consumers, and communities when multinational firms develop monopolistic control of cannabis markets? Cannabis as a commodity also reveals a key contradiction of neoliberalism insofar as its value is market driven yet profitability is severely constricted by prohibition policies. What is the nature of the relationship between legal and illegal markets? To what extent do taxation and strict control maintain illicit markets? How do cannabis business interests navigate post-prohibition market forces? What factors shape a business decision to either enter the regulated market or continue operating in the underground economy?

Reframing Industrial Cannabis as an Environmental Threat

Unregulated cannabis production, especially on public lands, has recently come to be viewed as an existential threat to natural ecosystems and the overall health of the planet. This represents a novel approach for vilifying the plant as it has passed in the past century from a "killer weed" to "dropout drug" (Himmelstein 1983) to existential environmental threat. The legitimacy of cannabis prohibition can be more easily rationalized by environmental harms from energy- and water-intensive growing methods using dangerous pesticides than it can be as a moral imperative. In fact, this strategy was shared with one of the authors by National Marijuana Initiative director Tommy LaNier during a community meeting in Humboldt County in 2012. In this respect, one dimension of cannabis prohibition continues as a matter of environmental health and safety. It is not just unregulated cannabis, however, that warrants research scrutiny; legal yet industrial cannabis markets have significant environmental impacts too. This reframing of cannabis as an environmental threat pushes us to ask what kinds of relationships might exist between cannabis and the environment? How do we identify and govern environmental impacts from cannabis? What is the role of the state and private industry in mitigating such impacts? Though cannabis liberalization provides the guardrails within which regulated cannabis is expected to operate, who creates and enforces those guidelines? How effective are cultivation regulations at discouraging environmentally harmful practices?

The institutional exception to prohibition that acknowledges state-level cannabis commerce also precludes federal acknowledgement of *legal cannabis* in the United States. Federal cannabis enforcement does not distinguish between state-licensed and unlicensed businesses or environmentally responsible and destructive operations. Painted with this broad-brush stroke, all cannabis producers represent unwanted encroachment and threat to the natural landscape, wildlife, and watersheds while contributing to global climate change. How are these false dichotomies, insofar as some unlicensed operations may leave a relatively smaller footprint on the environment than licensed cannabis businesses? As was argued separately by contributors to this handbook, cannabis cultivation (prohibited and not) also provides a revealing looking glass into the ongoing environmental harm and cultural degradations of colonial relationships with Native American communities and local farmers in Southern countries, respectively. Will cannabis production follow similar exploitative models of industrial agriculture? How can cannabis as a commodity be decolonized? How can legal cannabis markets be environmentally sustainable? In what ways can consumer politics—manifested in corporate social responsibility campaigns or home cultivation—resist the industrial agriculture model that strains ecosystems and harms workers and communities? How are cannabis liberalization campaigns embracing—or resisting—efforts to allow personal cultivation allowances?

Cannabis as Normatively Subversive

For cannabis to be accepted as a source of legitimate pleasure, we must reconcile cultural ambivalence about loss of control associated with altered states of consciousness. Resistance to pleasure-seeking behavior runs deep in many cultures (Schivelbusch 1992; Reinarman and Levine 1997). Cannabis consumers and workers must navigate shifting social norms regarding cannabis use and associations with the plant. These norms are fluid by population, place, and period. Post-prohibition cannabis reforms complicate the circumstances under which cannabis is normatively acceptable or subversive. While prohibition clearly defined all associations with cannabis as illegal, post-prohibition liberalization entitles some users the privilege of transcending legal sanctions and stigma while exposing others to greater social, legal, and physical risk. Privileges of race, class, gender, and physical ability insulate some from the added stigma of cannabis use.

Racial disparities also have lethal consequences for groups historically villainized by the drug war and victimized by racialized violence (Hart 2020). The presence of cannabis in their system or biography becomes the justification (Scully and Marolla 1984) for excessive and often lethal use of force by law enforcement. Cannabis, rather than racist policing, was added, for example, to the list of official justifications for the police killing of Trayvon Martin, Oscar Grant, Michael Brown, Sandra Bland, Philando Castile, and George Floyd, among many others. Ironically, the tax revenue generated by regulated cannabis helps support prohibition regimes of violent drug law enforcement. In California, for example, 20% of the originally anticipated $1 billion in annual tax revenue from passage of the state's legalization initiative in 2016 was earmarked for "public safety" (Roberts 2020). How do members of communities disproportionately targeted by the drug war understand the emergent legal cannabis industry?

There are many culture and social-change related directions for post-prohibition cannabis research to pursue. What is the relationship between cannabis, prohibition, and cultural change? To what extent does the prohibition stigma of cannabis persist following formal repeal? How might social relationships between users and nonusers change as a result of legalization? To what extent will commodification of cannabis, and commercialization of the culture surrounding its use, alter cannabis effects? Cannabis as a therapeutic drug is also politically and economically symbolic of racialized ambivalence, as allowances for medical cannabis have simultaneously excluded marginalized communities while reasserting the power and inclusion of dominant groups. Even if one is able to join the "green rush" of U.S. cannabis capitalism, how do existing hierarchies of race, class, and gender shape such experiences? What opportunities exist for making regulated cannabis an inclusive enterprise? What are the outcomes associated with creating pathways for equitable participation?

Post-Prohibition Cannabis Research Futures

These are exciting and significant times for new scholars developing cannabis-centered research agendas. Cannabis scholarship has developed rapidly over the past couple of decades, taking root globally in and across a variety of academic disciplines. As a rough indicator of growing scholarly interest in cannabis, we can consider the academic associations and scholarly journals that have formed and professional conferences convened since 1990. For example, the International Cannabinoid Research Society was incorporated in 1992 (International Cannabinoid Research Society n.d.), Cannabinoid Signalling Group (Complutense University, Madrid, Spain) was established by 1995, the Society of Cannabis Clinicians was founded in 1999, the Center for Medicinal Cannabis Research (UC San Diego) formed in 2000, the International Association for Cannabis as Medicine held its first meeting in 2001, and the Humboldt Institute for Interdisciplinary Marijuana Research (Humboldt State University) was established in 2012. The *Cannabis and Cannabinoid Research* journal launched, the Institute for Cannabis Research (Colorado State University), and the Center for

Medical Cannabis Education and Research at Thomas Jefferson University were all established in 2016. In subsequent years, cannabis research centers opened at UC Irvine and UCLA as well as the Multidisciplinary Center on Cannabinoid Research at the Hebrew University of Jerusalem (all in 2017), the journal *Cannabis* launched in 2018, and in 2019 the Berkeley Cannabis Research Center opened at UC Berkeley and the *Journal of Cannabis Research* released its first issue. University-affiliated cannabis research centers have also opened in Australia, Mexico, and Uruguay. There has also been a proliferation of academic degree programs established that are devoted to the study of cannabis. The creation of such infrastructure within academia for cannabis research makes it possible to more closely track rapidly unfolding global developments. These trends suggest increasingly accelerated attitudinal, behavioral, and policy shifts regarding cannabis on a global scale. Yet there remains considerable work to be done.

While we have argued that post-prohibition cannabis liberalization provides an opportunity to critique the ideology of free markets and neoliberal governance, it is also an invitation to describe what lies beyond the ideology and structure of prohibition. Future cannabis research must continue to be mindful of the ways in which both cultural acceptance and legality shape the integration and relative meaning and impact of cannabis in society. What might be the relationship between freedom and control in shaping cultivation, commerce, and consumption experiences? What role might cannabis play in the social and economic formation of daily life beyond the edge of prohibition? How will our relationships with other mind-altering substances adapt? How will attitudes towards cannabis and related consumption rituals be distributed across different communities? How will cannabis become integrated into broader systems of industrial agriculture, or alternatively, how will industrial agriculture be reconstituted? We hope that cannabis scholars can implement the research agendas presented in this handbook to inform cannabis policy going forward "to constitute cannabis markets that protect human rights, enhance social and racial justice and facilitate human flourishing" (Seddon 2020, 16).

References

ACLU. 2020. *A Tale of Two Countries Racially Targeted Arrests in the Era of Marijuana Reform*. American Civil Liberties Union. www.aclu.org/report/tale-two-countries-racially-targeted-arrests-era-marijuana-reform.

Alexander, Michelle. 2020. *The New Jim Crow: Mass Incarceration in the Age of Colorblindness*. Anniversary edition. New York: The New Press.

Anders, Jentri. 1990. *Beyond Counterculture: The Community of Mateel*. Pullman, WA: Washington State University Press.

Barry, Rachel Ann, and Stanton Glantz. 2016. "A Public Health Framework for Legalized Retail Marijuana Based on the US Experience: Avoiding a New Tobacco Industry." *PLoS Medicine* 13 (9): e1002131. https://doi.org/10.1371/journal.pmed.1002131.

Byrd, Renée M. 2016. "'Punishment's Twin': Theorizing Prisoner Reentry for a Politics of Abolition." *Social Justice* 43 (1): 1–22.

Central Valley California High Intensity Drug Trafficking Area [HIDTA]. 2010. "Marijuana Production in California." Accessed November 5, 2012. www.slocounty.ca.gov/Assets/DAS/DAAB/Marijuana Production in California.pdf.

Drug Enforcement Administration. 2016. "Denial of Petition To Initiate Proceedings To Reschedule Marijuana." *Federal Register* 81 (156) (August 12): 53688–766.

Gardner, Martha N., and Allan M. Brandt. 2006. """The Doctors' Choice Is America's Choice": The Physician in US Cigarette Advertisements, 1930–1953." *American Journal of Public Health* 96 (2): 222–32.

Gilmore, Ruth Wilson. 2007. *Golden Gulag: Prisons, Surplus, Crisis, and Opposition in Globalizing California*. Berkeley, CA: University of California Press.

Hansen, Helena, and Mary E. Skinner. 2012. "From White Bullets to Black Markets and Greened Medicine: The Neuroeconomics and Neuroracial Politics of Opioid Pharmaceuticals." *Annals of Anthropological Practice* 36 (1): 167–82.

Hart, Carl L. 2020. "Exaggerating Harmful Drug Effects on the Brain Is Killing Black People." *Neuron*. https://doi.org/10.1016/j.neuron.2020.06.019.

Himmelstein, Jerome L. 1983. "From Killer Weed to Drop-out Drug: The Changing Ideology of Marihuana." *Contemporary Crises* 7 (1): 13–38. https://doi.org/10.1007/BF00808341.

———. 2020. " 'Where Commerce Meets a Revolution:' The Complex Relationship Between the Marijuana Legalization Movement and the Cannabis Industry." *Journal of Drug Policy Analysis*.

International Cannabinoid Research Society. n.d. "About the ICRS." Accessed June 29, 2020. https://icrs.co/AboutUs.html#History.

Johnstad, Petter Grahl. 2020. "Cannabis as Entheogen: Survey and Interview Data on the Spiritual Use of Cannabis." *Journal of Cannabis Research* 2 (1): 30. https://doi.org/10.1186/s42238-020-00032-2.

Lynch, Sarah N. 2017. "U.S. Attorney General Says People Should Just 'Say No' to Opioids." Reuters, October 26. www.reuters.com/article/us-usa-trump-opioids-sessions-idUSKBN1CV2ZG.

Madras, Bertha K. 2017. "The Surge of Opioid Use, Addiction, and Overdoses: Responsibility and Response of the US Health Care System." *JAMA Psychiatry* 74 (5): 441. https://doi.org/10.1001/jamapsychiatry.2017.0163.

Meisel, Joshua. 2017. "Hidden in Plain Sight: Cannabis Cultivation in the Emerald Triangle." *California Geographer* 56: 13.

———. 2020. *'My Body is Literally Shutting Down and This Is My Last Night on Earth': Drug, Set, and Setting and Negative Cannabis Edible Experiences*. Arcata, CA: Humboldt Institute for Interdisciplinary Marijuana Research, Humboldt State University.

Meisel, Joshua, Tara Marie Watson, and Jared Wesley. 2019. "Eliminate Restrictions Preventing Cannabis Research." *Policy Options*, November 22. https://policyoptions.irpp.org/magazines/november-2019/eliminate-restrictions-preventing-cannabis-research/.

Miller, Char. 2018. *Where There's Smoke: The Environmental Science, Public Policy, and Politics of Marijuana*. Lawrence, KS: University Press of Kansas.

Moodie, A. Rob. 2014. "Big Alcohol: The Vector of an Industrial Epidemic." *Addiction* 109 (4): 525–26.

Newhart, Michelle, and William Dolphin. 2019. *The Medicalization of Marijuana: Legitimacy, Stigma, and the Patient Experience*. New York, NY: Routledge.

Piomelli, Daniele, Robert Solomon, Donald Abrams, Agnes Balla, Igor Grant, Thomas Marcotte, and John Yoder. 2019. "Regulatory Barriers to Research on Cannabis and Cannabinoids: A Proposed Path Forward." *Cannabis and Cannabinoid Research* 4 (1): 21–32.

Reinarman, Craig. 1994. "The Social Construction of Drug Scares." In *Constructions of Deviance: Social Power, Context, and Interaction*, edited by Patricia A. Adler and Peter Adler, 155–165. Boston, MA: Wadsworth Publishing.

Reinarman, Craig, and Harry G. Levine. 1997. *Crack In America: Demon Drugs and Social Justice*. Berkeley and London: University of California Press.

Roberts, Chris. 2020. "Why Marijuana Legalization Funds the Police." *Forbes*, June 8, 2020. https://www.forbes.com/sites/chrisroberts/2020/06/08/why-marijuana-legalization-funds-the-police/.

Rossman, Michael. 1971. *The Wedding Within the War*. New York: Doubleday.

Schivelbusch, Wolfgang. 1992. *Tastes of Paradise*. New York: Pantheon Books.

Scully, Diana, and Joseph Marolla. 1984. "Convicted Rapists' Vocabulary of Motive: Excuses and Justifications." *Social Problems* 31 (5): 530–44.

Seddon, Toby. 2020. "Immoral in Principle, Unworkable in Practice: Cannabis Law Reform, The Beatles, and the Wootton Report." *The British Journal of Criminology*, June. https://doi.org/10.1093/bjc/azaa042.

Sheeler, Andrew. 2020. "California Wants to Hire More Cannabis Cops to Get a Handle on Black Market Marijuana." *The Sacramento Bee*, June 2. www.sacbee.com/news/california/california-weed/article243061066.html.

Wallerstein, Immanuel. 2011. "Structural Crisis in the World-System: Where Do We Go from Here?" *Monthly Review*, March 1. Accessed October 17, 2020. https://monthlyreview.org/2011/03/01/structural-crisis-in-the-world-system/.

Index

Note: **Boldface** page references indicate tables. *Italic* references indicate figures and boxed text.